Immunochemical Protocols

METHODS IN MOLECULAR BIOLOGY™

John M. Walker, SERIES EDITOR

Immunochemical Protocols

SECOND EDITION

Edited by

John D. Pound

The University of Birmingham, UK

Humana Press ☀ Totowa, New Jersey

© 1998 Humana Press Inc.
999 Riverview Drive, Suite 208
Totowa, New Jersey 07512

This publication is printed on acid-free paper. ∞
ANSI Z39.48-1984 (American Standards Institute) Permanence of Paper for Printed Library Materials.

Cover illustration: Fig. 4 from Chapter 31, "Immunogold Probes in Electron Microscopy," by David J. P. Ferguson, David A. Hughes, and Julian E. Beesley .

Cover design by Jill Nogrady and Patricia F. Cleary.

For additional copies, pricing for bulk purchases, and/or information about other Humana titles, contact Humana at the above address or at any of the following numbers: Tel.: 973-256-1699; Fax: 973-256-8341; E-mail: humana@humanapr.com; or visit our Website: http://humanapress.com

Printed in the United States of America. 10 9 8 7 6 5 4 3 2 1

Library of Congress Cataloging in Publication Data

Main entry under title:

Methods in molecular biology™.
Immunochemical protocols/edited by John D. Pound—2nd ed.
p.   cm.—(Methods in molecular biology; v. 80)
Includes bibliographical references and index.
ISBN 0-89603-388-0 (combbound) (alk. paper); ISBN 0-89603-493-3 (hardcover) (alk. paper)
1.   Immunochemistry—Methodology.   II.   Pound, John D.   II.   Series:
Methods in molecular biology (Totowa, NJ); v. 80
QR183.6.I43   1998
616.07'56—dc21   97-39695
CIP

Preface

A working knowledge of basic immunochemical techniques is essential for all molecular biologists and most will occasionally call on more sophisticated immunochemical approaches to solve particular problems. Indeed, the great value of antibodies as reagents is underlined by the efforts made by molecular biologists themselves to make antibodies directly from DNA without immunization.

Developments in immunochemical techniques continue to meet the demands created by progress in molecular biology and many of these innovations are, of course, reported in specialist journals. However, locating such reports may not be easy and important refinements often are not published. This much anticipated 2nd edition of *Immunochemical Protocols* therefore aims to provide a user-friendly up-to-date handbook of reliable techniques selected to suit the needs of molecular biologists. It covers the full breadth of the relevant established immunochemical methods, from protein blotting and immunoassays through to visualization of cellular antigens and *in situ* hybridization, each with their latest refinements. Protocols for the production and purification of important classes of immunochemical reagents are also provided, including (of course) antibodies, fusion proteins, and their various conjugates. Prominence is given to the production of antibody chains in filamentous phage as a recent innovation that is now within the capabilities of most well-equipped laboratories. Phage antibodies represent a new generation of immunochemical reagents with exciting possibilities.

Each protocol is described in a step-by-step manner by a worker who had extensive experience with the technique. The majority of protocols treated here are therefore for specific applications rather than generic methods, although the possibilities for their wider application are indicated wherever relevant. A brief description of its rational basis and relative merits is given by way of introduction to each protocol. Concise but detailed Methods sections are underpinned by a Notes section to which the reader can refer for different options for particular steps, ways of monitoring progress, advice on how to avoid likely problems, and how to deal with them if they occur.

Immunochemical Protocols, 2nd edition, should be especially valuable to researchers and postgraduate students with no previous experience with a technique. It should also serve the occasional user of immunochemical methods as an update and perhaps, even as a source of inspiration.

John D. Pound

Contents

Contributors

JOHN R. ADAIR • *Axis Genetics Ltd., Cambridge, UK*

JULIAN E. BEESLEY • *Department of Molecular Pathology, Glaxo-Wellcome Medicines Research Centre, Stevenage, UK*

MAHESH K. BHALGAT • *Molecular Probes, Inc., Eugene, OR*

BHUPENDRA BHATT • *Bone and Joint Research Unit, London Hospital Medical College, London, UK*

KURT BIENZ • *Institute for Medical Microbiology, University of Basel, Switzerland*

VICTOR T.-W. CHAN • *Department of Obstetrics/Gynecology, Ohio State University, Columbus, OH*

ALAN J. CUMBER • *Institute of Cancer Research, London, UK*

CHRISTOPHER J. DEAN • *Institute of Cancer Research, McElwain Laboratories, Royal Cancer Hospital, Surrey, UK*

MONIQUE DIANO • *Laboratoire de Genetique, CNRS, Marseille, France*

RICHARD E. EDWARDS • *MRC Toxicology Unit, University of Leicester, UK*

DENISE EGGER • *Institute for Medical Microbiology, University of Basel, Switzerland*

GERARD I. EVAN • *Imperial Cancer Research Fund, London, UK*

DAVID J. P. FERGUSON • *Department of Molecular Pathology, Glaxo-Wellcome Medicines Research Centre, Stevenage, UK*

MICHAEL FINNEY • *Immunology Department, University of Birmingham, Birmingham, UK*

SIMON J. FORSTER • *Celsis International, Cambridge, UK*

RUTH R. FRENCH • *Lymphoma Research Unit, Tenovus Laboratory, Southampton General Hospital, Southampton, UK*

YVELINE FROBERT • *Section de Pharmacologie et D'Immunologie, Direction des Sciences du Vivant, Gif sur Yvette, France*

MARGARET GOODALL • *Immunology Department, University of Birmingham, Birmingham, UK*

JACQUES GRASSI • *Section de Pharmacologie et D'Immunologie, Direction des Sciences du Vivant, Gif sur Yvette, France*

JONATHAN A. GREEN • *MRC Toxicology Unit, University of Leicester, UK*

CHRISTOPHER D. GREGORY • *Immunology Department, University of Birmingham, Birmingham, UK*

MICHAEL J. HAAS • *Eastern Regional Research Center, US Department of Agriculture, Philadelphia, PA*

ANITA A. HAMILTON • *Eclagen Ltd., Auris Business Centre, Aberdeen, UK*

DAVID C. HANCOCK • *Imperial Cancer Research Fund, London, UK*

ROSARIA P. HAUGLAND • *Molecular Probes, Inc., Eugene, OR*

C. S. HERRINGTON • *Department of Pathology, Royal Liverpool University Hospital, University of Liverpool, UK*

J. MARK HEXHAM • *University of Texas-Southwestern, Dallas, TX*

MICHEL HIRN • *Laboratoire de Genetique, CNRS, Marseille, France*

STEPHEN M. HOBBS • *Institute of Cancer Research, Belmont, UK*

DAVID A. HUGHES • *Nuffield Department of Surgery, John Radcliffe Hospital, Oxford, UK*

SUSANNE F. IMRIE • *The Royal Marsden NHS Trust, London, UK*

PETER JONES • *Department of Biochemistry, University of Nottingham, UK*

SCOTT H. KAUFMANN • *Mayo Clinic, Rochester, MN*

UDO KELLNER • *Mayo Clinic, Rochester, MN*

ANDRÉ LE BIVIC • *Laboratoire de Genetique, CNRS, Marseille, France*

J. MICHAELA LEVENS • *Immunology Department, University of Birmingham, Birmingham, UK*

KITTIMA MAKARANANDA • *Department of Pharmacology, Faculty of Science, Mahidol University, Bangkok, Thailand*

MARGARET M. MANSON • *MRC Toxicology Unit, University of Leicester, UK*

ANNE E. MILNER • *Immunology Department, University of Birmingham, Birmingham, UK*

GLENN E. MORRIS • *MRC Biotechnology Group, NE Wales Institute, Deeside Clwyd, UK*

GORDON E. NEAL • *MRC Toxicology Unit, University of Leicester, UK*

DARIO NERI • *MRC Centre, Cambridge, UK*

AHUVA NISSIM • *MRC Centre, Cambridge, UK*

NICOLA J. O'REILLY • *Imperial Cancer Research Fund, London, UK*

MICHAEL G. ORMEROD • *Reigate, UK*

MARK PAGE • *Medeva Vaccine Research Unit, Department of Biochemistry, Imperial College of Science, Technology, and Medicine, London, UK*

ELIZABETH PHILP • *The Royal Marsden NHS Trust, London, UK*

ALESSANDRO PINI • *MRC Centre, Cambridge, UK*

R. ADRIAN ROBINS • *Division of Molecular and Clinical Immunology, University of Nottingham, UK*

TULIN SAHINOGLU • *Bone and Joint Research Unit, London Hospital Medical College, London, UK*

ANTHONY H. V. SCHAPIRA • *Department of Neurological Science, Royal Free Hospital School of Medicine, University of London, UK*

CLIFF STEVENS • *Bone and Joint Research Unit, London Hospital Medical College, London, UK*

RICHARD A. W. STOTT • *Department of Clinical Chemistry, Doncaster Royal Infirmary, Doncaster, UK*

JERRY STYLES • *MRC Toxicology Unit, University of Leicester, Leicester, UK*

DONALD F. SUMMERS • *Department of Biochemistry, University of Gdansk, Poland*

BOGUSLAW SZEWCZYK • *Department of Biochemistry, University of Gdansk, Poland*

ROBIN THORPE • *Medeva Vaccine Research Unit, Department of Biochemistry, Imperial College of Science, Technology, and Medicine, London, UK*

EDWARD J. WAWRZYNCZAK • *Rothschild Bioscience Unit, London, UK*

LUCINDA R. WEIR • *MRC Toxicology Unit, University of Leicester, UK*

GEORGE D. WILSON • *Gray Laboratory Cancer Research Trust, Mount Vernon Hospital, Northwood Middlesex, UK*

EDDIE C. Y. WANG • *Laboratory of Lymphocyte Molecular Biology, Imperial Cancer Research Fund, London, UK*

WENDY W. YOU • *Molecular Probes, Inc., Eugene, OR*

1

Production of Polyclonal Antisera

Jonathan A. Green and Margaret M. Manson

1. Introduction

All immunochemical procedures require a suitable antiserum or monoclonal antibody raised against the antigen of interest. Polyclonal antibodies are raised by injecting an immunogen into an animal and, after an appropriate time, collecting the blood fraction containing the antibodies of interest. In producing antibodies, several parameters must be considered with respect to the final use to which the antibody will be put. These include (1) the specificity of the antibody, i.e., the ability to distinguish between different antigens; (2) the avidity of the antibody, i.e., the strength of binding; and (3) the titer of the antibody, which determines the optimal dilution of the antibody in the assay system. A highly specific antibody with high avidity may be suitable for immunohistochemistry, where it is essential that the antibody remains attached during the extensive washing procedures, but may be less useful for immunoaffinity chromatography, as it may prove impossible to elute the antigen from the column without extensive denaturation.

To produce an antiserum, the antigen for the first immunization is often prepared in an adjuvant (usually a water-in-oil emulsion containing heat-killed bacteria), which allows it to be released slowly and to stimulate the animal's immune system. Subsequent injections of antigen are done with incomplete adjuvant that does not contain the bacteria. The species used to raise the antibodies depends on animal facilities, amount of antigen available, and the amount of antiserum required. Another consideration is the phylogenetic relationship between antigen and immunized species. A highly conserved mammalian protein may require an avian species in order to raise an antibody. Production of antibodies is still not an exact science and what may work for one antigen may not work for another.

From: *Methods in Molecular Biology, Vol. 80: Immunochemical Protocols, 2nd ed.*
Edited by: J. D. Pound © Humana Press Inc., Totowa, NJ

A simple, generally applicable protocol for raising polyclonal antiserum to a purified protein of >10,000 molecular weight is described. This method has been used to raise antibodies against a cytosolic protein, glutathione-*S*-transferase, and a membrane-bound glycosylated protein, gammaglutamyl transpeptidase. The latter was first solubilized by cleavage from the membrane with papain *(1)*. Variations to this basic procedure are discussed in Chapters 2, 3, and 8. For proteins or peptides of low molecular weight (<5–10 kDa), conjugation to a carrier protein is required for them to elicit antigenicity (*see* Chapter 7). Variations on this basic technique can be found in selected references *(2–5)*.

2. Materials

1. Phosphate-buffered saline (PBS), pH 7.4: 8 g of NaCl, 0.2 g of KH_2PO_4, 2.8 g of $Na_2HPO_4 \cdot 12H_2O$, and 0.2 g of KCl dissolved and made up to 1 L in distilled water.
2. Antigen: Purified protein diluted to about 100 µg/mL in PBS.
3. Complete and incomplete Freund's adjuvant.
4. Two glass luer lock syringes: 2 mL is the best size.
5. Three-way luer fitting plastic stopcock.
6. 19-g Needles, 0.7×22 mm Argyle medicut cannula.
7. Xylene.
8. Sterile glass universal tubes.
9. Up to four rabbits about 4–6 mo old. Various strains can be used, including half sandy lops or New Zealand whites (*see* Note 1).

3. Method

1. Take up 1 mL of complete adjuvant in one of the syringes and 1 mL of antigen solution containing approx 100 µg of the antigen in another. Attach both to the plastic connector (Fig. 1), making sure that the tap on the connector is open in such a way that only the two ports connecting the two syringes are open. Repeatedly push the mixture from syringe to syringe until it becomes thick and creamy (at least 5–10 min). Push all the mixture into one syringe, disconnect this, and attach it to a 19-g needle (*see* Notes 2 and 3).
2. Ensure that the rabbit to be injected is held firmly, but comfortably. For the primary immunization, inject 500 µL deeply into each thigh muscle and also inject 500 µL into each of two sites through the skin on the shoulders.
3. Repeat these injections biweekly for a further 4 wk, but make the emulsion with incomplete adjuvant.
4. Ten days after the last injection, test-bleed the rabbits from the marginal ear vein. Hold the animal firmly and gently swab the rear marginal vein with xylene to dilate the vein. Then cannulate the vein with an Argyle medicut cannula and withdraw the needle, leaving the plastic cannula in place. Draw blood out of the cannula with a syringe until the required amount has been collected. Transfer the collected blood into a sterile glass universal container.
5. Remove the cannula and stem the blood flow by sustained pressure on the puncture site with a tissue.

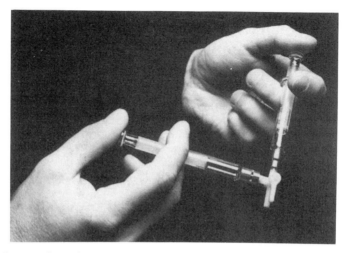

Fig. 1. Preparation of emulsion for immunization. Two luer lock glass syringes connected by a three-way plastic stopcock are used to form a stable emulsion of antigen and adjuvant.

6. Allow the collected blood to clot by letting it stand at room temperature for 2 h and then at 4°C overnight. Separate the serum from the blood by detaching the clot carefully with a spatula from the walls of the container and pouring the liquid into a centrifuge tube. Then centrifuge the clot at 2500g for 30 min at 4°C and remove any expressed liquid. Add this liquid to the clot-free liquid collected previously and centrifuge the whole pooled liquid as described above. Finally, remove the serum from the cell pellet with a Pasteur pipet (*see* Note 4).

7. At this stage, test the antiserum using an appropriate assay (*see* Note 5). If the antibody has the requirements for the use to which it will be put, up to three further bleeds on successive days may be performed. If the antiserum is unsatisfactory, i.e., the reaction is very weak, inject the rabbit again 1 mo after the test bleed, and again test-bleed 10 d after this injection.

8. St ore antibodies in small, preferably sterile, aliquots at a minimum of –20°C. Repeated freezing and thawing should be avoided. For long-term storage, aliquots may be freeze-dried and reconstituted when needed (*see* Note 6).

4. Notes

1. The production of antibodies in animals must be carried out in strict accordance with the legislation of the country concerned.

2. Emulsions containing antigens are just as immunogenic to humans as to the experimental animal. Great care should be exercised during all the procedures.

3. A stable emulsion has been produced when a drop of the preparation does not disperse when placed on water.

4. Serum should be straw colored; a pink coloration shows that hemolysis has taken place. This should not affect the performance of the antibodies during most assay procedures.

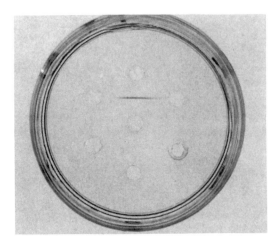

Fig. 2. Ouchterlony double-diffusion technique. The antigen is placed in the center well, cut in an agarose gel, and different antisera in a range of dilutions are placed in the surrounding wells. Antigen and antiserum diffuse toward each other and form a white precipitin line where an antibody recognizes the antigen.

5. This can be done by the Ouchterlony diffusion technique (*see* Fig. 2 and ref. *6*), by enzyme-linked immunosorbent assay (*see* Chapter 15), or by Western blot, either using the purified protein or a more complex mixture of proteins containing the antigen of interest separated on a sodium dodecyl sulfate-polyacrylamide gel electrophoresis gel (*see* Chapter 20).
6. Some freeze-dried antisera are difficult to reconstitute, or occasionally may lose activity. Test a small sample before drying the whole batch. Any cloudiness after reconstitution is denatured lipoprotein, and can be clarified by centrifugation and does not affect antibody binding.

References

1. Cook, N. D. and Peters, T. J. (1985) Purification of γ-glutamyl transferase by phenyl boronate affinity chromatography. *Biochim. Biophys. Acta* **828,** 205–212.
2. Catty, D. and Raykundalia, C. (1988) Production and quality control of polyclonal antibodies, in *Antibodies vol. 1—A Practical Approach* (Catty, D., ed.), IRL, Oxford.
3. Mayer, R. J. and Walker, J. H. (eds.) (1987) *Immunochemical Methods in Cell and Molecular Biology.* Academic, London.
4. Harlow, E. and Lane, D. (1988) *Antibodies. A Laboratory Manual.* Cold Spring Harbor Laboratory, Cold Spring Harbor, NY.
5. Langone, J. J. and Van Vunakis, H. (1983) *Methods in Enzymology,* vol. 93. Academic, New York.
6. Ouchterlony, O. and Nilsson, L. A. (1978) Immunodiffusion and immunoelectrophoresis, in *Handbook of Experimental Immunology,* 3rd ed. (Weir, D. H., ed.), Blackwell, Oxford, UK, pp. 19.1–19.44.

2

Raising Polyclonal Antibodies Using Nitrocellulose-Bound Antigen

Monique Diano, André Le Bivic, and Michel Hirn

1. Introduction

Highly specific antibodies directed against minor proteins, present in small amounts in biological fluids, or against nonsoluble cytoplasmic or membranous proteins, are often difficult to obtain. The main reasons for this are the small amounts of protein available after the various classical purification processes and the low purity of the proteins.

In general, a crude or partially purified extract is electrophoresed on a sodium dodecyl sulfate polyacrylamide gel (SDS-PAGE); then the protein band is lightly stained and cut out. In the simplest method, the acrylamide gel band is reduced to a pulp, mixed with Freund' s adjuvant, and injected. Unfortunately, this technique is not always successful. Its failure can probably be attributed to factors such as the difficulty of disaggregating the acrylamide, the difficulty with which the protein diffuses from the gel, the presence of SDS in large quantities resulting in extensive tissue and cell damage, and finally, the toxicity of the acrylamide.

An alternative technique is to extract and concentrate the proteins from the gel by electroelution (*see Methods in Molecular Biology*, Volume 1, Chapter 19), but this leads to considerable loss of material and low amounts of purified protein.

Another technique is to transfer the separated protein from an SDS-PAGE gel to nitrocellulose. The protein-bearing nitrocellulose can be solubilized with dimethyl sulfoxide (DMSO), mixed with Freund's adjuvant, and injected into a rabbit. However, although rabbits readily tolerate DMSO, mice do not, thus making this method unsuitable for raising monoclonal antibodies.

From: *Methods in Molecular Biology, Vol. 80: Immunochemical Protocols, 2nd ed.*
Edited by: J. D. Pound © Humana Press Inc., Totowa, NJ

The monoclonal approach has been considered as the best technique for raising highly specific antibodies, starting from a crude or partially purified immunogen. However, experiments have regularly demonstrated that the use of highly heterogenous material for immunization never results in the isolation of clones producing antibodies directed against all the components of the mixture. Moreover, the restricted specificity of a monoclonal antibody that usually binds to a single epitope of the antigenic molecule is not always an advantage. For example, if the epitope is altered or modified (i.e., by fixative, Lowicryl embedding, or detergent), the binding of the monoclonal antibody might be compromised, or even abolished.

Because conventional polyclonal antisera are complex mixtures of a considerable number of clonal products, they are capable of binding to multiple antigenic determinants. Thus, the binding of polyclonal antisera is usually not altered by slight denaturation, structural changes, or microheterogeneity, making them suitable for a wide range of applications. However, to be effective, a polyclonal antiserum must be of the highest specificity and free of irrelevant antibodies directed against contaminating proteins, copurified with the protein of interest and/or the proteins of the bacterial cell wall present in the Freund's adjuvant. In some cases, the background generated by such irrelevant antibodies severely limits the use of polyclonal antibodies.

A simple technique for raising highly specific polyclonal antisera against minor or insoluble proteins would be of considerable value.

Here, we describe a method for producing polyclonal antibodies, which avoids both prolonged purification of antigenic proteins (with possible proteolytic degradation) and the addition of Freund's adjuvant and DMSO. Two-dimensional gel electrophoresis leads to the purification of the chosen protein in one single, short step. The resolution of this technique results in a very pure antigen, and consequently, in a very high specificity of the antibody obtained. It is a simple, rapid, and reproducible technique for proteins present in sufficiently large quantities to be detected by Coomassie blue staining.

A polyclonal antibody, which by nature cannot be monospecific, can, if its titer is very high, behave like a monospecific antibody in comparison with the low titers of irrelevant antibodies in the same serum. Thus, this method is faster and performs better than other polyclonal antibody techniques while retaining all the advantages of polyclonal antibodies.

2. Materials

1. For isoelectric focusing (IEF) and SDS-PAGE gels, materials are those described by O'Farrell *(1,2)* and Laemmli *(3)*. It should be noted that for IEF, acrylamide and *bis*-acrylamide must be of the highest level of purity, and urea must be ultrapure (enzyme grade) *(see Methods in Molecular Biology*, Volume 3, Chapters 15–21).

2. Ampholines with an appropriate pH range, e.g., 5.0–8.0 or 3.0–9.0.
3. Transfer membranes: 0.45-μm BA 85 nitrocellulose membrane filters (from Schleicher and Schüll GmBH, Kassel, Germany); 0.22-μm membranes can be used for low-mol-wt antigenic proteins.
4. Transfer buffer: 20% methanol, 150 mM glycine, and 20 mM Tris base, pH 8.3.
5. Phosphate-buffered saline (PBS), sterilized by passage through a 0.22-μm filter.
6. Ponceau Red: 0.2% in 3% trichloroacetic acid.
7. Small scissors.
8. Sterile blood-collecting tubes, with 0.1M sodium citrate, pH 6.0, at a final concentration of 3.2%.
9. Ultrasonication apparatus, with 100 W minimum output. We used a 100-W ultrasonic disintegrator with a titanium exponential microprobe with a tip diameter of 3 mm (1/8 in.). The nominal frequency of the system is 20 kc/s, and the amplitude used is 12 μ.

3. Methods

This is an immunization method in which nitrocellulose-bound protein is employed and in which *neither DMSO nor Freund's adjuvant* are used, in contrast to the method described by Knudsen *(4)*. It is equally applicable for soluble and membrane proteins.

3.1. Purification of Antigen

Briefly, subcellular fractionation of the tissue is carried out to obtain the fraction containing the protein of interest. This is then subjected to separation in the first dimension by IEF using O'Farrell's technique *(1)*, or as described in *Methods in Molecular Biology*, Volume 3, Chapter 19. At this stage, it is important to obtain complete solubilization of the protein (*see* Note 1).

Separation in the second dimension is achieved by using an SDS polyacrylamide gradient gel (*see Methods in Molecular Biology*, Volume 1, Chapter 7 and refs. *1* and *4*; *see also* Note 2).

The proteins are then transferred from the gel to nitrocellulose (*Methods in Molecular Biology*, Volume 10, Chapters 24–26 and ref. *5*). It is important to work with gloves when handling nitrocellulose to avoid contamination with skin keratins.

3.2. Preparation of Antigen for Immunization

1. Immerse the nitrocellulose sheet in Ponceau red solution for 1–2 min, until deep staining is obtained, then destain the sheet slightly in running distilled water for easier detection of the spots. *Never let the nitrocellulose dry out.*
2. Carefully excise the spot corresponding to the antigenic protein. Excise inside the circumference of the spot to avoid contamination by contiguous proteins (*see* Fig. 1)
3. Immerse the nitrocellulose spot in PBS in an Eppendorf tube (1-mL size). The PBS bath should be repeated several times until the nitrocellulose is thoroughly

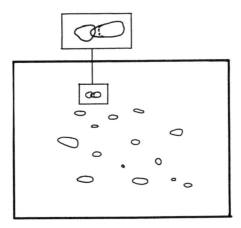

Fig. 1. Excision of the spot containing the antigen. Cut inside the circumference, for instance, along the dotted line for the right spot.

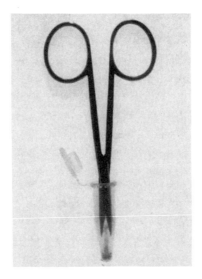

Fig. 2. Maceration of nitrocellulose.

destained. The last bath should have a volume of about 0.5 mL, adequate for the next step.
4. Cut the nitrocellulose into very small pieces with scissors. Then rinse the scissors into the tube with PBS to avoid any loss (*see* Fig. 2).
5. Macerate the nitrocellulose suspension by sonication. The volume of PBS must be proportional to the surface of nitrocellulose to be sonicated. For example, 70–80 μL of PBS is adequate for about 0.4 cm^2 of nitrocellulose (*see* Notes 3 and 4).

6. After sonication, add about 1 mL of PBS to the nitrocellulose powder to dilute the mixture, and aliquot it in 500, 350, and 250-µL fractions and freeze these fractions at –80°C until use. Under these storage conditions, the aliquots may be used for immunization for up to one year or, may be longer. Never store the nitrocellulose without buffer. Never use sodium azide because of its toxicity.

3.3. Immunization

1. Shave the backs of the rabbits. Routinely inject two rabbits with the same antigen.
2. Thaw the 500-µL fraction for the first immunization and add 1.5–2 mL of PBS to reduce the concentration of nitrocellulose powder.
3. Inoculate the antigen, according to Vaitukaitis et al. *(6),* into 20 or more sites (Vaitukaitis injects at up to 40 sites). Inject subcutaneously, holding the skin between the thumb and forefinger. Inject between 50 and 100 µL—a light swelling appears at the site of injection. As the needle is withdrawn, compress the skin gently. An 18-g hypodermic needle is routinely used, though a finer needle (e.g., 20- or 22-g) may also be used (*see* Note 5). Care should be taken over the last injection; generally, a little powder remains in the head of the needle. Thus, after the last injection, draw up 1 mL of PBS to rinse the needle, resuspend the remaining powder in the syringe, and position the syringe vertically to inject.
4. Three or four weeks after the first immunization, the first booster inoculation is given in the same way. The amount of protein injected is generally less, corresponding to two-thirds of that of the first immunization.
5. Ten days after the second immunization, bleed the rabbit (*see* Note 6). A few milliliters of blood suffice, i.e., enough to check the immune response against a crude preparation of the injected antigenic protein. The antigen is revealed on a Western blot with the specific serum diluted at 1:500 and a horseradish peroxidase-conjugated second antibody. We used 3,3'-Diaminobenzidine tetrahydrochloride (DAB) for color development of peroxidase activity (*see Methods in Molecular Biology*, Volume 10, Chapter 10). If the protein is highly antigenic, the beginning of the immunological response is detectable.
6. Two weeks after the second immunization, administer a third immunization in the same way as the first two, even if a positive response has been detected. If there was a positive response after the second immunization, one-half of the amount of protein used for the original immunization is sufficient.
7. Bleed the rabbits 10 d after the third immunization and every week thereafter. At each bleeding, check the serum as after the second immunization; but the serum should be diluted at 1:4000 or 1:6000. Bleeding can be continued for as long as the antibody titer remains high (*see* Note 7).
   Another booster should be given when the antibody titer begins to decrease if it is necessary to obtain a very large volume of antiserum (*see* Note 7).
8. After bleeding, keep the blood at room temperature until it clots. Then collect the serum and centrifuge for 10 min at 3000*g* to eliminate microclots and lipids. Store aliquots at –22°C.

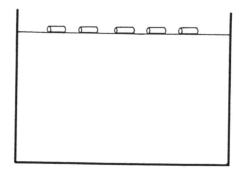

Fig. 3. Second dimension with several IEF gels. Several IEF gels are cut, 0.5 cm above and 0.5 cm below the isoelectric point of the protein of interest. They are placed side by side at the top of the second dimension slab gel. Thus, only one SDS gel is needed to collect several spots of interest.

4. Notes

1. To ensure solubilization, the following techniques are useful:
   a. The concentration of urea in the mixture should be $9.0–9.5M$, i.e., close to saturation.
   b. The protein mixture should be frozen and thawed at least six times. Ampholines should be added only after the last thawing because freezing renders them inoperative.
   c. If the antigenic protein is very basic and outside the pH range of the ampholines, it is always possible to carry out NEPHGE (nonequilibrium pH gradient electrophoresis) for the first dimension (*see* Section 3.1., and *see also Methods in Molecular Biology*, Volume 3, Chapter 17).
2. If the antigenic protein is present in small amounts in the homogenate, it is possible to save time by cutting out the part of the IEF gel where the protein is located and depositing several pieces of the first-dimension gel side by side on the second-dimension gel slab (*see* Fig. 3).
3. Careful attention should be paid to temperature during preparation of the antigen; always work between 2 and 4°C. Be particularly careful during sonication; wait 2–3 min between consecutive sonications.
4. This is a crucial point in the procedure. If too much PBS is added, the pieces of nitrocellulose will swirl around the probe and disintegration does not occur. In this case, the nitrocellulose pieces should be allowed to settle to the bottom of the tube before sonication and the excess buffer drawn off with a syringe or other suitable instrument (70–80 µL of PBS is sufficient for about 0.4 cm^2 of nitrocellulose). For these quantities, one or two 10-s cycles suffice to get powdered nitrocellulose. We mention the volume as a reference since the surface of nitrocellulose-bound antigen may vary. In every case the volume of PBS must be adjusted.

5. What is an appropriate amount of antigenic protein to inject? There is no absolute answer to this question. It depends both on the molecular weight of the protein, and also on its antigenicity. It is well known that if the amount of antigen is very low (0.5–1 µg for the classic method with Freund's adjuvant), there is no antibody production; if the amount of antigen is very high (e.g., several hundred micrograms of highly antigenic protein), antibody production might also be blocked.

It would appear that in our method, a lower amount of antigen is required for immunization; the nitrocellulose acts as if it progressively releases the bound protein, and thus, the entire amount of protein is used progressively by the cellular machinery.

Our experiments show that a range of 10–40 µg for the first immunization generally gives good results, although, in some cases, 5 µg of material is sufficient. The nitrocellulose powder has the additional effect of triggering an inflammatory process at the sites of injection, thus enhancing the immune response, as does Freund's adjuvant by means of the emulsion of the antigenic protein with the tubercular bacillus; macrophages abound in the inflamed areas.

6. It is perhaps worth noting that careful attention should be paid to the condition of the rabbit at time of bleeding. We bleed the rabbits at the lateral ear artery. When the rabbit is calm, 80–100 mL of blood may be taken. The best time for bleeding is early in the morning, and after the rabbit has drunk. Under these conditions, the serum is very clear. It is essential to operate in a quiet atmosphere. If the rabbit is nervous or under stress, the arteries are constricted so strongly that only a few drops of blood can be obtained. Note that to avoid clotting, the needle is impregnated with a sterile sodium citrate solution by drawing the solution into the syringe three times.

7. When the effective concentration required corresponds to a dilution of 1:2000, the titer is decreasing. Serum has a high titer if one can employ a dilution over 1:2000 and if there is a strong specific signal without any background.

8. We have also immunized mice with nitrocellulose-bound protein by intraperitoneal injection of the powder. This is convenient when time and material are very limited, since very little protein is needed to induce a response (three to five times less than for a rabbit) and since the time-lag for the response is shorter (the second immunization was 2 wk after the first, and the third immunization, 10 d after the second). Mice have a high tolerance for the nitrocellulose powder. Unfortunately, the small amount of serum available is a limiting factor. This technique for immunizing mice can, of course, be used for the preparation of monoclonal antibodies.

9. Utilization of serum. The proper dilutions are determined. We routinely use 1:4000 for blots, 1:300–1:200 for immunofluorescence, and 1:50 for immunogold staining. Serum continues to recognize epitopes on tissue proteins after Lowicryl embedding. Labeling is highly specific, and gives a sharp image of *in situ* protein localization. *There is no need to purify the serum.* IgG purified from serum by whatever means usually gives poorer results than those obtained with diluted serum. Purification procedures often give rise to aggregates and denaturation, always increase the background, and result in loss of specific staining.

10. Bacterial antigenic protein. When antibodies are used in screening cDNA libraries in which the host is *E. coli,* the antibodies produced against bacterial components of Freund's adjuvant may also recognize some *E. coli* components. An advantage of our technique is that it avoids the risk of producing antibodies against such extraneous components.
11. Is nitrocellulose antigenic? Some workers have been unable to achieve good results by immunization with nitrocellulose-bound protein. They reproducibly obtain antisera directed against nitrocellulose. We found that in every case, this resulted from injecting powdered nitrocellulose in Freund's adjuvant; using adjuvant actually increases the production of low affinity IgM that binds nonspecifically to nitrocellulose. We have never observed this effect in our experiments when the technique described here was followed strictly.
12. The purification step by 2-D electrophoresis implies the use of denaturing conditions (SDS), and thus, is not appropriate for obtaining antibodies directed against native structures. For that purpose, the protein should be transferred onto nitrocellulose after purification by classical nondenaturing methods and gel electrophoresis under nondenaturing conditions.

    However, it should be pointed out that, following the method of Dunn *(7),* it is possible partially to renature proteins with modifications of the composition of the transfer buffer.
13. Second dimension electrophoresis can be carried out with a first electrophoresis under native conditions, followed by a second electrophoresis under denaturing conditions, i.e., with SDS.

    Because the resolution provided by a gradient is better, it should always be used in the 2-D electrophoresis. Agarose may also be used as an electrophoresis support.
14. If only a limited amount of protein is available, and/or if the antigen is weakly immunogenic, another procedure may be used. The first immunization is given as a single injection, of up to 0.8 mL, into the popliteal lymphatic ganglion *(8),* using a 22-g needle, i.e., the finest that can be used to inject nitrocellulose powder. In this case, the antigen is delivered immediately into the immune system. If necessary, both ganglions can receive an injection. The small size of the ganglions limits the injected volume. The eventual excess of antigen solution is then injected into the back of the rabbit, as described above. The boosters are given in the classic manner, i.e., in several subcutaneous injections into the rabbit's back.

    If the amount of protein available is even more limited, a guinea pig may be immunized (first immunization in the lymphatic ganglion, and boosters, as usual).
15. The advantage of getting a high titer for the antibody of interest is that the amount of irrelevant antibodies is, by comparison, very low and, consequently, does not generate any background. Another advantage of using a crude serum with a high antibody titer, is that this serum may be used without further purification to screen a genomic bank *(9).*
16. The time required for transfer and the voltage used is dependent on the molecular weight and the nature of the protein to be transferred. During transfer, the electrophoresis tank may be cooled with tap water.

References

1. O'Farrell, P. H. (1975) High resolution two-dimensional electrophoresis of proteins. *J. Biol. Chem.* **250,** 4007–4021.
2. O'Farrell, P. Z., Goodman, H. M., and O'Farrell, P. H. (1977) High resolution two-dimensional electrophoresis of basic as well as acidic proteins. *Cell* **12,** 1133–1142.
3. Laemmli, U. K. (1970) Cleavage of structural proteins during the assembly of the head of bacteriophage T4. *Nature (London)* **227,** 680–685.
4. Knudsen, K. A. (1985) Proteins transferred to nitrocellulose for use as immunogens. *Anal. Biochem.* **147,** 285–288.
5. Burnette, W. N. (1981) Electrophoretic transfer of proteins from sodium dodecylsulfate polyacrylamide gels to unmodified nitrocellulose and radiographic detection with antibody and radioiodinated protein A. *Anal. Biochem.* **112,** 195–203.
6. Vaitukaitis, J., Robbins, J. B., Nieschlag, E., and Ross, G. T. (1971) A method for producing specific antisera with small doses of immunogen. *J. Clin. Endocrinol.* **33,** 980–988.
7. Dunn, S. D. (1986) Effects of the modification of transfer buffer composition and the renaturation of proteins in gels on the recognition of proteins on Western blots by monoclonal antibodies. *Anal. Biochem.* **157,** 144–153
8. Sigel, M. B., Sinha, Y. N., and Vanderlaan, W. P. (1983) Production of antibodies by inoculation into lymph nodes. *Methods Enzymol.* **93,** 3–12.
9. Preziosi, L., Michel, G. P. F., and Baratti, J. (1990) Characterisation of sucrose hydrolising enzymes of *Zymomonas mobilis. Arch. Microbiol.* **153,** 181–186.

3

Production and Characterization of Antibodies Against Synthetic Peptides

David C. Hancock and Gerard I. Evan

1. Introduction

1.1. Immunizations

Immunization protocols vary greatly among laboratories. In general, there are no hard and fast rules, and most protocols give satisfactory results. The methods described below are designed to give optimal results with minimal injury to the test animal, and we have used them extensively and successfully for several years *(1–6)*. Peptide immunizations differ from those where the immunogen is a larger macromolecule in that maximal antipeptide titers (which arise rapidly after two to three immunizations) do not always coincide with maximal titers against the intact protein (which tend to peak rather later at four to six immunizations). Thus, although antipeptide enzyme-linked immuno-sorbent assays (ELISAs) are useful gages of immune responsivity, there is no substitute for eventual screening on the intact protein (e.g., by immunoprecipitation, Western blotting, and so forth). Individual variation in antipeptide response is very marked, so it is advisable to use several animals (three to six) per immunogen. Rabbit responses are generally poorer in specific pathogen-free (SPF) animals, probably reflecting their greater immune naivity. Mouse responses are often best in F_1 crosses (e.g., Balb/c × C57Bl/6) rather than pure strains. Alternatively, SJL mice generally respond well.

Adjuvants stabilize immunogens so that they induce the immune system persistently over long periods. Oil–water adjuvants, such as Freund's, are extremely effective, but must be prepared properly as **stable** emulsions. Such emulsions are thick, do not separate even after standing for long periods, and do not disperse if pipeted onto the surface of water. Immunogens administered in Freund's adjuvant can persist for weeks, and there is thus no point in repeating

From: *Methods in Molecular Biology, Vol. 80: Immunochemical Protocols, 2nd ed.*
Edited by: J. D. Pound © Humana Press Inc., Totowa, NJ

immunizations too frequently. Freund's complete adjuvant (FCA), which contains killed pertussis bacteria to induce massive nonspecific inflammation, causes ulceration (resulting in loss of immunogen and considerable discomfort to the animal) if administered in too large a bolus in one place or if given more than once. For this reason, subsequent immunizations are given using Freund's incomplete adjuvant (FIA), which contains no pertussis. An effective alternative to oil–water adjuvants is to administer the immunogen on alum as a fine adsorbed suspension. Precipitation of peptide–carrier conjugates with acetone also renders them partially insoluble and thus more persistent immunogens. Acetone precipitates are particularly useful for priming prior to spleen fusions for the development of monoclonal antibodies (MAbs).

Immunizations prior to such fusions should not be done with persistent adjuvants, such as Freund's, because in this case the aim is to induce a rapid and transient immune response whose early (lymphoproliferative) stage coincides with fusion to myeloma cells.

1.2. ELISA for Antipeptide Antibodies

Because the peptide immunogen used to generate antibodies is available in comparatively large amounts, it is seldom necessary to use highly sensitive radioimmunoassays to check antibody titers. For almost all purposes, a peroxidase- or β-galactosidase-based enzyme-linked colorimetric assay is adequate. The target antigen is passively adsorbed to the walls of microtiter wells, either as free peptide or as peptide conjugated to an **irrelevant** carrier protein (e.g., bovine serum albumin [BSA]). Usually, the free peptide makes a perfectly effective antigenic target, but occasionally important determinants on some peptides are masked by adsorption to the plate, in which case peptide–carrier conjugates should be used. Thus, if antibody titer on free peptide is low, it is a good idea to try conjugated peptide as the target. Antibodies bound to the adsorbed peptide are detected with an appropriate enzyme-linked second-layer reagent, typically antiimmunoglobulin or protein A, and the assay developed with a colorimetric substrate.

1.3. Affinity Purification of Antipeptide Antibody

It can occasionally be necessary to purify an antibody preparation, perhaps in order to eliminate background "noise" in a particular assay. With a ready source of immunogen in the form of peptide, it is straightforward to purify antipeptide antibodies by affinity chromatography. The peptide is covalently coupled to agarose and the crude antibody passed down the column. Unbound material is washed away and the bound antibody eluted under denaturing conditions, for example, low pH (pH 2.5), high pH (pH 11.5), or $4M$ $MgCl_2$. Immunoglobulins are unusually resistant to permanent denaturation by pH extremes or chaotropic reagents, although there are always exceptions (especially with MAbs). $MgCl_2$ elution is the mildest, and therefore the first method to try; low pH followed by rapid neutralization is used most frequently in our laboratory.

The affinities of antibodies for their cognate peptides can be very high, so it is sometimes difficult to recover quantitatively the higher-affinity antibodies in a polyclonal serum from the peptide resin. For this reason, it is essential to use only low concentrations of peptide on the resin (typically 100–200 µg of peptide/mL of agarose gel) and to elute bound antibody in the **reverse** direction to which it was run into the column, so as not to drive eluting antibodies into a further excess of antigen. If both of these criteria are adhered to, yields are usually on the order of 60–80% recovery.

Suitable affinity resins are CNBr-activated Sepharose and similarly activated *N*-hydroxysuccinimide ester-based gels with spacer arms. These react with free amino groups on the peptide. If the peptide contains many lysine residues, alternative coupling systems may be used, for example, carbodiimide-activated agaroses. In our experience, however, even peptides with internal lysines make good immunoadsorbents, and we routinely use CNBr-activated Sepharose.

2. Materials

2.1. Immunizations

1. FCA and FIA: FCA is a suspension of killed pertussis in oil. This should be shaken well before use. FIA is just oil. Freund's adjuvants should be mixed with the aqueous immunogen solution/suspension at a ratio between 1:2 and 2:1 and mixed until set. This is most easily achieved by passage back and forth between two **glass** syringes connected by a three-way luer fitting. After a while (1–5 min) the mixture should become noticeably "stiffer," and may then be used.
2. Potassium aluminum sulfate (Alum) $AlK(SO_4)_2 \cdot 12H_2O$: The aqueous immunogen solution/suspension is mixed with 0.3 vol 10% aluminum. The pH is then adjusted to about 8.0 with sodium hydroxide solution, and the resultant precipitate washed in 0.9% NaCl solution and administered.
3. Acetone precipitates: The aqueous immunogen is precipitated with 4.5 vol acetone at –20°C. The precipitate is collected by centrifugation at 10,000*g* at **room temperature**, washed in 80% acetone, and air-dried. The pellet is resuspended in saline using a Dounce™ homogenizer, and then administered directly or in association with alum or Freund's adjuvants.
4. Bacillus Calmette-Guerin (BCG): An attenuated strain of bovine tubercle bacillus is available from Glaxo or from outdated hospital supplies as a lyophilized powder. Before use, it is suspended in sterile distilled water.
5. Saline: 0.9% NaCl.
6. Glass syringes (2 and 10 mL).

7. Disposable three-way luer fitting taps.
8. Peptide conjugate.

2.2. ELISA

1. 10X Adsorption buffer: $1M$ sodium bicarbonate, pH 9.6 (adjust with NaOH).
2. Peptide solution/suspension at 1 mg/mL in phosphate-buffered saline (PBS) stored at $-20°C$.
3. Antipeptide antibody.
4. "Immulon 2" **hard** plastic 96-well microtiter plates (Dynatech Ltd.).
5. Rabbit antimouse Ig-horseradish peroxidase conjugate (RaMIg-HRP), Donkey antirabbit Ig-horseradish peroxidase conjugate (DaRIg-HRP), swine antirabbit Ig-horseradish peroxidase conjugate (SwaRIg-HRP), protein A-peroxidase or appropriate β-galactosidase-conjugated second-layer reagent (DAKO [High Wycombe, UK] or Amersham International [Amersham, UK]).
6. Tris-buffered saline (TBS): 25 mM Tris-HCl/144 mM NaCl, pH 8.2.
7. Blocking buffer (TM): TBS containing 2% dried milk powder (Marvel).
8. Assay buffer (TMT): TBS containing 2% dried milk powder and 0.5% Tween-20.
9. Substrate solution for HRP: 1 mM 2,2' azinobis 3-ethylbenzthiazoline-6 sulfonic acid (ABTS) (Sigma, St. Louis, MO) in 0.1M sodium acetate, pH 5.0. Add 1 μL of 30% hydrogen peroxide/1 mL of ABTS solution **just before** use. Discard any old ABTS stocks that have a noticeable green color when dissolved in the absence of hydrogen peroxide.
10. Stop solution for peroxidase assays: 5% sodium dodecyl sulfate (SDS).
11. Substrate solution for β-galactosidase: 4 mg/mL dinitrophenyl-β-D-galactopyranoside (ONPG) dissolved in TBS containing 0.7% 2-mercaptoethanol and 1 mM MgCl$_2$.
12. Stop solution for β-galactosidase: $1M$ Na$_2$CO$_3$.

2.3. Affinity Purification

1. CNBr-activated Sepharose (Pharmacia, Uppsala, Sweden).
2. Sintered glass funnels.
3. Chromatography columns (Pharmacia C series).
4. Peristaltic pump.
5. Concentrated HCl.
6. PBS.
7. 100 mM Na acetate, pH 4.0.
8. $2M$ NaCl in PBS.
9. TBS.
10. TBS containing 0.1% sodium azide **(Caution: toxic)**.
11. TBS containing 0.1% NP40.
12. 250 mM EDTA, pH 8.0.
13. Saturated ammonium sulfate solution.
14. NP40 stock solution: 10% in water.
15. 100 mM Na citrate, pH 2.5.

16. $2M$ Tris base.
17. Saline: 0.9% NaCl.
18. $4M$ MgCl$_2$.
19. 10X TBS: 250 mM Tris-HCl/1.44M NaCl, pH 8.2.

3. Methods

3.1. KLH/Thyroglobulin-Peptide Conjugate Immunizations

1. Immunize rabbits as follows (*see* Note 2):
   a. Intradermally immunize with 50–200 µg of peptide conjugate in FCA at multiple sites.
   b. After 2–3 wk, immunize again intradermally with 50–100 µg of conjugate in FIA.
   c. Repeat step b at 2-wk intervals. Bleed 10 d after immunization. We usually test bleed (from the ear) after the third and fifth immunizations, and then completely exsanguinate after a further one to four immunizations as appropriate, depending on the efficacy of the antiserum.
2. Immunize mice as follows:
   a. Immunize in the tail-base with 20–100 µg of peptide conjugate in FCA.
   b. After 2 wk, immunize intramuscularly (e.g., in the base of the tail), or subcutaneously (in the flanks) with about 50 µg of conjugate in FIA.
   c. Repeat step b at 2–3-wk intervals until titers plateau (three to six immunizations in total). Test bleed (from the tail) 10 d after immunization.
   d. For fusions, 3–10 wk after last immunization, immunize intraperitoneally with about 50 µg of conjugate on alum or as an acetone precipitate in saline (d 0). Reimmunize 3 d later (d 3). Fuse 3 d later (d 6).
3. Immunization with PPD–peptide conjugates (*see* Note 1).
   a. Four to 6 wk before start of immunization, inoculate with two adult doses of BCG (all animals) in saline subcutaneously without adjuvant.
   b. Administer the first PPD–peptide immunization in FIA.
   c. Repeat step b at 3–4-wk intervals until titers plateau. Test bleed (from the tail) 10 d after immunization.
   d. For fusions, follow the same procedure used for KLH/thyroglobulin conjugates described in step 2d.

3.2. ELISA for Antipeptide Antibodies

3.2.1. Adsorption of Peptide to Microtiter Plates

1. If using free peptide as the antigenic target, dilute it to a final concentration of 50 pmol/mL in adsorption buffer (roughly a dilution of about 1 in 2000 for a 10-mer peptide). If using a peptide–carrier conjugate as the target, dilute the conjugate in adsorption buffer to a **peptide** concentration of about 10 µg/mL. The precise amount of peptide conjugate may need eventually to be titrated to give optimal signals.
2. Add 100 µL of diluted peptide solution to each well.

3. Leave at room temperature in a wet box overnight.
4. Shake out any unadsorbed peptide, and wash the plate three times in TBS by immersion of the plate in a TBS bath. Immerse the plate at an angle to avoid trapping air bubbles. Shake the plate dry.
5. Add 150 µL of TM buffer/well, and leave at room temperature for at least 30 min. If required, store the plates at this stage at –20°C.

3.2.2. ELISA

1. Empty the wells, and add 100 µL of antibody diluted in TMT/well. Suitable starting dilutions are 1 in 50 for antisera, 1 in 2 for hybridoma culture supernatants, and 1 in 500 for hybridoma ascites fluids. Serially dilute antibody in doubling dilutions down one row of the microtiter plate (i.e., eight dilutions).
2. Leave for 30 min at room temperature.
3. Wash the wells three times in TBS as before.
4. Add 100 µL/well of appropriate second-layer reagent diluted in TMT. Dilute the stock HRP–anti-Ig conjugates (from the manufacturer) 1 in 200, stock protein A-HRP solution (1 mg/mL) 1 in 200, and stock β-galactosidase conjugates 1 in 100 (*see* Note 3).
5. Leave for 30 min at room temperature.
6. Wash three times in TBS as before.
7. Add 100 µL of substrate solution/well.
8. Incubate at room temperature. Peroxidase reactions take about 5–30 min to develop. β-galactosidase reactions can take longer. Judge the reaction time by eye (*see* Notes 4 and 5). Reactions may be stopped by adding 100 µL of appropriate stop solution to each well (5% SDS for peroxidase, $1M$ Na_2CO_3 for β-galactosidase). The SDS also solubilizes any precipitated products formed in the HRP reaction.
9. Read the optical density (OD) on an ELISA plate reader. Green ABTS reaction product and yellow ONPG reaction product may both be read at a wavelength of 406 nm.

3.3. Affinity Purification

3.3.1. Preparation of Peptide Agarose

1. Mix 1.5 g of CNBr-Sepharose and 200 mL of 1 mM HCl, and leave for 15 min at room temperature.
2. Collect the slurry on a sinter funnel, and drain until a moist cake is formed. Add the cake (typically ~ 5 mL vol) to 5 mL of PBS (pH 7.5–8.0) containing ~ 500 µg of peptide. Agitate **gently** for about 2 h at room temperature. **Note: Do not** use a magnetic stirrer, since this fragments the resin and generates fines, which then slow or block the column flow.
3. Pour the slurry onto a sinter, and wash sequentially with 20 mL of the following: PBS; 100 mM sodium acetate, pH 4.0; $2M$ NaCl in PBS; TBS. Store as a 50% slurry in TBS containing 0.1% sodium azide at 4°C.

3.3.2. Preparation of Serum or Ascites Fluid

1. Allow clots to form. Ring the tube to prevent the clot adhering and leave overnight at 4°C.
2. Remove the supernatant, and clarify the serum/ascites by centrifugation at 1000g for 5 min.
3. Adjust the sample to 5 mM EDTA, add 0.82 vol of saturated ammonium sulfate solution while stirring, and leave for 15 min at room temperature.
4. Collect the pellet by centrifugation (10 min, 10,000g, 4°C).
5. Redissolve the pellet in its original volume using TBS. Add 10% NP40 to a final concentration of 0.1%, and spin in a microfuge to clarify.

3.3.3. Affinity Chromatography

1. Use a Pharmacia reversible column. Pack 2 mL of affinity matrix into the column (keep moist) in running buffer (TBS containing 0.1% NP40). Wash with 20 mL of running buffer over 20 min.
2. Run in the antibody solution as prepared earlier. The flow rate should be about 1–2 mL/min (a peristaltic pump is useful to control the flow rate). Run in the equivalent of about 1 mL of antiserum/mL of gel.
3. Wash with 10 column volume of running buffer.
4. Reverse the direction of flow. Wash with 10 column volume of TBS containing 0.1% NP40 over 10 min 5 column volume of TBS at the same flow rate and 5 column volume of 0.9% NaCl.
5. Elution of antibody may be achieved by either one of the following two procedures.
   a. Low pH elution: Elute the bound antibody with 4-column volume of 100 mM sodium citrate, pH 2.5, over 10 min, collecting the eluate and immediately neutralizing to pH 5.0–8.0 with 2M Tris base. This can be achieved by prealiquoting into the collecting tubes the amount of Tris base necessary to neutralize a given fraction volume. Fractions may be assayed by ELISA (*see* Section 3.2.) diluted 1 in 5 to 1 in 50. Pool the most strongly positive fractions. Adjust the pooled fractions to pH 6.0, and add 1 vol of saturated ammonium sulfate solution. Leave for 10 min at room temperature, and pellet the antibody at 10,000g for 10 min at 4°C. Resuspend the antibody in water at about 1–5 mg/mL (OD$_{280}$ of IgG is about 1.4 for a 1 mg/mL solution). Either dialyze against TBS containing 0.1% sodium azide or add 1/10 vol 10X TBS (*see* Note 6). Store in aliquots at –20°C.
   b. Elution with 4M MgCl$_2$: Elute the bound antibody with 4 column volumes of 4M MgCl$_2$. Dilute the eluate 10 times with distilled water. Add an equal volume of saturated ammonium sulfate and pellet the immunoglobulin at 10,000g. Resuspend the pellet in water. Either dialyze against TBS containing 0.1% sodium azide or add 1/10 vol 10X TBS (*see* Note 6). Store in aliquots at –20°C.

4. Notes

1. If PPD is used as the carrier for peptide immunizations, the animals must first be primed with live attenuated tubercle bacteria (BCG strain), which express PPD on their surface. This priming step elicits a strong T-cell helper response against subsequent PPD-linked immunogens. FCA actually appears to interfere with this priming process and so **must** be avoided if using this method.
2. A "preimmunization" serum sample from the test animal serves as an excellent negative control serum. This can conveniently be taken at the time of the first immunization.
3. Protein A only binds certain Ig subclasses at neutral pH (for example, many mouse antibodies of the IgG1 subclass fall into this category). Its binding range can, however, be greatly extended by using high-pH (pH 8.5) buffers and high salt (1–2M NaCl), although these conditions can be inconsistent with antibody binding to peptide. For this reason, anti-Ig detection reagents are advised for primary testing of antipeptide antibodies.
4. If the ELISA color development takes more than a few minutes, continue the incubation in the dark. β-galactosidase reactions tend to have a lower spontaneous background than peroxidase reactions, but take longer to develop. β-galactosidase reactions can be sped up by incubation at 37°C.
5. Avoid contamination of substrate solutions by skin contact, since this can sometimes increase background activity. Read HRP reactions immediately, since atmospheric oxidation will gradually react with substrate in all wells.
6. Ammonium sulfate precipitation of IgG inevitably leads to residual ammonium sulfate in the pellet. Dialysis will remove this, but may also lead to a significant loss of antibody. For most purposes, addition of 10X TBS to the resuspended pellet is an acceptable alternative.

References

1. Evan, G. I., Hancock, D. C., Littlewood, T. D., and Gee, N. S. (1986) Characterization of human *myc* proteins. *Curr. Top. Micro. Immunol.* **132**, 362–374.
2. Evan, G. I., Lewis, G. K., Ramsay, G., and Bishop, J. M. (1985) Isolation of monoclonal antibodies specific for the human c-*myc* protooncogene product. *Mol. Cell. Biol.* **5**, 3610–3616.
3. Hunt, S. P., Pini, A., and Evan, G. I. (1987) Induction of c-*fos*-like protein in spinal cord neurons following sensory stimulation. *Nature (Lond.)* **328**, 632–634.
4. Moore, J. P., Hancock, D. C., Littlewood, T. D., and Evan, G. I. (1987) A sensitive and quantitative enzyme-linked immunosorbence assay for the c-*myc* and N-*myc* oncoproteins. *Oncogene Res.* **2**, 65–80.
5. Waters, C. M., Hancock, D. C., and Evan, G. I. (1990) Identification and characterization of the *egr-1* gene product as an inducible, short-lived, nuclear phosphoprotein. *Oncogene* **5**, 669–674.
6. Littlewood, T. D., Amati, B., Land, H., and Evan, G. I. (1992) Max and c-Myc/Max DNA-binding activities in cell extracts. *Oncogene* **7**, 1783–1792.

4

Preparation and Testing of Monoclonal Antibodies to Recombinant Proteins

Christopher J. Dean

1. Introduction

Monoclonal antibodies (MAbs) are essential reagents for the isolation, identification, and cellular localization of specific gene products and for aiding in
the determination of their macromolecular structure. They can also help in
identifying the function of the protein. Although the ability to clone and
sequence specific genes has revolutionized our understanding of cellular structure and function, the preparation of recombinant proteins and the synthesis of
peptides based on protein sequences derived from cDNA clones have provided
sufficient material for generating specific antibodies. The proteins may be isolated and purified directly from cells, or recombinant proteins may be derived
from prokaryotic systems, such as *Escherichia coli*, or from eukaryotic expression systems, such as Chinese hamster ovary (CHO) cells, or insect cells
expressing constructs in *baculovirus*. The eukaryotic systems are being used
increasingly for expression of glycoproteins, because the recombinant material
is glycosylated. It should be remembered, however, that glycosylation may be
species-specific and if one of the functions of the protein depends on carbohydrate, then the function of a recombinant glycoprotein may be altered depending on the species used for expression.

A number of protocols will be described here that have been used successfully with both rat (Y3 and IR983F) and mouse (SP2/0) myelomas to generate
MAbs to cellular proteins, recombinant proteins, or peptides based on cDNA
sequences. Successful hybridoma production relies on the ability to:

1. Generate specific B-cells;
2. Fuse them with a myeloma cell line;
3. Identify the antibodies that are sought in culture supernatants; and
4. Isolate and clone the specific hybridoma.

From: *Methods in Molecular Biology, Vol. 80: Immunochemical Protocols, 2nd ed.*
Edited by: J. D. Pound © Humana Press Inc., Totowa, NJ

Of particular importance is the elicitation of the specific B-cells required for fusion, and several protocols to achieve this aim will be described. It should be remembered that the presence of specific antibody in serum is not necessarily a guarantee of success, nor is its absence a surety for failure.

The second important requirement is for a quick, reliable assay(s) for the specific antibody that can be applied to the large numbers of culture supernatants (≥ 96) that may be generated. Usually, the assays make use of a labeled second antibody (e.g., rabbit, sheep, or goat antibodies directed against the F[ab']$_2$ of mouse or rat immunoglobulins) to identify the binding of MAb to antigen. The second antibody can be detected because it is conjugated to a fluorescent marker, e.g., fluorescein or a radiolabel, such as ^{125}I. Alternatively, conjugates of second antibody with enzymes, such as alkaline phosphatase, peroxidase, or β-galactosidase, may be employed.

Persistence is an absolute requirement for the hybridoma producer; fusions can fail for many reasons, and it is essential not to give up because of early failures. The methods described in this chapter include techniques for:

1. Preparation of antigen;
2. Immunization;
3. Hybridoma production; and
4. Assaying the MAb-producing hybridomas.

2. Materials
2.1. Generation of Immune Spleen or Lymph Node Cells

1. Rats of any strain aged 10–12 wk, or Balb/c mice aged 6–8 wk (*see* Notes 1 and 2).
2. Phosphate-buffered saline (PBS), pH 7.4: 1.15 g of Na_2HPO_4, 0.2 g of KH_2PO_4, 0.2 g KCl, 8.0 g of NaCl dissolved in water, and make up to 1 L.
3. Antigen: One of the following sources of antigen can be used to raise MAbs.
   a. Cells, e.g., mouse 3T3-cells expressing recombinant human membrane protein (*see* Note 3).
   b. Soluble protein dissolved in PBS at a concentration of 1.0–4.0 mg/mL.
   c. Soluble recombinant protein extracted from cells or supernatants of eukaryotic cells (e.g., CHO cells or insect cells expressing recombinant *baculovirus*), or bacteria, such as *E. coli*, harboring plasmids or recombinant viruses. In *E. coli*, recombinant material is often generated as a fusion protein with β-galactosidase or glutathione transferase (*see* Notes 3 and 4).
   d. Proteins separated electrophoretically in sodium dodecyl sulfate containing polyacrylamide gels (SDS-PAGE), and eluted electrophoretically from gel slices. Often, β-galactosidase fusion proteins are prepared in this way because of their poor solubility.
   e. Peptide conjugated to a protein carrier and dissolved in PBS.
4. Freund's complete adjuvant (FCA).
5. Freund's incomplete adjuvant (FIA).

2.1.1. Conjugation to Carriers

1. Ovalbumin, bovine serum albumin (BSA), or Keyhole lympet hemocyanin (KLH), at 20 mg/mL in PBS.
2. PPD-kit (tuberculin-purified protein derivative, Cambridge Research Biochemicals Ltd., Macclesfield, UK).
3. Glutaraldehyde (specially purified grade 1): 25% solution in distilled water.
4. $1M$ Glycine-HCl, pH 6.6.

2.2. Hybridoma Production

1. Dulbecco's Modified Eagle's Medium (DMEM) containing glucose (1 g/L), sodium bicarbonate (3.7 g/L), glutamine ($4 \times 10^{-3}M$), penicillin (50 U/mL), streptomycin (50 µg/mL), and neomycin (100 µg/mL) stored at 5–6°C and used within 2 wk of preparation.
2. Fetal calf serum (FCS): inactivated by heating for 30 min at 5–6°C and tested for ability to support growth of hybridomas (*see* Note 5).
3. HAT selection medium: Prepare 100X HT by dissolving 136 mg of hypoxanthine and 38.75 mg of thymidine in 100 mL of $0.02M$ NaOH prewarmed to 60°C. Cool, filter-sterilize, and store at –20°C in 1- and 2-mL aliquots. Prepare 100X A by dissolving 1.9 mg aminopterin in 100 mL $0.01M$ NaOH, and then filter-sterilize and store at –20°C in 2-mL aliquots. HAT medium is prepared by adding 2 mL of HT and 2 mL of A to 200 mL of DMEM containing 20% FCS.
4. HT medium: Add 1 mL of HT to 100 mL DMEM containing 10% FCS.
5. Feeder cells for fusion cultures (*see* Note 6): essential for fusions employing rat myelomas. Quickly thaw irradiated rat fibroblasts, prepared as described in Note 6, just before commencing the cell fusion. Add the cells to 10 mL of serum-free DMEM, centrifuge, and wash once in serum-free DMEM. Resuspend feeders in HAT medium just before addition of the fusion mixture. Alternatively, use thymocytes from spleen donors (mouse).
6. Polyethylene glycol (PEG) solution: Weigh 50 g of PEG (1500 molecular weight) into a capped 200-mL bottle, add 1 mL water, and then autoclave for 30 min at 120°C. Cool to about 70°C, add 50 mL of DMEM, mix, and after cooling to ambient temperature, adjust the pH to about 7.2 with $1M$ NaOH (the mixture should be colored orange). Store as 1-mL aliquots at –20°C.
7. Freezer medium: Freshly prepared 5% dimethyl sulfoxide in FCS.
8. Myeloma cell line: Mouse SP2/0–Ag14 or rat IR 983F cells growing exponentially in 25- or 75-cm² flasks containing DMEM/10% FCS (dilute to $2–3 \times 10^5$ cells/mL the day before fusion). The rat myeloma Y3 Ag1.2.3. has to be grown in spinner culture to fuse well. Seven to 10 d before cells are required, about 5×10^6 cells, stored frozen in liquid nitrogen as 1-mL aliquots in freezer medium, are thawed quickly at 37°C, diluted with 10 mL DMEM-10% FCS, centrifuged ($500g$ for 2 min), then resuspended in 100 mL of the same medium, and placed in a 200-mL spinner flask. Let stand for 2 d at 37°C to allow cells to attach to the base of the vessel. Then place the spinner flask on a magnetic stirrer (e.g., Bellco)

running at about 160 rpm. The Y3 myeloma has a generation time of about 10 h, and exponentially growing cultures require feeding daily by fourfold dilution with fresh medium.

2.3. Screening Culture Supernatants

1. PBSA: PBS containing 0.02% NaN_3. (NaN_3 should be handled with care. It is an inhibitor of cytochrome oxidase, and is highly toxic and mutagenic. Aqueous solutions release HN_3 at 37°C.)
2. PBST: PBSA containing 0.4% Tween-20.
3. PBS-BSA: PBSA containing 0.5% BSA.
4. PBS-Marvel: PBSA containing 3% Marvel (skimmed milk powder). Centrifuge or filter through Whatman No. 1 paper to remove undissolved solids. This is cheaper to use and just as effective as PBS-BSA.
5. Plate-coating buffer (PCB), pH 8.2: $0.01M$ Na_2HPO_4, $0.01M$ KH_2PO_4, and $0.14M$ NaCl.
6. Alkaline sarkosyl: 1% Sodium dodecyl sarkosinate in $0.5M$ NaOH.
7. Plates containing cell-bound antigens: Monolayers of cells grown in 96-well polystyrene (PS) plates (*see Methods in Molecular Biology*, Volume 5, Chapter 54 for detailed instructions).
   a. Rodent cells expressing a recombinant protein, e.g., CHO or 3T3 cells transfected with genes for human transmembrane proteins;
   b. Tumor cell lines overexpressing transmembrane proteins, e.g., the receptor for EGF or the product of the *c-erbB-2* gene;
   c. Adherent cell line expressing high cytoplasmic levels of the specific antigen, which can be accessed following fixation and permeabilization with methanol. Wash the cells with ice-cold DMEM and then add to each well 200 µL of methanol that has been precooled to –70°C by standing in cardice-ethanol. Leave at ambient temperature for 5 min, "flick" off the methanol, and wash twice with medium containing 5% FCS (live cells), or PBS-Marvel (fixed cells); and
   d. Control cell line that either does not express the specific antigen (e.g., normal 3T3 cells), or in which expression is at the normal one gene copy level. This will act as the negative control.
8. Plates coated with purified soluble antigen. As an alternative to step 7 above, and providing purified soluble antigen is available, 96-well PS or polyvinyl chloride (PVC) plates can be coated with protein, recombinant protein, peptide, or peptide conjugated to a carrier protein. Plates are coated as follows:
   a. Dissolve the antigen at 1 µg/mL in PCB.
   b. Coat by incubation with 50 µL of antigen per well for 2 h at 37°C or overnight at 4–6°C.
   c. Block the remaining reactive sites by incubation for 2 h at 37°C with 200 µL/ well of PBS-Marvel.
   d. Wash the plates with PBST before use.
   In many cases, the coated plates can be stored at 4–6°C for several weeks (fill wells with PBST), but it is wise to check their antibody-binding capacity before use.

9. Plates for antibody-capture assays: Where a specific antibody is available, this may be a better assay to use than step 8 above, because the antigen is less likely to be subject to denaturation.
    a. Coat wells first by incubating for either 2 h at 37°C or overnight at 4–6°C with 50 μL (1–5 μg/mL in PCB) of a polyclonal antibody or MAb to the specific antigen. Where peptides coupled to BSA are used, the plates can be coated first with rabbit antibodies to BSA.
    b. Block the wells with PBS-Marvel for 2 h at 37°C.
    c. Incubate with the specific antigen (50 μL/well of a 0.1–1 μg/mL solution in PBST) for 2 h at 37°C, or overnight at 4–6°C, and then wash with PBST. For antigens that are not readily soluble, e.g., membrane proteins extracted in nonionic detergents, the extract in 0.5–1% Triton X-100 or Nonidet-P40 can be used after suitable dilution with PBSA containing 0.5% of the detergent. All subsequent procedures should be carried out using buffers containing detergent at 0.1–0.5%. These plates are best prepared within a day of use.

2.3.1. Immunoprecipitations

1. Protein A/G or specific anti-immunoglobulin covalently linked to Sepharose 4B or similar bead support for preparing immunoprecipitates (*see* Note 14).
2. CNBr-activated Sepharose 4B.
3. Radiolabeled (^{3}H, ^{14}C, ^{35}S, or ^{125}I) protein or cell extract prepared in PBSA containing $10^{-3}M$ phenyl methyl sulfonyl fluoride (PMSF) as proteinase inhibitor, and 0.5–1.0% nonionic detergent.
4. Specific MAb either purified or as culture supernatant.
5. Polyclonal antibody to mouse or rat immunoglobulins depending on the species in which the MAb was raised.

2.3.2. Western Blotting (see also Chapter 20)

1. Blotting membrane: Nitrocellulose or PVDF membrane.
2. Equipment for wet or semidry blotting.

2.3.3. Second Antibodies

1. Sheep, rabbit, or goat antibodies to rat or mouse F[ab']$_2$, IgG, IgA, and IgM for labeling with ^{125}I to carry out radioimmunoassay (RIA), or conjugated to alkaline phosphatase or biotin for an enzyme-linked immunosorbent assay (ELISA).
2. 1.5-mL polypropylene microcentrifuge tubes coated with 10 μg of IODO-GEN (Pierce Chemical, Rockford, IL) by evaporation, under a stream of nitrogen, from a 100 μg/mL solution in methylene chloride (*see* Note 8).
3. Carrier-free ^{125}I, radioactive concentration 100 mCi/mL (e.g., code IMS.30, Amersham International, Amersham, UK).
4. γ-Counter.
5. UB: 100 mM phosphate-buffer (Na$_2$HPO$_4$/KH$_2$PO$_4$), pH 7.4, containing 0.5M NaCl and 0.02% NaN$_3$.

6. 30 × 0.7 cm Disposocolumn (Bio-Rad, Hercules, CA) containing Sephadex G25, equilibrated before use with UB and pretreated with 100 µL of FCS to block sites that bind protein nonspecifically.
7. 3-mL Tubes for collection of samples.
8. Lead pots for storage of ^{125}I-labeled antibodies.
9. Streptavidin labeled with ^{125}I or conjugated to alkaline phosphatase or to fluorescein.
10. 96-Well plate reader for ELISA.

2.3.4. Buffers and Substrates for Alkaline Phosphatase Used in ELISA

1. 10 mM Diethanolamine, pH 9.5, containing 0.5M NaCl.
2. 100 mM Diethanolamine, pH 9.5, containing 100 mM NaCl, and 5 mM MgCl$_2$.
3. Substrate to give a soluble product (plate assays): 0.1% p-nitrophenyl phosphate in 10 mM diethanolamine, pH 9.5, containing 0.5 mM MgCl$_2$.
4. Substrate to give an insoluble product (Western blots):
   a. NBT stock: 5% nitroblue tetrazolium in 70% dimethyl formamide.
   b. BCIP stock: 5% disodium bromochloroindolyl phosphate in dimethyl formamide.
   c. Alkaline phosphatase buffer: 100 mM diethanolamine, pH 9.5, containing 100 mM NaCl, and 5 mM MgCl$_2$.
   Just before use, add 66 µL NBT stock solution to 10 mL of alkaline phosphatase buffer, mix well, and add 33 µL of BCIP stock solution.

3. Methods
3.1. Conjugation of Peptides to Carriers

Peptides that do not bear epitopes recognized by T-cells are poor immunogens and must be conjugated to carrier proteins or PPD to elicit good immune responses.

1. Protein carriers, such as BSA or KLH: Mix the peptide and carrier in a 1:1 ratio, e.g., pipet 250 µL of each into a 5-mL glass beaker on a magnetic stirrer. Small fleas can be made from pieces of paper clip sealed in polythene tubing by heating. Add 5 µL 25% glutaraldehyde and continue stirring for 15 min at room temperature. Block excess glutaraldehyde by adding 100 µL of 1M glycine and stirring for a further 15 min. Use directly or dialyze overnight against PBS, and store at –20°C.
2. PPD kit: **Read instructions supplied with the kit very carefully.** Inhalation of the ether-dried tuberculin PPD is dangerous for tuberculin-sensitive people to handle. Follow specific instructions to couple 2 mg of peptide to 10 mg PPD and, after dialysis, store at –20°C.

3.2. Antigens for Immunization

1. Suspend whole cells in PBS or DMEM at 5 × 10^6–10^7 cells/mL.
2. Mix proteins, peptide conjugates, or eluates from polyacrylamide gels in PBS 1:1 with adjuvant (FCA for the first immunization, subsequently with FIA) in a

capped plastic tube (LP3 [Luckham Ltd., Burgess Hill, UK]), "bijou," or 30-mL universal bottle by vortexing until a stable emulsion is formed. Check that phase separation does not occur on standing at 4°C for >2 h. Alternatively, allow drop to fall from a Pasteur pipet onto a water surface. The drop should contract, remain as a droplet, and not disperse.

3.3. Immunization Procedures

1. Anesthetize animals (*see* Note 1), and take a blood sample from the jugular or tail vein into a capped 0.5- or 1.5-mL microcentrifuge tube to act as a preimmune sample. Allow it to clot, centrifuge at 1500g, remove the serum, and store at –20°C.
2. For fusions that will use spleen cells, immunize at 5 sites (4 times subcutaneously and 1 time intraperitoneally) with a total of 50–500 µg of antigen in FCA/animal. Test bleed 14 d later and reimmunize using the same protocol, but with antigen in FIA. Test bleed and reimmunize at monthly intervals until sera are positive for antibodies to the antigen (*see* Section 3.5.). Three days before the fusions are done, rechallenge the animals intravenously with antigen in PBS alone.
3. For fusions that will use mesenteric lymph nodes of rats, the antigens are injected into the Peyer's patches that lie along the small intestine. The surgical procedures are described in *Methods in Molecular Biology*, Volume 5, Chapter 54. Again, test bleed the rats and then immunize two or three times at 1-mo intervals, and use the mesenteric nodes 3 d after the final immunization. This protocol has resulted in good yields of specific IgG- and IgA-producing hybridomas *(1,2)*.

3.4. Hybridoma Production

3.4.1. Preparation of Cells for Fusion

1. Centrifuge exponentially growing rat or mouse myeloma cells in 50-mL aliquots for 3 min at 400g, wash twice by resuspension in serum-free DMEM, count in a hemocytometer, and resuspend in this medium to 1–2 × 10^7 cells/mL.
2. Kill immune animals by cervical dislocation or CO_2 inhalation, test bleed, and open abdominal cavity. Remove spleens or mesenteric nodes by blunt dissection.
3. Disaggregate spleens or nodes by forcing through a fine stainless-steel mesh (e.g., tea strainer) into 10 mL of serum-free DMEM using a spoon-head spatula (dipped into ethanol and flamed to sterilize it).
4. Centrifuge cells for 5 min at 400g, wash twice in serum-free DMEM, and resuspend in 10 mL of the same medium.
5. Count viable lymphoid cells in a hemocytometer. Spleens from immune mice yield about 10^8 cells, from rats 3–5 × 10^8 cells, and the mesenteric nodes of rats up to 2 × 10^8 cells.

3.4.2. Fusion Protocol

1. Mix 10^8 viable lymphocytes with 5 × 10^7 rat myeloma cells or 2 × 10^7 mouse myeloma cells in a 10-mL sterile capped tube, and centrifuge for 3 min at 400g.
2. Pour off the supernatant, drain carefully with Pasteur pipet, and then release cell pellet by gently tapping tube on bench.

3. Stir 1 mL of PEG solution, prewarmed to 37°C, into the pellet over a period of 1 min. Continue mixing for a further minute by gently rocking the tube.
4. Dilute the fusion mixture with DMEM (2 mL over a period of 2 min, and then 5 mL over 1 min).
5. Centrifuge for 3 min at 400g, and then resuspend the cells in 200 mL HAT selection medium, and add irradiated fibroblast or thymocyte feeder cells. Plate 2-mL aliquots into four 24-well plates or, if necessary, five 96-well plates (fusions with SP2/0 myeloma) (*see* Note 6).
6. Screen culture supernatants for specific antibody 6–14 d after commencement of incubation at 37°C in 5% CO_2–95% air (*see* Section 3.5.).
7. With a Pasteur pipet, pick individual colonies into 1 mL of HT medium contained in 24-well plates. Feed with 1 mL of HT medium, and split when good growth commences. Freeze samples in liquid nitrogen.
8. Rescreen the picked colonies and expand positive cultures. Freeze samples of these in liquid nitrogen and clone twice.

3.4.3. Cloning of Hybridomas

1. Prepare a suspension of mouse thymocytes or irradiated rat fibroblasts as feeders (5×10^5/20 mL of HT or DMEM containing 10% FCS).
2. Centrifuge cells from at least two wells of a 24-well plate that contain confluent layers of hybridoma cells. Count the number of cells, and then dilute to give about 50 cells in 20 mL of HT or DMEM containing 10% FCS-containing feeder cells.
3. Carefully "flick off" the supernatant medium from the rat feeder cells, and plate 0.2-mL aliquots of hybridoma cells into each of the 96-wells.
4. Examine the plates 5–10 d later and screen those wells that contain only single colonies.
5. Pick cells from positive wells into 24-well plates, expand, and freeze in liquid nitrogen.
6. Reclone the best antibody producing colonies (*see* Section 3.5.).

3.5. Assays for Specific MAb

In most of the assays described, the detection of rat or mouse MAb depends on the use of a second antibody reagent specific for F[ab']$_2$ or heavy-chain isotype (*see* Note 14). These second antibodies are detected because they have either a radiolabel (^{125}I) or fluorescent tag (fluorescein), or are conjugated to an enzyme (e.g., alkaline phosphatase, peroxidase, or β-galactosidase) either directly or indirectly via a biotin–streptavidin bridge. As examples of these procedures, two alternative types of methodology, i.e., RIA using ^{125}I-labeled antibodies and ELISA using alkaline phosphatase conjugates, will be described. It is assumed that in most cases the second antibodies will be bought either as purified material for radiolabeling or already conjugated to fluorescein, biotin, or the enzyme of choice (*see* ref. *3* for additional methods).

3.5.1. Radiolabeling with ^{125}I

All of the following manipulations should be carried out in a Class I fume hood according to local safety regulations.

1. Add 50 μg purified antibody in 0.1 mL PBS to an IODO-GEN-coated tube followed by 500 μCi of ^{125}I (e.g., 5 μL of IMS-30, Amersham International). Cap and mix immediately by "flicking," and keep on ice with occasional shaking (*see* Note 11).
2. After 5 min, transfer the contents of the tube with a polythene, capillary ended, Pasteur pipet to a prepared Sephadex G-25 column, then wash in, and elute with, UB.
3. Collect 0.5-mL fractions by hand, count 10-μL aliquots, and pool the fractions containing the first peak of radioactivity.
4. Store at 4°C in an enclosed lead pot (e.g., ^{125}I container).

3.5.2. RIA Using Antigens Bound Directly to PVC Multiwell Plates

1. Add 50 μL of antibody containing culture supernatant, purified antibody, or ascites, diluted to 1–10 μg/mL in PBS-Marvel, to each of the antigen-coated wells.
2. Incubate for 1 h at ambient temperature, and then wash three times with 200 μL of PBST/well.
3. Add 50 μL of ^{125}I-labeled second antibody (10^5 cpm/50 μL in PBS-Marvel) to each well, and incubate for a further 1 h at ambient temperature.
4. Carefully discard the radioactive supernatant by inverting the plate over a sink, designated for aqueous radioactive waste, and then wash the wells three times with PBST.
5. Cut the plates into individual wells with scissors, and determine the ^{125}I-bound in a γ-counter.

3.5.3. RIA Using Antigens Bound via Antibody to PVC Multiwell Plates

The assays are done as described in Section 3.5.2. with the modification that, if the antigens require the presence of a nonionic detergent to retain their solubility or native conformation, the detergent should be added to the PBS-Marvel diluent/wash solution.

3.5.4. Assay Using Live Adherent Cells Grown in Multiwell PS Plates

All solutions should be prepared in DMEM or other suitable growth medium containing 5% FCS (or newborn calf serum [NBS], which, if tested for nontoxicity, may be used as a cheaper alternative). If the effect of antibody binding on the behavior of the membrane protein is unknown, then all incubations should be carried out at 4°C (float plates on ice bath and precool diluents). Monolayers of cells vary widely in their adhesion to plastic, and also, they may roundup after prolonged incubation at 4°C owing to depolymerization of microtubules (*see* Note 7).

1. Wash cell monolayers with DMEM containing 5% FCS or NBS to remove non-adherent/dead cells. Then proceed as described for antigens bound to PVC plates (*see* Section 3.5.2.), but using DMEM containing 5% FCS/NBS for all diluents, and washings.
2. After the final wash, lyse the cells by incubating for 15 min at room temperature with 200 µL/well of alkaline sarkosyl.
3. Transfer lysates to LP2 tubes (Luckham Ltd.), or similar, and determine the amount of ^{125}I present. Depending on the cells used, the background binding will vary from 50–200 cpm/well, whereas positive wells will be at least five times this value.

3.5.5. Competitive Assays

These are useful for mapping epitopes, determining whether two antibodies crossreact, and for comparing antibody affinities. They are the basis of quantitative assays (RIA), and use multiwell plates coated either with antigen or antibody as described in Section 2.3. The principle is either to compete the test antibody with ^{125}I-labeled specific MAb (*see* Section 3.5.1. for preparation), or polyclonal antibody for binding to antigen bound to a plastic surface (antibody-capture can be used to secure antigen to the plastic well, and this form of assay is useful where it is necessary to retain the antigen in its native conformation), or compete test antibody with ^{125}I-labeled antigen for binding to a specific antibody bound to a plastic surface.

1. Make doubling dilutions in PBS-Marvel of culture supernatant or of purified antibody starting at 20 µg/mL to give 50 µL final volume.
2. Add to each well 50 µL ^{125}I-labeled specific antibody or antigen ($2–4 \times 10^4$ cpm/mL in PBS-Marvel).
3. Transfer 50-µL aliquots of the mixtures to the antibody or antigen-coated PVC multiwell plate so that each well contains $1–4 \times 10^4$ cpm of radiolabel.
4. After 1–4 h at ambient temperature, wash the plates three times with PBST, and determine the ^{125}I bound. Controls to determine maximum binding should be included together with a standard curve prepared from dilutions of unlabeled specific antibody or antigen. Comparison of the inhibition curve produced with the test antibody with that of the control yields information on the crossreactivity of the two antibodies and their relative affinities for antigen. Expect to obtain a maximum binding of between 1 and 5×10^3 cpm/well, depending on the purity and quality of the labeled antigen or antibody. Hybridoma supernatants containing good competing antibodies (1–10 µg/mL) will reduce binding to the background (50–100 cpm/well).

3.5.6. Immunoprecipitation

This is an essential procedure for the isolation of antigens from complex sources (e.g., cells) and for their subsequent separation by electrophoresis in SDS-containing polyacrylamide gels and analysis by Western blotting.

1. Label cellular proteins metabolically by incubating cultures for 4–24 h with ^{35}S-methionine, ^{3}H-lysine, or ^{14}C-amino acids in medium deficient in the relevant amino acid.
2. Wash the cells three times with complete medium, and then incubate for a further hour in the same medium.
3. Wash the cells in ice-cold PBSA containing $10^{-3}M$ PMSF, and then lyse with minimum volume (1–2 mL/25-cm^2 flask) of PBSA containing $10^{-3}M$ PMSF and 0.5% Triton X-100 by incubating for 30 min on ice.
4. Transfer the lysate to a centrifuge tube, and spin at 30,000g for 30 min to remove cell debris.
5. Prepare immunoabsorbent beads by linking 5–15 mg of purified MAb or polyclonal antibody to mouse or rat F[ab']$_2$ to Sepharose 4B (about 3 mL of swollen gel). Alternatively, use protein A/G-beads for mouse antibodies (*see* Note 14).
6. Incubate 1 mL of cell lysate (~3 × 10^6 cells) with either 10 μg of MAb or 100 μL (packed volume) Ab-beads overnight at 4°C.
7. When soluble MAb is used, add 50 μL (packed volume) of protein A-beads or anti-Ig beads, and incubate for a further hour at 4°C.
8. Wash the beads three times with PBSA containing 0.5% Triton X-100 and PMSF, pelleting the beads by centrifugation.
9. Elute the antigen (±MAb) by heating beads (5 min at 95°C) with equal volume of SDS-sample buffer, and apply to an SDS-containing polyacrylamide gel. Run prestained markers on these gels, because they will transfer to blots and assist in determining the molecular size of the proteins.

3.5.7. Western Blotting

This procedure is particularly useful where an antibody recognizes an amino acid sequence or carbohydrate moiety, but may be unsuitable for antibodies that bind to a conformational epitope on the protein.

1. Follow the instructions of the suppliers of the blotting equipment for the electrophoretic transfer of proteins from SDS-containing polyacrylamide gels to either nitrocellulose or PVDF membranes (*see* ref. *4* and Chapter 20 for detailed instructions).
2. Carefully separate the membrane from the polyacrylamide gel. Block the blot by placing it in a polythene bag, add 20 mL PBS-Marvel + 3% BSA/180 × 150 cm blot, and then after sealing the bag, incubate for 2 h at 37°C on a rocking platform.
3. Wash the blot twice with PBST, and then cut into strips when necessary (after labeling the individual strips in pencil), using the gel comb as a guide. Alternatively, use a proprietary manifold that allows staining of individual tracks without the need for cutting the blot into individual strips.
4. Place each blot strip in a suitably sized polythene bag, and add 1 mL of neat culture supernatant or purified antibody (10 μg/mL in PBS-Marvel) for every 20 cm^2 of membrane.
5. Seal the bags, and incubate for 1 h at room temperature on a rocking platform.

6. Cut off one end of each bag, discard the contents, and wash the blot strips three times with PBST. Transfer the strips to "communal" bags, and add 1 mL/20 cm² blot of ^{125}I-labeled antibodies to rat or mouse F[ab']₂ (10^6 cpm/mL in PBS-Marvel containing 3% normal rabbit, sheep, or goat serum).
7. After rocking for 1 h at room temperature, open the bags, dispose of the radioactive supernatant safely, and then wash the blots four times with PBST, and dry at 37°C.
8. Secure the blot strips to a sheet of Whatman 3MM paper using Photomount or other spray-on adhesive, and then autoradiograph at –70°C using prefogged X-ray film and an intensifying screen *(5)*.

3.5.8. ELISAs

As an alternative to the use of ^{125}I, most, if not all of the procedures described in the preceding section can be done using antibodies conjugated to an enzyme that converts a substrate into a colored or fluorescent product (*see also* Chapter 24) that is either soluble (plate assays) or insoluble (Western blots) (*see* Note 12). The protocols for the use of either radiolabeled or enzyme-conjugated antibodies are the same until the completion of washing following treatment with the second antibody or, in the case of competitive assays, the specific antibody. At this time, the substrate for the enzyme is added, the samples are incubated at room temperature or 37°C for a suitable time, and then the reaction is terminated. Plates coated with proteins, peptides, or conjugated peptides, and those used in antibody-capture assays can usually be read directly in a multiwell plate reader (e.g., Titertek multiscan). For this reason, it is better to use flat-bottom PS multiwell plates because of their better optical qualities. Alternatively, as with tests using cell monolayers, the supernatants can be transferred to a new plate for reading. The final steps for use with alkaline phosphatase conjugates are given below (*see* Note 10).

3.5.8.1. PLATE ASSAYS

1. Wash the plate once with PBS, and then twice with 10 m*M* diethanolamine, pH 9.5, containing 500 m*M* NaCl.
2. Add 50 µL of *p*-nitrophenyl phosphate substrate solution to each well, and incubate at room temperature for 10–30 min.
3. Stop the reaction by addition of 50 µL of 100 m*M* EDTA/well.
4. Read at 405 nm (positive wells appear bright yellow).

3.5.2. Western Blots

1. Wash the blots twice with 100 m*M* diethanolamine, pH 9.5, containing 100 m*M* NaCl and 5 m*M* MgCl₂.
2. Add 1 mL of BCIP-NBT substrate/20 cm² of membrane, and incubate at room temperature on a rocking platform until the purplish-black bands/spots are suitably developed.
3. Rinse the membrane in PBS containing 20 m*M* EDTA to stop the reaction.

3.6. Isotyping of MAbs

1. Coat PVC plates with MAbs or polyclonal antibodies (5 μg/mL of PBS, pH 8.0) specific for rat or mouse heavy-chain isotypes using the protocol described in Section 2.3., item 8.
2. Block with PBS-Marvel.
3. Add 50 μL of test MAb to each well at 1 μg/mL in PBS-Marvel or as neat supernatant, and incubate for 1–4 h at room temperature or overnight at 4°C.
4. Wash three times with PBS-Marvel.
5. Add 50 μL/well (10^5 cpm in PBS-Marvel) of ^{125}I-labeled antibodies to rat or mouse F[ab']$_2$, and incubate for 1 h at room temperature.
6. Wash three times with PBST, and determine the amount of radioactivity bound. Include MAbs of known isotype as controls (*see* Note 13).

4. Notes

1. The use of animals for experimental purposes is under strict control in many countries, and licences are necessary before surgical procedures can be performed.
2. For growth of rat hybridomas as ascites, we recommend the use of nude rats, since these have low levels of endogenous immunoglobulins (<1 mg/mL) and can yield up to 30 mL of ascitic fluid/rat (1–5 mg/mL specific antibody).
3. Problems may be encountered when using recombinant fusion proteins (with β-galactosidase or glutathione transferase) as immunogens, because the response is directed predominantly against the bacterial enzyme. In this case, it is advisable where possible to cleave off and isolate the specific protein.
4. Immune responses in rats and mice can be elicited by direct transfer of DNA, e.g., by injecting an expression plasmid containing the specific gene directly into muscle or other tissue. Some of the muscle cells will express the specific gene that may activate the host immune system. Alternatively, naked DNA or gold particles coated with low concentrations of the plasmid DNA can be transferred into the tissue using a pneumatic gun or by particle bombardment. These procedures circumvent the need to express in vitro and then purify the recombinant protein, but as yet they have not been widely used for hybridoma production. Details of these procedures are given in refs. 6 and 7.
5. Some batches of FCS are toxic to hybridomas, and it is important to test all new batches for their ability to support hybridoma growth. Alternatively, obtain samples of FCS that have been tested by the supplier.
6. Feeder cells are essential when the Y3 myeloma is the fusion partner. We use cell lines derived by trypsinization of the xiphoid cartilage that terminates the xiphisternum of adult rats. Chop the cartilage from six to eight adult rats into 2–3 mm pieces with a scalpel, and then transfer into 15 mL of DMEM containing 0.5% trypsin (bovine pancreas type III) and 1% collagenase (type II), and stir for 45 min at room temperature. Add FCS to 10% and filter through sterile gauze to remove debris. Wash the cells in DMEM containing 10% FCS, and plate into the same medium. Passage the cells in DMEM containing 10% FCS after removing

the cells by incubation for 2–3 min in PBS containing 0.05% Na$_2$EDTA and 0.2% trypsin. Irradiate the cells in DMEM with 30 Gy of X- or γ-rays, then wash once in DMEM, and freeze the cells in liquid nitrogen as aliquots of 10^6 cells in 5% DMSO/95% FCS.

7. Cell monolayers fixed with glutaraldehyde or paraformaldehyde can overcome the problem of loss of cells from the wells, but the effect of fixative on the binding of antigen should be determined. Wash cells in PBS, and then add to each well 50 μL of freshly prepared 0.5% glutaraldehyde in PBS, containing 2 mM CaCl$_2$, 2 mM MgCl$_2$, and 300 mM sucrose or, alternatively, 50 μL of 0.4% paraformaldehyde. After incubating on ice for 30 min, "flick off" the fixative and replace with 200 μL PBS containing 0.1M glycine to block excess glutaraldehyde. Leave for 30 min, and then wash twice with PBS-Marvel. Fixed cells can be handled in the same way as antigens bound to PVC plates.

8. IODO-GEN (1,3,4,6–tetrachloro-3-6–diphenylglycouril) is a better reagent for the iodination of proteins than chloramine-T, is less damaging, and has fewer side reactions than the latter. The insolubility of IODO-GEN in water means that tubes can be precoated with the reagent dissolved in methylene chloride or chloroform. Then the tubes are stored in the dark until required. The reaction is started by adding the protein and radioiodide, and terminated by removing the sample from the reaction vessel.

9. Pristane (2,6,10,14-tetramethylenedecanoic acid) acts as an irritant, and as a result, macrophages and monocytes are recruited into the peritoneal cavity. The nutrients secreted by these cells provide a good environment for the growth of hybridomas in suspension.

10. When unfixed cells or frozen sections are used for ELISA, it may be necessary to block endogenous alkaline phosphatase activity, and in this case, include 0.1 mM levamisole in the substrate solution.

11. Iodination reactions employing either chloramine-T or IODO-GEN are particularly sensitive to the presence of thiocyanate ions and, if antibodies are required for this purpose, it is essential that they be dialyzed thoroughly after elution from affinity columns with thiocyanate ions.

12. The use of biotinylated antibodies provides perhaps the greatest versatility and sensitivity of all methods. The affinity of biotin for avidin or the more usually used streptavidin is very high, and the latter can be conjugated to radioisotope, fluorescent moiety, or enzyme. Again, the basic procedures are the same as outlined for ^{125}I-labeled antibodies with the additional steps required for streptavidin binding and subsequent incubation with enzyme substrate (*see also* Chapters 17 and 18).

13. Only occasionally will an MAb show reactivity with more than one anti-isotypic antibody in this capture assay. In this case, try immunoprecipitation in agarose gels (Ouchterlony procedure; *see* ref. *8*) using polyclonal reagents. Because a crosslinked lattice must be formed among several different epitopes on the antigen and several antibodies to give an immunoprecipitate, the Ouchterlony procedure gives few false positives.

14. Unlike their murine counterparts, rat antibodies bind poorly, if at all, to protein A, but some isotypes will bind to protein G. For this reason, we use a sheep antirat F[ab']$_2$ as a general reagent both for immunoprecipitations and for screening hybridoma supernatants.

References

1. Dean, C. J., Gyure, L. A., Hall, J. G., and Styles, J. M. (1986) Production of IgA-secreting rat × rat hybridomas. *Methods Enzymol.* **121,** 52–59.
2. Modjtahedi, H., Styles, J. M., and Dean, C. J. (1993) The human EGF receptor as a target for cancer therapy: six new rat Mabs against the receptor on the breast carcinoma MDA-MB 468. *Br. J. Cancer* **67,** 247–253.
3. Harlow, E. and Lane, D. P. (1988) *Antibodies, A Laboratory Manual.* Cold Spring Harbor Laboratory, Cold Spring Harbor, NY.
4. Towbin, H., Staehlin, T., and Gordon, J. (1979) Electrophoretic transfer of proteins from polyacrylamide gels to nitrocellulose sheets: procedures and some applications. *Proc. Natl. Acad. Sci. USA* **76,** 4350–4354.
5. Laskey, R. A. (1980) The use of intensifying screens or organic scintillators for visualizing radioactive molecules resolved by gel electrophoresis. *Methods Enzymol.* **65,** 363–371.
6. Tang, D., DeVit, M., and Johnston, S. A. (1992) Genetic immunization is a simple method for eliciting an immune response. *Nature* **356,** 152–154.
7. Vahlsing, H. L., Yankauckas, M. A., Sawdey, M., Gromkowski, S. H., and Manthorpe, M. (1994) Immunization with plasmid DNA using a pneumatic gun. *J. Immunol. Methods* **175,** 11–22.
8. Ouchterlony, O. and Nilsson, L. A. (1986) Immunodiffusion and Immunoelectrophoresis, in *Handbook of Experimental Immunology,* 4th ed. (Weir, D. M., ed.), Blackwell Scientific, Oxford, pp. 32.1–32.50.

5

A Simple Hollow-Fiber Bioreactor for the "In-House" Production of Monoclonal Antibodies

Margaret Goodall

1. Introduction

Monoclonal antibodies (MAbs) have traditionally been produced in quantity by transfer of the hybridomas to the peritoneal cavity of mice and subsequent recovery of MAb from the ascitic fluid. Legislation in many countries, however, now limits the use of animals for such purposes. Although it is possible to produce MAbs in vitro by maintenance of hybridomas under standard cell-culture conditions, this requires the processing of large volumes of supernatant and is expensive. This chapter describes a simple method for culturing hybridomas in vitro in renal dialysis cartridges, which allows several hundred milligrams of MAb to be recovered at high concentration.

The apparatus is modified from that of Klerx et al. (1) and is represented diagrammatically in Fig. 1. High cell densities can be maintained by constant perfusion of medium through the hollow fibers of dialysis membrane (molecular weight cutoff usually ~10,000) with minimal dilution of the MAb. The assembled apparatus, which can be moved readily around the laboratory on a small trolley, is designed for use in a controlled 37°C "warm" room, but can also be set up in an incubator that has the appropriate access ports. The equipment is inexpensive, and is simple to assemble and operate.

2. Materials

1. Pump (302S/RL, Watson Marlow, Falmouth, UK) (see Note 1).
2. Pump head and adapter (303D/A, Watson Marlow).
3. Pump head extension (303X, Watson Marlow).
4. Marprene tubing, 15 m, 4.8-mm bore/1.6-mm wall (Watson Marlow).

From: *Methods in Molecular Biology, Vol. 80: Immunochemical Protocols, 2nd ed.*
Edited by: J. D. Pound © Humana Press Inc., Totowa, NJ

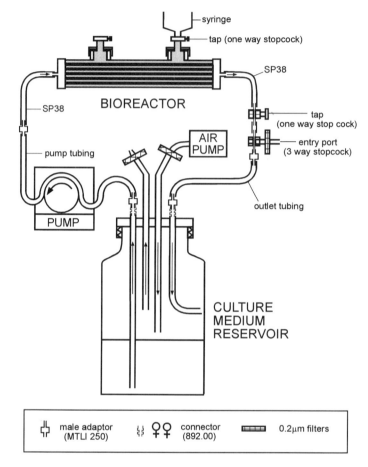

Fig. 1. Circuit diagram of a hollow-fiber production unit.

5. Renal dialysis cartridge (e.g., Disscap 180SE, Hospal Ltd., Rugby, UK) (*see* Note 2).
6. In-line adapters, 2/cartridge (SP38, Hospal Ltd.).
7. Air pump (e.g., Whisper 800, Interpet Ltd. [Dorking, UK] or tropical fish suppliers) (*see* Note 1).
8. Reservoirs: Duran Schott glass without caps and rings, 5- and 2-L capacity.
9. Screw caps and PTFE pouring rings for reservoirs (*see* Note 3).
10. Silicone rubber inserts for reservoir caps (*see* Note 4).
11. Air filters, hydrophobic, 2/reservoir (Acro 50, 0.2 μm, 50-mm diameter, Gelman Sciences, Ann Arbor, MI).
12. Spring loading dialysate hose connectors, 2/cartridge (Cobe 500218, Hospal Ltd.).
13. 50-mL Male luer lock syringes.
14. Lockable stopcocks: one-way tap (cat. no. 872.10) and three-way tap (cat. no. 876.00, Vygon Ltd. Cirencester, UK).

15. Luer lock connectors: double female (cat. no. 892.00, Vygon Ltd.).
16. Long adapter: male/female adapter (R90, Sims Distribution, Dudley, UK).
17. Plug, male/female (R94, Sims Distribution).
18. Luer lock cap, male (R96, Sims Distribution).
19. Luer lock male adapter (MTLI 250, Value Plastics Inc., Fort Collins, CO).
20. RPMI 1640 culture medium containing penicillin (200 U/mL), and streptomycin (100 µg/mL). Store at 4°C, and use within 7 d (*see* Note 5).
21. Fetal calf serum (FCS) for bioreactor medium (*see* Note 6). Batch test before purchase (*see* Note 7). Inactivate the complement by heating to 56°C for 30 min and store in 100-mL aliquots at –20°C.
22. 5 L Saline.
23. Media filtration capsules, 0.2-µm pore size (Gelman Sciences) (*see* Note 8).
24. Class II laminar air flow cabinet.
25. Clamp stands and clamps.
26. 5 in./127-mm Kwill extension tubes (Sims Distribution).
27. Portex blue nylon layflat sheeting for bags (BDH-Merck Ltd., Poole, UK).
28. Glucose test BM Test 1-44 (Boehringer-Mannheim, Diagnostics and Biochemicals, Lewes, UK).
29. Aluminum foil.
30. 50 mL Polypropylene conical tubes.
31. Disinfectant spray for hard surfaces: chlorhexidine gluconate 0.1% (w/v), e.g., Aerocide (De Puy Healthcare, Leeds, UK.).
32. In-line filters, 0.2 µm pore size (e.g., Sterivex GP.1015, Millipore, Bedford, MA) (*see* Note 9).
33. 10-cm Glass Pasteur pipet tubing with 90° bend 3 cm from one end.
34. Sterile tryptose phosphate broth (TPB).

3. Methods
3.1. Assembly of Equipment
3.1.1. Tubing and Connectors

Tubing and connectors are preassembled as described below, stored sterile in nylon bags cut from Portex nylon sheeting, and sealed with autoclave tape.

1. Pump tubing: Cut 1 m of Marprene tubing, and fit a male adapter MTLI 250 into each end. Loosely attach plug R94 to each MTLI 250 for additional protection during manipulation. Prepare several of these, since one is used for each hollow-fiber production unit and for the filtration circuit.
2. Outlet tubing: Cut 35 cm Marprene tubing, and push a male adapter MTLI 250 into each end. Protect ends with R94 plugs to prevent accidental contamination.
3. Product access port connectors (2/cartridge): Push a male/female adapter R90 into the barb hose part of the dialysate hose connector and reinforce with 2 cm of tubing (*see* Fig. 2). Protect adapter end with a male luer lock cap R96.
4. Washing port connector tubes (2/cartridge): Attach 20-cm tubing to barb hose end of dialysate hose connector. Fit male adapter MTLI 250 to free end, and protect with R94 plug.

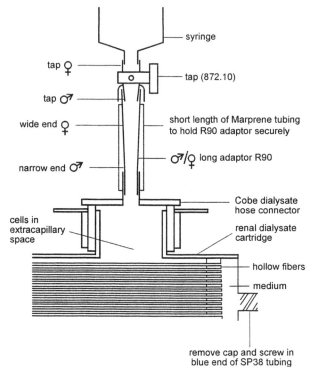

Fig. 2. Dialysis cartridge fittings.

3.1.2. Reservoirs

The arrangement of fittings for the reservoirs is shown in Fig. 3.

1. Drill four holes each 8-mm diameter in the lids equidistant from one another (*see* Note 10).
2. Cut circles of silicone rubber to fit inside the lids, and punch out four holes of 7.8-mm diameter to marry up with those in the lid (*see* Note 10).
3. Through the holes in the lid and rubber seal, pass four pieces of tubing as follows:
   a. Medium output tubing: 40-cm tubing for 5-L bottles, 30-cm tubing for 2-L bottles with 10 cm of it protruding outside the lid. Push a double female connector (892.00) into this end, and protect with male cap R96. Cover the tubing end and fittings with aluminum foil to prevent accidental displacement of the cap. Inside the bottle, the tubing should extend almost to the bottom.
   b. Medium input tubing: 20 cm with 10 cm of it protruding through the lid. Push a double female connector (892.00) into the tubing end on the outside, and protect with a male cap R96. Cover with aluminum foil. Push the bent Pasteur

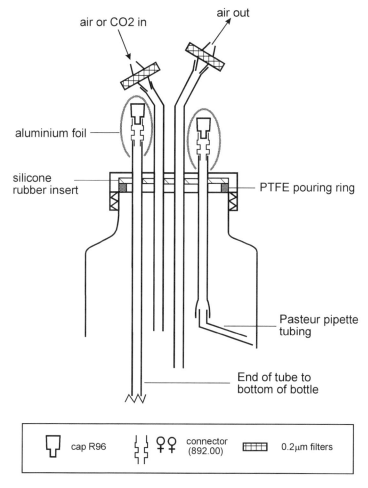

Fig. 3. Fittings for top of reservoir.

pipet glass tubing into the end that will be inside the bottle so that it will touch the inside wall (*see* Note 11).

c. Air input tubing: 20-cm tubing with 5 cm protruding outside the lid. Attach an air filter (Acro 50) by pushing the barb hose into the tubing. Number and/or label filter for ease of identification (*see* Note 12).

d. Air output tubing: 15-cm tubing with 5 cm on the outside of the cap. Attach the second Acro 50 air filter. Number and/or label as in step c.

4. Assemble the bottle, but unscrew the lids by a half-turn to allow free access of steam during autoclaving. Tighten and store sterile.

5. Allocate two small (2-L) reservoirs to the cartridge washing procedure.

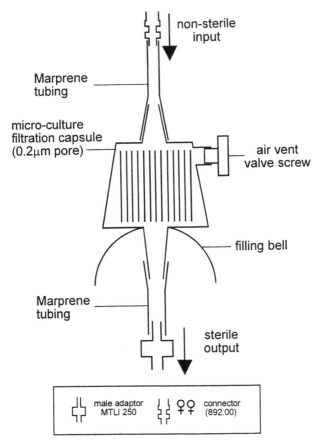

Fig. 4. Filtration unit fittings.

3.1.3. Filtration Unit Fittings

Figure 4 shows the necessary modifications to the filtration capsules.

1. Mark each for identification purposes, and record its lot number.
2. Push 10 cm of tubing onto each barb hose end of the filtration capsule.
3. Attach a double female connector 892.00 to the input tubing and a male adapter MTLI 250 to the output tubing.
4. Cover the output end with two layers of aluminum foil (no plug), and autoclave the filter in a nylon bag. Separate the air vent valve screw from the unit to facilitate the circulation of steam around the filter.
5. Prepare one or more adapter tubes by cutting 30 cm Marprene tubing, and attaching a double female connector 892.00 to one end and a male adapter MTLI 250 to the other. Sterilize each in a nylon bag.

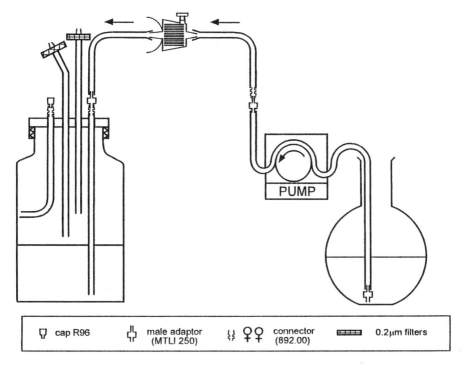

⊔ cap R96	male adaptor (MTLI 250)	connector (892.00)	0.2μm filters

Fig. 5. Circuit diagram for filtration.

3.2. Filtration of Media

Addition of serum to the medium in the reservoirs is not necessary for the growth of most hybridomas. The filtration circuit is shown in Fig. 5.

1. Work in a laminar air flow cabinet.
2. Remove filtration unit from autoclave pack, replace vent valve loosely, and mount on a clamp with the vent at the top.
3. To the input tubing on the filter, attach adapter tube and pump tubing in series.
4. Fix pump tubing in pump head and put the free end into the medium. Pump tubing can be extended using additional adapter tubing. Remove the aluminum foil and take care not to touch the exposed end.
5. Switch on the pump, fill the filter, and screw down the vent valve. Pump 100 mL of medium into a small sterile bottle as the "start" sterility control (*see* Note 13).
6. Attach the filter output tubing to the longer tubing in the first reservoir (i.e., not the one with the Pasteur pipet tubing attached: *see* Fig. 3). Keep the cap sterile for reuse later.
7. Filter 3.5 L of medium into the 5-L bottles and 1.5 L of medium into the 2-L bottles.

8. Replace the sterile cap, but not the aluminum foil. This identifies the output port for the pump tubing when changing the reservoirs.
9. Label and date the reservoir.
10. Fill the other reservoirs, and record the sequence of filling (*see* Note 14). Other than after the last 100 mL (*see* Note 13), do not allow the filter to dry out, since the buildup of pressure may push through contaminants.
11. Filter the last 100 mL into a small sterile bottle as the "finish" sterility control (*see* Note 13).
12. Continue to pump for about 10 s after all of the medium has passed through to confirm integrity of the filter by disconnecting the pump tubing from the filter at the luer lock and releasing the pressure. If the pressure is not considerable, then the integrity of the filter is in doubt, and the media must be refiltered.
13. Wash the filter and tubing by pumping through 200 mL of deionized water. Circulate a further 1 L of deionized water for 15 min. Continue to pump until empty, and then repack for sterilization.
14. Store the filled reservoirs in a refrigerated room (*see* Note 13).

3.3. Preconditioning the Bioreactor

Before seeding, the renal dialysis cartridges must be washed through with saline to remove preservative and then recirculated with fresh saline until ready for use. The circuit diagram for washing the bioreactor is shown in Fig. 6.

1. Work in a laminar air flow cabinet.
2. Take out the dialysis cartridge from its packaging, check that all ports are capped, and fix horizontally to a clamp stand.
3. Take out an in-line adapter SP38 from its packaging, and remove the plug from its color-coded end. Remove the plug from one end of the cartridge, and screw the SP38 onto the cartridge until tight.
4. Affix the second SP38 onto the other end of the cartridge as above.
5. Remove the protector from the right-hand access port. Take out a washing port connector tubing from its bag (ensure that the male adapter is protected with the R94 plug). Fix it to the access port with the spring loading connector (*see* Fig. 2 and Note 15).
6. Fix the second access port connector tubing to the left-hand port in the same way.
7. Remove the safety cap from the right-hand SP38, and remove the R94 from the right-hand access port connector tubing. Lock the two together (*see* Note 16).
8. Remove the aluminum foil and cap from either the output tubing or the input tubing of a sterile empty small reservoir. This will collect the discarded washings. Remove the R94 plug from the left access port connector tubing and lock the tubing onto the reservoir.
9. Filter-sterilize 1.5 L of saline into a second small reservoir as shown in steps 1–6 of Section 3.2. This is the recirculation reservoir.
10. Carefully detach the filter from the reservoir.
11. Remove the safety cap from the left-hand SP38, and place it on the exposed end of the tubing of the reservoir for protection.

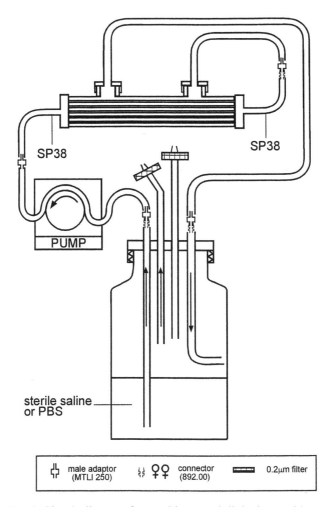

Fig. 6. Circuit diagram for washing renal dialysis cartridge.

12. Attach the filter to the SP38, and pump a further 1.5 L of saline through the dialysis cartridge. The saline will pass through the fibers and then through the extracapillary space before pouring into the discard bottle. Tilt the cartridge to displace as much air as possible.
13. Detach the filter from the left SP38, and filter a further 100 mL of saline into a sterile bottle for the sterility check.
14. Attach sterile pump tubing to the exposed SP38.
15. Attach the other end of the pump tubing to the recirculation reservoir via the tubing capped with the SP38 safety cap (*see* step 11).
16. Detach the washings reservoir by removing the left dialysate hose connector from the dialysis cartridge, and replace it with a product access port connector. Ensure that the end is protected with an R96 cap before opening the bag.

17. Detach the right dialysate hose connector, and replace it with the second product access port connector (capped).
18. Check that the outlet tubing has its plugs in place before opening the bag. Attach one end to the medium input tubing of the saline reservoir (i.e., that with the Pasteur pipet tubing, the outlet of which is covered with aluminum foil).
19. Remove the washing port connector tubing from the right-hand SP38.
20. Attach a one way stopcock 872.10 (*see* Note 17) onto the exposed end of the SP38.
21. Join the free end of the outlet tubing onto the stopcock. Check that the stopcock is open.
22. The circuit is now complete, and the apparatus can be lifted from the laminar air cabinet onto a bench. Fix the pump tubing into the pump head and switch on.
23. Check that the saline flows from the long tubing of the reservoir and returns by the glass tubing. The flow rate should be about 1 L in 10 min.
24. Circulate the saline for at least 2 h, but preferably overnight.
25. Add 2 mL TPB or serum to each sterility control sample, incubate at 37°C for 2–3 d, and monitor.

3.4. Preparation of Cells

Although 10^8 viable cells will generally be sufficient to establish growth in the bioreactor, the use of greater numbers allows the product to be harvested sooner (*see* Section 3.7.). Ideally, the cells should be in midlog phase and their viability 100%. Harvest the cells and resuspend in 50 mL of culture medium containing serum (*see* Note 18).

3.5. Loading the Cartridge

1. Disconnect the pump head from the pump. Transfer the apparatus into a laminar air flow cabinet.
2. With the cartridge mounted horizontally, replace each male cap R96 with a one-way tap (872.10). Ensure that this is in the "off" position, and that the free end is protected by its own cap.
3. Tilt the cartridge into the vertical position with the ports on the right side.
4. Remove the cap from the lower access port tap. Lock on a 50-mL syringe (*see* Fig. 2).
5. Open the tap at the top access port, and loosen the cap to allow air to pass into the cartridge.
6. Open the bottom tap, and gently draw into the syringe as much of the saline as possible. Close the tap, remove the syringe, and discard the saline aseptically. If necessary, replace the syringe, and repeat this procedure until the bioreactor is as empty as possible.
7. Fill the syringe with the cell suspension using a Kwill extension tubing. Inject the cells into the cartridge, and chase them through with a further 50 mL or more of medium, as required to fill the cartridge. Take care not to overfill, since this will

result in loss of medium through the upper tap. The cartridge can be tilted backward slightly so that as much air as possible can be displaced.

8. Close the upper tap, and tighten its cap.
9. Close the lower tap but leave the empty syringe in place.

3.6. Changing Reservoirs

Exchange the saline reservoir for one containing culture medium (*see* Note 19) as follows:

1. Transfer a reservoir containing culture medium (*see* Note 20) into the laminar air flow cabinet.
2. Remove the cap from the longer tubing (from which the aluminum foil has been removed).
3. Close the stopcock, remove the pump tubing from the saline reservoir, and lock it onto the medium reservoir via the long medium output tubing (*see* Fig. 1).
4. Remove the cap from the input tubing of the reservoir (which should still be protected with aluminum foil).
5. Disconnect the outlet tubing from the saline reservoir (connected to the Pasteur pipet), and reconnect it to the medium reservoir (again to tubing attached to the Pasteur pipet). The circuit is now complete.
6. Spray the access port taps with disinfectant or alcohol.
7. Transfer the apparatus into a warm room or incubator, and fix the pump head onto the pump.
8. Open the in-line stopcock and start pump.
9. Check that the medium flows in the correct direction. Move the bioreactor to a horizontal position (*see* Note 21).

3.7. Maintenance

3.7.1. General Maintenance

1. Periodically check the bioreactor for air bubbles. Tilt the bioreactor to the vertical to allow the air to be pumped out of the fibers and headspaces.
2. If there are air bubbles in the extracapillary space, tilt the bioreactor to the vertical, so that they accumulate at the syringe access port (which will now be at the top). Open the tap of the syringe port only, and gently draw the air into the syringe. Close the tap. The reduced pressure created within the bioreactor will be compensated for by the flow of medium through the membranes (*see* Note 22).
3. Check for signs of contamination: gross bacterial contamination of the reservoir is potentially hazardous (*see* Section 3.7.2.).
4. If bacterial contamination is suspected, the bioreactor may be saved by adding Gentamycin (*see* Note 23).
5. If fungal contamination is suspected, add Nystatin to the bioreactor (*see* Note 24).
6. The pH of the bioreactor should be about 7.0. If the pH rises above 7.5, run 5% CO_2 into the headspace (*see* Note 25); if the pH falls to 6.8, change the medium if low nutrient concentration is suspected (*see* Note 26), or attach the air pump and increase aeration of the medium (*see* Note 27).

The bioreactor is allowed to become established without interference for about 4 d or until the pH of the medium begins to fall (color change of the phenol red indicator), whichever is sooner. This time limit is critical, because glutamine levels fall rapidly and the antibiotic cover deteriorates.

3.7.2. Contamination

In the event of contamination, wear gloves and transfer the apparatus to a wash-up area.

1. If the reservoir medium is contaminated, carefully unscrew the reservoir from the cap, and drop a chlorine tablet (e.g., Haztab) into the medium. Rest the cap in place, and leave at least 2 h before dismantling.
2. Remove the port connectors and tubing, and immerse in detergent. Carefully dispose of the cartridge with its SP38 adapters still attached in a hazard bag, and autoclave.
3. Remove cap from the reservoir, and sluice away the medium. Wash the bottle and the tubes several times. Leave the reservoir full of water (change frequently) with the fittings in place to remove the chlorine, which may be absorbed by the Marprene. The fittings may have to be replaced. Rinse with deionized water, set up for autoclaving, and reuse.
4. Spent medium can be sluiced away without further treatment. The bottle is rinsed several times with tap water and then deionized water, drained, and prepared for autoclaving and reuse.
5. In the event of the cartridge alone becoming contaminated, carry out steps 2 and 4, only.

3.8. Harvesting

The earliest time at which product can be harvested from the bioreactor depends on:

1. The number of cells used for seeding.
2. The number of cells remaining viable.
3. The growth rate of the cells.
4. The rate at which the bioreactor culture becomes established.

Generally the first harvest can be made within 4–7 d, but it is important to ensure that as few cells as possible are removed. Proceed as follows:

1. Detach the head from the pump, close the stopcock, and lift the whole unit into the laminar flow cabinet.
2. Tilt the bioreactor to the vertical so that the syringe is at the bottom right side.
3. Open the upper tap, and loosen the protective cap.
4. Open the lower tap, and gently withdraw 50 mL.
5. Close the lower tap, unlock the syringe, and expel the syringe contents into a sterile conical centrifuge tube.

6. Replace the syringe on the cartridge, and repeat steps 4 and 5 as required to empty the cartridge.
7. Refill the cartridge with fresh culture medium containing 10% heat-inactivated FCS (aliquoted in 50- or 100-mL volumes, depending on the size of the cartridge) as in Section 3.5., steps 7–9.
8. Change the reservoir as in Section 3.6.
9. Take a sample of the hollow-fiber product, determine cell viability by trypan blue exclusion (*see* Note 28), and assess the glucose level using the BM-Test 1-44 strips (*see* Note 26).
10. Centrifuge the cells and decant the supernatant for further processing (*see* Note 29).
11. Assay the supernatant for product content and concentration, since cells may cease production or other changes may occur.

3.9. Records

Records can be most informative when problems occur and can save much time and expense. The format shown in Table 1 has been found to be useful, and this also allows detailed costing to be obtained.

4. Notes

1. These pumps have been found to function reliably under warm room conditions.
2. The hollow-fiber bioreactor is a sterile renal dialysis cartridge, and may be obtained from distributors or hospital supplies departments. There are various sizes, but we find the most useful to have an internal volume of 50 or 150 mL. Not all dialysis cartridges are suitable for growing cells. The fibers should be of regenerated cellulose, about 10,000 in number, and approx 200-µm diameter and 8–10-µm wall thickness.
3. It is recommended that the more durable PTFE rings and screw caps be fitted to the reservoirs, since they withstand successive autoclaving and are more resistant to chemicals, such as hypochlorite. It is, however, more difficult to bore holes in these caps.
4. The rubber inserts in the caps for the bottles can be cut from silicone rubber sheet (~2-mm thickness). These ensure a very close fit with the Marprene tubing to maintain an airtight seal
5. Usually extra glucose (1 g/L) should also be added to the medium because there is a danger of glucose starvation at high cell densities. Extra glutamine may be required for some cell lines.
6. FCS is added to the bioreactor medium only; serum is not added to the medium in the reservoir.
7. Some batches of FCS do not support cell growth well and may even be toxic. Test several batch samples for ability to support cell growth. Take two representative clones, and set up duplicates in 2 mL RPMI with 10% heat-inactivated FCS at a starting seeding density of 10^3 cells/mL. Record cell counts and viability every 48 h. Choose the serum that supports the highest viable number for the longest period, which may not necessarily be that which gives the steepest log-

Table 1
Example of Hollow-Fiber Log

CLONE: MG7 (2a)	Run No.: HF#1		Date loaded: 1.7.95		Date terminated: 15.7.95

Cells Seeded: 1.5x10^8 Source of cells: tissue culture re-clone a9 Total No. days run: 16

Reservoir medium: RPMI 1640+pen/strep

Bioreactor medium: RPMI 1640+10% HIFCS (90107S)

	Bioreactor: Hospal Disscap 180SE					Reservoir						HA* titre/concn.
Date	pH	glucose	viability (%)	replace vol (mL)	comments	pH	glucose added (g/L)	vol (L)	ID	air	comments	
30.6.95					wash with saline; filter 33			1.5	66&67			
1.7.95	7.4	18	90	100	loaded	7.4	1	1.5	90&91	0		9
4.7.95	7.0	17	90	100	gentle harvest	7.4	1	3.0	72&73	0		9
7.7.95	6.9	12	95	100	harvest	7.4	1	3.5	74&75	0		12
9.7.95	6.9									+		
10.7.95	6.8	6	95	100	harvest. Cells returned.	7.4	1	3.5	76&77	+		14
12.7.95	6.8	6	100	100	harvest	7.4	1	3.5	80&81	+		15
13.7.95	6.8	7	100	100	harvest	7.4	1	3.5	68&69	+	10mg Gentamycin	15
14.7.95	6.8	8	95	100	harvest	7.4	1	3.5	70&71	+	10mg Gentamycin	15
15.7.95	6.8	6	95		harvest; terminate; yield sufficient							15
				700	total			23.5				>250mg

HA, Hemagglutination assay.

growth phase. This may be important for maximum production levels: For many cell lines, optimum MAb production occurs as the cells enter the stationary phase with little occurring during the early and midlog phases of growth.

8. To reduce costs, the filtration capsules should be autoclavable. Normally, they can be used five times before their efficiency is reduced, but this depends on the clarity of the medium, the throughput volume, and the size of the capsule.

9. Many types of in-line filter are available, but few have a luer lock fitting for both the inlet and outlet. Wherever possible, the use of luer lock fittings is recommended for ease of manipulation and greatest adaptability.

10. The holes in the cap should be evenly spaced, not too near the rim. They should be slightly smaller than the tubing, so that they form a tight seal, but not a stranglehold, which may impede the flow. The diameter of the holes in the silicone rubber is much more critical, since gaps may become apparent during storage or manipulation, and consequently become a source of infection.

11. The glass tubing allows medium to drip down the inside of the bottle. This helps in mixing and aeration, and also minimizes frothing.

12. Identification (by numbering) of the filters helps to monitor their use, and replacement as well as identifying the bottle. The air input tubing is longer and thus closer to the medium to maximize aeration. Take care to avoid the possibility of medium splashing into the tubing during transportation.

13. The samples of medium taken for sterility checks may require the presence of protein or peptides to allow growth of potential contaminants. Thus, about 2 mL of sterile serum or tryptose phosphate broth (TPB) are added before leaving the samples at 37°C for as long as possible. Because the rate of contamination may be very low or the presence of antibiotics retard growth, 100-mL samples may not be sufficient to detect this. Therefore, the last bottle of a batch of medium should be left at 37°C and monitored.

14. Contamination is potentially the most serious problem. Therefore, it is prudent to compile a detailed record of media preparation and sterilization. For example, the filter may fail toward the end of a run, but the level of contamination is too low to be detected by the normal quality-control protocol, yet this may become apparent later.

15. Several access port or dialysate hose connectors are available. Most have a spring lock fitting. Ensure that the fitting is secure. Otherwise, fluid will leak from the port or air will enter and the cartridge will slowly empty owing to differential pressures set up during pumping.

16. When joining tubes together with a luer lock connection, care must be taken that the tubes have a degree of twist that is always ensuring that the luer fittings remain locked. They can work loose because of the movement in the apparatus generated by the peristaltic pump.

17. Optional devices, such as the in-line filter, can be introduced at the junction of the stopcock and outlet tubing. Two filters in series incorporate extra protection against contamination. If the first is observed to be contaminated, then it can be removed, the second filter replaces it, and a new filter is introduced in-line. Close the

stopcock before carrying out any procedures to prevent loss of medium. Alternatively or additionally, a three-way stopcock (876.00) can be introduced at this point together with a 0.2-μm syringe filter attached to the free arm. Through this entry port can be introduced any additives into the reservoir. Mix well after pumping has been restarted.

18. For routine production of MAbs and for initial assessment of the product, RPMI 1640 with 10% heat-inactivated FCS is the standard culture medium. Ideally, however, the medium is that in which the cells are usually cultured. Only the biorector itself requires the presence of proteins of molecular weight significantly greater than the hollow-fiber cutoff point of 10,000. It may be an advantage for the initial loading of cells to be in medium containing 20% heat-inactivated FCS to allow the coating of all surfaces with protein.

19. At the beginning of a production run, it is preferable to use small reservoirs of medium, and replace them more frequently. This maintains the levels of glutamine and antibiotic. As the cells grow and nutrients are consumed more rapidly, then the large reservoirs can be used. It is advisable to prewarm the medium before use.

20. The medium should be warm. Leave the filled reservoir in a warm room or incubator (this will also act as a sterility control). If glutamine concentration is critical for a hybridoma, make up medium without glutamine, and add it when changing the reservoirs. Alternatively, warm the reservoir in running warm water, taking care to protect the sterility of lid fittings.

21. The growth characteristics of the cells govern the optimum mounting position of the bioreactor at any given time. If the cells are adherent, e.g., Chinese Hamster Ovary (CHO) cells, then they will spread to occupy the whole surface area independent of the position of the bioreactor. Having chased the cells through when loading, most are found toward the top, and the cartridge can be left in the vertical position. However, cells that are weak or nonadherent will fall to the bottom of the cartridge. Overcrowding of cells leads to necrosis of those areas not receiving adequate nutrition or gaseous exchange. Thus, turning and tilting of the cartridge at frequent intervals will help to maintain dispersion and maximum viability.

22. The presence of air in the bioreactor will not jeopardize the cells in the initial phase of growth, but as the cells become established and increase in numbers, the bioreactor must be kept full or cell death of adherent cells will occur in the air pockets.

23. If infection is suspected, Gentamycin may control it. This is not recommended, since resistant organisms may develop. However, in trying to salvage a bioreactor, the addition of 20 mg Gentamycin to a new large reservoir in the first instance and the addition of 10 mg to subsequent reservoirs may prolong the life of the bioreactor sufficiently to complete a production run. Add the Gentamycin with a syringe into the inlet tubing of the new reservoir before locking into the unit. When the pump is engaged, swirl the reservoir to mix the contents.

24. If fungal contamination is suspected in the bioreactor (which indicates failure of a filter), then the addition of Nystatin to the replacement medium on harvesting

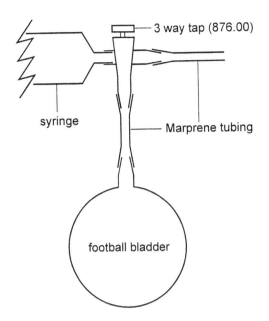

Fig. 7. Gas delivery system.

may prove helpful. Nystatin is not very effective for fungal contamination of CHO cells, since it is phagocytosed. Yeast contamination usually swamps the bioreactor before effective steps can be taken to eradicate it. Fungal or yeast contamination of the reservoir may be arrested by putting a sterile magnetic bar into a new reservoir, adding Nystatin, and maintaining the antifungal agent in suspension by rapid mixing.

25. A simple device for measuring and delivering gas can be made from a football bladder, tubing, and a three-way tap as shown in Fig. 7: Fill the bladder with CO_2, close the tap, and detach from the cylinder. Turn the tap so that the syringe can be filled with the gas. Attach the tubing to the input filter on the reservoir, and turn the tap so that the CO_2 can be injected into the reservoir. In this fashion, a predetermined volume can be delivered.

26. For some cell lines, the glucose concentration needs to be monitored, since glucose starvation can occur. The use of blood glucose strips is very effective. A drop of spent medium after a reservoir has been changed or a drop of harvested supernatant is placed on the reaction site of the strip, and left for 1 min. This is wiped off, and after a further minute, the color change is compared with a reference chart.

27. By pumping air through the reservoir, CO_2 is blown off and the pH of the medium will rise. However, if the air is pumped in too soon, the pH may rise too high; this tends to occur with clones that utilize glutamine preferentially. The input of air or CO_2 to adjust pH is learned by experience of the growth characteristics of the clone.

28. With an adherent cell line, initially there will be few cells in the harvest and those that are recovered may be nonviable. This is not necessarily a cause for concern, since viable cells will remain attached to the fibers. With a nonadherent cell line, the first 50 mL of the initial harvests may yield a higher proportion of dead cells, because these tend to fall more rapidly to the bottom of the cartridge.

29. In the early stages with a nonadherent cell line, too many cells may inadvertently be removed during harvesting. After centrifugation, these cells may be suspended in the replacement medium and reintroduced into the bioreactor. It is also possible to use cells from a well-established bioreactor to seed another.

Reference

1. Klerx, J. P. A. M., Jansen Verplanke, C., Blonk, C. G., and Twaalfhoven, L. C. (1988) In vitro production of monoclonal antibodies under serum-free conditions using a compact and inexpensive hollow fibre cell culture unit. *J. Immunol. Methods* **111,** 179–188.

6

Screening of Monoclonal Antibodies Using Antigens Labeled with Acetylcholinesterase

Yveline Frobert and Jacques Grassi

1. Introduction

The production of large quantities of monoclonal antibodies (MAbs) of pre-determined specificity has been rendered possible by the pioneering work of Köhler and Milstein *(1)*. These workers have shown that lymphocytes can be immortalized and subsequently cultured after somatic fusion with genetically selected myeloma cells. Usually, once fusion between spleen cells and myeloma cells has been performed, cells are suspended in a large volume of selective medium and distributed in culture wells, so that hybridomas are brought to clonal dilution. If fusion is successful, the first hybridoma colonies will be detectable within a few days (5–15 d). Because fusion is a random process, most clones code for MAbs of unknown specificity, characterizing the immunological past of the host. It is then necessary to select the different colonies that secrete MAbs of the desired specificity. Owing to the great number of wells to be tested (often a few hundred), and to the small quantities of MAbs available (at best, 300 µL at a few µg/mL), it is not easy at this stage to characterize the fine specificity of the antibodies (i.e., recognition of a precise epitope, inhibitory effect on a biological system, properties suitable for purifying antigen, or for histochemical characterization, and so on). Initially, it is generally preferable to use a simple method to select all the hybridomas producing MAbs directed against the immunizing antigen. Further characterization of these MAbs is performed later, after expansion of the clones. Of the different steps involved in the production of MAbs, this "screening" step is certainly one of the most critical, since this is the moment when the good clones are kept or lost. Screening is preferably performed on all the culture supernatants regardless of whether hybridoma colonies are visible. This obviates the need for time-

From: *Methods in Molecular Biology, Vol. 80: Immunochemical Protocols, 2nd ed.*
Edited by: J. D. Pound © Humana Press Inc., Totowa, NJ

consuming microscopic examination of each well and limits the risk of losing a slowly growing clone.

An ideal screening method would include the following characteristics: (i) sufficient sensitivity to allow detection of antibodies below the μg/mL range; (ii) high specificity, resulting in strict and reliable characterization of clones secreting the expected antibodies, avoiding both underestimation and false positives; and (iii) simple methodology, since primary screening and cloning involve many assays (up to 4000 for the entire procedure, including recloning and final expansion of the clones).

Most of the methods described in the literature *(2–4)* are based on the use of solid-phase immobilized antigens. Specific antibodies in culture supernatants are bound to the solid phase coated with the specific antigen, and then detected by a reaction with a labeled reagent specific to mouse immunoglobulins (antimouse second-antibody or protein A from *Staphylococcus aureus*). One advantage of this approach is the use of a single-labeled reagent, regardless of the specificity of the MAbs. On the other hand, an appropriate solid phase must be developed for each antigen. This requires large amounts of purified antigen, which might be problematic in some cases. In addition, this approach may lead to the selection of falsely positive clones if one particular MAb is nonspecifically adsorbed on the solid phase.

We have developed a contrasting strategy based on the use of a solid phase coated with a universal reagent of mouse immunoglobulins (i.e., a second antibody). MAbs bound to this solid phase are detected by their ability to bind the labeled antigen specifically (*see* Fig. 1). This approach appears more specific in that nonspecific adsorption of unrelated MAbs on the solid phase will not be detected. In this method, the solid phase represents a universal reagent, but the appropriate antigen must be labeled for each particular screening.

The aim of this chapter is to describe simple methods allowing the labeling of small quantities of antigen (or hapten) with the enzyme acetylcholinesterase (AChE). We show that this can be achieved in every case by using either covalent labeling methods or noncovalent coupling through avidin–biotin interactions. Depending on the labeling method used, three different screening procedures are described (*see* Fig. 1).

Acetylcholinesterase was chosen as the labeling enzyme because it presents many advantageous properties. First, AChE can be assayed at extremely low levels because of its very high turnover (amol amounts of the enzyme can be detected using a one-step, 1-h colorimetric assay *(5)*. This detection limit is lower than that observed for ^{125}I and other enzymes currently used in immunoassays (i.e., horseradish peroxidase, β-galactosidase, or alkaline phosphatase) *(5)*. In addition, AChE provides a continuous signal for many hours (at least 24 h under the usual conditions), thus offering the possibility of increasing the

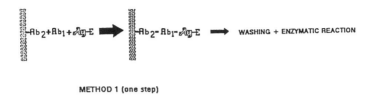

METHOD 1 (one step)

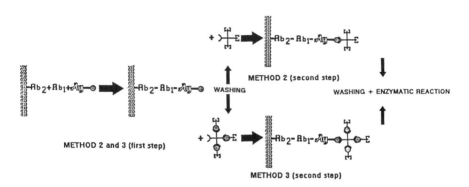

Fig. 1. Schematic representation of screening procedures. MAbs contained in culture supernatants are bound to a solid phase coated with a second antibody. The presence of MAbs on the solid phase is revealed by their ability to bind antigen labeled with the enzyme acetylcholinesterase (AChE). Three different methods for labeling antigens with AChE are described in this chapter. Depending on the labeling method, three different screening procedures are used. Method 1: This is a one-step procedure using an antigen–AChE covalent conjugate as tracer. After completion of immunoreaction between MAb and tracer, the solid phase is extensively washed and the enzymatic activity immobilized on the solid phase is measured, using a colorimetric assay (Ellman's method). Methods 2 and 3: These are two-step procedures using a biotinylated antigen (biot-antigen) as tracer. In the first step the biot-antigen is reacted with MAbs. After washing, biot-antigen immobilized on the solid phase is revealed by reaction with either an avidin–AChE conjugate (Method 2) or an avidin/biot-AChE complex (Method 3). Washing and enzymatic steps are performed as for Method 1.

sensitivity of the test by allowing the enzymatic reaction to proceed for a longer period. Finally, it has been shown that AChE can be used efficiently for labeling various molecules, including haptens *(6–9)*, antigens *(10,11)*, or antibodies *(11)*, coupling with the enzyme always being achieved without significant loss of enzyme activity. The corresponding conjugates are stable for years when kept frozen (–20 or –80°C) or lyophilized (+4°C) under suitable conditions. Screening of MAbs using AChE-labeled antigens has already been described *(12)*.

2. Materials

1. Acetylcholinesterase (AChE): This is purified from the electric organs of the electric eel, *Electrophorus electricus,* using one-step affinity chromatography *(13)*. The resulting preparation has a specific activity of 10^5 Ellman U/mg of protein and shows the electrophoretic pattern characteristic of the pure enzyme. This preparation contains mainly asymmetric molecular forms of the enzyme (A_8 and A_{12} forms) and a small proportion of the G_4 globular form. Details of these molecular forms of AChE are reviewed in Massoulié and Toutant *(14)*. The major fraction of asymmetric forms is converted into the tetrameric form (G_4) by reaction with trypsin for 18 h at 25°C in $0.1M$ phosphate buffer, pH 7.0 (enzyme/protein ratio [w/w] 1/2000). This mixture of AChE forms is used for labeling without further purification (*see* Notes 1 and 2). For the measurement of AChE activity, *see* Note 3.
2. *N*-succinimidyl-4-(*N*-maleimidomethyl)-cyclohexane-1-carboxylate (SMCC) and *S*-succinimidyl-*S*-acetyl-thioacetate (SATA) are marketed by various companies.
3. *N*-hydroxysuccinimide ester of biotin (NHS-biotin).
4. Egg avidin.
5. Biogel A 0.5 m, A 1.5 m, and A 15 m are used for molecular sieve fractionation.
6. G25 gel.
7. $0.05M$ Potassium phosphate buffer, pH 7.4.
8. Enzyme immunoassay (EIA) Buffer: $0.1M$ potassium phosphate buffer, pH 7.4, containing 0.1% BSA, $0.4M$ NaCl, $0.001M$ EDTA, and 0.01% sodium azide (toxic).
9. Washing buffer: $0.01M$ potassium phosphate-buffer, pH 7.4, containing 0.05% Tween-20.
10. $0.1M$ Sodium phosphate buffer, pH 6.0, containing $0.005M$ EDTA.
11. Polyspecific antimouse Ig antibodies are available from different commercial sources (use only affinity-purified quality).
12. 96-Well microtiter plates (Immunonunc I 96F, NUNC, Denmark).
13. Anhydrous dimethylformamide (DMF).
14. $0.1M$ Sodium borate buffer, pH 9.0.
15. $1M$ Tris-HCl buffer, pH 7.4.
16. *N*-ethyl-maleimide 12.5 mg/mL ($0.1M$) in $0.1M$ potassium phosphate buffer, pH 7.4.
17. $1M$ Hydroxylamine in $0.1M$ potassium phosphate buffer, pH 7.0.
18. $0.001M$ 5-5'-Dithio-*bis*-nitrobenzoate (DTNB) in $0.1M$ potassium phosphate buffer, pH 7.0.
19. Multidispenser (8 or 12 pipets)
20. Ellman medium: $7.5 \times 10^{-4}M$ acetylthiocholine and $5 \times 10^{-4}M$ DTNB in $0.1M$ phosphate buffer, pH 7.0.

3. Methods

3.1. Immobilization of Antimouse Immunoglobulins on the Solid Phase

The principle of the screening test implies that the antimouse immunoglobulin solid phase has the capacity to recognize all mouse immunoglobulin classes and subclasses (*see* Note 4).

1. Fill the wells of microtiter plates with 200 µL of a 10 µg/mL solution of affinity-purified second antibodies in $0.05M$ phosphate buffer, pH 7.4.
2. Leave overnight at room temperature, then wash the plates extensively with washing buffer.
3. Saturate the solid phase by adding 300 µL of EIA buffer in each well and store the plates at +4°C. They can be used 8 h later or kept under these conditions at +4°C for at least 6 mo.

3.2. Labeling of Antigens with AChE

Two methods for labeling antigens with AChE are presented.

3.2.1. Labeling of Antigens Through Avidin–Biotin Interactions

In this method, antigen and AChE (Fig. 1, Method 3) are covalently labeled with biotin molecules. AChE and antigen are coupled during the course of the screening test via high-affinity avidin interactions (*see* principle in Fig. 1, Methods 2 and 3). Biotin is covalently linked to AChE or antigen by reaction of an activated *N*-hydroxysuccinimide ester of biotin (NHS-biotin) with the primary amino groups of the proteins. NHS-biotin is quickly hydrolyzed in presence of water and is then dissolved in anhydrous DMF a few minutes before use. Ideally, the reaction is performed in basic medium (borate buffer, pH 9.0), but can be realized at reduced efficiency in neutral medium (phosphate buffer, pH 7.0). (*See* further recommendations in Note 5.)

3.2.1.1. LABELING OF ANTIGENS WITH BIOTIN

1. To 100 µg of antigen dissolved in 200 µL of $0.1M$ borate buffer, pH 9.0 (10 nmol of a 10-kDa antigen), add 17 µL of a 1 mg/mL solution of NHS-biotin in anhydrous DMF (50 nmol). Allow the reaction to proceed for 30 min at room temperature.
2. Stop the reaction by adding 100 µL of $1M$ Tris-HCl buffer, pH 7.4.
3. After a further 15-min reaction period, dilute biotinylated antigen (biot-Ag) in EIA buffer up to a concentration of 100 to 10 µg/mL. Store concentrated biotinylated antigen at –20°C.

3.2.1.2. LABELING OF AChE WITH BIOTIN

1. To 500 µL of a 250 µg/mL solution of AChE (31.000 Ell.U/mL, 0.4 nmol of G_4-AChE) in $0.1M$ borate buffer, pH 9.0, add 5 µL of a 8.5 mg/mL solution of NHS-biotin in anhydrous DMF (125 nmol). Allow the reaction to proceed for 30 min at room temperature.

2. Add 100 µL of 1*M* Tris-HCl buffer.
3. Add 1 mL of EIA buffer 15 min later.
4. Then purify biotinylated AChE (biot-AChE) on a Biogel A 0.5 m column (1.5 × 90 cm) equilibrated in EIA buffer. The enzymatic profile is established using Ellman's method, and fractions corresponding to the G_4 form (major peak) are pooled. Store concentrated biot-AChE at −20°C.

3.2.2. Covalent Labeling of Antigens with AChE

Antigens can be covalently coupled to AChE using the heterobifunctional reagent SMCC. This method involves the reaction of thiol groups (previously introduced into antigen) with maleimido groups incorporated into AChE after reaction with SMCC. This method has been applied successfully to the labeling of various haptens *(7,8)* and antigens *(10,11)*.

3.2.2.1. INTRODUCING MALEIMIDO GROUPS INTO ACHE

Maleimido groups are introduced into AChE by reaction of their primary amino groups with the *N*-hydroxy-succinimide moiety of SMCC in neutral medium. This reaction is very similar to that used for incorporation of biotin molecules into proteins. Prior to this reaction, the enzyme is treated with *N*-ethyl maleimide in order to block any thiol groups. Finally, SMCC-AChE is purified by molecular sieve chromatography on a Biogel A 1.5 m column.

1. To 100 µL of a 2 mg/mL solution of G_4-AChE (0.62 nmol), add 10 µL of a 12.5 mg/mL solution of *N*-ethyl-maleimide in phosphate buffer, pH 7.0. Allow the reaction to proceed for 30 min at room temperature.
2. Add 10 µL of a 15 mg/mL solution of SMCC (449 nmol) in anhydrous DMF.
3. After a further 30-min reaction period at 30°C, chromatograph the mixture on a Biogel A 1.5 m column (1 × 30 cm) equilibrated in phosphate buffer, pH 6.0, containing EDTA.
4. Collect fractions of about 1 mL and determine their enzymatic activity using the Ellman method (*see* Note 3). Pool the fractions corresponding to the G_4 form (second major peak) and determine the AChE concentration of the pool enzymatically. G_4-SMCC can be used immediately. It can also be kept frozen at −80°C for at least 6 mo.

3.2.2.2. INTRODUCING THIOL GROUPS INTO ANTIGENS

Thiol groups are introduced into antigens by reaction of their primary amino groups with SATA. This is the same kind of reaction as that used for incorporation of biotin molecules into antigens or of SMCC into AChE and requires the same precautions. The thioester function of SATA is then hydrolyzed in the presence of hydroxylamine in order to reveal the thiol groups. Excess reagents (SATA, hydroxylamine) are finally eliminated by molecular sieve chromatography. As an example, we shall describe the procedure used for the thiolation of egg–avidin (preparation of an avidin–AChE conjugate).

1. To 500 μg of avidin (8.7 nmol) dissolved in 250 μL of 0.1M borate buffer, pH 9.0, add 14 μL of a 2.5 mg/mL solution of SATA (150 nmol) in anhydrous DMF. Allow to react for 30 min at room temperature.
2. Add 250 μL of a 1M solution of hydroxylamine in 0.1M phosphate buffer, pH 7.0.
3. After a further 30-min reaction period, chromatograph the mixture on a G25 column (1 × 10 cm). Elute with phosphate buffer, pH 6.0, containing EDTA. Before and during chromatography, the eluant is kept under a continuous stream of nitrogen to eliminate dissolved oxygen and avoid any oxidation of thiol groups. Collect fractions of about 1 mL and pool the fractions corresponding to the void volume (identified by measuring the absorbance at 280 or at 412 nm after reaction of thiol groups with DTNB) *(see below)*.
4. Measure the thiol content of the pool by mixing 100 μL of the solution with 100 μL of a 0.001M solution of DTNB in 0.1M phosphate buffer, pH 7.0 (reaction performed in wells of a microtiter plate).
5. After 5 min, read the absorbance at 412 nm and calculate the thiol concentration ([SH]) according the following equation:

$$[SH] = (A \times 2)/(\varepsilon \times 1)$$

where (A) is the measured absorbance, (ε) is the molar extinction coefficient of reduced DTNB (13600), and (l) the optical pathlength (0.439 cm if a microtiter plate is used).

Ideally, thiolated avidin will be coupled immediately to G_4-SMCC, although it can be kept for a few weeks at –80°C. If thawed, check its SH content as described above.

3.2.2.3. COUPLING THIOLATED ANTIGEN WITH MALEIMIDO-AChE

Coupling of AChE with the antigen is achieved by mixing G_4-SMCC (immediately after isolation by molecular sieve chromatography or from storage at –80°C) with an excess of thiolated antigen. We generally use a molar ratio (moles of SH/moles of G_4-SMCC) ranging from 10 to 50. Depending on the efficiency of the coupling reaction, the ideal ratio can be determined empirically.

In the case of avidin, we currently use a ratio of 50. In one typical experiment, this corresponded to a mixture of 395 μL of thiolated antigen (measured as containing 6.3 × 10^{-5}M of SH groups) with 755 μL of a 26200 Ell.U/mL solution of G_4-SMCC.

1. Perform the coupling reaction at 30°C for 3 h.
2. Purify the enzymatic conjugate on a Biogel A 0.5 m column (Bio-Rad, USA, 1.5 × 90 cm) equilibrated in EIA buffer.
3. Collect fractions of about 2 mL, pool those containing AChE activity, and store the conjugate (at –20 or –80°C) for months or years, depending on the stability of the antigen.

3.3. Performing the Screening

The screening procedure differs slightly according to whether the antigen is labeled with biotin or directly coupled to AChE (*see* Fig. 1). The use of biotinylated antigen requires one more step. In both cases, the first step consists of transferring an aliquot of the culture supernatant to second antibody-coated plates. This operation is straightforward since culture plates and coated plates are geometrically equivalent and the transfer can be performed using a multidispenser (8 or 12 pipets). Under these conditions, up to 2000 supernatants can be transferred in 1 h by a single experimenter. Usually, 50 µL of culture supernatants are used for the screening test.

3.3.1. Screening Using Covalent Antigen–AChE Conjugates (Method 1)

1. Transfer 50 µL of culture supernatants to second antibody-coated plates.
2. Add to each well 50 µL of the antigen–AChE conjugate previously diluted in EIA buffer. This tracer is generally used at a concentration of 2–10 Ell.U/mL. Allow the reaction to proceed overnight at +4°C.
3. Wash the plates extensively, using washing buffer. We recommend at least three washing cycles, including 3-min soaking for each step.
4. Add 200 µL of Ellman medium to each well. Allow the enzymatic reaction to proceed at room temperature.
5. Read the plates when a strong yellow color appears in any well. This usually occurs within 30 min or 1 h, but longer enzymatic reaction periods (up to 6 h) can be used.

3.3.2. Screening Using Biotin-Labeled Antigens (Methods 2 and 3)

1. After the transfer of culture supernatants, add 50 µL of biotin-antigen (0.1–1 µg/mL diluted in EIA buffer) to each well.
2. After overnight reaction at +4°C, wash the plates as described above (*see* Section 3.3.1.).
3. At this point, the presence of biotinylated antigen on the solid phase can be revealed in two ways:
   a. Method 2: Add 100 µL of avidin–AChE conjugate (2–5 Ell.U/mL diluted in EIA buffer), or
   b. Method 3: Add 100 µL of a prereacted mixture of avidin and biot-AChE. This mixture is obtained as follows (quantity for 100 tests): add 40 µL of a 15 µg/mL solution of avidin (in EIA buffer) to 80 µL of a 300 Ell.U/mL solution of biot-AChE (in EIA buffer) and allow to react for 30 min at room temperature. Then dilute the mixture with 10 mL of EIA buffer before adding 100 µL to each well.
4. After a further 2–4 h of reaction at room temperature with stirring, wash the plates, develop, and read as described above. For an example, *see* Note 6.

4. Notes

1. All the procedures described in this chapter have been especially optimized in terms of AChE labeling. We recommend the use of this enzyme that we feel is particularly well suited to this application. However, the same basic principles can be applied (with appropriate modifications) to the labeling of antigens with other enzymes (peroxidase, alkaline phosphatase, β-galactosidase). This is particularly true for those labeling methods involving the use of biotinylated antigens, since biotinylated enzymes as well as avidin–enzyme conjugates are available from numerous commercial sources.

2. It is not advisable to use AChE from commercial sources (Sigma, USA or Boehringer, RFA), since these preparations are largely impure and possess a specific activity about tenfold lower than our preparations. Pure AChE can be obtained on request from our laboratory.

3. AChE activity is measured using the method of Ellman et al. *(15);* final concentrations of acetylthiocholine and DTNB are $7.5 \times 10^{-4} M$ and $5 \times 10^{-4} M$, respectively. One Ellman unit (Ell.U) is defined as the amount of enzyme producing an absorbance increase of 1 absorbance unit (AU) in 1 min, in 1 mL of medium and for an optical pathlength of 1 cm. It corresponds to about 8 ng of enzyme. AChE concentrations are determined enzymatically using a turnover number of 4.4×10^7 mol/h/site *(16)* and a molecular mass of 80 kDa for the catalytic subunit (G_4 = 320 kDa). According to these values, a detection limit of 1.8 amol of enzyme may be calculated for the G_4 form (i.e., the quantity of AChE producing an absorbance increase of 0.01 AU in 1 h, in 200 μL of Ellman medium, 0.44 cm pathlength *[5]*).

4. Polyspecific antimouse immunoglobulin antibodies may be obtained by immunizing rabbits with an appropriate mixture of MAbs. Ideally, this immunizing preparation should contain equivalent amounts of IgG_1, IgG_{2a}, IgG_{2b}, IgG_3, and IgM, some of these antibodies bearing λ light chain. Primary immunization and booster injections are performed as described by Vaitukatis *(17)* in the presence of Freund's complete adjuvant. A dose of 50 μg is used for each injection. The first booster injection is given 6 wk after immunization, and the rabbits are bled weekly from this date. Booster injections can be given every 2 mo. The presence of antimouse Ig directed against the different classes and subclasses can be checked using conventional immunological techniques *(12)*. Specific antibodies from pooled sera will be further purified by affinity chromatography in order to prepare a solid phase with maximum binding capacity. Purification can be performed using an affinity column composed of mouse immunoglobulins (either polyclonal immunoglobulins or a mixture of MAbs) covalently linked to a solid matrix. In a previous paper, we described a method based on the use of polyclonal immunoglobulins immobilized on cyanogen bromide-activated Sepharose 4B *(12)*.

5. For the labeling of antigens with biotin, it is essential to avoid the presence of other compounds containing primary amino groups (Tris-HCl buffer, for instance), since they interfere with the labeling reaction. Interfering substances may be eliminated by dialyzing the antigen preparation against borate buffer prior to

labeling. In order to preserve the immunoreactive properties of the antigen, it is advisable to introduce only a few biotin molecules into the antigen. This can be achieved by using low NHS-biotin to antigen ratios. We usually recommend a molar ratio of 5 mol of NHS-biotin for each 10 kDa of antigen (e.g., 15 mol of NHS-biotin/1 mol of a 30-kDa antigen). This ratio can be modified within the range of 100 to 1 if, for any reason, the efficiency of the reaction is particularly low (poorly concentrated antigen, neutral pH) or high (highly concentrated antigen, primary amine enriched antigen).

6. As an example, we present the results of screening tests performed for detecting anti-interleukin 1β (IL1β) MAbs. The three methods described above have been tested, i.e., the use of an IL1β–AChE conjugate (Method 1), the use of biotinylated IL1β associated with either an avidin–AChE conjugate (Method 2), or a complex of avidin and biot-AChE (Method 3). Biot-IL1β was prepared using a NHS-biotin/IL1β ratio of 10 and was used at a concentration of 1 µg/mL. The preparation of IL1β–AChE conjugate has been described elsewhere *(11)*.

    IL1β–AChE and avidin–AChE conjugates were used at a concentration of 2 and 4.5 Ell.U/mL, respectively. The enzymatic reaction was allowed to proceed for 13 min in all three methods. The 96-wells of one entire plate were tested. Fifteen wells appeared clearly positive regardless of the method used. The signal observed with each method for these 15 wells is represented in Fig. 2. For each method, the "blank" was estimated by averaging the signal measured for the other 81-wells (*see* corresponding values in the legend of Fig. 2). These results show that Methods 1 and 2 provide an absolute signal significantly superior to that of Method 3. In terms of specific signals (signal/blank ratio), Method 1 is better than Method 2 because of lower nonspecific binding. In addition, from a practical point of view, the use of a covalent conjugate appears advantageous in that it requires one step fewer, thus simplifying the screening. The hierarchy observed in this test (Method 1 > Method 2 > Method 3) is representative of our general experience. It is worth noting, however, that the three methods allow correct selection of positive clones, and that methods using biotinylated antigens are more easily accessible to the experimenter because of a greatly simplified labeling procedure. The weaker signal observed with Method 3 cannot be regarded as a major drawback, since taking advantage of the enzymatic properties of AChE, a stronger signal, can be obtained using a longer reaction time (up to 6 h).

7. Maximum efficiency of the screening methods described in this chapter will be obtained by optimizing the different steps of the labeling procedure and of the screening test itself. This includes:
    a. Optimization of the NHS-biot/antigen ratio for the biotin labeling of antigens.
    b. Optimization of the SATA/antigen ratio and of the thiolated-antigen/AChE-SMCC ratio for the preparation of covalent conjugates.
    c. Determination of the optimal concentration of the different reactants used in the screening test (biot-antigen, antigen–AChE conjugate, G4-avidin, and so on).
        These prefusion operations can be performed using the sera of immunized mice. In addition, the availability of an optimized method will allow the

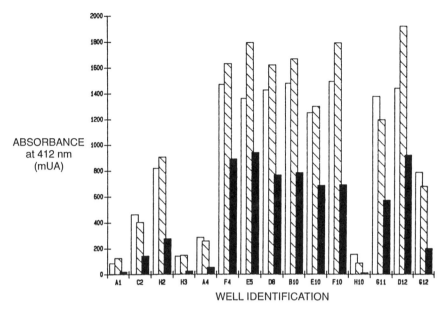

Fig. 2. Comparative results of screening tests performed with the three methods. The 96 culture supernatants of one entire plate were tested using the three screening procedures described in Fig. 1. Fifteen wells appeared clearly positive regardless of the method used. The signal observed with each method for these 15 wells is represented in this figure. For each method, the "blank" was estimated by averaging the signal measured for the other 81 wells and expressed in terms of mean ± 1σ. □, Method 1, blank = 12.5 ± 19 mUA; ▨, Method 2, blank = 37 ± 19 mUA; ■, Method 3, blank = 4 ± 4 mUA.

       experimenter to control the effectiveness of immunization and to select for fusion the mouse presenting the most marked immune response.

8. When optimized, the screening test can detect very low concentrations of antibodies (up to a few ng/mL *[12]*). This could lead to the detection of antibodies secreted by lymphocytes still present in the culture medium during the few days following fusion. We thus recommend that the screening test be performed at least 10 d after fusion and that the culture medium be changed at least twice during this period.

References

1. Köhler, G. and Milstein, C. (1975) Continuous cultures of fused cells secreting antibody of predefined specificity. *Nature* **256,** 495–497.
2. Lane, D. P. and Lane, E. B. (1981) A rapid antibody assay system for screening hybridoma cultures. *J. Immunol. Methods* **47,** 303–307.
3. Huet, J., Phalente, L., Buttin, G., Sentenac, A., and Fromageot, P. (1982) Probing yeast RNA polymerase A subunits with monospecific antibodies. *EMBO J.* **1,** 1193–1198.

4. Hawkes, R., Niday, E., and Gordon, J. (1982) A dot immunoblotting assay for monoclonal and other antibodies. *Anal. Biochem.* **119,** 142–147.

5. Grassi, J., Maclouf, J., and Pradelles, P. (1987) Radioiodination and other labeling techniques, in *Handbook of Experimental Pharmacology,* vol. 82 (Patrono, C. and Peskar, B. A., eds.), Springer-Verlag, Berlin, pp. 91–141.

6. Pradelles, P., Grassi, J., and Maclouf, J. (1985) Enzyme immunoassay of eicosanoids using acetylcholinesterase as label. *Anal. Chem.* **57,** 1170–1173.

7. McLaughlin, L., Wei, Y., Stockmann, P. T., Leahy, K. M., Needleman, P., Grassi, J., and Pradelles, P. (1987) Development, validation and application of an enzyme immunoassay of atriopeptin. *Biochem. Biophys. Res. Commun.* **144(1),** 469–476.

8. Renzi, D., Couraud, J. Y., Frobert, Y., Nevers, M. C., Gepetti, P., Pradelles, P., and Grassi, J. (1987) Enzyme immunoassay for substance P using acetylcholinesterase as label, in *Trends in Cluster Headache* (Sicuteri, F., Vecchiet, L., and Fanciullaci, M., eds.), Elsevier, Amsterdam, pp. 125–134.

9. Pradelles, P., Grassi, J., Chabardes, D., and Guiso, N. (1989) Enzyme immunoassay of cAMP and cGMP using acetylcholinesterase. *Anal. Chem.* **61,** 447–453.

10. Caruelle, D., Grassi, J., Courty, J., Groux-Muscatelli, B., Pradelles, P., Barritault, D., and Caruelle, J. P. (1988) Development and testing of radio and enzyme immunoassays for acidic fibroblast growth factor. *Anal. Biochem.* **173,** 328–339.

11. Grassi, J., Frobert, Y., Pradelles, P., Chercuite, F., Gruaz, D., Dayer, J. M., and Poubelle, P. (1989) Production of monoclonal antibodies against interleukin 1α and 1β. *J. Immunol. Methods* **123,** 193–210.

12. Grassi, J., Frobert, Y., Lamourette, P., and Lagoutte, B. (1988) Screening of monoclonal antibodies using antigens labeled with acetylcholinesterase: application to the peripheral proteins of photosystem 1. *Anal. Biochem.* **168,** 436–450.

13. Massoulié, J. and Bon, S. (1976) Affinity chromatography of acetylcholinesterase. *Eur. J. Biochem.* **68,** 531–539.

14. Massoulié, J. and Toutant, J. P. (1988) Vertebrate cholinesterases: structure and types of interactions, in *Handbook of Experimental Pharmacology* (Whitaker, V. P., ed.), Springer-Verlag, Berlin, pp. 167–224.

15. Ellman, G. L., Courtney, K., Andres, V., and Featherstone, R. (1961) A new and rapid colorimetric determination of acetylcholine esterase activity. *Biochem. Pharmacol.* **7,** 88–95.

16. Vigny, M., Bon, S., Massoulié, J., and Leterrier, F. (1978) Active site, catalytic efficiency of acetylcholinesterase molecular forms in electrophorus, torpedo, rat and chicken. *Eur. J. Biochem.* **85,** 317–323.

17. Vaitukaitis, L. (1981) Production of antisera with small doses of immunogen: multiple intradermal injections, in *Methods in Enzymology,* vol. 73 (Langone, J. J. and Van Vunakis, H., eds.), Academic, New York, pp. 46–52.

7

Synthesis of Peptides for Use as Immunogens

David C. Hancock, Nicola J. O'Reilly, and Gerard I. Evan

1. Introduction

An increasing problem in cell and molecular biology is the preparation of antibodies specific to proteins that are present in minute quantities within cells or tissues. With the advent of recombinant DNA technology, it is now often possible to deduce the primary amino acid sequence of a polypeptide without its purification. Two strategies then exist to raise appropriate antibodies. The gene can be expressed in a heterologous species, usually bacteria, and the resultant purified protein used as an immunogen. Glutathione S-transferase fusion proteins, for example, have been extensively used as immunogens. Alternatively, small synthetic peptides can be made that contain amino acid sequences inferred from that of the gene. Such antipeptide antibodies crossreact with the intact native protein with surprisingly high frequency and have the additional advantage that the epitope recognized by the antibody is already well defined (1,2). In this way, antibodies can be raised against novel gene products that are specifically directed against sites of interest, for example, unique regions, highly conserved regions, active sites, or extracellular or intracellular domains. Moreover, the ready availability of the pure peptide immunogen against which the antibody was raised means that sera can be rapidly and easily screened, e.g., using an enzyme-linked immunosorbent assay (ELISA) for antipeptide activity. Free peptide can also be used to block antibody binding and so demonstrate immunological specificity, and it may be coupled to a solid support (e.g., agarose) to generate an affinity matrix for antibody purification. In this chapter, we describe the basic principles behind the design, synthesis, and use of synthetic peptides as immunogens, and in this and Chapter 3, give some of the basic methods used in our laboratories. These

From: *Methods in Molecular Biology, Vol. 80: Immunochemical Protocols, 2nd ed.*
Edited by: J. D. Pound © Humana Press Inc., Totowa, NJ

methods have been used for several years with a considerable degree of success by many groups, both in our institute and elsewhere.

1.1. Choosing Peptide Sequences

Many peptide sequences are immunogenic, but not all are equally effective at eliciting antibodies that crossreact with the intact cognate protein (we term these crossreactive peptides). Many factors can influence the success of using peptide immunogens to raise antiprotein antibodies. They include such elements as the number of peptides from one protein sequence to be used and the number of animals available for immunization (both of which may be determined by the existing facilities), the availability of sequence data, the predicted secondary structure of the intact protein, and finally, the ease of synthesis of specific sequences. Continual improvements to synthesis methodologies means that the latter aspect is less significant than in the past, although certain sequences can still be problematic (*see* Section 1.2.). There is no guarantee that antibodies raised against a particular synthetic peptide will crossreact with the intact protein from which the sequence is derived. In our experience, the probability of generating a successful antiprotein antibody by these methods may be somewhat <50%. Nonetheless, there are a number of ways of improving one's chances of success (*see* Sections 1.1.1.–1.1.4.).

1.1.1. Predicted Structure of the Whole Protein

There are several predictive algorithms available, for both mainframe and personal computers, that can provide data on antigenicity, hydrophilicity, flexibility, surface probability, and charge distribution over a given amino acid sequence. In addition, the seasoned algorithms of Chou and Fasman and of Garnier et al. *(3,4)* give a good idea of where regions of particular secondary structure, such as α-helix, β-sheet, turns, and coils, are likely to form. Primary sequences can also indicate consensus sequences that may be sites of post-translational modification (e.g., O- and N-linked glycosylation sites and sites of phosphorylation) and that may therefore be immunologically unavailable in the mature protein. Clearly, accessibility on the external surface of the intact protein is, overall, the most important requirement for a crossreactive peptide.

Very frequently, the C-terminus of a protein, although often not a region of strongly predicted secondary structure, is exposed, and this sequence makes a good first choice. However, the C-terminus occasionally forms the membrane-anchoring region of some membrane-bound proteins and is therefore generally too hydrophobic to consider. The N-terminus of a protein can also prove to be a good candidate sequence, but in our experience, is a less reliable choice than the C-terminus and may be modified or truncated. Regions with too high a charge or hydrophilicity are sometimes not as effective as might be expected, probably because almost all known antibody-combining sites make contact with their epitope by polar and Van der Waal's bonds, and not ionic interactions. Hydrophilic α-helical regions can be good peptide epitopes, because provided the synthetic peptide is itself long enough to form a helix, it often assumes an identical conformation to that in the intact protein.

1.1.2. Specific Requirements

By their nature, peptide-specific antibodies are **site-directed** probes for proteins. Both the sequence and position of the antibody epitope are predefined. Indeed, the technique of "epitope tagging" exploits the existence of an antibody with specificity for a given linear peptide epitope that can be expressed in the context of a fusion protein *(5)*. It is therefore possible to target antipeptide antibodies to specific regions of interest in the intact protein, such as areas of high conservation in order to identify additional members of a protein family, or areas of hypervariability in order to unambiguously identify a particular family member. The increasing reliability of synthesis of, for example, phosphopeptides means that sites of posttranslational modification can also be analyzed. Other functional regions of a protein, such as binding sites, transmembrane domains, or signal sequences, may also be targeted in this way. However, the factors mentioned above may affect the success of any given peptide immunogen.

1.1.3. Immunological Requirements

Peptides of 10–20 amino acids are optimal as antigens. Our standard is around 15 residues. Short peptides (below about seven residues) are probably of insufficient size to function as epitopes. Larger peptides may adopt their own specific conformation (which is often immunodominant over any primary structural determinants), which may not be reflected in the conformation of the sequence within the intact protein. Given the above criteria, it is fair to say that almost all peptide sequences are immunogenic if presented to the immune system in the right way (*see* Section 1.3.), but that not all will generate crossreactive antibodies. Probably the single most important factor in optimizing one's chances of making useful antibodies is to use several peptides from different regions of the protein sequence and immunize several animals with each. Different animals within the same group frequently respond differently to the same immunogen. Often a given antipeptide antibody may work well in one assay, e.g., Western blotting, but not in another, e.g., immunoprecipitation.

1.1.4. Synthesis Requirements

The chemical difficulties of synthesizing certain amino acid sequences are complex and briefly dealt with in the next section (Section 1.2.). In general, hydrophilic sequences are easier to synthesize, more soluble, and more likely to be exposed on the surface of the intact molecule. There appears to be little requirement for a high degree of purity for peptide immunogens. Our experience is that peptides of 75% purity (sometimes even less) generate effective polyclonal antisera, although criteria may need to be more stringent when making monoclonal antibodies (MAbs).

1.2. Peptide Synthesis

Once a requirement for synthetic peptides has been identified, the major decision to be made is how to obtain them. The options are either to have them made commercially or to attempt to synthesize them in-house. Whichever option is chosen depends largely on current and future needs, local expertise, and funding. Peptides may be purchased from several companies specializing in contract synthesis, and if only a few are required, this is clearly the most straightforward way to obtain the desired reagents. However, custom synthesis of peptides can be expensive, with many specific sequences or modifications costing even more. On the other hand, in-house synthesis is labor-intensive, requires significant knowledge of peptide chemistry, and if carried out using an automated machine, involves large capital expenditure. In general, acquisition of an automated peptide synthesizer is probably best suited to laboratories or institutes with substantial and ongoing requirements for synthetic peptides, and preferably with their own dedicated personnel. An in-house peptide synthesis facility is a particularly attractive alternative to custom synthesis, because it allows much greater flexibility in the design and production of peptides. This can be particularly important if specially derivatized peptides, such as phosphopeptides, are needed, or if, for example, chemically defined immunogens, such as multiple antigen peptides (MAPs) *(6)*, mimotopes *(7,8)*, or epitope mapping *(9,10)*, are envisaged.

1.2.1. Principles of Peptide Synthesis

A wide choice of peptide synthesizers is currently available, ranging from manual to fully automated. They are all based on solid-phase peptide synthesis methodologies in which either *t*-butoxy carbonyl (*t*-boc) *(11)*, or 9-fluorenylmethoxycarbonyl (Fmoc) *(12)* is the major protecting group during synthesis. A detailed description of peptide synthesis is clearly beyond the scope of this chapter, and further information on practical and theoretical approaches to this chemistry may be found elsewhere *(13–15)*. However, a brief outline of solid-phase synthesis may prove useful.

The peptide is synthesized on a derivatized solid support, often a polyamide or polystyrene resin, and synthesis proceeds from C-terminus to N-terminus. The linker group, which provides the link between the resin and the peptide chain, varies and depends on the type of C-terminus desired, e.g., C-terminal acid or amide. In addition, resins are available that already have the first protected amino acid attached. This is often desirable, since the bond between the first amino acid and the resin linker is not a peptide bond and therefore requires a different reaction to the subsequent peptide chain assembly steps.

Each amino acid has its primary amine group protected (with either a *t*-boc or an Fmoc group). In addition, the amino acid side chain may need protection. Commercially available amino acids are supplied either as free acids or with derivatized carboxyl groups, as required by the particular synthetic chemistry being used. After cleavage of the amine-protecting group on the resin, the incoming amino acid is solubilized, activated in a polar solvent, and then allowed to react with the deprotected amine group of the growing peptide chain. After washing, usually with the same solvent, the peptide resin is ready for another round of N-terminal deprotection and amino acid addition. Automated synthesis is generally performed in the 0.025–0.5 mmol range. The time taken to perform addition of each amino acid is on the order of 1 h, although smaller-scale procedures can use shorter coupling times. The stepwise percentage yield is typically >95%. Recent developments in automated synthesis include on-line monitoring and feedback control of synthesis. This allows automatic analysis of each chain assembly step in real time, with the option to "double-couple" any amino acid that falls below a predetermined coupling efficiency. As a result, stepwise yield is improved, and the number of failed syntheses is reduced.

When chain assembly has been completed and the final N-terminal-protecting group removed, the peptide is cleaved from the resin with strong acid (typically hydrogen fluoride [HF], or trifluoromethanesulfonic acid [TFMSA] with *t*-boc chemistry and trifluoroacetic acid [TFA] with Fmoc chemistry) to give a free acid C-terminus. This acid treatment also cleaves most side chain-protecting groups. Frequently, various scavengers have to be added during acid cleavage in order to minimize side reactions and protect certain moieties: for example, thiols are used to preserve free sulfhydryl groups on cysteine and protect methionine side chains during Fmoc acid cleavages. Where possible, amino acid side chain-protecting groups are chosen to allow the use of less odorous scavengers, such as triisopropyl silane. It may be necessary to perform pilot cleavages to determine the optimum conditions for a particularly difficult sequence. Once liberated from the resin, the peptide may be desalted, precipitated, and lyophilized. Clearly, the nature of the reagents used in these organic syntheses requires access to a good fume cupboard (in particular, hydrogen fluoride demands great care), and the postsynthesis workup typically utilizes a rotary evaporator and lyophilizer. The final product is usually evaluated by reverse-phase HPLC (C_8 or C_{18} columns with water/acetonitrile gradients) and amino acid analysis/protein sequencing or mass spectrometry. For a synthesis scale of 0.1 mmol, the typical yield is in the region of 10 mg/residue, i.e., approx 100 mg for a 10-mer, which is more than sufficient for antisera production and characterization.

The synthesis of most peptide sequences in the region of 20 residues in length may nowadays be considered quite routine. There are, however, always exceptions. Certain sequences can be extremely difficult to synthesize and often dictate the choice of chemistry used. For example, tryptophan residues are often problematic with *t*-boc synthesis because of their instability during the harsher acid treatment during synthesis and deprotection. Peptides containing multiple arginine residues often present difficulties with Fmoc chemistry owing to poor substitution and incomplete deprotection. Alternative side-chain-protecting groups for problematic amino acids are, however, increasingly commercially available and can sometimes solve a particular synthesis problem. Very hydrophobic peptides may require unusual solvents to maintain their solubility during synthesis, and longer peptides (above, say, 25 residues) can prove progressively more difficult to solvate adequately, and therefore give low yields, although improvements in chain assembly efficiency mean that peptides of 50 or 60 residues can now be reliably made. Other problems encountered are frequently peculiar to a specific sequence made with a specific chemistry. Sometimes changing chemistries (i.e., *t*-boc to Fmoc or vice versa) solves the problem. Occasionally, it proves impossible to synthesize directly a pure peptide of the appropriate sequence, and the correct species has to be identified from among the reaction products and subsequently purified with concomitant loss of yield.

1.3. Conjugation of Peptides to Carrier Proteins

In general, short oligopeptides are poor immunogens, so it is necessary to conjugate them covalently to immunogenic carrier proteins in order to raise effective antipeptide antibodies. These carrier proteins provide necessary MHC Class II/T-cell receptor epitopes, whereas the peptides can then serve as B-cell determinants. Keyhole limpet hemocyanin (KLH) and thyroglobulin are examples of carriers that we have used successfully to generate polyclonal antipeptide antibodies. We generally avoid using bovine serum albumin (BSA), because the high levels of anti-BSA antibody generated can interfere with subsequent studies on cells grown in media containing bovine sera.

The peptides are covalently conjugated to the carrier molecule using an appropriate bifunctional reagent—the most straightforward coupling methodologies involve the amine or sulfhydryl groups of the peptide. Not surprisingly, substantial antibody titers are also frequently generated against determinants present on these carrier molecules. In general, such anticarrier antibodies present few problems in polyclonal antipeptide antibodies and may, anyway, be adsorbed out on a matrix of carrier bound to agarose. When making MAbs, however, the substantial anticarrier response may mask the frequently weaker antipeptide response, resulting in few, if any, peptide-specific hybridomas being isolated. For the preparation of MAbs, therefore, we advise the use of the carrier tuberculin-purified protein derivative (PPD) *(16)*. The advantage of PPD is that it is an extremely poor B-cell antigen, yet elicits a strong helper T-cell response. Using PPD as the carrier thus gives an antibody response that is predominantly directed against the peptide of interest. The only drawback with routinely using PPD as a carrier is that animals have first to be primed with live attenuated tubercle bacilli at least 3 wk before immunization (*see* Chapter 3). An alternative approach to the use of peptide–carrier conjugates has been developed by Tam *(6)*. The MAP system makes use of the ε-amino group of lysine residues to generate a branched core matrix that can be used as a scaffold for subsequent peptide synthesis. This system can be employed to deliver high densities of single, defined peptide antigens, or to generate B-cell and T-cell epitopes attached to the same MAP scaffold *(17)*. MAP synthesis products can be difficult to analyze by HPLC and mass spectrometry owing to their large mass. However, in our experience, MAPs can be successfully used to generate good antisera where conventional peptide–carrier conjugates have failed.

The most straightforward carrier–peptide conjugation procedure uses glutaraldehyde as the bifunctional reagent, which crosslinks amino groups on both carrier and peptide. In our experience, glutaraldehyde conjugation is reliable, easy, and effective, and generates good antipeptide antibodies even with short peptides containing internal lysine residues, doubtless reflecting the haphazard manner in which complex antigens are processed by the immune system. *m*-Maleimidobenzoyl-*N*-hydroxysuccinimide ester (MBS) can be used to crosslink the thiol group of cysteine on the peptide to an amino group on the carrier. The MBS method generates a somewhat better-defined conjugate, but it involves a slightly more complicated procedure and requires the presence of a **reduced** cysteine residue within the peptide (this is frequently added to the sequence during synthesis for conjugation purposes).

2. Materials

2.1. Conjugation of Peptides

1. KLH: purchased as a solution in 50% glycerol (Calbiochem, La Jolla, CA), and stored at 4°C. If obtained as an ammonium sulfate suspension, the KLH will require extensive dialysis against borate-buffered saline (20 mM Na borate/ 144 mM NaCl) containing 50% glycerol.
2. Porcine thyroglobulin: obtained as a partially purified powder (Sigma, St. Louis, MO).
3. BSA: purified and essentially globulin-free (Sigma).

4. PPD of tuberculin: derived from the tubercle bacillus and available from Statens Serum Institut (Copenhagen, Denmark) as a 1 mg/mL solution in PBS. Store at 4°C.

5. Glutaraldehyde (Sigma, Grade 1) stock: a 25% solution divided into 1-mL aliquots. It is stored at −20°C and never refrozen.

6. Sodium bicarbonate stock (10X): a 1M solution adjusted to pH 9.6 with HCl.

7. Glycine ethyl ester (Sigma): make up as a 1M stock, and adjust to pH 8.0 with NaOH.

8. MBS: "Sulfo" version of this reagent is water-soluble and, therefore, preferable (Pierce, Rockford, IL).

9. 0.1M Sodium phosphate-buffer, pH 6.0: mix 12 mL of 1M disodium hydrogen phosphate with 88 mL of 1M sodium dihydrogen phosphate, and make up to 1 L with water.

10. Sephadex G25.

11. Sodium borohydride.

12. Borate buffer: 0.1M boric acid solution adjusted to pH 8.0 with NaOH.

13. 1M HCl.

14. 1M NaOH.

15. Acetone.

16. Saline: 0.9% NaCl.

17. Ammonium hydrogen carbonate, pH 7.5.

3. Methods

3.1. Glutaraldehyde Conjugation Procedure (see Note 1)

1. Weigh out the peptide and an equal weight of KLH or thyroglobulin carrier. This gives an approximate ratio of 40–150 mol of peptide to each molecule of carrier (2 mg of peptide/animal is ample). If using PPD as carrier, weigh out at a molar peptide:PPD ratio of about 2:1 assuming the molecular weight of PPD to be about 10 kDa (i.e., for a 15 amino acid peptide, use 3 mg peptide for each 10 mg of PPD).

2. Dissolve the peptide and carrier protein in 0.1M (1X) sodium bicarbonate using 1 mL for every 2 mg of carrier protein.

3. Thaw out a fresh vial of glutaraldehyde, and add to the peptide–carrier solution to a final concentration of 0.05%. Mix in a glass tube, stirring with a magnetic stirring bar at room temperature overnight in the dark. The solution will usually turn a pale yellow color. Occasionally the solution will turn pale brown or orange— this reflects the fact that peptide preparations often contain traces of scavenger reagents used in cleavage from the resin and is not a cause for concern.

4. Either dialyze against double-distilled water for 12 h and lyophilize the coupled carrier (N.B. for PPD conjugates, use low molecular weight cutoff dialysis tubing) to assess the yield, weigh the lyophilized material, and determine the percentage of peptide coupled, or, because coupling efficiency is usually reasonable and not too critical, it is easier to do the following: Add 1M glycine ethyl ester to a final concentration of 0.1M, and leave for 30 min at room temperature. Then, precipitate the coupled carrier with 4–5 vol of ice-cold acetone at −70°C for 30 min.

Briefly warm at room temperature, and pellet the protein at 10,000g for 10 min at room temperature, pour off the acetone, air-dry the pellet, and redisperse it in saline at 1 mg carrier/mL. Since the pelleted protein is rather sticky, this is best done using a Dounce™ homogenizer. If necessary, store the immunogen at −20°C and rehomogenize before use.

3.2. MBS Coupling Method (see Note 2)

1. Dissolve 15–20 mg of carrier protein in minimum amount of PBS (about 1 mL).
2. Dissolve 5 mg of MBS in minimum amount of dimethylformamide (about 0.75 mL), or if crosslinker is sulfo type, dissolve in minimum amount of sterile water.
3. When crosslinker and carrier are completely dissolved, mix well and leave at room temperature for 1 h.
4. Desalt on a 20 mL Sephadex G25 column using 0.1M sodium phosphate-buffer, pH 6.0. Collect 2-mL fractions. Read the optical density (OD) of the fractions at 280 nm. Keep the two fractions with the highest OD_{280}.
5. Meanwhile reduce the peptide.
   a. Make up fresh 5 mg/mL solution of sodium borohydride, and store on ice.
   b. Dissolve 15–20 mg of peptide in minimum amount of 0.1M borate buffer, pH 8.0.
   c. Add 100 mL sodium borohydride to the dissolved peptide, mix well, and stand on ice for 5 min.
   d. Lower pH by adding 1M HCl (approx 5 drops), mix, and leave on ice for a further 5 min.
   e. Add equal number of drops of 1M NaOH, and check that the pH is between 6.0 and 7.0. If not, then adjust with 1M NaOH or 1M HCl. **Note:** 10 mL are approx 0.5 of a pH unit.
6. Add desalted crosslinker to reduced peptide, and leave overnight.
7. If the conjugate becomes insoluble, precipitate completely with 4–5 vol of ice-cold acetone at −70°C for 30 min. Briefly warm at room temperature. Pour off the supernatant and air-dry. Resuspend in saline as in Section 3.1., step 4. Alternatively, if the conjugate remains soluble, desalt the solution on a 20-mL Sephadex G25 column using ammonium hydrogen carbonate buffer, pH 7.5. Collect 2-mL fractions, and pool those of $OD_{280} > 0.4$. Store at −20°C.

4. Notes

1. During glutaraldehyde conjugation, it is vital to exclude any buffers containing amino, imino (e.g., Tris), ammonium, or azide moieties, since these will inhibit the crosslinking reaction. If the peptide or carrier is insoluble in coupling buffer, sodium dodecyl sulfate (SDS) may be added to 0.1% without affecting the conjugation.
2. It is often worth adding a cysteine residue at the C-terminus of the peptide to give the option of MBS coupling. This method couples the −NH_2 groups on KLH to −SH groups of cysteine in the peptide molecules.

3. During MBS coupling, the DMF concentrations should never exceed 30% or KLH will come out of solution. KLH concentrations in excess of 20 mg/mL will also cause it to come out of solution. If possible, use the sulfo derivative.

References

1. Lerner, R. A., Green, N., Alexander, H., Liu, F. T., Sutcliffe, J. G., and Schinnick, T. M. (1981) Chemically synthesized peptides predicted from the nucleotide sequence of the hepatitis B virus genome elicit antibodies reactive with the native envelope protein of Dane particles. *Proc. Natl. Acad. Sci. USA* **78,** 3403–3407.
2. Niman, H. L., Houghten, R. A., Walker, L. E., Reisfeld, R. A., Wilson, I. A., Hogle, J. M., and Lerner, R. A. (1983) Generation of protein-reactive antibodies by short peptides is an event of high frequency: implications for the structural basis of immune recognition. *Proc. Natl. Acad. Sci. USA* **80,** 4949–4953.
3. Chou, P. Y. and Fasman, G. D. (1978) Prediction of the secondary structure of proteins from their amino acid sequence. *Adv. Enzymol. Related Areas Mol. Biol.* **47,** 45–158.
4. Garnier, J., Osguthorpe, D. J., and Robson, B. (1978) Analysis of the accuracy and implications of simple methods of predicting the secondary structure of globular proteins. *J. Mol. Biol.* **120,** 97–120.
5. Munro, S. and Pelham, H. R. B. (1986) An HSP70-like protein in the ER: identity with the 78kD glucose-regulated protein and immunoglobulin heavy chain binding protein. *Cell* **46,** 291–300.
6. Tam, J. P. (1988) Synthetic peptide vaccine design: synthesis and properties of a high-density multiple antigenic peptide system. *Proc. Natl. Acad. Sci. USA* **85,** 5409–5413.
7. Geysen, H. M., Rodda, S. J., Mason, T. J., Tribbick, G., and Schoofs, P. G. (1987) Strategies for epitope analysis using peptide synthesis. *J. Immunol. Methods* **102,** 259–274.
8. Geysen, H. M., Rodda, S. J., and Mason, T. J. (1986) *A priori* delineation of a peptide which mimics a discontinuous antigenic determinant. *Mol. Immunol.* **23,** 709–715.
9. Geysen, H. M., Meloen, R. H., and Barteling, S. J. (1984) Use of peptide synthesis to probe viral antigens for epitopes to a resolution of a single amino acid. *Proc. Natl. Acad. Sci. USA* **81,** 3998–4002.
10. van't Hof, W., van den Berg, M., and Aalberse, R. C. (1993) The use of T bag synthesis with paper discs as the solid-phase in epitope mapping studies. *J. Immunol. Methods* **161,** 177–186.
11. Merrifield, R. B. (1963) Solid-phase peptide synthesis. 1. The synthesis of a tetrapeptide. *J. Am. Chem. Soc.* **85,** 2149–2154.
12. Atherton, E., Gait, M. J., Sheppard, R. C., and Williams, B. J. (1979) The polyamide method of solid-phase peptide and oligonucleotide synthesis. *Bioorg. Chem.* **8,** 351–370.
13. Bodanszky, M. (1984) *The Principles of Peptide Synthesis.* Springer-Verlag, Berlin, Heidelberg.

14. Bodanszky, M. (1988) *Peptide Chemistry: A Practical Approach.* Springer-Verlag, Berlin, Heidelberg.
15. Atherton, E. and Sheppard, R. C. (1989) *Solid-Phase Peptide Synthesis: A Practical Approach.* IRL, Oxford.
16. Lachmann, P. J., Strangeways, L., Vyakarnam, A., and Evan, G. I. (1984) *Raising Antibodies by Coupling Peptides to PPD and Immunising BCG-Sensitized Animals.* CIBA Foundation Symposium. Wiley, Chichester, UK.
17. Calvo-Calle, J. M., de Oliveira, G. A., Clavijo, P., Maracic, M., Tam, J. P., Lu, Y.-A., Nardin, E. H., Nussenzweig, R. S., and Cochrane, A. H. (1993) Immunogenicity of multiple antigen peptides containing B and nonrepeat T-cell epitopes of the circumsporozoite protein of *Plasmodium falciparum. J. Immunol.* **150,** 1403–1412.

8

Use of Proteins Blotted to Polyvinylidene Difluoride Membranes as Immunogens

Boguslaw Szewczyk and Donald F. Summers

1. Introduction

The great analytical power of sodium dodecyl sulfate-polyacrylamide gel electrophoresis (SDS-PAGE) makes it one of the most effective tools of protein chemistry and molecular biology. In the past, there have been many attempts to convert the technique from analytical to preparative scale, because by SDS-PAGE, one can resolve more than 100 protein species in 5–6 h. The number of papers that describe preparative elution from polyacrylamide gels is immense (for example, *see* refs. *1–5*). In spite of the numerous variations in the procedure of elution, none of the available methods is entirely satisfactory. Some of the methods are very laborious, and others lead to loss of resolution or poor recovery.

In general, the elution of proteins above 100 kDa from polyacrylamide gels always presents considerable problems. Another of the serious limitations of elution from gels is owing to the elastic nature of preparative polyacrylamide gels. The precise excision of a protein band from a complex mixture is difficult, and the slice may contain portions of other protein bands located close to the band of interest. To overcome some of the limitations of elution from gels, Parekh et al. *(6)* and Anderson *(7)* attempted to elute proteins from nitrocellulose replicas of SDS-PAGE gels. Binding of proteins to nitrocellulose is, however, so strong that the dissociating reagents (acetonitrile, pyridine) partly or completely dissolve the membrane. When such preparations are used for immunization, they may cause adverse effects in animals. We have found that when a polyacrylamide gel replica is made on polyvinylidene difluoride (PVDF) membrane, then the conditions for elution are much milder *(8)*. In this method,

From: *Methods in Molecular Biology, Vol. 80: Immunochemical Protocols, 2nd ed.*
Edited by: J. D. Pound © Humana Press Inc., Totowa, NJ

proteins are first separated by SDS-PAGE, then electroblotted to PVDF membrane, and stained with amido black or Ponceau S. The protein bands of interest are excised and are then eluted from the membrane with detergent-containing buffers at pH 9.5. Elution from PVDF membranes is nearly independent of protein molecular weight and recoveries of 70–90% are routinely obtained.

2. Materials

1. Transfer buffer: Tris-glycine (25 mM Tris/192 mM glycine), pH 8.3.
2. Methanol.
3. Protein stains:
   a. 0.01% Amido black in water.
   b. 0.5% Ponceau S in 1% acetic acid.
4. Elution buffer: 1% Triton X-100/2% SDS in 50 mM Tris-HCl, pH 9.5.
5. PVDF membrane (e.g., Immobilon P™ from Millipore Corp., Bedford, MA).
6. Whatman 3MM filter paper.
7. Scotch Brite pads.
8. SDS-PAGE apparatus.
9. Transfer apparatus (e.g., Trans Blot Cell from Bio-Rad Laboratories, Hercules, CA).
10. Glass vessels with flat bottom.
11. Rocker platform.
12. Microfuge.
13. Small dissecting scissors.

3. Method

1. Apply a mixture of proteins containing antigen to be purified (*see* Notes 1 and 2) to an SDS-PAGE gel, and run the gel (*see* Methods in Molecular Biology, Volume 1, Chapter 6).
2. Prepare transfer buffer (about 4 L for Bio-Rad Trans Blot Cell) and five glass vessels, one of them large enough to accommodate the gel holder.
3. Pour methanol (around 50 mL) into one of the vessels, and 100–200 mL of transfer buffer into the other vessels.
4. Place the gel holder and Scotch Brite pads in the biggest vessel, and six sheets of Whatman paper in another vessel. The size of the Whatman sheets should be slightly smaller than the size of the Scotch Brite pads.
5. Using gloves, cut the PVDF membrane to a size slightly bigger than the size of the resolving gel. Put the sheet into a vessel with methanol for 1 min and then place it in one of the vessels containing transfer buffer.
6. Put a wetted Scotch Brite pad on one side of the gel holder, and then three sheets of Whatman paper saturated with transfer buffer on top of the pad.
7. On completion of electrophoresis, carefully remove the upper stacking gel because it may stick to the membrane.
8. Place the lower resolving gel on Whatman paper in the gel holder. Pour a few milliliters of transfer buffer on top of the gel.

9. Place a sheet of a PVDF membrane on the gel. Roll over the membrane with a glass rod to remove air bubbles from between the gel and the membrane.
10. Next place three Whatman sheets prewetted with Tris-glycine buffer on top of the PVDF membrane and finally a prewetted second Scotch Brite pad. Close the holder.
11. Place the holder in the transfer tank bearing in mind that the membrane should face the anode.
12. Begin electroblotting. Apply 20 V for overnight runs. It is not necessary to use methanol in the transfer buffer, since it does not improve the binding of proteins to this membrane (*see* Note 3).
13. After transfer, stain the membrane with amido black solution for 20–30 min or with Ponceau S for 5 min (*see* Notes 4 and 5).
14. Destain the membrane with distilled water.
15. Excise the band(s) of interest with scissors, and place it in an Eppendorf tube containing 0.2–0.5 mL of elution buffer/cm^2 of the membrane.
16. Mix well by vortexing, or centrifuge the tube at low revolutions in a microfuge for 10–20 min.
17. Spin down the membrane in a microfuge at maximum revolutions for 2 min.
18. Transfer the supernatant to a new tube.
19. Add 0.2–0.5 mL of fresh elution buffer to the tube with the PVDF membrane.
20. Break up the crumpled PVDF membrane into a few pieces using a disposable needle.
21. Mix well by vortexing, or centrifuge the tube at low revolutions in a microfuge for 5–10 min.
22. Centrifuge the membrane in a microfuge at maximum revolutions for 2 min.
23. Combine the supernatant with the supernatant from step 18.
24. Pierce the bottom of the tube containing the membrane with a hot needle.
25. Place this tube on top of another open Eppendorf tube, and cut off caps of both tubes.
26. Centrifuge the tubes at maximum speed for a few seconds to remove the residual eluent from the membrane.
27. Transfer the residual eluent to the combined supernatants (step 23).
28. Centrifuge the last traces of PVDF membrane from the combined supernatants in a microfuge at maximum revolutions for 5 min.
29. Collect the supernatant.
30. Divide the supernatant into the appropriate number of tubes, and add 4 vol of cold acetone (–20°C) to 1 vol of protein solution.
31. Leave the tubes overnight at –20°C or in a dry-ice bath for 1 h.
32. Centrifuge the tubes in a microfuge at maximum revolutions for 10 min at 4°C.
33. Discard the supernatant.
34. Wash the pellets twice with 0.5 mL of acetone.
35. Resuspend the pellets in a small volume of water, phosphate-buffered saline, or 20 mM Tris-HCl, pH 7.5.
36. Prepare a stable emulsion with adjuvant and inject into animals by standard procedures (*see* Chapter 1).

4. Notes

1. The method has been used to obtain a variety of sera against bacterial, viral, and eukaryotic proteins. The amount of immunogen needed to stimulate high levels of antibodies varies for different proteins, but generally, 50–500 μg of protein are sufficient to induce the formation of high levels of specific antibodies.
2. The PVDF membrane should not be overloaded with protein to prevent its deep penetration into the matrix. The protein band excised from a single electrophoretic lane (about 1 cm in length) should not contain more than 10–20 μg of protein.
3. Transfer of proteins from the gel to PVDF membrane should not be performed at elevated temperatures (above 30°C), since the force of protein binding to the membrane apparently increases with temperature. Therefore, it is advisable to make transfers in a cold room at 4°C or use precooled transfer buffer.
4. Depending on the supplier and batch of amido black, the sensitivity of protein detection with this reagent may vary. If the sensitivity of staining is not satisfactory, it is advisable to dilute the amido black solution 5–10 times with water rather than to increase its concentration. In our hands, amido black purchased from Research Organics (Cleveland, OH) or Sigma Chemical Co. (St. Louis, MO) gives optimum results.
5. The sensitivity of staining with amido black in water or with Ponceau S is not very high (about 0.5–5 μg depending on protein species). The advantage of these stains is their reversibility.
6. With some experience, no staining of the membrane is necessary. When the PVDF membrane is illuminated with white light immediately after transfer, protein bands appear as white, opaque areas surrounded by translucent protein-free membrane. Taking care not to dry the membrane, a protein band to be eluted can be marked with a pencil.
7. The elution from PVDF membranes is strictly pH-dependent. At pH 7.0, there is practically no elution; the maximum efficiency of elution is reached at 8.5–9.5.
8. Often SDS can be omitted from the elution buffer. The eluted proteins can be injected then without necessity of Triton X-100 removal. However, depending on the batch and supplier of the membrane, elution efficiency with Triton X-100 alone may vary, and some proteins are eluted poorly with this eluent.
9. The membrane should not be allowed to dry before the completion of the elution procedure.
10. When semidry apparatus is used, the manufacturer's suggestions for transfer of proteins to the PVDF membrane should be followed.

References

1. Tuszynski, N. Y., Damsky, C. H., Fuhrer, J. P., and Warren, L. (1977) Recovery of concentrated protein samples from sodium dodecyl sulfate-polyacrylamide gels. *Anal. Biochem.* **83,** 119–129.
2. Nguyen, N. Y., DiFonzo, J., and Chrambach, A. (1980) Protein recovery from gel slices by steady-state stacking: an apparatus for the simultaneous extraction and concentration of ten samples. *Anal. Biochem.* **106,** 78–91.

3. Hager, D. A. and Burgess, R. R. (1980) Elution of proteins from sodium dodecyl sulfate-polyacrylamide gels, removal of sodium dodecyl sulfate, and renaturation of enzymatic activity: results with sigma subunit of *Escherichia coli* RNA polymerase, wheat germ DNA topoisomerase, and other enzymes. *Anal. Biochem.* **109,** 76–86.

4. Stralfors, P. and Belfrage, P. (1983) Electrophoretic elution of proteins from polyacrylamide gel slices. *Anal. Biochem.* **128,** 7–10.

5. Hunkapiller, M. W., Lujan, E., Ostrander, F., and Hood, L. E. (1983) Isolation of microgram quantities of proteins from polyacrylamide gels for amino acid sequence analysis. *Methods Enzymol.* **91,** 227–236.

6. Parekh, B. S., Mehta, H. B., West, M. D., and Montelaro, R. C. (1985) Preparative elution of proteins from nitrocellulose membranes after separation by sodium dodecyl sulfate-polyacrylamide gel electrophoresis. *Anal. Biochem.* **148,** 87–92.

7. Anderson, P. J. (1985) The recovery of nitrocellulose-bound protein. *Anal. Biochem.* **148,** 105–110.

8. Szewczyk, B. and Summers, D. F. (1988) Preparative elution of proteins blotted to Immobilon membranes. *Anal. Biochem.* **168,** 48–53.

9

Purification of Glycoproteins and Their Use as Immunogens

Boguslaw Szewczyk and Donald F. Summers

1. Introduction

Glycosylation is a major posttranslational modification that produces heterogeneity in a protein and results in a group of structurally different species called glycoforms. Protein-associated oligosaccharides are large, structurally diverse molecules, and the biological roles ascribed to them are numerous. Some of these functions include the following: intercellular adhesion, adhesion of microorganisms, including viruses to target cells, and modulation of immunological activity of polypeptide chains.

The isolation of individual glycoforms for immunological studies is usually a very difficult task. Molecular-weight heterogeneity of glycoforms is responsible for the diffuse or multiple bands on a gel for glycoproteins analyzed by sodium dodecyl sulfate-polyacrylamide gel electrophoresis (SDS-PAGE). Potentially, glycoforms could be eluted from gel slices. However, the direct elution from gels is very often ineffective. Hence, the elution from replicas of gels would be an attractive alternative. The elution procedure described here is a modification of the method described in Chapter 8. It follows from our experience that the elution of glycoproteins with a mixture of guanidinium hydrochloride and lysolecithin is superior to other methods of elution of this class of biological macromolecules from SDS-PAGE replicas. Additionally, this method of elution does not interfere with the subsequent structural studies of oligosaccharides, which are very often required for the correlation of the immunological activity with the extent and complexity of modifications of polypeptide chains with carbohydrates.

From: *Methods in Molecular Biology, Vol. 80: Immunochemical Protocols, 2nd ed.*
Edited by: J. D. Pound © Humana Press Inc., Totowa, NJ

2. Materials

1. 100 mM Sodium acetate, pH 5.5.
2. 30 mM Sodium m-periodate in 100 mM sodium acetate, pH 5.5.
3. 80 mM Sodium bisulfite in 100 mM sodium acetate, pH 5.5.
4. 5 mM Biotin hydrazide in 100 mM sodium acetate, pH 5.5.
5. Prestained protein molecular weight standards.
6. TBS buffer: 0.47 g of Tris-base, 2.54 g of Tris-HCl, 29.25 g of NaCl made up to 1 L with distilled water.
7. Transfer buffer: Tris-glycine buffer (25 mM Tris/192 mM glycine), pH 8.3.
8. Methanol.
9. Blocking solution: 1% (w/v) bovine serum albumin (BSA) in TBS buffer.
10. Avidin (or streptavidin)-alkaline phosphatase complex: Dilution in TBS supplemented with 1% (w/v) BSA as suggested by manufacturer for immunodetection on membranes.
11. Alkaline phosphatase buffer: 100 mM Tris-HCl, pH 9.5, containing 50 mM MgCl$_2$.
12. Nitrotetrazolium blue (NBT): 50 mg/mL in deionized dimethylformamide.
13. 5-Bromo-4-chloro-3-indolylphosphate (BCIP), toluidine salt: 75 mg/mL in deionized dimethylformamide.
14. Protein stains: 0.01% (w/v) amido black in water or 0.5% (w/v) Ponceau S in 1% (v/v) acetic acid.
15. Elution buffer: 7M guanidinium hydrochloride (GuHCl) in 100 mM Tris-HCl, pH 8.0, containing 0.5% (w/v) lysophosphatidylcholine (Sigma [St. Louis, MO] catalog no. L-5254).
    The eluent is prepared just before the elution by adding solid lysophosphatidylcholine (lysolecithin) to the buffered 7M GuHCl (pH should be checked and, if necessary, adjusted before the addition of lysophosphatidylcholine).
16. Absolute ethanol.
17. Freund's complete and incomplete adjuvants. Alternatively, other adjuvants can be used in countries where the use of Freund's adjuvants is not allowed.
18. PBS buffer, pH 7.4, 8 g of NaCl, 0.2 g of KH$_2$PO$_4$, 2.8 g Na$_2$HPO$_4 \cdot$ 12H$_2$O, and 0.2 g of KCl, dissolved and made up to 1 L in distilled water.
19. Sodium azide or thiomersal for preservation of antisera.
20. Xylene.
21. 96% Ethanol (v/v).
22. PVDF membrane (e.g., Immobilon P from Millipore Corp., Bedford, MA).
23. Whatman 3MM filter paper.
24. Scotch Brite pads.
25. SDS-PAGE apparatus.
26. Transfer apparatus.
27. Glass vessels with flat bottom.
28. Rocker platform.
29. Microfuge.
30. Small scissors.

31. Ultrasonification apparatus (100 W minimum output) fitted with a titanium microprobe with a tip diameter around 3 m*M*.
32. Syringes.
33. Short thin needles (22-gage or thinner) for injections.
34. Short thick needles for bleeding.
35. Sterile tubes for blood.
36. Rabbits.
37. Bench centrifuge for the removal of blood clots.

3. Methods
3.1. Biotinylation of Glycoproteins with Biotin Hydrazide (1)

1. Mix 10 µg of a glycoprotein (in approx 20 µL of 100 m*M* sodium acetate, pH 5.5) with 10 µL of 30 m*M* sodium *m*-periodate in the same buffer, and incubate the mixture for 20 min at room temperature in dark.
2. Remove the excess of periodate by adding 10 µL of sodium bisulfite solution, and leaving the mixture for 5 min at room temperature.
3. Add 10 µL of biotin hydrazide solution, and leave for 1 h at room temperature.
4. Store at –20°C until ready to run an SDS-PAGE gel.

3.2. Transfer of Glycoproteins onto PVDF Membrane and Detection of Glycoproteins on the Membrane

1. Prepare an SDS-PAGE gel (*see Methods in Molecular Biology*, Volume 1, Chapter 6). The number of sample application wells in a stacking gel should allow for running the samples in duplicates.
2. Boil the original and the respective biotinylated glycoproteins in SDS-PAGE sample buffer. Apply samples to the gel. Start with the original underivatized glycoproteins, then apply prestained protein molecular weight standards, and finally apply the biotinylated glycoproteins. The prestained markers can be applied also on one end of the gel to eliminate the ambiguity when cutting the membrane after transfer.
3. Run the gel (*see Methods in Molecular Biology*, Volume 1, Chapter 6).
4. On completion of electrophoresis, proceed with transfer of glycoproteins onto a polyvinylidene difluoride (PVDF) membrane. Remember to discard the upper stacking gel and to wet the PVDF membrane in methanol before use. "Wet" transfer may be done according to the procedure described in Chapter 8. For "semidry" blotting, follow the procedure described in Chapter 20.
5. After transfer, cut the membrane along the lane of prestained protein standards. Keep the piece of PVDF membrane with original, underivatized glycoproteins in a buffer for future elutions. Proceed with the detection of biotinylated glycoproteins.
6. Block the piece of PVDF membrane containing biotinylated glycoproteins with 1% (w/v) BSA in TBS for 1 h on a platform shaker.
7. Incubate the membrane in solution of avidin (or streptavidin)–alkaline phosphatase complex in 1% (w/v) BSA in TBS for 30 min (the dilution of the complex will vary depending on a manufacturer; usually it is about 1:1000).

8. Remove the excess of the complex by three consecutive washes with TBS (10 min each wash, 200 mL of TBS each time).
9. Wash the membrane with 100 mL of alkaline phosphatase buffer once for 10 min.
10. Add 66 µL of NBT solution to a plastic tube containing 15 mL of alkaline phosphatase buffer, and mix it by gentle swirling. Then add 50 µL of BCIP (toluidine salt) solution, and mix it again.
11. Place the membrane in the solution of substrates. The membrane should be completely covered with liquid.
12. Incubate the membrane for at least 10 min in the solution of substrates. The vessel should be wrapped with aluminum foil to protect the solution from light. The incubation time can be much longer (up to 12 h), but this leads to higher background.
13. Wash the membrane twice with distilled water for 5 min.
14. Dry the membrane on air, and store it in a place protected from light.

3.3. Elution of Glycoproteins with Guanidinium Hydrochloride Solution

1. Wash the piece of membrane containing transferred underivatized glycoproteins with distilled water for 5 min.
2. Stain the membrane with amido black solution for 10–30 min or with Ponceau S for 5 min.
3. Destain the membrane with distilled water until the bands are clearly visible.
4. Locate the glycoprotein band of interest on the membrane by comparing the total protein pattern with glycoprotein pattern obtained as described in the previous subsection.
5. Mark the position of glycoprotein band(s) with pencil, excise it with scissors, and place it in an Eppendorf tube containing 0.2 mL of GuHCl/lysolecithin eluent/ cm^2 of the membrane.
6. Proceed with steps 16–29 of the procedure described in Chapter 8.
7. Divide the supernatant into small aliquots (about 0.1 mL/tube).
8. Add enough cold absolute ethanol to each tube to obtain at least 90% final ethanol concentration, and leave the tubes at –20°C overnight.
9. Centrifuge the tubes in a microfuge at maximum speed for 5 min.
10. Discard the supernatant, and wash the pellet twice with absolute ethanol.
11. Resuspend the pellet in a small volume of distilled water or a buffer (e.g., PBS).

3.4. Preparation of Monospecific Polyclonal Antisera

1. Prepare a stable 1:1 (v/v) emulsion of an eluted glycoprotein (20–250 µg in a buffer, preferably PBS) and an adjuvant. If Freund's complete adjuvant is used for the first intradermal injection, this can be done by subjecting the mixture in an Eppendorf tube to a short ultrasonic treatment (usually three to four pulses for 10–20 s each time). During sonication, the tube should be placed on ice.
2. Check the stability of the emulsion by placing a small drop on the surface of cold water. The drop should stay as a discrete globule.
3. Inject about 1 mL of the emulsion intradermally at a few sites at the back of the rabbit.

4. Three weeks after the first injection, immunize the animal subcutaneously. The emulsion is prepared in the same quantity and in the same way as before, but instead of Freund's complete adjuvant, use Freund's incomplete adjuvant (or an alternative adjuvant of the "new generation" of adjuvants).
5. Two weeks after the second injection, test bleed the rabbit from an ear vein. Swab the ear with xylene to dilate the vein before bleeding.
6. Collect no more than 15 mL of blood from a mature, middle-sized rabbit.
7. Stem the blood flow by pressing the puncture with a tissue.
8. Remove xylene by washing the ear with an ample volume of ethanol.
9. Keep blood at room temperature for 2 h and then at 4°C overnight.
10. Detach the clot carefully, and transfer it to a centrifuge tube. Transfer the serum to another centrifuge tube.
11. Centrifuge the clot at $2500g$ for 10–15 min. Remove any supernatant and combine it with the serum of the previous step.
12. Centrifuge the pooled serum at $3000g$ for 15 min. Collect the supernatant.
13. Add sodium azide (0.02% w/v final concentration) to the serum to prevent microbial growth. Thiomersal can be used for inhibition of bacteria in cases where use of sodium azide is not compatible with subsequent application of the serum (e.g., sodium azide is a potent inhibitor of horseradish peroxidase, which is often used in enzymatic detection of antigen–antibody complexes).
14. Aliquot, and store the antiserum at –20°C.
15. Check the antiserum titer. Repeat the booster injection, and proceed with the protocol if the titer is not satisfactory.

4. Notes

1. The method was used for elution of many glycoproteins of a wide range of molecular weights and of different degrees of glycosylation. The data for a number of common glycoproteins are shown in Table 1. The elution from the membrane is practically complete in each case; lower overall yields are owing to losses during the steps of precipitation with ethanol. Figure 1 shows SDS-PAGE analysis of human IgG heavy chain eluted from PVDF membrane.
2. Usually, 0.1 mg of the sample is sufficient for raising the monospecific sera. Sometimes, especially for smaller proteins, more glycoprotein is needed to obtain high-titer sera. In very rare cases, no humoral response is observed after repeated injections with an immunogen of low molecular weight. In these cases, it is advisable to prepare immunogen conjugates with keyhole limpet hemocyanin (KLH) or with other highly immunogenic proteins that do not interfere with future assays. The method for preparation of conjugates is described in *Methods in Molecular Biology*, Volume 10, Chapter 4.
3. For membrane proteins, the derivatization with biotin hydrazide can be done in the presence of SDS *(1)*.
4. Derivatization with biotin hydrazide can be done directly on blots after transfer of proteins from SDS-PAGE gels. In general, a method described in ref. *2* can be followed with the exception that biotin hydrazide is used instead of

Table 1
Recoveries of Glycoproteins from PVDF Membranes

Glycoprotein	Recovery, %
Human IgG, heavy chain	70
Ovalbumin	63
Horseradish peroxidase	52
Fetuin	60
Ribonuclease B	42
Human α acid glycoprotein	61
Bovine α acid glycoprotein	68
Ovomucoid	59
Transferrin	37
Fibrinogen	
α chain	40
β chain	53
γ chain	38

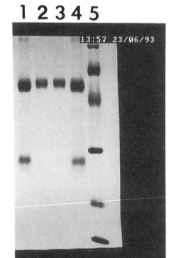

Fig. 1. SDS-PAGE pattern of human IgG heavy chain eluted from PVDF membrane. Human IgG (10 μg) was resolved by SDS-PAGE and transferred to a PVDF membrane. The proteins on the membrane were stained with amido black in water, and the heavy chain was excised and eluted with guanidinium hydrochloride/lysophosphatidylcholine. After precipitation with absolute alcohol, the glycoprotein was subjected to analytical SDS-PAGE, and the gel was stained with Coomassie brilliant blue to ascertain its purity. Lanes 1 and 4: original commercial preparation of human IgG; lanes 2 and 3: IgG heavy chain eluted from the PVDF membrane; lane 5: mixture of molecular mass standards, from top to bottom: phosphorylase b (94 kDa), BSA (67 kDa), ovalbumin (43 kDa), carbonic anhydrase (30 kDa), soybean trypsin inhibitor (20 kDa), α-lactalbumin (14.4 kDa).

digoxigenin hydrazide. However, lower sensitivity than for derivatization before SDS-PAGE is to be expected.

5. The purified glycoprotein can be used not only for amino acid microsequencing, but also for the determination of the structure of oligosaccharide chains.
6. The removal of eluent from the sample can be also achieved by dialysis. When dialyzing the concentrated GuHCl solution in a dialysis bag, it is important to leave some space in the bag, since there is a significant increase in volume with the decrease of GuHCl concentration.
7. The recovery of a glycoprotein should be checked before injection into animals by applying a part of the glycoprotein suspension (before the addition of an adjuvant) to an SDS-PAGE gel (Fig. 1).
8. A rabbit may be bled every week provided that booster injections are administered every 8–12 wk. When this schedule is followed a large volume of antiserum can be collected from a single animal.

Acknowledgments

The authors thank Z. Pilat for his assistance. This work was supported by Grant No. 5P06K04110 from Polish Committee for Science.

References

1. O'Shannessy, D. J., Voorstad, P. J., and Quarles, R. H. (1987) Quantitation of glycoproteins on electroblots using the biotin–streptavidin complex. *Anal. Biochem.* **163,** 204–209.
2. Haselbeck, A. and Hosel, W. (1990) Description and application of an immunological detection system for analyzing glycoproteins on blots. *Glycoconjugate J.* **7,** 63–74.

10

IgG Purification

Mark Page and Robin Thorpe

1. Introduction

Several immunological procedures can be successfully carried out using nonpurified antibodies, such as unfractionated antisera or ascitic fluid/culture supernatant containing monoclonal antibodies (MAbs). However, a much "cleaner" result can often be obtained if some form of enrichment or isolation of immunoglobulin (Ig) is employed. Some procedures, such as conjugation with isotopes, fluorochromes, or enzymes, and preparation of immunoaffinity columns cannot usually be efficiently performed with nonpurified immunoglobulin; other procedures may yield artifactual results if whole antiserum or ascitic fluid is used as a source of antibody. Purification of immunoglobulin is therefore at least useful and sometimes essential for a range of immunological methods. This process may consist of purification of total IgG or subpopulations (e.g., subclasses) of IgG from antisera/ascitic fluid/culture supernatant or the isolation of a particular antigen-binding fraction of Ig from such fluids. The former can be achieved by biochemical procedures, whereas the latter usually requires some type of affinity purification.

Many biochemical methods can be used for immunoglobulin purification. They range from simple precipitation techniques yielding an immunoglobulin-enriched preparation to more complex chromatographic techniques for the production of "pure" immunoglobulin. Most of these procedures can be applied to the purification of immunoglobulin from the more commonly used species; however, mouse and rat IgGs are less stable than immunoglobulin from higher mammals and are generally less easily purified. Avian antibodies may require special conditions for efficient purification (1).

From: *Methods in Molecular Biology, Vol. 80: Immunochemical Protocols, 2nd ed.*
Edited by: J. D. Pound © Humana Press Inc., Totowa, NJ

2. Materials

2.1. Precipitation Techniques

1. Saturated ammonium sulfate solution: Add excess $(NH_4)_2 SO_4$ to distilled water (about 950 g to 1 L), and stir overnight at room temperature. Chill at 4°C, and store at this temperature.
2. Phosphate-buffered saline (PBS): $0.14M$ NaCl, 2.7 mM KCl, 1.5 mM KH_2PO_4, 8.1 mM Na_2HPO_4. Store at 4°C.
3. Sodium sulfate.
4. 20% (w/v) Polyethylene glycol (PEG) 6000 in PBS.
5. $0.6M$ Sodium acetate buffer, pH 4.6. Adjust pH with $0.6M$ acetic acid.
6. Caprylic acid (free acid).

2.2. Chromatography Techniques

1. Diethylaminoethyl (DEAE) Sepharose CL-6B.
2. $0.07M$ Sodium phosphate-buffer, pH 6.3: Prepare by mixing $0.07M$ Na_2HPO_4 and $0.07M$ NaH_2PO_4 until required pH is obtained.
3. $1M$ NaCl.
4. Sodium azide.
5. Anion-exchange HPLC.
   a. Anion exchanger (e.g., Anagel TSK DEAE, Anachem, Luton, UK).
   b. $0.05M$ Tris-HCl buffer, pH 8.5.
   c. $0.5M$ Na_2SO_4.
   d. $0.3M$ NaOH.
6. Anion-exchange FPLC.
   a. Anion exchanger (e.g., Mono-Q, Pharmacia Biotech, Uppsala, Sweden).
   b. $0.02M$ Triethanolamine, pH 7.7.
   c. $1M$, $2M$ NaCl.
   d. $2M$ NaOH.
7. Gel-filtration column matrices, e.g., Bio-gel P 200, Sephacryl, Ultrogel AcA 44, TSK G3000.
8. $0.2M$ Sodium phosphate-buffer, pH 6.0, containing $0.1M$ sodium sulfate.

2.3. Affinity Chromatography Techniques

1. Sepharose 4B.
2. $0.5M$ Sodium carbonate, pH 10.5. Adjust pH with $0.1M$ NaOH.
3. Cyanogen bromide (CNBr). **(WARNING: CNBr is toxic and should be handled only in a fume hood.)**
4. $1M$, $4M$ NaOH.
5. $0.1M$ Trisodium citrate, pH 6.5. Adjust pH with $0.1M$ citric acid.
6. Ligand solution (2–10 mg/mL in $0.1M$ sodium citrate buffer, pH 6.5).
7. $2M$ Ethanolamine.
8. PBS: $0.14M$ NaCl, 2.7 mM KCl, 1.5 mM KH_2PO_4, 8.1 mM Na_2HPO_4.
9. 0.1% Sodium azide.

10. 0.1M Glycine, pH 2.5. Adjust pH with 1M HCl.
11. 1M Tris-HCl buffer, pH 8.8. Adjust pH with 1M HCl.
12. Divinylsulfone.
13. 0.1M, 0.5M Sodium carbonate, pH 9.0. Adjust pH with 0.1M NaOH.
14. β-Mercaptoethanol.
15. 0.1M Tris-HCl, pH 7.6, containing 0.5M K$_2$SO$_4$.
16. 0.1M Ammonium bicarbonate.

2.4. SDS-PAGE Technique

1. Gel solution: 1M Tris/1M Bicine (2.0 mL), 50% (w/v) acrylamide containing 2.5% (w/v) bisacrylamide (4.0 mL), 1.5% (w/v) ammonium persulfate (0.4 mL), 10% (w/v) sodium dodecyl sulfate (SDS) (0.2 mL). Make up to 20 mL with distilled water.
2. Gel running buffer: 1M Tris/1M Bicine (2.8 mL), 10% (w/v) SDS (1.4 mL). Make up to 140 mL with distilled water.
3. Sample buffer: sucrose (1.0 g), 1M Tris/1M Bicine (0.2 mL), 10% (w/v) SDS (1.0 mL), 2-mercaptoethanol (0.25 mL). Make up to 3 mL with distilled water, and add 0.001% (w/v) bromophenol blue. Store at –20°C.
4. Coomassie Blue R stain: Add Coomassie brilliant blue R (0.025 g) to methanol (50 mL), and stir for 10 min. Add distilled water (45 mL) and glacial acetic acid (5 mL). Use within 1 mo.
5. Destain solution: Glacial acetic acid (7.5 mL), methanol (5 mL). Make up to 100 mL with distilled water.
6. N,N,N',N'-Tetramethylethylenediamine (TEMED).
7. Molecular weight markers (range 200,000–14,000 M_r).

3. Methods
3.1. Prepurification Techniques
3.1.1. Separation of Serum from Whole Blood

Separating the IgG-containing serum from cells and other insoluble components of whole blood can be simply achieved by allowing the blood to clot and then centrifuging to yield serum as a supernatant. This should be carried out as soon as possible after collection to avoid hemolysis and degradation of IgG (*see* Note 1).

1. Allow blood to clot at room temperature (this takes approx 1 h). Leave overnight at 4°C—this allows the clot to contract (*see* Notes 2 and 3).
2. Detach the clot from the walls of the container using a wooden or plastic rod, and pour off all liquid into a centrifuge tube or vessel (leave the clot and adhering substances behind).
3. Pour the clot into a separate centrifuge tube and centrifuge for 30 min at 1500g at 4°C. Remove any expressed liquid, and add this to the previously aspirated clot-free liquid.

4. Centrifuge the pooled liquid for 15–20 min at 1500*g* at 4°C. Aspirate the clear serum, and store in aliquots at –20°C (or –70°C). Alternatively, serum can be stored at 4°C if an antibacterial agent (e.g., 0.02% [w/v] NaN$_3$) is added. Do not freeze chicken serum.

3.2. Preliminary Purification (Precipitation) Techniques

Addition of appropriate amounts of salts, such as ammonium or sodium sulfate *(2)*, or other chemicals, such as PEG, cause precipitation of IgG from serum. Caprylic acid can also be used to fractionate proteins from serum. Although such IgG is usually contaminated with other proteins, the ease of these precipitation procedures coupled with the high yield of IgG produced has led to them being very widely used to produce enriched IgG preparations suitable for many immunochemical procedures, e.g., production of immunoaffinity columns, and as a starting point for further purification. The precipitated IgG is usually very stable and such preparations are ideally suited for long-term storage or distribution and exchange between laboratories.

Ammonium sulfate precipitation is the most widely used and adaptable procedure, yielding up to 75% pure preparation.

3.2.1. Ammonium Sulfate Precipitation

1. Prepare saturated ammonium sulfate at least 24 h before the solution is required for fractionation.
2. Centrifuge serum for 20–30 min at 10,000*g* at 4°C. Discard the pellet.
3. Cool the serum to 4°C, and stir slowly. Add saturated ammonium sulfate solution dropwise to produce 35–45% final saturation (*see* Note 4). Alternatively, add solid ammonium sulfate to give the desired saturation (2.7 g of ammonium sulfate/10 mL of fluid = 45% saturation). Stir at 4°C for 1–4 h or overnight.
4. Centrifuge at 2000–4000*g* for 15–20 min at 4°C (alternatively for small volumes of 1–5 mL, microfuge for 1–2 min). Discard the supernatant, and drain the pellet (carefully invert the tube over a paper tissue).
5. Dissolve the precipitate in 10–20% of the original volume in PBS or other physiological buffer by careful mixing with a spatula or drawing repeatedly into a wide-gage Pasteur pipet. When fully dispersed, add more buffer to give 25–50% of the original volume, and dialyze against the required buffer (e.g., PBS) at 4°C overnight with 2–3 buffer changes. Alternatively, the precipitate can be stored at 4 or –20°C if not required immediately.

3.2.2. Sodium Sulfate Precipitation

Sodium sulfate may be used for precipitation of IgG instead of ammonium sulfate. The advantage of the former salt is that a purer preparation of IgG can be obtained for some species, e.g., human. The disadvantages are that yield may be reduced and that fractionation must be carried out at a precise temperature (usually 25°C), since the solubility of Na_2SO_4 is very temperature-dependent. Sodium sulfate is usually employed only for the purification of rabbit or human IgG, but it can be used for other species.

1. Centrifuge the serum at 10,000g for 20–30 min. Discard the pellet, warm the serum to 25°C, and stir.
2. Add solid Na_2SO_4 to produce a 18% (w/v) solution (i.e., add 1.8 g/10 mL), and stir at 25°C for 30 min to 1 h.
3. Centrifuge at 2000–4000g for 30 min at 25°C.
4. Discard the supernatant, and drain the pellet. Redissolve in the appropriate buffer as described for ammonium sulfate precipitation.

3.2.3. Precipitation with PEG

PEG precipitation works well for IgM, but is less efficient for IgG, and salt precipitation methods are usually recommended for the latter. PEG precipitation may be preferred in multistep purifications that use ion-exchange columns, because the ionic strength is not altered and therefore does not require dialysis before ion-exchange chromatography. Furthermore, it is a very mild procedure that usually results in little denaturation of antibody. This procedure is applicable to both polyclonal antisera and most MAb-containing fluids.

1. Cool 20% (w/v) PEG 6000 solution to 4°C.
2. Prepare serum/ascitic fluid for fractionation by centrifugation at 10,000g for 20–30 min at 4°C. Discard the pellet. Cool to 4°C.
3. Slowly stir the antibody containing fluid, and add an equal volume of 20% PEG dropwise (*see* Note 5). Continue stirring for 20–30 min.
4. Centrifuge at 2000–4000g for 30 min at 4°C. Discard the supernatant, and drain the pellet. Resuspend in PBS or other buffer as described for ammonium sulfate precipitation.

3.2.4. Caprylic Acid Precipitation

Caprylic (octanoic) acid can be used to isolate mammalian IgG from serum, plasma, ascites fluid, and hybridoma culture supernatant by precipitation of non-IgG protein *(3)* (*see* Note 6). Other methods have been described in which caprylic acid has been used to precipitate immunoglobulin depending on the concentration used. The concentration of caprylic acid required to purify IgG varies according to species (*see* step 2 *below*).

1. Centrifuge the serum at 10,000g for 20–30 min. Discard the pellet, and add twice the volume of $0.06M$ sodium acetate buffer, pH 4.6.
2. Add caprylic acid dropwise while stirring at room temperature. For each 25 mL of serum, use the following amounts of caprylic acid: human and horse, 1.52 mL; goat, 2.0 mL; rabbit, 2.05 mL; cow, 1.7 mL. Stir for 30 min at room temperature.
3. Centrifuge at 4000g for 20–30 min. Collect the supernatant, and discard the pellet.

3.3. Chromatography Techniques Based on Charge or Size Separation

3.3.1. DEAE Sepharose Chromatography

IgG may be purified from serum from several species by a simple one-step ion-exchange chromatography procedure. The method is widely used and works on the principle that IgG has a higher or more basic isoelectric point than most serum proteins. Therefore, if the pH is kept below the iso-electric point of most antibodies, the immunoglobulins do not bind to an anion exchanger and are separated from the majority of serum proteins bound to the column matrix. The high-capacity of anion-exchange columns allows for large-scale purification of IgG from serum. The DEAE anion-exchange group, covalently linked to Sepharose (e.g., DEAE Sepharose CL-6B, Pharmacia) is particularly useful for this purpose, because it is provided preswollen and ready for packing into a column. Furthermore, it is relatively stable to changes in ionic strength and pH. Other matrices (e.g., DEAE cellulose) are provided as solids, and therefore require preparation and equilibration *(4)*.

This procedure does not work well for murine IgG or preparations containing mouse or rat Mabs, since these do not generally have the high-pI IgGs of other species. Other possible problems are that some immunoglobulins (e.g., mouse IgG_3) are unstable at low-ionic strength, and precipitation may occur during the ion-exchange procedure.

1. Dialyze the serum (preferably ammonium sulfate fractionated) against $0.07M$ sodium phosphate buffer, pH 6.3, exhaustively (at least two changes over a 24 h period) at a ratio of at least 1 vol of sample to 100 vol of buffer.
2. Apply the sample to the column, and wash the ion exchanger with 2 column volumes of sodium phosphate buffer. Collect the wash, which will contain IgG, and monitor the absorbance of the eluate at 280 nm (A_{280}). Stop collecting fractions when the A_{280} falls to baseline.
3. Pool the wash fractions from step 2, and measure the A_{280} *(see* Note 7).
4. Regenerate the column by passing through 2–3 column volumes of phosphate-buffer containing $1M$ NaCl.
5. Wash thoroughly in phosphate-buffer (2–3 column volumes), and store in buffer containing 0.1% (w/v) sodium azide.

3.3.2. Conventional Ion-Exchange Chromatography

Conventional ion-exchange chromatography separates molecules by adsorbing proteins onto the ion-exchange resin that are then selectively eluted by slowly increasing the ionic strength (this disrupts ionic interactions between the protein and column matrix) or by altering the pH (the reactive groups on the proteins lose their charge). Anion-exchange groups (DEAE) covalently linked to a support matrix (such as Sepharose) can be used to purify IgG in which the pH of the mobile phase buffer is raised above the pI of IgG, thus allowing most of the antibodies to bind to the DEAE matrix. Compare this method with that above (Section 3.3.1.) in which the IgG passes through the column. The procedure can be carried out using a column that is washed and eluted under gravity *(4)*. However, high-performance liquid chromatography (HPLC) provides improved reproducibility (because of the sophisticated pumps and accurate timers), speed (because of the small, high-capacity columns), and increased resolution (because of the fine resins and control systems). Fast-performance liquid chromatography (FPLC) is a variant of HPLC that has proven useful in the purification of murine MAbs, although the technique is applicable to IgG preparations from all species.

3.3.2.1. ANION-EXCHANGE HPLC

1. Prepare IgG fraction from serum by ammonium sulfate precipitation (45% saturation). Dialyze the sample against $0.05M$ Tris-HCl, pH 8.5. Dilute the sample at least 1:1 in $0.05M$ Tris-HCl and filter (0.2 μm) before use (*see* Note 8).
2. Assemble the HPLC system according to the manufacturer's instructions.
3. Wash the column (e.g., TSK DEAE 5PW) with buffer A ($0.05M$ Tris-HCl, pH 8.5), at an optimal flow rate (1.0 mL/min) until absorbance at 280 nm is stable.
4. Run a blank salt gradient 0–100% buffer B (buffer A + $0.5M$ Na_2SO_4) over 20 min to complete preparation of the matrix. Finally, re-equilibrate the column with buffer A before sample application, so that the A_{280} is at baseline.
5. Add the sample manually using a 1–5 mL loop, and allow at least 10 min before applying the salt gradient.
6. Apply salt gradient from 0–100% (buffer B) over 45 min collecting protein peaks. The length of the run will depend on column size. A larger column will take longer to apply the salt gradient at the same flow rate.
7. Purge the column with 100% $0.5M$ Na_2SO_4 for 10 min.
8. Wash the column with $0.3M$ NaOH for 10 min. Other columns (e.g., silica-based) may require different wash buffers.
9. Wash the column with sample buffer until absorbance is stable, and store in distilled water containing 0.02% sodium azide.

3.3.2.2. FPLC PURIFICATION OF IgG

1. Prepare serum by ammonium sulfate precipitation (45% saturation). Redissolve the precipitate in $0.02M$ triethanolamine buffer, pH 7.7, and dialyze overnight against this buffer at 4°C. Filter (0.2 μm) the sample before use (*see* Note 8).
2. Assemble the FPLC system according to the manufacturer's instructions for use with the Mono-Q ion-exchange column.
3. Equilibrate the column with $0.02M$ triethanolamine buffer, pH 7.7 (buffer A). Run a blank gradient from 0–100% buffer B (buffer A + $1M$ NaCl). Use a flow rate of 4–6 mL/min for this and subsequent steps.

4. Load the sample depending on column size by reference to the manufacturer's instructions for loading capacities of the columns.
5. Equilibrate the column with buffer A for at least 10 min.
6. Set the sensitivity in the UV monitor control unit to a suitable value that will enable peak detection at a given concentration of protein. Zero the baseline or chart recorder.
7. Apply a salt gradient from 0–28% buffer B for about 30 min (*see* Note 9), and collect protein peaks. Follow with 100% 1*M* NaCl for 15 min to purge the column of remaining proteins.
8. Wash the Mono-Q ion-exchange with at least 3 column volumes each of 2*M* NaOH followed by 2*M* NaCl.
9. Store the Mono-Q ion-exchange column in distilled water containing 0.02% NaN$_3$.

3.3.3. Gel-Filtration Chromatography

In gel filtration, a protein mixture (the mobile phase) is applied to a column of small beads with pores of carefully controlled size (the stationary phase). The movement of the solute is dependent on the flow of the mobile phase, and the Brownian motion of the solute molecules causes their diffusion into and out of the chromatographic bed. Large proteins, above the "exclusion limit" of the gel, cannot enter the pore and are hence eluted in the "void volume" of the column (*see* Note 10). Small proteins enter the pores and are therefore eluted in the "total volume" of the column, and intermediate-size proteins are eluted between the void and total volumes. Proteins are therefore eluted in order of decreasing molecular size. Column matrices or ready-made columns are available in a number of fractionation ranges, allowing users to select the appropriate column for their particular application. Columns may also be incorporated into HPLC equipment giving the user greater control over flow rates and peak monitoring.

Gel-filtration is not especially effective for the purification of IgG, which tends to elute in a broad peak and is usually contaminated with albumin (mainly derived from dimeric albumin, $M_r \sim 135,000$). The technique is more useful for the purification of IgM or may be used as an adjunct to ion-exchange chromatography. Some IgGs (monoclonal), however, possess pIs that make them difficult to purify using ion-exchange chromatography. In such cases using gel filtration as a method of fractionation may be desirable (5).

3.3.3.1. Preparation and Equilibration of Gel-Filtration Column (*see* Note 11)

1. Gently stir the filtration medium (enough to fill the column plus 10%) into 2X the column volume of buffer.
2. Degas the slurry using a Büchner side arm flask under vacuum for 1–2 h with periodic swirling. Do not use a magnetic stirrer, since this may damage the beads.

3. Resuspend the slurry in approx 5X its volume of buffer, and leave to stand until most of the beads have settled. Remove the fines by aspirating the supernatant down to about 1.5X the settled slurry volume.

4. Carefully pack a clean column by first filling with a third column volume of buffer (0.2M sodium phosphate, pH 6.0, containing 0.1M sodium sulfate). Swirl the slurry to resuspend it evenly, and pour it down a glass rod onto the inside wall to fill the column. Allow to settle under gravity for 0.5–1 h and to let air bubbles escape (*see* Note 12).

5. Adjust the height of the outlet end of the column, so that the vertical distance between it and the top of the column is less than the maximum operating pressure for the gel (*see* Note 13). Unclamp the bottom of the column, and allow the gel to pack under this pressure.

6. Top up the column periodically by siphoning off excess supernatant, stirring the top of the gel (if it has settled completely), and filling the column up to the top with resuspended slurry.

7. Once the column is packed (gel bed just runs dry), connect the top of the column to a buffer reservoir, remove any air bubbles in the tube, and allow one column volume of buffer to run through the column.

3.3.3.2. Sample Application and Elution (*see* Note 14)

1. Disconnect the top of the column from the buffer reservoir, and allow the gel just to run dry.

2. Apply the IgG sample (*see* Note 15) carefully by running it down the inside wall of the column so that the gel bed is not disturbed.

3. When the sample has entered the bed, gently overlay the gel with buffer, and reconnect the column to the buffer reservoir.

4. Collect fractions (4–6 mL), and monitor the absorbance at 280 nm (A_{280}) (*see* Notes 7 and 16).

3.4. Affinity Chromatography

Affinity chromatography is a particularly powerful procedure that can be used to purify IgG, subpopulations of IgG, or the antigen-binding fraction of IgG present in serum/ascitic fluid/hybridoma culture supernatant. This technique requires the production of a solid matrix to which a ligand that has either affinity for the relevant IgG or vice versa has been bound. Examples of ligands useful in this context are:

1. The antigen recognized by the IgG (for isolation of the antigen-specific fraction of the serum/ascitic fluid, and so forth).

2. IgG prepared from an anti-immunoglobulin serum, e.g., rabbit antihuman IgG serum, or murine antihuman IgG MAb for the purification of human IgG (*see* Note 17).

3. IgG-binding proteins derived from bacteria, e.g., protein A (from *Staphylococcus aureus* Cowan 1 strain) or proteins G or C (from *Streptococcus; see* Note 18).

The methods for production of such immobilized ligands and for carrying out affinity purification of IgG are essentially similar whatever ligand is used. Sepharose 4B is probably the most widely used matrix for affinity chromatography, but there are other materials available. Activation of Sepharose 4B is usually carried out by reaction with CNBr; this can be carried out in the laboratory before coupling or ready-activated lyophilized Sepharose can be purchased. The commercial product is obviously more convenient than "homemade" activated Sepharose, but it is more expensive and may be less active.

3.4.1. Activation of Sepharose with CNBr and Preparation of Immobilized Ligand

Activation of Sepharose with CNBr requires the availability of a fume hood and careful control of the pH of the reaction—failure to do this may lead to the production of dangerous quantities of hydrogen cyanide (HCN) as well as compromising the quality of the activated Sepharose. CNBr is toxic and volatile. All equipment that has been in contact with CNBr and residual reagents should be soaked in $1M$ NaOH overnight in a fume hood, and washed before discarding/returning to the equipment pool. Manufacturers of ready-activated Sepharose provide instructions for coupling (*see* Note 19).

1. Wash 10 mL (settled volume) of Sepharose 4B with 1 L of water by vacuum filtration. Resuspend in 18 mL of water (do not allow the Sepharose to dry out).
2. Add 2 mL of $0.5M$ sodium carbonate buffer, pH 10.5, and stir slowly. Place in a fume hood and immerse the glass pH electrode in the solution.
3. **Carefully** weigh 1.5 g of CNBr into an airtight container (**N.B. Weigh in a fume hood; wear gloves)**—remember to decontaminate equipment that has contacted CNBr in $1M$ NaOH overnight.
4. Add the CNBr to the stirred Sepharose. Maintain the pH between 10.5 and 11.0 by dropwise addition of $4M$ NaOH until the pH stabilizes and all the CNBr has dissolved. If the pH rises above 11.5, activation will be inefficient, and the Sepharose should be discarded.
5. Filter the slurry using a sintered glass or Büchner funnel, and wash the Sepharose with 2 L of cold $0.1M$ trisodium citrate buffer, pH 6.5. Do not allow the Sepharose to dry out. Carefully discard the filtrate. (**Caution: This contains CNBr.**)
6. Quickly add the filtered, washed Sepharose to the ligand solution (2–10 mg/mL in $0.1M$ sodium citrate, pH 6.5) and gently mix on a rotator ("windmill") at 4°C overnight (*see* Note 20).
7. Add 1 mL of $2M$ ethanolamine solution, and mix at 4°C for a further 1 h—this blocks unreacted active groups.
8. Pack the Sepharose into a suitable chromatography column (e.g., a syringe barrel fitted with a sintered disk), and wash with 50 mL of PBS. Store at 4°C in PBS containing 0.1% sodium azide.

3.4.2. Purification of IgG Using Affinity Chromatography on Antigen-Ligand or Protein A/G Columns

Isolation of IgG by affinity chromatography involves application of serum to a column of matrix-bound ligand, washing to remove non-IgG components and elution of IgG by changing the conditions such that the ligand–IgG interaction is disrupted.

1. Wash the affinity column with PBS. "Pre-elute" with dissociating buffer, e.g., $0.1M$ glycine-HCl, pH 2.5. Wash with PBS; check that the pH of the eluate is the same as the pH of the PBS (*see* Note 21).
2. Apply the sample to the column (filtered through a 0.45-µm membrane). As a rule, add an equivalent amount of sample to that of the ligand coupled to the column. Close the column exit and incubate at room temperature for 15–30 min (*see* Note 22).
3. Wash non-IgG material from the column with PBS; monitor the A_{280} as an indicator of protein content.
4. When the A_{280} reaches a low value (approx 0.02), disrupt the ligand–IgG interaction by eluting with dissociating buffer (*see* step 1). Monitor the A_{280} and collect the protein peak into tubes containing $1M$ Tris, pH 8.8 (120 µL for a 1 mL fraction). If eluting with an alkali buffer, then neutralize with acid.
5. Wash the column with PBS until the eluate is at pH 7.4. Store the column in PBS containing 0.1% azide. Dialyze the IgG preparation against a suitable buffer (e.g., PBS) to remove glycine/Tris.

3.4.3. Thiophilic Chromatography

Immunoglobulins recognize sulfone groups in close proximity to a thioether group *(6)* and therefore thiophilic adsorbents provide an additional chromatographic method for the purification of immunoglobulin that can be carried out under mild conditions preserving biological activity. A thiophilic gel is prepared by reducing divinylsulfone (coupled to Sepharose 4B) with β-mercaptoethanol.

Caution: Divinylsulfone is highly toxic, and the column preparation procedures should be carried out in a well-ventilated hood.

1. Wash 100 mL Sepharose 4B (settled volume) with 1 L of water by vacuum filtration.
2. Resuspend in 100 mL of $0.5M$ sodium carbonate, and stir slowly.
3. Add 10 mL of divinylsulfone dropwise over a period of 15 min with constant stirring. After addition is complete, slowly stir the gel suspension for 1 h at room temperature.
4. Wash the activated gel thoroughly with water until the filtrate is no longer acidic (*see* Note 23).
5. Wash activated gel with 200 mL of coupling solution ($0.1M$ sodium carbonate, pH 9.0) using vacuum filtration, and resuspend in 75 mL of coupling solution.
6. In a well-ventilated hood, add 10 mL of β-mercaptoethanol to the gel suspension with constant stirring, and continue for 24 h at room temperature (*see* Note 24).

7. Filter, and wash the gel thoroughly. The gel may be stored at 4°C in 0.02% sodium azide.
8. Pack 4 mL of the gel in a polypropylene column, and equilibrate with 25 mL of binding buffer (0.1M Tris-HCl buffer, pH 7.6, containing 0.5M K$_2$SO$_4$).
9. Perform chromatography at 4°C. Mix 1 mL of clarified IgG preparation with 2 mL of binding buffer, and load onto the column. Clarification of IgG is carried out by high-speed centrifugation using a small bench centrifuge (microfuge) for about 5 min.
10. After the sample has entered the gel, wash non-IgG from the column with 20 mL of binding buffer; monitor the A$_{280}$ as an indicator of protein content in the wash until the absorbance returns to background levels.
11. Elute the bound IgG with 0.1M ammonium bicarbonate, and collect into 2-mL fractions. Monitor the protein content by absorbance at 280 nm, and pool the IgG-containing fractions (i.e., those with protein absorbance peaks). Dialyze against an appropriate buffer (e.g., PBS) with several changes.

3.5. Analysis of IgG Fractions

After the purification procedure, obtaining some index of sample purity is necessary. One of the simplest methods for assessing purity of an IgG fraction is by sodium dodecyl sulfate-polyacrylamide gel electrophoresis (SDS-PAGE). Although "full-size" slab gels can be used with discontinuous buffer systems and stacking gels, the use of a "minigel" procedure (*see* Note 25), using a Tris-bicine buffer system *(4)* rather than the classical Tris-glycine system, is quicker and easier, and gives improved resolution of immunoglobulin light chains (these are usually smeared with the Tris-glycine system). Gel heights can be restricted to about 10 cm, and are perfectly adequate for assessing purity and monitoring column fractions.

1. Prepare sample buffer.
2. Adjust antibody preparation to 1 mg/mL in 0.1M Tris, 0.1M bicine (*see* Note 7).
3. Mix the sample in the ratio 2:1 with sample buffer.
4. Heat at 100°C for 2–4 min.
5. Prepare gel solution and running buffer as described in Section 2.
6. Assemble gel mold according to manufacturers' instructions.
7. Add 30 μL TEMED to 10 mL of gel solution, pour this solution between the plates to fill the gap completely, and insert the comb in the top of the mold (there is no stacking gel with this system). Leave for 10 min for gel to polymerize.
8. Remove comb and clamp gel plates into the electrophoresis apparatus. Fill the anode and cathode reservoirs with running buffer.
9. Load the sample(s) (30–50 μL/track), and run an IgG reference standard and/or molecular weight markers in parallel.
10. Electrophorese at 150 V for 1.5 h.
11. Remove gel from plates carefully and stain with Coomassie blue R stain for 2 h (gently rocking) or overnight (stationary) (*see* Note 26).

12. Pour off the stain, and rinse briefly in tap water.
13. Add excess destain to the gel. A piece of sponge added during destaining absorbs excess stain. Leave until destaining is complete (usually overnight with gentle agitation).

4. Notes

1. Mouse and rat IgGs are less stable than IgG from higher mammals; it is best to separate mouse/rat serum from whole blood when clotting has occurred.
2. If an anticoagulant has been added to the blood and the plasma isolated, it may be advisable to defibrinate the plasma to yield a serum analog. The method for this varies according to the anticoagulant; for citrate, add 1/100 volume of thrombin solution (100 IU/mL in $1M$ $CaCl_2$), to warmed (37°C) plasma, stir vigorously, and incubate for 10 min at 37°C followed by 1 h at room temperature to ensure completion. For heparin, add 1/100 vol of 5 mg/mL protamine sulfate solution and thrombin (as above) to warmed plasma.
3. Blood clots more quickly in glass than in plastic containers and contracts more readily.
4. The use of 35% saturation will produce a fairly pure IgG preparation but will not precipitate all the IgG present in serum or ascitic fluid. Increasing saturation to 45% causes precipitation of nearly all IgG, but this will be contaminated with other proteins, including some albumin. Purification using $(NH_4)_2SO_4$ can be improved by repeating the precipitation, but this may cause some denaturation, especially of MAbs. Precipitation with 45% $(NH_4)_2SO_4$ is an ideal starting point for further purification steps, e.g., ion-exchange or affinity chromatography and FPLC purification.
5. Although the procedure works well for most antibodies, it may produce a fairly heavy contamination with non-IgG proteins with some samples; if this is the case, reduce the concentration of PEG. Consequently, carrying out a pilot-scale experiment before fractionating all of the sample is best.
6. The method can be used before ammonium sulfate precipitation to yield a product of higher purity.
7. The extinction coefficient ($E_{280}^{1\%}$) of human IgG is 13.6 (i.e., a 1 mg/mL solution has an A_{280} of 1.36).
8. It is essential that the sample to be loaded and all buffers are filtered using 0.2-μm filters. For HPLC, all buffers must be degassed by vacuum.
9. For FPLC, using the Mono Q system, IgG elutes between 10 and 25% buffer B and usually around 15%. When IgG elutes at 25% (dependent on pI), it will tend to coelute with albumin, which elutes at around 27%. When this occurs, alternative purification methods should be employed. For HPLC, IgG elutes between 15 and 25% buffer B.
10. The "void-volume" of the column is the volume of liquid between the beads of the gel matrix and usually amounts to about one-third of the total column volume.
11. There are a number of criteria to consider when setting up a gel-filtration system, e.g., choice of gel, column, and buffer. The gel of choice may be composed of

beads of carbohydrate or polyacrylamide, and is available in a variety of pore sizes and therefore fractionation ranges. Useful gels for the separation of IgG include Ultrogel AcA 44 (mixtures of dextran and polyacrylamide), Bio-Gel P 200 (polyacrylamide), and G3000 SW (silica-based). For IgM fractionation, Sephacel S-300 (crosslinked dextran) is useful. When selecting a column for gel-filtration, the column should be of controlled diameter glass with as low a dead space as possible at the outflow. Column tubing should be about 1 mm in diameter, which helps reduce dead space volume. A useful length for a gel-filtration column is about 100 cm and the choice of cross-sectional area is governed by sample size, both in terms of volume and amount of protein. As a rough rule of thumb, the sample volume should not be >5% of the total column volume (1–2% gives better resolution). Between 10 and 30 mg of protein/cm^2 cross-sectional area is a satisfactory loading. More protein will increase the yield, but decrease resolution and therefore purity, whereas less protein loaded improves resolution, but reduces the yield. Commercial columns suitable for gel-filtration are available from a number of manufacturers. Ensure columns are clean before use by washing with a weak detergent solution and rinsing thoroughly with water. Gel-filtration can be performed using a variety of buffers generally of physiological specification, i.e., pH 7.0, 0.1*M*.

12. Gel-filtration columns may also be packed by using an extension reservoir attached directly to the top of the column. Here the total volume of gel and buffer can be poured and allowed to settle without continual topping up. When using an extension reservoir, leave the column to pack until the gel bed just runs dry, and then remove excess gel.

13. The operating pressure of the gel is the vertical distance between the top of the buffer in the reservoir and the outlet end of the tube; this should never exceed the manufacturer's recommended maximum for the gel.

14. When loading commercial columns with flow adapters touching the gel bed surface, the most satisfactory way to apply the sample is by transferring the inlet tube from the buffer reservoir to the sample. The sample enters the tube and gel under operating pressure, and then the tube must be returned to the buffer reservoir. Ensure no air bubbles enter the tube. In homemade columns it is also possible to load the sample directly onto the gel bed by preparing it in 5% (w/v) sucrose. Elution of samples is either by pressure from the reservoir (operating pressure) or by a peristaltic pump between the reservoir and the top of the column. Overall the flow rate should be the volume contained in 2–4 cm height of column/h. To prevent columns without pumps from running dry, the inlet tube should be arranged so that part of it is below the outlet point of the column. Eluted fractions should be collected by measured volume rather than time (this prevents fluctuations in flow rate from altering fraction size). In general for a 100-cm column, a column volume of eluent should be collected in about 100 fractions. The void volume is eluted at fraction 30–35.

15. The choice of column size will depend on the sample size. As a rule, the sample size should not exceed 5% of the total column volume: 10–30 mg of protein/cm^2

cross-sectional area is a suitable loading (equivalent to 10–30 mg of protein/100 mL of gel for a 100-cm column).

16. The protein yield for gel-filtration chromatography should be >80% and is often as high as 95%. The yield will improve after the first use of a gel, because new gel adsorbs protein nonspecifically in a saturable fashion. When very small amounts of protein are being fractionated, the column should be saturated with an irrelevant protein, e.g., albumin, before use.

17. The use of subclass-specific antibodies or MAbs allows the immunoaffinity isolation of individual subclasses of IgG.

18. Some strains of *S. aureus* synthesize protein A, a group-specific ligand that binds to the Fc region of IgG from many species *(7,8)*. Protein A does not bind all subclasses of IgG, e.g., human IgG3, mouse IgG3, and sheep IgG1, and some subclasses bind only weakly, e.g., mouse IgG1. For some species, IgG does not bind to protein A at all, e.g., rat, chicken, goat, and some MAbs show abnormal affinity for the protein. These properties make the use of protein A for IgG purification limited in some cases, although it can be used to advantage in separating IgG subclasses from mouse serum *(9)*. Protein G (derived from groups C and G *Streptococci*) also binds to IgG Fc with some differences in species-specificity from protein A. Protein G binds to IgG of most species, including rat and goat, and recognizes most subclasses (including human IgG3 and mouse IgG1 and IgG3), but has a lower binding capacity. Protein G also has a high affinity for albumin, although recombinant DNA forms now exist in which the albumin-binding site has been spliced out and are therefore very useful for affinity chromatography.

Another bacterial IgG binding protein (protein L) has been identified *(10)*. Derived from *Peptostreptococcus magnus,* it binds to some κ (but not λ) chains. Furthermore, protein L binds to only some light-chain domains, although Igs from many species are recognized. Its full potential is yet to be established.

Finally, hybrid molecules produced by recombinant DNA procedures, comprising the appropriate regions of IgG-binding proteins (e.g., protein L/G, protein L/A), also have considerable scope in immunochemical techniques. These proteins are therefore very useful in the purification of IgG by affinity chromatography. Columns are commercially available (MabTrap G II, Pharmacia) or can be prepared in the laboratory.

19. Coupling at pH 6.5 is less efficient than at higher pH , but is less likely to compromise the binding ability of immobilized ligands (especially antibodies).

20. Check the efficiency of coupling by measuring the A_{280} of the ligand before and after coupling. Usually at least 80% of the ligand is bound to the matrix.

21. Elution of bound substances is usually achieved by a reagent that disrupts noncovalent bonds. These vary from "mild" procedures, such as the use of high salt or high or low pH, to more drastic agents, such as $8M$ urea, 1% SDS, or $5M$ guanidine hydrochloride. Chaotropic agents, such as $3M$ thiocyanate or pyrophosphate, may also be used. Usually an eluting agent is selected that is efficient, but does not appreciably denature the purified molecule; this is often a compromise between the two ideals. In view of this, highly avid polyclonal antisera obtained

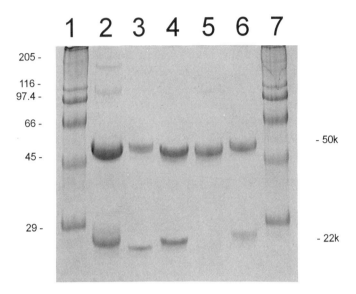

Fig. 1. SDS-PAGE minigel depicting purified IgG preparations derived from human serum (lane 2), mouse ascitic fluid (lanes 3 and 4), rabbit serum (lane 5), and sheep serum (lane 6). Samples are electrophoresed under reducing conditions and stained with Coomassie blue. All IgGs consist predominantly of two bands comprising heavy (50,000 M_r) and light (22,000 M_r) chains with no major contaminating proteins. Molecular weight markers are shown in lanes 1 and 7 and their molecular weights given on the left.

     from hyperimmune animals are often not the best reagents for immunoaffinity purification, since it may be impossible to elute the IgG in a useful form. The 0.1M glycine-HCl buffer, pH 2.5, will elute most IgGs from immunoaffinity and protein A and G columns, but may denature some MAbs. Most IgGs can be eluted from protein A by using pH 3.5 buffer. Preelution of the column with dissociating reagent just before affinity chromatography ensures that the isolated immunoglobulin is minimally contaminated with ligand.

22. Incubation of the IgG-containing sample with the ligand matrix is not always necessary, but will allow maximal binding to occur. Alternatively, slowly pump the sample through the column. Flow rate depends on the IgG concentration in the sample, and the binding capacity and size of the affinity column.

23. The activated gel can be stored by washing thoroughly in acetone and kept as a suspension in acetone at 4°C.

24. Immobilized ligands prepared by the divinylsulfone method are unstable above pH 8.0.

25. The "minigel" is easily and quickly prepared, consisting of a resolving (separating) gel only, and takes approx 1.5 h to run once set up. The IgG sample is prepared for electrophoresis under reduced conditions, and is run in parallel with either a reference IgG preparation or standard molecular weight markers. The heavy chains have a characteristic M_r of approx 50,000 and the light chains an M_r of 22,000 (Fig. 1).

26. Mark the gel uniquely before staining so that its orientation is known. By convention, a **small** triangle of the bottom left- or right-hand corner of the gel is sliced off.

Acknowledgments

We would like to thank Chris Ling for technical assistance and Deborah Richards for help in preparing the manuscript.

References

1. Jensenius, J. C., Andersen, I., Hau, J., Crone, M., and Koch, C. (1981) Eggs: conveniently packaged antibodies. *J. Immunol. Methods* **46**, 63–68.
2. Heide, K. and Schwick, H. G. (1978) Salt fractionation of immunoglobulins, in *Handbook of Experimental Immunology,* 3rd ed. (Weir, D. M., ed.), Blackwell Scientific, Oxford, UK.
3. Steinbuch, M. and Audran, R. (1969) The isolation of IgG from mammalian sera with the aid of caprylic acid. *Arch. Biochem. Biophys.* **134**, 279–284.
4. Johnstone, A. and Thorpe, R. (1996) *Immunochemistry in Practice,* 3rd ed., Blackwell Scientific, Oxford, UK.
5. Guse, A. H., Milton, A. D., Schulze-Koops, H., Müller, B., Roth, E., Simmer, B., Wächter, H., Weiss, E., and Emmrich, F. (1994) Purification and analytical characterization of an anti-CD4 MAb for human therapy. *J. Chromatogr.* **661**, 13–23.
6. Porath, J., Maisano, F., and Belew, M. (1985) Thiophilic adsorption—a new method for protein fractionation. *FEBS Lett.* **185**, 306–310.
7. Lindmark, R., Thorén-Tolling, K., and Sjöquist, J. (1983) Binding of immunoglobulins to protein A and immunoglobulin levels in mammalian sera. *J. Immunol. Methods* **62**, 1–13.
8. Hermanson, G. T., Mallia, A. K., and Smith, P. K. (1992) *Immobilized Affinity Ligand Techniques.* Academic, London.
9. Ey, P. L., Prowse, S. J., and Jenkin, C. R. (1978) Isolation of pure IgG1, IgG2a and IgG2b immunoglobulins from mouse serum using protein A-sepharose. *Immunochemistry* **15**, 429–436.
10. Kerr, M. A., Loomes, L. M., and Thorpe, S.J. (1994) Purification and fragmentation of immunoglobulins, in *Immunochemistry Labfax* (Kerr, M. A. and Thorpe, R., eds.), Bios Scientific, Oxford, UK, pp. 83–114.

11

Purification of Monoclonal Antibodies

Mark Page and Robin Thorpe

1. Introduction

Hybridoma technology has made possible the production of specific homogeneous antibodies (monoclonal antibodies [MAbs]) with predefined binding characteristics that can be produced in large amounts from immortal cell lines. MAbs can be exquisitely specific, but preparations containing these may be contaminated with tissue-culture additives and nonimmunoglobulin secretion products when produced in vitro, and by host animal proteins when prepared as an ascitic fluid. These contaminants may give rise to artifactual results in immunological methods and will preclude the use of applications that require purified immunoglobulin, such as labeling with radioisotopes, enzymes, and fluorochromes, and coupling to gels for production of immunoaffinity columns. Therefore, some form of purification may be required.

IgG MAbs may be purified using a variety of methods as described in Chapter 10, but these may require some modification to make them applicable for a single molecular species rather than for a mixture that is present in serum. A reliable method for a highly pure product is ion-exchange chromatography preceded by a precipitation step (usually 45% ammonium sulfate). Murine MAbs, however, are not readily purified using a generic method for conventional ion-exchange chromatography because of the relatively lower isoelectric points (pIs) of these antibodies compared with those of higher mammals, e.g., humans and rabbits (*see* Chapter 10). Also, each MAb is unique and has a distinct isoelectric point, and thus the ion-exchange conditions need to be tailored for each individual MAb. This is laborious, but can usually be avoided by the use of strong anion exchangers (e.g., Mono-Q, Pharmacia [Uppsala, Sweden];

From: *Methods in Molecular Biology, Vol. 80: Immunochemical Protocols, 2nd ed.*
Edited by: J. D. Pound © Humana Press Inc., Totowa, NJ

Hydropore SAX, Rainin [Woburn, MA]) in which conditions may be set so that a general method is used for more or less any IgG MAb.

IgM MAbs require different purification procedures from IgG MAbs because of the contrast in both size and charge. Ion-exchange chromatography can be used, but a more simple and reliable method is gel-filtration chromatography because the large molecular size of IgM facilitates the isolation. Precipitation methods with polyethylene glycol (PEG) and ammonium sulfate may also be used either alone or in conjunction with gel filtration. Affinity chromatography on protamine sulfate, the complement protein C1q, or mannan binding protein can also be used.

Purification from culture supernatants can be problematic because of the low concentration of IgG/IgM. However, some in vitro culture systems that utilize dialysis bubble chambers *(1)* and hollow-fiber supports (*see* Chapter 5) can produce immunoglobulin concentrations in excess of 0.5 mg/mL, and are therefore suitable for enrichment by precipitation techniques or direct purification using chromatographic methods. If these systems are not used, it may be necessary to reduce the supernatant volume to about 5–10 mL using ultrafiltration membranes under nitrogen pressure or centrifugation. Another useful preliminary procedure is a euglobin precipitation step in which IgM is precipitated by low-ionic strength dialysis.

2. Materials

1. Ultrafiltration cell fitted with a membrane having an M_r cutoff ~500, e.g., from Amicon.
2. Nitrogen pressure source.
3. 2 mM Sodium phosphate buffer, pH 6.0.
4. Phosphate-buffered saline (PBS): 0.14M NaCl, 2.7 mM KCl, 1.5 mM KH_2PO_4, 8.1 mM Na_2HPO_4.
5. Dialysis tubing.
6. Protamine sulfate.
7. Cyanogen bromide (CNBr)-activated Sepharose 4B (*see* Chapter 10, Section 3.4.1.).
8. 0.1M Sodium phosphate buffer, pH 7.5, containing 1M sodium chloride.
9. 10 mM Tris-HCl buffer, pH 7.4, containing 65 mM NaCl.
10. 50 mM Sodium phosphate buffer, pH 7.4, containing 150 mM NaCl, 2 mM EDTA, and 0.02% sodium azide.
11. 10 mM Tris-HCl buffer, pH 7.4, containing 1.2M NaCl, 20 mM $CaCl_2$, and 0.02% sodium azide.
12. 10 mM Tris-HCl buffer, pH 7.4, containing 1.25M NaCl.
13. 10 mM Tris-HCl buffer, pH 7.4, containing 1.25M NaCl, 2 mM EDTA, and 0.02% (w/v) sodium azide.
14. C1q (Sigma, St. Louis, MO) (*see* Note 1).
15. Silicone dioxide.
16. PEG 6000.

3. Methods

3.1. Prepurification Techniques

3.1.1. Concentration of MAbs in Culture Supernatants

The low concentration of MAbs in conventionally produced culture supernatants entails the need for use of large volumes of supernatant and large amounts of precipitant to yield useful quantities of antibody. If ascitic fluid cannot be made (as with human MAbs; *see* Note 2) then the precipitation step can often be more easily managed if the culture supernatant is reduced in volume. This is readily carried out by using ultrafiltration membranes that remove water and small molecular weight solutes from the supernatant.

1. Assemble the ultrafiltration cell according to the manufacturer's instructions, inserting a membrane with an M_r cutoff of 500 (*see* Note 3).
2. Add the supernatant (*see* Note 4). Place the cell on a magnetic stirring table, and pressurize the system to the recommended nitrogen pressure for a given membrane (usually about 55 psi).
3. Stir continuously at 4°C until the sample is reduced to the desired volume (5–10 mL).
4. Turn off the nitrogen pressure source, turn off the stirrer, and slowly release the pressure in the system (*see* manufacturer's instructions).
5. Dialyze the concentrated supernatant against PBS, pH 7.4.

3.1.2. Euglobin IgM Precipitation

Most IgM molecules are insoluble at low-ionic strength, and therefore, dialysis of the IgM preparation against a weak salt solution will cause precipitation. However, some IgM molecules are not precipitated by this means, and other methods must be employed.

1. Dialyze the IgM hybridoma culture supernatant or ascites fluid against at least three changes of 10 vol of 2 mM phosphate, pH 6.0, at 4°C.
2. Centrifuge at 2000g for 10 min at 4°C, discard the supernatant, resuspend the precipitate in cold phosphate buffer, and recentrifuge. Repeat this washing procedure immediately.
3. Dissolve the final euglobin precipitate in ~1/10 of the starting volume of PBS.

3.1.3. Clarification of Ascitic Fluid

Ascitic fluid derived from the peritoneal cavity of mice or rats that have been injected with hybridomas contain high concentrations of MAb (2–10 mg/mL), but this is usually mixed with variable amounts of blood cells, proteins, and fatty materials. It is therefore necessary to separate these components from the ascitic fluid before attempting purification of the MAb.

1. Allow the ascitic fluid to clot at room temperature (some samples will not clot; in this case, proceed as in step 2). Detach the clot from the sides of the container using a wooden or plastic spatula.

2. Pour the ascitic fluid into a centrifuge tube, and spin for 10–15 min at 2500*g* at 4°C. Aspirate the clear supernatant, and store at –20°C or below (*see* Note 5).

3.2. Preliminary Purification

As with serum IgG (*see* Chapter 10), enrichment of MAbs by precipitation is a useful starting point for further purification. The use of ammonium sulfate, sodium sulfate, PEG, and caprylic acid, as described in Chapter 10, is applicable to hybridoma culture supernatants and ascitic fluid.

3.2.1. Ammonium and Sodium Sulfate Precipitation

Sodium sulfate precipitation is not usually recommended for most murine MAbs because mouse/rat IgG can be degraded by the relatively high temperature (25°C) used during this procedure. If lipid contamination of ascitic fluids is a particular problem, add silicone dioxide powder (15 mg/mL), and centrifuge for 20 min at 2000*g*. Use the method described in Chapter 10, Section 3.2.1.

3.2.2. PEG Precipitation

Use the method described in Chapter 10, Section 3.2.3. For IgG MAbs, use 20% PEG, and for IgM MAbs, use 6% PEG.

3.2.3. Caprylic Acid Precipitation

It is necessary to determine experimentally the quantity of caprylic acid required for a given volume of MAb to produce the desired purity and yield. This will vary for each MAb.

Use the method described in Chapter 18, Section 3.2.4. **N.B.** The supernatant contains the immunoglobulin.

3.3. Chromatography Techniques

3.3.1. Ion-Exchange Chromatography

Fractionation using diethylaminoethyl (DEAE) (or several other anion exchangers) does not work well for murine MAbs, because each MAb has a different isoelectric point that often overlaps with many other proteins present in the MAb-containing preparation, except of course for those MAbs that happen to have a suitable charge. However, conditions can be tailored if necessary. Strong anion exchangers may be used as a generic method for any MAb. Two methods are described in Chapter 10, Section 3.3.2.

3.3.2. Gel-Filtration Chromatography

Use the method described in Chapter 10, Section 3.3.3. This method is appropriate for MAbs that possess pIs, which are unsuitable for fractionation by ion-exchange chromatography, but it is also useful for MAb preparations that have been derived from cultures propagated in serum-free medium that do not contain albumin (the albumin fraction and other serum proteins may be coeluted during ion-exchange chromatography). It is helpful to calibrate the column beforehand with a reference IgG or IgM preparation, so that the retention time for the immunoglobulin can be identified and the appropriate peak collected during sample fractionation. Choice of column with an appropriate fractionation range will also be important. IgG has a molecular weight of approx 156,000. Therefore, columns, such as Anagel TSK G3000, Ultrogel AcA, and Bio-Gel P200, would be suitable. IgM has a molecular weight of approx 900,000, and therefore a column with a higher fractionation range will be required, e.g., Anagel TSK G4000 and Sephacel S-300.

3.3.3. Affinity Chromatography

MAbs can be readily purified by affinity chromatography using ligands that are bound to a solid matrix, such as Sepharose. Such ligands are protein A, protein G, or protein L, an antimouse immunoglobulin, the antigen recognized by the MAb, or some other reagent that specifically reacts with the immunoglobulin.

Special mention should be made of the binding properties of proteins A and G. Protein A does not bind mouse or human IgG3 and only weakly binds mouse IgG1 and human IgM. Protein G will recognize all mouse and human IgG subclasses, but has a lower binding capacity (it does not bind human IgM). Protein G also has a high affinity for albumin, although recombinant forms are available in which the albumin binding site has been spliced out and are therefore very useful for IgG MAb purification. Protein L is able to bind Ig molecules of all classes, but is restricted to molecules containing some κ chains (it does not bind λ chains). A further restriction is its ability to bind human κ chain regions; the protein binds well to the VκI, VκIII, and VκIV subgroups, but does not seem to recognize VκII. Use the method described in Chapter 10, Section 3.4.2.

3.3.4. Thiophilic Chromatography

Use the method described in Chapter 10, Section 3.4.3.

3.3.5. Purification of IgM MAb Using Immobilized Protamine Sulfate

Protamine sulfate has a low affinity for IgM and is only recommended for producing small amounts of immunoglobulin. Some form of enrichment procedure before chromatography is advised.

1. Couple the protamine sulfate to CNBr-activated Sepharose 4B using the method described in Chapter 10, Section 3.4.1. (*see* Note 6).
2. Equilibrate the column with PBS until the absorbance of the washings is below 0.02 (at 280 nm).

3. Apply IgM MAb sample to the column (*see* Note 7), and recirculate through the column with a peristaltic pump for at least 2 h.
4. Wash sample through with PBS until the absorbance drops to 0.02.
5. Elute IgM with 0.1*M* sodium phosphate, pH 7.5, containing 1*M* sodium chloride.
6. Collect protein peaks, and dialyze into PBS or buffer of choice (*see* Note 8).

3.3.6. Purification of IgM Using Immobilized C1q

The complement protein, C1q, has an 18-fold higher affinity for pentameric IgM than IgG. This property may be used to purify IgM selectively from MAb ascites. Immobilized C1q binds IgM at 4°C, and the immunoglobulin is eluted simply and isocratically (using the same buffer) by bringing the column to room temperature for 2 h.

1. Couple purified C1q to CNBr-activated Sepharose 4B as described in Chapter 10, Section 3.4.1. Approximately 2.8 mg of C1q are coupled/mL of matrix (*see* Note 1).
2. Perform the chromatography at 4°C. Equilibrate the column with 10 m*M* Tris-HCl buffer, pH 7.4, containing 65 m*M* NaCl (binding buffer).
3. Apply the IgM MAb culture supernatant to the C1q column.
4. When the sample has entered the column matrix, wash with binding buffer until the absorbance falls to baseline (<0.02).
5. Bring the column to room temperature, and incubate for 2 h. Do not let the column dry out. Elute the IgM with 50 m*M* sodium phosphate buffer, pH 7.4, containing 150 m*M* NaCl, 2 m*M* EDTA, and 0.02% sodium azide (elution buffer).
6. Collect 2-mL fractions, and measure the absorbance at 280 nm to identify those containing IgM (*see* Note 8).
7. The IgM sample may be stored in the elution buffer.

3.3.7. Purification of IgM
Using Immobilized Mannan-Binding Protein (MBP)

MBP is present in various mammalian sera and activates the complement system through the classical pathway. It also specifically binds to murine monoclonal IgM and, hence, can be used to purify IgM MAb from mouse ascitic fluids. The binding reaction is calcium-dependent, so that IgM can be specifically eluted with a buffer containing a calcium chelator (e.g., EDTA).

1. MBP is purified from rabbit serum using affinity chromatography on immobilized mannan *(3)*. The resulting dialyzed MBP may be used directly to couple to activated Sepharose 4B.
2. Couple MBP to CNBr-activated Sepharose 4B using the method described in Chapter 10, Section 3.4.1.
3. Equilibrate the MBP column at 4°C with 10 m*M* Tris-HCl buffer, pH 7.4, containing 1.25*M* NaCl, 20 m*M* CaCl$_2$, and 0.02% sodium azide (binding buffer).

4. Dialyze mouse ascitic fluid (clarified) containing IgM against 10 mM Tris-HCl, pH 7.4, containing 1.25M NaCl.
5. Following dialysis, mix the ascitic fluid with an equal volume of binding buffer, and apply to the column.
6. When the sample has entered the column matrix, wash the column with binding buffer until the absorbance falls to baseline (<0.02 at 280 nm).
7. Bring the column to room temperature, and incubate for 2 h.
8. Elute bound IgM using 10 mM Tris HCl, pH 7.4, containing 1.25M NaCl, 2 mM EDTA, and 0.02% (w/v) sodium azide.
9. Collect fractions, and measure the absorbance at 280 mM to identify those containing IgM.
10. Dialyze pooled fractions against PBS, pH 7.4, and concentrate using an ultrafiltration membrane if required (*see* Section 3.1.1.).

4. Notes

1. C1q is available commercially (Sigma), but is expensive. Alternatively, it can be isolated from plasma *(2)*.
2. In cases where the cell line is a heterohybrid, that is, a human/mouse hybrid, it may be possible to grow the cell line as a tumor in sublethally irradiated mice and produce ascitic fluid.
3. Some ultrafiltration membranes must be used in the correct orientation.
4. Centrifuge or prefilter the supernatants to remove any particulate matter, such as cell debris or precipitates. This will prevent the filter from becoming clogged.
5. Do not store ascitic fluids at 4°C, because they contain proteolytic enzymes, which will digest immunoglobulin at this temperature. Always store aliquots at −20 or −70°C.
6. 10 mg Protamine sulfate will bind about 2 mg of pentameric IgM.
7. Only dilute solutions of IgM are required, i.e., culture supernatants, obviating the need to produce ascites.
8. The extinction coefficient ($E_{280}^{1\%}$) of human IgM is 11.8 (i.e., a 1 mg/mL solution will have an A_{280} of 1.18). This may vary for each MAb.

References

1. Pannell, R. and Milstein, C. (1992) An oscillating bubble chamber for laboratory scale production of monoclonal antibodies as an alternative to ascitic tumors. *J. Immunol. Methods* **146,** 43–48.
2. Tenner, A. J., Lesavre, P. H., and Cooper, N. R. (1981) Purification and radiolabelling of human C1q. *J. Immunol.* **127,** 648–653.
3. Kozutsumi, Y., Kawasaki, T., and Yamashima, I. (1980) Isolation and characterization of a mannan-binding protein from rabbit serum. *Biochem. Biophys. Res. Commun.* **95,** 658–664.

12

Production of Bispecific and Trispecific F(ab)$_2$ and F(ab)$_3$ Antibody Derivatives

Ruth R. French

1. Introduction

Bispecific antibodies (BsAbs) are hybrid molecules designed to combine two antibodies with different specificities. This dual specificity has led to their application in a variety of diagnostic situations that require the crosslinking of two protein surfaces, for example, antigen and detecting agent in immunohistochemistry or immunoassays. More interestingly, BsAbs have been shown to have considerable therapeutic potential when used as targeting reagents to deliver pharmacological substances (drugs or toxins) or cellular effectors (T-cells, monocytes, or NK cells) to tumor cells (1,2). A relatively new development is the design of BsAbs to deliver chelated radiometals for the diagnostic imaging of tumors and for radioimmunotherapy (1).

The first BsAb derivatives were described in the early 1960s by Nisonoff and Rivers (3), who showed that a mixture of reduced Fab fragments from two rabbit IgG antibodies could reoxidize via their hinge region SH-groups to produce F(ab)$_2$ heterodimers. Over the past few years, two main approaches have been adopted for the production of BsAbs, chemical conjugation and hybrid-hybridoma technology. Chemical conjugation, in which two antibodies are joined using a chemical crosslinking reagent, has allowed the construction of a variety of BsAb derivatives. Lysyl reactive crosslinkers with free SH-groups, such as N-succinimidyl-3-(-2-pyridyldithio)-propionate (SPDP), have been used to produce disulfide-linked IgG- and F(ab)$_2$-heterodimers (4,5), and F(ab)$_2$/Fab (6) and IgG/Fab (7) conjugates. Smaller bispecific F(ab)$_2$ derivatives have been constructed using thiol-reactive reagents to disulfide- (8) or, as in this laboratory, thioether-link the hinge region SH-groups of two antibodies (9). The second approach, hybrid-hybridoma technology, involves the fusion

From: *Methods in Molecular Biology, Vol. 80: Immunochemical Protocols, 2nd ed.*
Edited by: J. D. Pound © Humana Press Inc., Totowa, NJ

of two antibody-producing hybridoma cell lines to give a hybrid-hybridoma or quadroma cell line secreting bispecific IgG *(10)*. The application of genetic engineering has allowed the construction of a range of new BsAb derivatives. Humanized Fab fragments with a single cysteine residue introduced at the hinge region have been produced in *Escherichia coli* and then chemically conjugated to obtain fully humanized $F(ab)_2$ BsAb *(11)*. As a possible alternative to chemical conjugation, dimerization domains, such as "leucine zippers," have been genetically fused to pairs of antibody Fab fragments to promote the formation of heterodimers *(12)*. Recently two types of derivatives combining just the Fv regions of two antibodies have been described, small dimeric bispecific antibody fragments known as "diabodies" *(13)* and single-chain BsAbs *(14,15)*, generated by joining two single-chain Fv regions via a flexible tanker.

This chapter describes the procedures developed in the laboratory of Martin Glennie at the Lymphoma Research Unit, Tenovus Laboratory, Southampton, UK, for preparing bispecific $F(ab)_2$ and $F(ab)_3$ and trispecific antibody (TsAb) $F(ab)_3$ derivatives from antibody Fab fragments using the crosslinker o-phenylenedimaleimide (o-PDM).

1.1. Production of Multispecific F(ab)$_2$ and F(ab)$_3$ from Fab Fragments

1.1.1. Preparation of IgG and F(ab)$_2$

First, the IgG fraction is isolated from mouse ascites, hybridoma, or bioreactor culture supernatant as described in Chapter 10. The $F(ab)_2$ fragment of IgG is then obtained by limited proteolysis *(16)*. $F(ab)_2$ can be produced from IgG1 and IgG2a antibodies' digestion at pH 4.0–4.2. Some IgG1 antibodies that are resistant to pepsin can be digested with the enzymes ficin or bromelain *(17,18)*. Pepsin will break down a few antibodies to smaller peptides and, provided they are of IgG1 isotype, ficin or bromelain may again present a useful alternative (*see* Notes 1 and 2).

1.1.2. Bispecific F(ab)$_2$

Bispecific $F(ab)_2$ derivatives are produced by using the bifunctional crosslinker o-PDM to join two Fab fragments via their hinge region SH-groups. The procedure is illustrated in Fig. 1. First, Fab fragments are obtained from the two parent $F(ab)_2$ species by reduction with thiol, thus exposing free SH-groups at the hinge region (three SH-groups for mouse IgG1 and IgG2a antibodies). One of the Fab species (Fab-A) is selected for alkylation with o-PDM. Because o-PDM has a strong tendency to crosslink adjacent intramolecular SH-groups *(19)*, two of the three hinge SH-groups will probably be linked together, leaving a single reactive maleimide group available for conju-

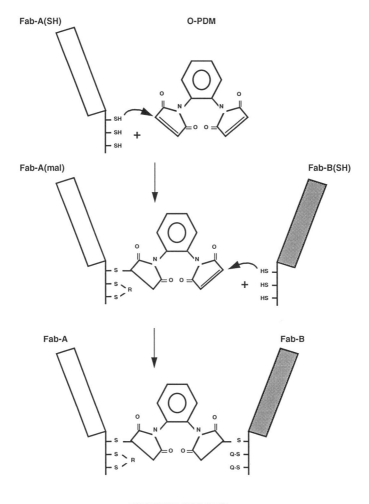

BISPECIFIC ANTIBODY

Fig. 1. Preparation of BsAb using *o*-PDM as crosslinker. BsAb production is described in Sections 1.1.2. and 3.2. The F(ab)$_2$ BsAb illustrated is produced from Fab fragments derived from mouse IgG1 or IgG2a antibody. Two adjacent hinge SH-groups of Fab-A are crosslinked by *o*-PDM (R, *o*-phenylenedisuccinimidyl linkage) leaving one with a free maleimide group for crosslinking with an SH-group at the hinge of Fab-B. Unconjugated SH-groups at the Fab-B hinge are blocked by alkylation (Q, carboxyamidimethyl). Increasing the ratio of Fab-A (mal) to Fab-B(SH) will favor the production of bispecific F(ab)$_3$ in which 2 mol of Fab-A(mal) are linked to 1 mol of Fab-B (Sections 1.1.3. and 3.3.).

gation (*see* Section 1.1.5.). When excess *o*-PDM has been removed, the Fab-A(mal) is mixed with the second reduced Fab, Fab-B(SH), under conditions favoring the crosslinking of the maleimide and SH-groups. When equal amounts of Fab-A(mal) and Fab-B(SH) are used, the major product is bispecific F(ab)$_2$ resulting from the reaction of one Fab-A(mal) with one of the SH-groups at the hinge of Fab-B. Remaining free SH-groups on Fab-B are alkylated, and the F(ab)$_2$ BsAb product (Fab-A × Fab-B) is separated by gel-filtration chromatography.

In addition to the hinge region SH-groups, each reduced Fab fragment may also contain two SH-groups resulting from the reduction of the heavy (H)–light (L) chain S–S bond. However, these are less likely to be involved in conjugation than those at the hinge region for three reasons. First, under the conditions used, it has been shown that only around 50% of the H–L S–S bonds are reduced *(9);* second, the *o*-PDM will tend to crosslink the interchain SH-groups on Fab-A, so that they are not available for conjugation, and finally, the SH-groups on Fab-B will be buried between the H and L chains. Therefore, they will be less likely than exposed hinge SH-groups to react with the Fab-A(mal).

1.1.3. Bispecific F(ab)$_3$

Increasing in the proportion of Fab-A(mal) in the reaction mixture results in a significant amount of F(ab)$_3$ product by the reaction of two molecules of Fab-A(mal) with two free SH-groups at the hinge of a single Fab-B molecule. By selecting the appropriate parent Fab to be Fab-A, F(ab)$_3$ with two arms from either of the parent antibodies can be produced. These derivatives have proven useful in cellular retargeting studies because they can be designed with either two Fab arms binding to the effector and one to the target or vice versa *(20)*.

1.1.4. Trispecific F(ab)$_3$

The protocol for the preparation of a BsAb can be extended to allow the preparation of a F(ab)$_3$ TsAb, with each Fab arm having different specificity. This is illustrated in Fig. 2. The BsAb product (Fab-A × Fab-B) is isolated, but not alkylated and so still has free SH-groups at the Fab-B hinge. This reduced BsAb can then be used in a second conjugation step in which maleimidated Fab from a third antibody, Fab-C(mal), is linked to one of the remaining SH-groups at the Fab-B hinge, thus giving trispecific F(ab)$_3$ as the major product.

1.1.5. Selection of F(ab)$_3$ for BsAb Preparation

Since this procedure relies on one SH-group remaining free for conjugation after the intramolecular crosslinking of adjacent SH-groups at the hinge with *o*-PDM (Fig. 1), the Fab species chosen to be maleimidated must be derived from IgG with an odd number of hinge region disulfide bonds. Mouse IgG1

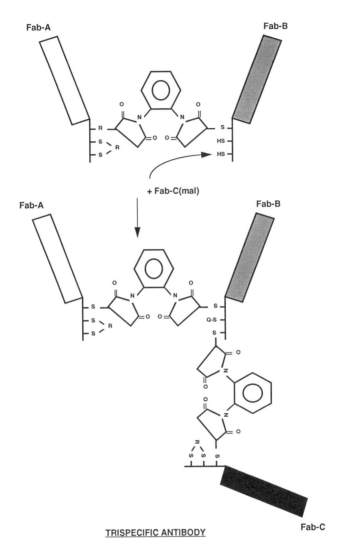

Fig. 2. Preparation of TsAb using *o*-PDM. TsAb production is described in Sections 1.1.4. and 3.4. The BsAb (Fab-A × Fab-B)(SH) is conjugated to Fab-C(mal), giving trispecific F(ab)$_3$ as the major product.

and IgG2a antibodies are both suitable in this respect, since they each have three SH-groups at the hinge. Rabbit Fab-SH (one SH-group) and rat IgG1 (three hinge disulfide bonds) can likewise be employed. However, rat IgG2a and IgG2c have two and rat IgG2b has four such bonds *(21)* and, therefore, cannot be used to make a rat/rat F(ab)$_2$ by this method. On the other hand, rat

IgG2a, 2b, and 2c can be used to produce a rat/mouse BsAb derivative if used as the unmaleimidated partner. If F(ab)$_3$ derivatives are required, the number of SH-groups at the hinge of the unmaleimidated partner must be considered, since this determines the number of Fab(mal) arms that can be conjugated. Thus, mouse IgG1 and IgG2a (three SH-groups) can be used to construct F(ab)$_3$. If rabbit Fab(SH) is the unmaleimidated partner, the major product is always F(ab)$_2$. We have found that a few antibodies give a consistently low yield of BsAb when used as the maleimidated partner. If large quantities of derivative are required, it is worthwhile performing small-scale pilot preparations to determine which maleimidated partner gives the optimal yield.

1.1.6. Removal of Residual Fc

The bispecific and trispecific derivatives produced by these procedures are almost always contaminated with trace amounts of intact IgG antibody or Fc fragments, which are coharvested with the parent F(ab)$_2$ and, accordingly, with the final product. In derivatives to be used for immunohistochemistry or drug/ toxin targeting, this trace contamination is unimportant. However, even small amounts (<1%) of contaminating Fc can cause a major problem if BsAbs are to be used in cell proliferation studies or in redirected cellular cytotoxicity assays *(2,20)*. If this is likely to be a problem, preparations can be checked for Fc by ELISA and, if necessary, Fc removed by immunoaffinity chromatography *(22)*.

1.1.7. Advantages of this Procedure
for Preparing Multispecific Derivatives

Using these procedures, well-defined derivatives are produced with good yield, and the products are easily isolated; starting with 10 mg each of two parent F(ab)$_2$ species, expect to obtain 5–10 mg of BsAb. The derivatives can be produced at relatively low cost and quickly: It is possible to obtain the BsAb product from the parent IgG in five working days. The protocols can be scaled up to produce larger amounts (100–150 mg) of derivative for therapeutic applications.

2. Materials
2.1. Reagents

1. TE8, 2M stock, pH 8.0: 2M Tris-HCl, 100 mM EDTA. Prepare 0.2M TE8 and 20 mM TE8 from 2M stock.
2. Acetate buffer, 2M, pH 3.7: 103 mL glacial acetic acid, 17.2 g sodium acetate, made up to 1 L.
3. 70 mM Acetate/50 mM NaCl, pH 4.0: 3.22 mL acetic acid, 1.15 g sodium acetate, 2.92 g NaCl, made up to 1 L.
4. Tris base, 1M, pH 9.2.
5. TE7, 50 mM, pH 7.0: 50 mM Tris-HCl, 2 mM EDTA.

6. 2-Mercaptoethanol (2-ME).
7. $F(ab)_2$ reducing solution: 220 mM 2-ME, 1 mM EDTA. Make up 10 mL.
8. Sephadex G25, Sephacryl S200 (Pharmacia, Uppsala, Sweden), and Ultrogel ACA44 (BioSepra S.A., Villeneuve la Garenne, France) gel-filtration media.
9. Sepharose 4B (Pharmacia).
10. Human albumin, e.g., Zenalb 20 (BPL, Elstree, Herts, UK).
11. Polymixin B sulfate (Sigma, St. Louis, MO).
12. G25 column buffer (AE, 0.05M): 3.35 g sodium acetate, 0.526 mL glacial acetic acid, 0.186 g EDTA, made up to 1 L. Degas before use, e.g., under vacuum (*see* Chapter 10) or by using nitrogen.
13. S200 Buffer (NAE, 0.5M): 0.5M NaCl, 0.1M sodium acetate, 9 mM EDTA. For therapeutic applications, use sterile pyrogen-free water.
14. HPLC buffer (0.2M phosphate, pH 7.0): Add 0.2M Na_2HPO_4 to 0.2M NaH_2PO_4 to obtain required pH.
15. *o*-PDM/DMF for Fab(SH) alkylation: 12 mM *o*-PMD in DMF. Make up 5 mL just prior to use (*see* Note 3).
16. NTE8, 1M, pH 8.0: 1M NaCl, 0.2M Tris-HCl, 10 mM EDTA.
17. Iodoacetamide.
18. Ammonium thiocyanate for cleaning Polymixin column: 1M potassium thiocyanate, 0.5M ammonia in sterile, pyrogen-free water.
19. Limulus Amebocyte Lysate test kit (Pyrogen Plus, BioWhittaker Inc., Walkersville, MD).

2.2. Equipment

1. Two peristaltic pumps capable of rates between 15 and 200 mL/h for column chromatography.
2. Columns of approx 1.6-, 2.6-, and 5-cm diameter. Pharmacia K series columns are suitable. These must be fitted with two end-flow adapters and water jackets to allow chilling throughout the preparation of Fab(SH) and Fab(mal) (*see* Section 3.2.).
3. Chiller/circulator to cool chromatography columns (*see* Note 4).
4. UV monitor, chart recorder, and fraction collector.
5. Amicon stirred concentrating cell (Series 8000, 50 or 200 mL) with a 10,000 M_r cutoff filter for concentration $F(ab)_2$ and products.
6. HPLC system fitted with a Zorbex Bio series GF250 column (Du Pont Company, Wilmington, DE) or equivalent gel-permeation column capable of fractionation up to ~250,000 M_r.
7. Pyrogen-free water for therapeutic preparations.

3. Methods
3.1. Preparation of Parent F(ab)₂
3.1.1. Pepsin Digestion

A routine digestion would employ 50–200 mg of IgG. However, for new antibodies, a pilot digestion using 5–10 mg is recommended.

1. Concentrate the mouse IgG1 or IgG2a antibody to approx 10–15 mg/mL using the Amicon concentration cell and dialyze into $0.02M$ TE8 buffer.
2. Adjust pH to 4.0–4.2 with $2M$ acetate buffer, pH 3.7.
3. Make up a 10 mg/mL solution of pepsin in 70 mM acetate/50 mM NaCl, pH 4.0. Add pepsin to anybody solution to give a final concentration of 3% (w/w).
4. Incubate at 37°C in a water bath. At hourly intervals, take 10-μL samples for size fractionation by HPLC (*see* Note 5). As the digestion proceeds, the profile will change from a single IgG peak to a doublet. When <10% remains as intact IgG, or when the size of the $F(ab')_2$ peak ceases to increase, stop the digestion by adjusting the pH to 8.0 with $1M$ Tris. Under these conditions, most IgG1 digestions take 6–12 h (*see* Note 6).
5. Fractionate the digestion mixture on Ultrogel AcA44 in $0.2M$ TE8 buffer. For digestions up to about 150 mg (not more than 10 mL), use two 2.6-cm diameter columns connected in series, with a gel bed height of 80 cm and a flow rate of ~30 mL/h. For larger preparations (up to 200 mg, more than 10 mL), use a single 5-cm diameter column and a gel bed height of 90 cm. Harvest the $F(ab')_2$ peak ($M_r \sim 100,000$).

3.1.2. Bromelain Digestion

1. Concentrate IgG as described above, and dialyze into 50 mM TE7.
2. Make up a 10 mg/mL solution of bromelain in 50 mM TE7, and add 2-ME to a final concentration of 0.5 μM to activate the enzyme. Incubate for 15 min at 37°C. Add bromelain to the antibody solution to a final concentration of 0.5–4% (w/w) depending on the susceptibility of the antibody to this enzyme.
3. Incubate at 37°C in a water bath. At hourly intervals, remove 10-μL aliquots and analyze by HPLC as described in Section 3.1.1. (*see* Note 7). Stop the digestion by adding iodoacetamide to a final concentration of 0.5 mM when intact IgG represents <10% of the mixture.
4. Fractionate on AcA44 columns in series as described in Section 3.1.1.

3.2. Preparation of Bispecific $F(ab)_2$ Derivatives

The following procedures describe the small-scale preparation of BsAb, starting with between 5 and 20 mg of each $F(ab)_2$ species to obtain 1–8 mg of BsAb. Large-scale preparations for therapy require the scaling up of the columns as described in Section 3.5.

1. Start with equal amounts of $F(ab)_2$ from the two parent antibodies. If necessary, dialyze into $0.2M$ TE8. The samples should be concentrated to between 5 and 12 mg/mL in a final volume of 1–3 mL.
2. Reduce both $F(ab)_2$ preparations to Fab(SH) by the addition of 1/10 vol of $F(ab)_2$ reducing solution (*see* Section 2.1.). Incubate for 30 min at 30°C and then keep on ice. **The temperature must be maintained at 0–4°C for the remainder of the procedure.**

3. Select the Fab(SH) to be maleimidated (referred to hereafter as Fab-A[SH]). Remove 2-ME by running through a cooled Sephadex G25 column (1.6-cm diameter, bed height 25 cm) in 0.05M AE buffer at a flow rate of approx 60 mL/h. Collect the protein peak (eluted after 8–10 min) in a graduated glass tube in an ice bath. Take a 45-µL sample from the top of the peak for HPLC analysis. Contamination of the Fab-A(SH) with 2-ME must be avoided. Therefore, stop collecting when the chart recorder pen has returned between half and two-thirds of the way to the baseline. Keep the Fab-A(SH) on ice. Leave the column running to remove all 2-ME, which elutes as a small second peak.

4. While on the HPLC column, Fab(SH) fragments can reoxidize to give F(ab)$_2$. Alkylation of free SH-groups by the addition of 5 µL of 50 mM iodoacetamide in 1M NTE8 to the 45 µL of peak sample prevents this. Incubate for 10 min at room temperature before applying a 10-µL sample to the HPLC column.

5. While Fab-A(SH) is on the Sephadex G25 column, make up o-PDM/DMF, making sure that all of the o-PDM is dissolved. Immediately chill solution in a methylated spirit/ice bath.

6. When the 2-ME has eluted from Sephadex G25 column (chart recorder has returned to baseline), load the second reduced Fab, Fab-B (SH), and separate as for Fab-A(SH), again taking a peak sample for HPLC analysis.

7. While Fab-B(SH) is on the column, quickly add 1/2 vol (normally 4–5 mL) of cold o-PDM/DMF to Fab-A(SH). Cover the tube with Parafilm or something similar, and invert two to three times to mix. Leave in an ice bath for 30 min.

8. When Fab-B(SH) has been eluted, connect a second, larger Sephadex G25 column (2.6-cm diameter, bed height 20 cm) to the chart recorder. After the 30 min-incubation, load the Fab-A(SH)/o-PDM/DMF mixture onto this second G25 column, and elute at a flow rate of approx 200 mL/h. Collect the Fab-A(mal) protein peak (elutes after 8–10 min), taking a 45-µL sample for HPLC analysis. Stop collecting when the chart recorder pen has returned half way to baseline to avoid contamination with o-PDM/DMF, which elutes as a large second peak.

9. Pool Fab-A(mal) and Fab-B(SH) and concentrate rapidly at 0–5°C in a stirred Amicon cell until approximately equal to the starting volume of the two parent F(ab)$_2$ fragments (around 5 mL). Remove the mixture from the cell, and leave at 4°C overnight. To avoid loss of product, slightly overconcentrate and then wash residue from the cell with a small volume of chilled buffer.

10. To reduce any homodimers produced, add 1/10 vol of 1M NTE8 to increase the pH and then 1/10 vol of F(ab)$_2$ reducing solution. Incubate at 30°C for 30 min and then alkylate by adding 1/10 vol of 250 mM iodoacetamide in 0.2M TE8. Check the composition of the mixture by HPLC.

11. Fractionate the mixture on two AcA44 columns run in series as in step 5, Section 3.1.1. Collect 10–15 min fractions (5–7.5 mL). A typical elusion profile is shown in Fig. 3.

12. Pool the BsAb product. To minimize contamination, only take the middle two-thirds of the peak. Check the final product by HPLC.

13. Concentrate in an Amicon, and dialyze into the appropriate buffer.

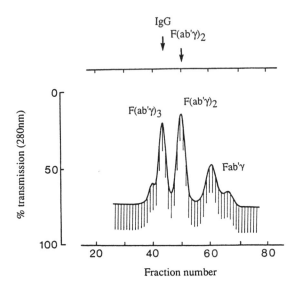

Fig. 3. Chromatography profile showing the separation of parent Fab and bispecific F(ab)₂ and F(ab)₃ products on AcA44 columns. The preparation of bispecific F(ab)₂ and F(ab)₃ is described in Sections 3.2. and 3.3. In this case, Fab-A(SH) and Fab-B(mal) were mixed at a ratio of 2:1 to increase the formation of bispecific F(ab)₃. The unreacted Fab fragments and the F(ab)₂ and F(ab)₃ products are indicated. The arrows show the points at which protein standards eluted from the same columns.

3.3. Preparation of Bispecific F(ab)₃ Derivatives

This is as for the preparation of bispecific F(ab)₂ (*see* Section 3.2.), except that the ratio of Fab(mal) to Fab(SH) is increased from 1:1 to 2:1 or greater. Therefore, start with at least twice as much of the F(ab)₂ species, which is to provide two arms of the F(ab)₃ product.

3.4. Preparation of Trispecific F(ab)₃ Derivatives

Preparation of trispecific F(ab)₃ (Fab-A × Fab-B × Fab-C) should be carried out over two consecutive days.

1. Day 1: Prepare the BsAb (Fab-A × Fab-B) as described in Section 3.2., but with the following modifications:
    a. If possible, start with 10–20 mg each of F(ab)₂-A and F(ab)₂-B since smaller quantities can lead to problems during the second stage of the preparation.
    b. The alkylation with iodoacetamide described in step 10 **must be omitted**. This leaves SH-groups at the hinge region of (Fab-A × Fab-B) onto which a third Fab (Fab-C) can be coupled. After concentration of the Fab-A(mal) and Fab-B(SH) described in Section 3.2., step 9, **immediately** load the mixture

onto the AcA44 columns. The BsAb (Fab-A × Fab-B) will thus be available for use on d 2 of the preparation.

2. Day 2: Pool the (Fab-A × Fab-B) peak from the columns and concentrate to 3 mL or less. Check the protein concentration.

3. $F(ab)_2$ from the required third arm, $F(ab)_2$-C, should be at 5–12 mg/mL (max. 3 mL in $0.2M$ TE8). For each 1 mg of the BsAb (Fab-A × Fab-B) use 2 mg of $F(ab)_2$-C for the second stage.

4. Reduce both $F(ab)_2$-C and (Fab-A × Fab-B) with 1/10 vol of 220 mM 2-ME for 30 min at 30°C, and then keep on ice. Maintain at 0–4°C

5. The remainder of the procedure is as described for the preparation of BsAb in Section 3.2., steps 3–8, but with Fab-C substituted for Fab-A, and (Fab-A × Fab-B) substituted for Fab-B. Thus, remove 2-ME from Fab-C and (Fab-A × Fab-B) on a 1.6-cm diameter Sephadex G25 column (25-cm bed height, flow rate ~60 mL/h) maleimidate Fab-C and separate Fab-C(mal) on larger Sephadex G25 column (2.6-cm diameter, bed height 20 cm, flow rate ~200 mL/h).

6. Pool and rapidly concentrate Fab-C(mal) with (Fab-A × Fab-B) back to the starting volume. Remove the concentrated mixture from the cell, and leave overnight at 4°C.

7. Increase the pH of the mixture, reduce, and alkylate as described in Section 3.2., step 10. Take a sample for HPLC analysis, and then separate on AcA44 columns as described in Section 3.2., step 11.

3.5. Modifications for Large-Scale Preparations for Therapeutic Applications

For a large-scale preparation of BsAb starting with 100–150 mg of each parent $F(ab)_2$, the columns are scaled up appropriately: Use Sephadex G25 columns of 2.6-cm diameter (25-cm bed height, flow rate 200 mL/h) and 5-cm diameter (30-cm bed height, flow rate 500–800 mL/h) (*see* Note 8).

For therapeutic preparations, subsequent stages are carried out as "cleanly" as possible. Sephacryl S200 columns (5-cm diameter, 80-cm bed height, flow rate 100–200 mL/h) are used instead of AcA44 for the separation of the products, because they can be cleaned up easily by running through with $0.2M$ NaOH for 1 h and then washing with 2 column volumes of S200 buffer ($0.5M$ NAE). In order to minimize contamination with pyrogens, the running buffer should be prepared in sterile, pyrogen-free water and fractions collected in disposable, sterile plastic tubes.

After concentration in a concentration cell washed with $0.2M$ NaOH, preparations are passed through a Sepharose-human albumin/Sepharose-polymixin column in $0.5M$ NAE buffer to remove pyrogens (*see* Note 9).

Use a 2.6-cm diameter column containing a 10-cm bed of Sepharose-human albumin over a 10-cm bed of Sepharose-Polymixin and a flow rate 25–50 mL/h.

The pyrogen-depleted preparation passes through a sterile filter before being collected in a transfusion bag. The column is cleaned between uses with 1 column volume of ammonium thiocyanate followed by washing with 2 column volumes of S200 buffer.

Preparations are pyrogen-tested using a Limulus Amebocyte Lysate test kit.

4. Notes

1. The "prime" character ('), as in F(ab')$_2$ and Fab', indicates that the fragments have been produced by pepsin digestion.
2. None of the proteolytic enzymes alluded to in Section 1.1.1. will produce F(ab)$_2$ from mouse IgG2b antibodies.
3. **Caution:** *o*-PDM is reported to be carcinogenic and should be handled with due caution.
4. A polystyrene box containing water and crushed ice and a submersible garden pond pump (rate approx 10 L/min) can be used in place of purpose-built chillers.
5. For a Zorbax Bio series GF250 column, equilibrate the gel with 0.2M phosphate buffer, pH 7.0, and use a flow rate of 0.5 mL/min. Each run takes about 30 min.
6. Since the activity of pepsin is highly pH-sensitive, the digestion rate can be increased by reducing the pH slightly (just 0.1 pH unit may be sufficient) or decreased by increasing the pH. Digestions not completed in a working day can be left overnight at 4°C and continued the next day.
7. As the digestion proceeds, some Fc and Fab may be apparent on the HPLC trace.
8. Care must be taken to avoid the buildup of back-pressure in 5-cm diameter Sephadex G25 columns.
9. Human albumin and polymixin B sulfate are each coupled to Sepharose according to the manufacturer's instructions.

Acknowledgments

This work was supported by Tenovus Cardiff, Tenovus Solentside, and the Cancer Research Campaign.

References

1. Glennie, M. J. and French, R. R. (1995) Targeting drugs, toxins and radionuclides with bispecific antibodies, in *Bispecific Antibodies* (Fanger, M. W., ed.), Landes, Georgetown, TX, pp. 107–120.
2. Tutt, A., Stevenson, G. T., and Glennie, M. J. (1991) Trispecific F(ab')$_3$ derivatives that use cooperative signalling via the TCR/CD3 complex and CD2 to activate and redirect resting cytotoxic T cells. *J. Immunol.* **147**, 60–69.
3. Nisonoff, A. and Rivers, M. M. (1961) Recombination of a mixture of univalent antibody fragments of different specificity. *Arch. Biochem. Biophys.* **93**, 460–462.
4. Karpovsky, B., Titus, J. A., Stephany, D. A., and Segal, D. M. (1984) Production of target-specific effector cells using hetero-cross-linked aggregates containing anti-target cell and anti-Fcγ receptor antibodies. *J. Exp. Med.* **160**, 1686–1701.
5. Jung, G., Freimann, U., and von Marschall Z. (1991) Target-cell induced T-cell activation with bi- and trispecific antibody fragments. *Eur. J. Immunol.* **21**, 2431–2435.

6. Mabondzo, A., Aussage, P., Bartholeyns, J., Lenaour, R., Raoul, H., Rometlemonne, J. L., and Dormont, D. (1992) Bispecific antibody targeting of human immunodeficiency virus type I (HIV-1) glycoprotein 41 to human macrophages through the Fc IgG receptor I mediates neutralizing effects in HIV-1 infection. *J. Infect. Dis.* **166,** 93–99.
7. Mabondzo, A., Boussin, F., Raoul, H., Lenaour, R., Gras, G., Vaslin, B., Bartholeyns, J., Rometlemonne, J. L., and Dormont, D. (1994) Antibody-dependent cellular cytotoxicity and neutralization of human immunodeficiency virus type I by high affinity cross-linking of gp41 to human macrophage Fc IgG receptor using bispecific antibody. *J. Gen. Virol.* **75,** 1451–1456.
8. Nitta, T., Yagita, H., Azuma, T., Sato, K., and Okomura, K (1989) F(ab')$_2$ monomer prepared with anti-CD3 and anti-tumor monoclonal antibodies is most potent in induction of cytolysis of human T cells. *Eur. J. Immunol.* **19,** 1437–1441.
9. Glennie, M. J., McBride, H. M., Worth, A. T., and Stevenson, G. T. (1987) Preparation and performance of bispecific F(ab'γ)$_2$ antibody containing thioether-linked Fab'γ fragments. *J. Immunol.* **139,** 2367–2375.
10. Milstein, C. and Cuello, A. C. (1983) Hybrid hybridomas and their use in immunochemistry. *Nature* **305,** 537–540.
11. Shalaby, M. R., Shepard, H. M., Presta, L., Rodrigues, M. L., Beverley, P. L. C., Feldmann, M., and Carter, P. (1992) Development of humanized bispecific antibodies reactive with cytotoxic lymphocytes and tumor cells overexpressing the HER2 protooncogene. *J. Exp. Med.* **175,** 217–225.
12. Kostelney, S. A., Cole, M. S., and Tso, J. Y. (1992) Formation of bispecific antibody by the use of leucine zippers. *J. Immunol.* **148,** 1547–1553.
13. Holliger, P., Prospero, T., and Winter, G. (1993) "Diabodies": small bivalent and bispecific antibody fragments. *Proc. Natl. Acad. Sci. USA* **90,** 6444–6448.
14. Gruber, M., Schodin, B. A., Wilson, E. R., and Kranz, D. M. (1994) Efficient tumor cell lysis mediated by a bispecific single-chain antibody expressed in *Escherichia coli. J. Immunol.* **152,** 5368–5374.
15. Mack, M., Riethmuller, G., and Kufer, P. (1995) A small bispecific antibody construct expressed as a functional single-chain molecule with high tumor-cell cytotoxicity. *Proc. Natl. Acad. Sci. USA* **92,** 7021–7025.
16. Lamoyi, E. and Nisonoff, A. (1983) Preparation of F(ab')$_2$ fragments from mouse IgG of various subclasses. *J. Immunol. Methods* **56,** 235–243.
17. Milenic, D. E., Estaban, J. M., and Colcher, D. (1989) Comparison of methods for the generation of immunoreactive fragments of a monoclonal-antibody (B72.3) reactive with human carcinomas. *J. Immunol. Methods* **120,** 71–83.
18. Mariani, M., Camagna, M., Tarditi, L., and Seccamani, E. (1991) A new enzymatic method to obtain high yield F(ab)$_2$ suitable for clinical use from mouse IgG1. *Mol. Immunol.* **28,** 69–77.
19. Stevenson, G. T., Pindar, A., and Slade, C. J. (1989) A chimeric antibody with dual Fc regions (bisFabFc) prepared by manipulations at the IgG hinge. *Anti-Cancer Drug Design* **3,** 219–230.

20. Tutt, A., Greenman, J., Stevenson, G. T., and Glennie, M. J. (1991) Bispecific F(ab'γ)₃ antibody derivatives for redirecting unprimed cytotoxic T cells. *Eur. J. Immunol.* **21,** 1351–1358.

21. Kabat, E. A., Wu, T. T., Perry, H. M., Gottesman, K. S., and Foeller, C. (1991) in Sequences of Proteins of Immunological Interest, vol. I. US Department of Health and Human Services, Public Health Service, National Institute of Health, Bethesda, MD, p. 675.

22. Glennie, M. J., Tutt, A. L., and Greenman, J. (1993) in *Tumor Immunobiology, A Practical Approach* (Gallagher, G., Rees, R. C., and Reynolds, C. W., eds.), Oxford University Press, Oxford, UK, pp. 225–244.

13

Preparation of Cytotoxic Antibody–Toxin Conjugates

Alan J. Cumber and Edward J. Wawrzynczak

1. Introduction

Conjugates of antibodies with plant toxins, such as ricin and abrin, are potent cytotoxic agents that selectively eliminate target cells from mixed cell cultures in vitro, and have great promise as antitumor agents in cancer therapy *(1)*. Ricin and abrin are protein toxins consisting of two different polypeptide subunits, the A and B chains, which are of similar size (between 30 and 34 kDa) and are joined by a single disulfide bond. The A chain is a ribosome-inactivating protein (RIP) that inactivates eukaryotic ribosomes by a specific irreversible covalent modification of the ribosomal RNA *(2)*. The B chain binds to cell surface galactose-containing oligosaccharide residues. Following receptor-mediated endocytosis of toxin bound to the cell surface, the A chain gains access to the cytosol and destroys the ability of the cell to make protein *(3)*.

Antibody–toxin conjugates prepared with intact toxins are invariably cytotoxic, and their preparation and use requires special care owing to the hazardous nature of the toxins *(4)*. An alternative way to construct conjugates is to couple the isolated A chain directly to the antibody. This is conveniently achieved by using the single free sulfhydryl group of the A chain, which is revealed when the B chain is removed. Such conjugates, also referred to as immunotoxins, retain the catalytic activity of the A chain and possess a target specificity conferred solely by the antibody component. Many constructs of this type are highly potent and specific cytotoxins *(5)*.

The preparation of cytotoxic antibody-A chain conjugates using chemical crosslinking methods has two main requirements. First, the number of crosslinkers introduced per antibody molecule should be low. This minimizes the risk that the antigen-binding capability of the antibody will be compro-

From: *Methods in Molecular Biology, Vol. 80: Immunochemical Protocols, 2nd ed.*
Edited by: J. D. Pound © Humana Press Inc., Totowa, NJ

mised by modification. Second, the subsequent reaction of the derivatized antibody with the A chain should lead to the formation of a disulfide bond between the two components. This disulfide linkage is necessary for maximal expression of cytotoxic activity by the conjugate *(6)*.

The most commonly used crosslinking reagent is *N*-succinimidyl 3-(2-pyridyldithio)propionate (SPDP). This heterobifunctional agent attaches covalently to the antibody at lysyl ε-amino groups introducing an *S*-pyridyl group that is attached to the linker by a disulfide bond *(7)*. In the conjugation step, the derivatized antibody is mixed with an excess of freshly reduced A chain. The sulfhydryl group of A chain molecules displaces *S*-pyridyl groups with concomitant formation of a disulfide bond between A chain and antibody. A useful feature of the SPDP reagent is the formation of pyridine-2-thione, which is a chromophore, on release of the *S*-pyridyl group. Therefore, the level of derivatization and the degree of reaction can be measured spectrophotometrically.

RIPs, which act in a fashion identical to the toxin A chains and are similar in size (about 30 kDa), also occur naturally in plants as single chain polypeptides *(8)*. A variety of RIPs of this type, including gelonin and momordin, have been used to make cytotoxic conjugates *(9,10)*. The single chain RIPs differ from the toxin A chains and from one another in primary structure, isoelectric point, and glycosylation. They also lack cysteinyl residues because they are not associated with the equivalent of a cell-binding toxin B chain. For conjugation to antibody, such RIPs must first be reacted with SPDP. Subsequently, free sulfhydryl groups are revealed by treating the derivatized RIP with a reducing agent to detach the *S*-pyridyl group.

The methods described below for the preparation of antibody–toxin conjugates containing A chains isolated from toxins or single-chain RIPs are generally applicable to the synthesis of conjugates using any type of antibody and all known RIPs of plant origin.

2. Materials

1. Antibody solution in PBSE (*see* item 6) containing between 10 and 15 mg at a concentration of 5–10 mg/mL (*see* Notes 6–8).
2. Solution of toxin A chain or RIP in PBSE, containing between 5 and 7.5 mg, at a concentration of about 1.5 mg/mL (*see* Notes 1–5).
3. *N*-Succinimidyl 3-(2-pyridyldithio)propionate (SPDP) (Pharmacia, Uppsala, Sweden).
4. Dimethylformamide (DMF) (Sequanal grade, Pierce [Rockford, IL]).
5. Dithiothreitol (DTT) (Sigma, St. Louis, MO).
6. Phosphate/saline buffer (PBSE): 28.4 g of Na_2HPO_4, 11.7 g of NaCl, 0.744 g of EDTA disodium salt. Adjust to pH 7.5 with $1M$ HCl and make up to a final vol of 2 L in distilled water.

7. Acetate/saline buffer: 16.4 g of CH_3COONa, 11.7 g of NaCl, 0.744 g EDTA disodium salt. Adjust to pH 4.5 with $1M$ HCl and make up to a final vol of 2 L in distilled water.

8. Column chromatography apparatus, including a suitable low-pressure pump, on-line UV monitoring at 280 nm and a fraction collector.

9. Chromatography media: Sephacryl S-200 (SF), Sephadex G-25 (SF) (Pharmacia).

10. Chromatography columns:
    a. Sephacryl S-200 (SF): dimensions, 80 cm × 1.6 cm internal diameter (id); bed vol, 160 mL; equilibrated with PBSE (for purification of antibody and antibody–toxin conjugate).
    b. Sephadex G-25 (SF): dimensions, 30 cm × 1.6 cm (id); vol, 60 mL; equilibrated with PBSE (for purification of derivatized antibody).
    c. Sephadex G-25 (SF): dimensions, 30 cm × 1.6 cm (id); vol, 60 mL; equilibrated with acetate/saline buffer (for purification of derivatized RIP).
    d. Sephadex G-25 (SF): dimensions, 45 cm × 1.6 cm (id); vol, 90 mL; equilibrated with PBSE (for purification of reduced RIPs).

11. N_2 cylinder.

12. Ultrafiltration cell (10 mL vol) containing a suitable membrane with a cut-off of $M_r > 10,000$ for globular proteins (PM10 membrane, Amicon [Beverley, MA]).

13. Low protein binding 0.22-μm filtration units (Millex GV, Millipore [Bedford, MA]).

3. Methods

3.1. Derivatization of Antibody

1. Apply the antibody solution at a concentration between 5 and 10 mg/mL to the S-200 column (*see* Section 2., item 10a) and elute with PBSE at a flow rate of between 10 and 20 mL/h as a preliminary purification step (*see* Notes 6–8).

2. Pool all the fractions contained within the main antibody peak, i.e., corresponding to an M_r of 150,000 relative to protein standards. Discard any flanking fractions that may contain aggregated protein or contaminants of lower molecular weight.

3. Concentrate the antibody solution to about 10 mg/mL in the ultrafiltration cell under N_2 pressure and transfer the solution to a suitable reaction vessel holding 10 mL of solution.

4. Make up a fresh solution of SPDP at 2 mg/mL in DMF in a glass vessel (*see* Note 9).

5. To 1 mL of the antibody solution at 10 mg/mL (a total of 67 nmol), slowly add 42 μL of the SPDP solution (a total of 0.27 μmol, i.e., a fourfold molar excess of reagent added) while stirring rapidly. Once the addition is complete, stir the mixture gently for 30 min at room temperature (*see* Note 10).

6. Apply the reaction mixture to the G-25 column (*see* Section 2., item 10b) and elute with PBSE at a flow rate of 30 mL/h to remove low molecular weight byproducts of the reaction. Collect the protein peak that elutes at the void vol of the column (total vol, about 7 mL).

7. Remove 0.5 mL of the pooled protein solution to measure the loading of *S*-pyridyl groups on the antibody (*see* Notes 11 and 12).
8. Concentrate the remainder of the derivatized antibody solution to a final vol of about 1 mL by ultrafiltration. Store in the ultrafiltration cell at 4°C in preparation for the conjugation procedure.

3.2. Derivatization of Single-Chain RIPs

1. Make up a fresh solution of SPDP at 2 mg/mL in DMF.
2. To a solution (about 3 to 5 mL) of the single-chain RIP in PBSE containing 7 mg (a total of 0.22 µmol), slowly add 67 µL of the SPDP solution (a total of 0.43 µmol, i.e., a twofold molar excess of reagent added) while stirring rapidly. Once the addition is complete, stir gently for 30 min at room temperature.
3. Apply the reaction mixture to the G-25 column (*see* Section 2., item 10c) and elute with acetate/saline buffer at a flow rate of 30 mL/h to remove the low molecular weight byproducts of the reaction (*see* Note 13). Collect the protein peak that elutes at the void vol of the column (total vol, about 5 mL).
4. Remove 0.25 mL of the pooled RIP solution to measure the extent of modification with SPDP (*see* Note 14). Use the remainder of the derivatized RIP preparation for conjugation to the antibody.

3.3. Conjugation

1. Prepare a fresh solution of 1*M* DTT in PBSE.
2. To the solution of toxin A chain or derivatized single-chain RIP, add DTT solution to a final concentration of 50 m*M*. Leave the solution for 30 min at room temperature.
3. Apply the solution of reduced RIP to the G-25 column (*see* Section 2., item 10d) and elute with PBSE at a flow rate of 30 mL/h to remove the excess DTT and low molecular weight byproducts of the reaction (*see* Notes 15 and 16). Collect the protein that elutes at the void vol of the column (total vol, about 7 mL).
4. Determine the protein concentration of the RIP solution by measuring the optical density of the solution at 280 nm.
5. Add the appropriate vol of the freshly reduced RIP solution that contains a total of 5 mg of RIP to the solution of derivatized antibody in the ultrafiltration cell. Stir gently to mix and then leave overnight at room temperature, without stirring, under a gentle stream of N_2.
6. Concentrate the reaction mixture, with gentle stirring, to about 3.5 mL and leave for between 4 and 6 h at room temperature under a gentle stream of N_2 (*see* Note 17).
7. Pass the reaction mixture through a 0.22-µm filtration unit.
8. Apply the filtered reaction mixture to the S-200 column (*see* Section 2., item 10a) and elute with PBSE at a flow rate of between 10 and 20 mL/h to separate the antibody–toxin conjugate from the excess of the RIP and the pyridine-2-thione released during the reaction. Collect fractions of approx 2 mL in vol (*see* Notes 18 and 19).
9. Remove samples from the column fractions making up the broad band containing conjugate and unconjugated antibody, and subject to SDS-PAGE in the absence of reducing agent to determine their content (*see* Note 20).

10. Pool fractions according to the determined content of conjugate and unconjugated antibody (*see* Note 21).
11. Pass the final conjugate preparation through a 0.22-µm filtration unit in a sterile hood and store in suitable containers at 4°C for short-term use, or at –70°C for long-term storage following rapid freezing.

4. Notes
4.1. Toxin A-Chains and Single-Chain RIPs

1. Toxin A chains are isolated from ricin and abrin by reductive cleavage of the toxin, followed by separation of the chains. These procedures are hazardous and should not be undertaken without the proper safeguards *(4)*.
2. Commercially obtained preparations of ricin A chain and abrin A chain may require further purification to eliminate traces of contaminating toxin B chains. The simplest procedure is to pass the A chain preparation over a column of Sepharose-linked asialofetuin, to which the B chains bind avidly *(4,11)*.
3. RIPs should generally appear as a single band on SDS-PAGE. The presence of additional bands is a clear indication of impurity, and may complicate the interpretation of electrophoretic analysis of conjugate products. The exception is ricin A chain that has been isolated from the native toxin. Native ricin A chain exists as a mixture of two differently glycosylated forms giving the appearance of a doublet on SDS-PAGE: Bands with apparent M_rs of about 32,000 and 34,000 occur in the approximate ratio of 2:1.
4. Caution must be exercised with the handling of ricin A chain which has a tendency to form "stringy" precipitates. The concentration of ricin A chain in solution should not exceed about 1.5 mg/mL. At higher concentration, even gentle agitation will cause aggregation. Frothing of the solution should also be avoided. Ricin A chain is much less prone to precipitation following conjugation to antibody.
5. The single-chain RIPs are generally more stable to a wider range of experimental conditions than ricin A chain. However, loss of material can occur in the course of procedures based on selective passage through membranes. Ultrafiltration may be performed using a membrane with a lower M_r cut-off.

4.2. Derivatization of Antibody

6. The method described has been used to prepare antibody–toxin conjugates containing mouse and rat monoclonal antibodies of various IgG subtypes and polyclonal antibody from several animal species. Modifications of this method have also been used to prepare conjugates with antibodies of other classes.
7. The starting antibody preparation should be as highly purified as possible, e.g., by using ion-exchange chromatography, affinity chromatography, or protein A chromatography, as appropriate. The gel filtration of the antibody on Sephacryl S-200 before derivatization removes protein aggregates that are frequently present even in the most carefully prepared antibody samples, and any low molecular weight contaminants that may interfere with the subsequent derivatization reaction. Precise knowl-

edge of the elution position of the antibody at this step also assists in the analysis of the chromatographic profile of the conjugation reaction mixture *(see below)*.

8. The method is readily adapted for the preparation of conjugates starting with between 20 and 50 mg of antibody by using columns of the same length but increased id (2.6 cm) and an ultrafiltration cell with 50 mL capacity. For preparations using less than 5 mg of antibody, HPLC gel filtration apparatus is more suitable for purification purposes.

9. SPDP is very stable when stored dry. As a solution in DMF, it is hydrolyzed only slowly, provided that moisture is rigorously excluded from the solution. It is advisable to prepare this solution freshly before each conjugation.

10. The *S*-pyridyl group on the derivatized antibody is also relatively stable. In practice, the conjugation procedure can be completed comfortably within a day. If this proves to be impossible, the antibody solution may be stored under nonreducing conditions for a few days at 4°C with little loss of *S*-pyridyl groups.

11. The level of substitution of the antibody after reaction with SPDP is determined spectrophotometrically. A sample of the derivatized antibody is treated with DTT at a final concentration of 5 m*M,* and the optical density measured at 280 nm and 343 nm. The pyridine-2-thione released by reduction has a molar extinction coefficient at 343 nm of $8.08 \times 10^3 M/cm$ *(12).* This product also absorbs at 280 nm with a molar extinction coefficient of $5.1 \times 10^3 M/cm$. The true protein absorbance is determined from the formula:

$$A_{280}(\text{protein}) = A_{280}(\text{observed}) - (C \times 5.1 \times 10^3)$$

where C is the molar concentration calculated for the pyridine-2-thione from the absorbance at 343 nm. The molar extinction coefficient for antibody at 280 nm is $2.1 \times 10^5 M/cm$.

The sample used for this analysis must be discarded and not returned to the bulk of the derivatized antibody because of the presence of the added DTT.

12. Using the conditions described, i.e., a fourfold molar excess of SPDP over antibody, the level of derivatization should be between 1.5 and 2.0 *S*-pyridyl groups per antibody molecule on average. At higher levels of modification, there is an increased risk of inactivating or precipitating the antibody.

4.3. Derivatization of Single-Chain RIPs

13. The acetate/saline buffer was originally used for the column chromatography of the derivatized RIP because the *S*-pyridyl group is easily displaced by sulfhydryl reagents under the conditions of low pH at which protein disulfide bonds are relatively stable. Most single-chain RIPs are stable to these conditions.

14. The level of substitution of the single-chain RIPs obtained using the method described should be close to 1.0 *S*-pyridyl group per RIP molecule on average. Slight impairment of the enzymic function of several RIPs has been reported as a result of derivatization with SPDP. Alternative procedures for the introduction of sulfhydryl groups using different crosslinkers (e.g., 2-iminothiolane) may be used to circumvent this problem *(8,13).*

4.4. Conjugation

15. It is essential that all traces of DTT should be removed from the RIP after the reduction step. The presence of even very low concentrations of DTT at this stage will release *S*-pyridyl groups from the antibody in preference to the formation of conjugate. For this reason, the G-25 column should be rigorously cleaned before use. EDTA in the column buffer inhibits disulfide bond formation, catalyzed by trace amounts of metal ions.

16. The number of reactive sulfhydryl groups following reduction and chromatography can be measured by mixing a sample of the RIP with Ellman's reagent. Reaction of sulfhydryl groups with Ellman's reagent leads to the quantitative release of the 3-carboxylato-4-nitrothiophenolate anion, a chromophore with a molar extinction coefficient of $1.36 \times 10^4 M/cm$ at 412 nm *(14)*.

    The sample used for this analysis should be discarded. The remaining RIP solution should then be added to the derivatized antibody solution without delay.

17. The final reaction mixture should not be stirred overnight to avoid the risk of precipitating the RIP. The course of the reaction between the derivatized antibody and the RIP can be followed by monitoring the release of pyridine-2-thione spectrophotometrically. The reaction mixture can be stored at 4°C for several days without deleterious effect.

18. The conjugate product consists of a mixture of antibody molecules crosslinked to one or more RIP molecules. Using the conditions described, the 1:1 conjugate is obtained in the highest yield. On S-200 column chromatography, the 1:1 conjugate elutes at a position well separated from unreacted RIP and released pyridine-2-thione. Any aggregated protein and the multiple-substituted conjugates elute near the void volume of the column. This procedure does not efficiently separate the 1:1 conjugate from unconjugated antibody (*see* Fig. 1 and also Chapter 14).

19. In the case of ricin A chain, a proportion of unreacted RIP binds irreversibly to the S-200 column during the final purification. The column can be cleaned by washing with $0.1M$ NaOH before further chromatography.

20. The pooled conjugate preparation contains the 1:1 conjugate as the major product and unconjugated antibody as the major contaminant. Smaller amounts of multiple-substituted conjugates are also present. The composition of the conjugate preparation can be determined by densitometric analysis of the pattern of bands on SDS-PAGE before and after reduction of the sample (Figs. 2 and 3). An alternative procedure involves trace radiolabeling of the RIP component before conjugation to allow a precise measurement of the RIP content of the conjugate *(15)*.

21. Antibody–toxin conjugates made with ricin A chain, abrin A chain, gelonin, and momordin can be stored for at least 4 yr at –70°C without detectable loss of activity. The bond between the antibody and the RIP breaks down very slowly at 4°C in PBSE but, provided that care is taken to ensure the sterility of the solution, conjugates can be stored under these conditions for up to one year with little deterioration in quality.

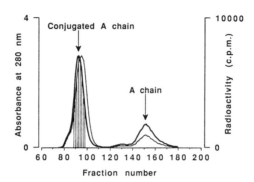

Fig. 1. Gel permeation chromatography of an antibody–toxin conjugate reaction mixture. The reaction mixture obtained following the conjugation of a mouse monoclonal antibody (50 mg) and [^{125}I]-labeled abrin A chain was chromatographed on a column of Sephacryl S-200 (SF), dimensions: 80 cm × 2.6 cm (id). Fractions eluting from the column were monitored spectrophotometrically at 280 nm (—) to measure total protein, and by gamma counting (—) to measure the A chain in its free or conjugated form. The hatched area indicates a typical pooled conjugate preparation.

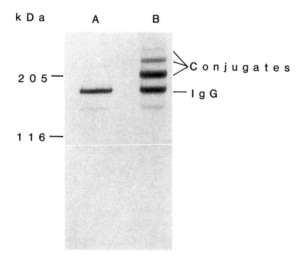

Fig. 2. SDS-PAGE of an antibody–toxin conjugate preparation. **(A)** Antibody (starting material). **(B)** Abrin A chain conjugate (pooled fractions shown in Fig. 1). Samples were prepared under nonreducing conditions and run on a 2–27% gradient polyacrylamide gel.

142

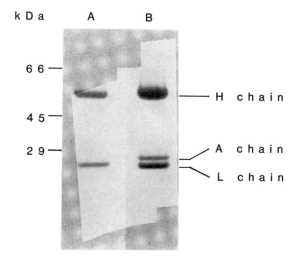

Fig. 3. SDS-PAGE of reduced antibody–toxin conjugate. (**A**) Antibody (starting material). (**B**) Abrin A chain conjugate (as in Fig. 2). Samples were prepared in the presence of 5% w/v DTT and run on a 2–27% gradient polyacrylamide gel.

References

1. Blakey, D. C., Wawrzynczak, E. J., Wallace, P. M., and Thorpe, P. E. (1988) Antibody toxin conjugates: a perspective, in *Monoclonal Antibody Therapy* (Waldmann, H., ed.), Karger, Basel, pp. 50–90.
2. Endo, Y. (1988) Mechanism of action of ricin and related toxins on the inactivation of eukaryotic ribosomes, in *Immunotoxins* (Frankel, A. E., ed.), Kluwer Academic, Boston, pp. 75–89.
3. Olsnes, S. and Sandvig, K. (1988) How protein toxins enter and kill cells, in *Immunotoxins* (Frankel, A. E., ed.), Kluwer Academic, Boston, pp. 39–73.
4. Cumber, A. J., Forrester, J. A., Foxwell, B. M. J., Ross, W. C. J., and Thorpe, P. E. (1985) Preparation of antibody–toxin conjugates. *Methods Enzymol.* **112,** 207–225.
5. Thorpe, P. E. (1985) Antibody carriers of cytotoxic agents in cancer therapy: a review, in *Monoclonal Antibodies '84: Biological and Clinical Applications* (Pinchera, A., Doria, G., Dammacco, F., and Bargellesi, E., eds.), Editrice Kurtis s. r. l., Milan, pp. 475–506.
6. Wawrzynczak, E. J. and Thorpe, P. E. (1988) Effect of chemical linkage upon the stability and cytotoxic activity of A chain immunotoxins, in *Immunotoxins* (Frankel, A. E., ed.), Kluwer Academic Publishers, Boston, pp. 239–251.
7. Carlsson, J., Drevin, H., and Axen, R. (1978) Protein thiolation and reversible protein–protein conjugation. *N*-succinimidyl 3-(2-pyridyldithio)propionate, a new heterobifunctional crosslinking reagent. *Biochem. J.* **173,** 723–737.

8. Lambert, J. M., Blattler, W. A., McIntyre, G. D., Goldmacher, V. S., and Scott, C. F., Jr. (1988) Immunotoxins containing single chain ribosome-inactivating proteins, in *Immunotoxins* (Frankel, A. E., ed.), Kluwer Academic, Boston, pp. 175–209.

9. Thorpe, P. E., Brown, A. N. F., Ross, W. C. J., Cumber, A. J., Detre, S. I., Edwards, D. C., Davies, A. J. S., and Stirpe, F. (1981) Cytotoxicity acquired by conjugation of an anti-Thy1.1 monoclonal antibody and the ribosome-inactivating protein, gelonin. *Eur. J. Biochem.* **116,** 447–454.

10. Stirpe, F., Wawrzynczak, E. J., Brown, A. N. F., Knyba, R. E., Watson, G. J., Barbieri, L., and Thorpe, P. E. (1988) Selective cytotoxic activity of immunotoxins composed of a monoclonal anti-Thy1.1 antibody and the ribosome-inactivating proteins bryodin and momordin. *Br. J. Cancer* **58,** 558–561.

11. Fulton, R. J., Blakey, D. C., Knowles, P. P., Uhr, J. W., Thorpe, P. E., and Vitetta, E. S. (1986) Purification of ricin A_1, A_2, and B chains and characterization of their toxicity. *J. Biol. Chem.* **261,** 5314–5319.

12. Stuchbury, T., Shipton, M., Norris, R., Malthouse, J. P. G., Brocklehurst, K., Herbert, J. A. L., and Suschitsky, H. (1975) A reporter group delivery system with both absolute and selective specificity for thiol groups and an improved fluorescent probe containing the 7-nitrobenzene-2-oxa-1,3-diazole moiety. *Biochem. J.* **151,** 417–432.

13. Wawrzynczak, E. J. and Thorpe, P. E. (1987) Methods for preparing immunotoxins: effect of the linkage on activity and stability, in *Immunoconjugates: Antibody Conjugates in Radioimaging and Therapy of Cancer* (Vogel, C.-W., ed.), Oxford University Press, New York and Oxford, pp. 28–55.

14. Ellman, G. L. (1959) Tissue sulphydryl groups. *Arch. Biochem. Biophys.* **82,** 70–77.

15. Thorpe, P. E. and Ross, W. C. J. (1982) The preparation and cytotoxic properties of antibody–toxin conjugates. *Immunol. Rev.* **62,** 119–158.

14

Immunoaffinity Purification and Quantification of Antibody–Toxin Conjugates

Edward J. Wawrzynczak and Alan J. Cumber

1. Introduction

Cytotoxic antibody–toxin conjugates made using antibodies and ribosome-inactivating proteins (RIPs) are prepared using chemical crosslinking methods (*1,2* and Chapter 13). Gel permeation chromatography is used as a first step to purify conjugate molecules from the reaction mixture. This procedure removes protein aggregates, the excess of RIP employed in the conjugation reaction, and low molecular weight byproducts. However, a significant fraction of the resulting conjugate preparation consists of unconjugated antibody that cannot be completely separated from the conjugate on the basis of size discrimination alone (*see* Chapter 13).

The efficient separation of some antibody–toxin conjugates from unconjugated antibody can be achieved using methods exploiting the physico-chemical properties of the RIP. Separation by ion-exchange chromatography is possible in cases where the RIP and the antibody have sufficiently distinct iso-electric points *(3)*. Affinity chromatography on Blue Sepharose CL-6B can be used to purify conjugates containing ricin A chain or abrin A chain *(4)*. However, these methods are not certain to succeed with different antibody-RIP combinations because the chromatographic properties of RIPs may be altered following their attachment to antibody *(5)*.

An alternative approach to purification is immunoaffinity chromatography using RIP-specific antibody immobilized on a column matrix. Affinity chromatography using soft gel matrices leads to poor recoveries and large sample dilution. An effective high performance immunoaffinity chromatography procedure that purifies antibody–toxin conjugates free from contaminating antibody and overcomes the problems associated with soft gel chromatography is

From: *Methods in Molecular Biology, Vol. 80: Immunochemical Protocols, 2nd ed.*
Edited by: J. D. Pound © Humana Press Inc., Totowa, NJ

described below. This generally applicable method is based on the selective binding of antibody-conjugated RIP molecules to affinity-purified anti-RIP antibody immobilized on a silica matrix.

The concentration of antibody–toxin conjugates made with mouse monoclonal IgG antibodies and a number of different RIPs can be accurately measured, even in the presence of free antibody and serum proteins by means of a highly sensitive enzyme-linked immunosorbent assay (ELISA). The noncompetitive indirect ELISA procedure presented below uses immobilized affinity-purified rabbit anti-RIP antibody to capture conjugate molecules by binding to the RIP component. The conjugate bound to the anti-RIP antibody is then detected using an enzyme-linked reagent that specifically recognizes the mouse antibody component of the conjugate.

2. Materials
2.1. Production of RIP-Specific Antiserum
1. New Zealand white rabbits.
2. Filtration units: 0.45 μm (Millex HA, Millipore) and 0.22 μm (Millex GV, Millipore).
3. Dulbecco's phosphate-buffered saline, solution A (PBSA): 0.2 g of KCl, 0.2 g of KH_2PO_4, 8.0 g of NaCl, 2.16 g of $Na_2HPO_4 \cdot 7 H_2O$ in 1 L of distilled, deionized water. Sterile.
4. Freund's complete adjuvant.
5. RIP solution: 1 mg in PBSA.
6. Sodium azide. **Care: Toxic.**

2.2. Affinity Purification of Anti-RIP Antibody
1. CNBr-activated Sepharose 4B (Pharmacia, Uppsala, Sweden).
2. Low protein binding 0.22-μm filtration units (Millex GV, Millipore, Bedford, MA).
3. Glass sinter (No. 1).
4. $1M$ Ethanolamine solution in distilled water (50 mL).
5. 1 mM HCl (1 L).
6. Bicarbonate buffer: 8.4 g of $NaHCO_3$, 29.2 g of NaCl. Make up to a final vol of 1 L in distilled water. The pH should be 8.3.
7. Acetate/saline buffer: 8.2 g of CH_3COONa, 29.2 g of NaCl. Adjust to pH 4.0 with CH_3COOH and make up to a final vol of 1 L in distilled water.
8. Borate/saline buffer: 6.18 g of H_3BO_3, 29.2 g of NaCl. Adjust to pH 8.0 with $1M$ NaOH and make up to a final vol of 1 L in distilled water.
9. Phosphate/saline buffer: 1.42 g of Na_2HPO_4, 8.53 g of NaCl. Adjust to pH 7.4 with $1M$ HCl and make up to a final vol of 1 L in distilled water.
10. Saline solution: 8.53 g of NaCl in 1 L of water.
11. Eluting solution: 71.2 g of $MgCl_2 \cdot 6H_2O$ in 100 mL of distilled water.
12. RIP solution: 10–20 mg in 10 mL of bicarbonate buffer.

2.3. High Performance Immunoaffinity Chromatography

1. High performance liquid chromatography (HPLC) apparatus (isocratic system) fitted with a 2-mL sample loop.
2. Ultraffinity-EP HPLC column; dimensions, 50 mm × 4.6 mm id (Beckman, High Wycombe, UK).
3. Loading buffer: 78.0 g of $NaH_2PO_4.2H_2O$. Adjust to pH 6.8 with $1M$ NaOH and make up to a final vol of 1 L in distilled water.
4. Running buffer: 2.84 g of Na_2HPO_4, 11.7 g of NaCl. Adjust to pH 6.8 with $1M$ HCl and make up to a final vol of 1 L in distilled water. This buffer should be degassed before use.
5. Eluting buffer: 0.751 g of glycine. Adjust to pH 2.5 with $1M$ HCl and make up to a final vol of 100 mL in distilled water.
6. Neutralizing buffer: $1M$ Tris-HCl, pH 7.5 (100 mL).
7. Affinity-purified rabbit anti-RIP antibody solution: 6 mg in 6 mL of loading buffer.
8. RIP solution: 1 mg in 1 mL of running buffer.

2.4. ELISA

1. Flat-bottomed microtiter plates (96-well) treated to enhance protein binding (Immulon2, Dynatech).
2. Humidified chamber, e.g., a sandwich box containing a wet tissue.
3. Sheep antimouse immunoglobulin–horseradish peroxidase (SAMIg-HRP), (Amersham).
4. Casein (hammersten grade) (BDH, Atherstone, UK).
5. *O*-Phenylenediamine (OPD). **Mutagenic: Handle with care**.
6. Thimerosal. **Highly toxic: Handle with care**.
7. Conc.HCl.
8. 12.5% (v/v) H_2SO_4 solution in distilled water. Make up by adding conc.H_2SO_4 slowly to excess water.
9. 100 vol H_2O_2 solution.
10. PBSA (*see* Section 2.1.3.).
11. Carbonate/bicarbonate buffer: 0.159 g of Na_2CO_3, 0.294 g of $NaHCO_3$. Adjust the pH to 9.6 and make up to 100 mL in distilled water. Make up the solution freshly before each assay.
12. Casein buffer: 25 g of casein, 6.05 g of Tris base, 45 g of NaCl, 1 g of thimerosal in 5 L of distilled water. Warm the buffer briefly to 60°C with gentle stirring and leave stirring overnight at room temperature. Add conc.HCl to adjust the pH of the buffer to 7.6 and keep stirring until any precipitates that appear on addition of the acid have redissolved. Store at 4°C and use within 1 mo. Warm to room temperature before use.
13. Substrate buffer: 12 mL of $0.1M$ citric acid (stock solution stored at 4°C), 13 mL of $0.2M$ Na_2HPO_4 (stock solution), and 25 mL of distilled water. Check that the pH of the solution is 5.0. Add 20 mg of OPD and shake to dissolve. Then add 10 μL of 100 vol H_2O_2 solution and mix well. Prepare this solution shortly before use and cover to protect from light.

14. Affinity-purified rabbit anti-RIP antibody solution in carbonate/bicarbonate buffer, 20–40 μg per microtiter plate.

3. Methods
3.1. Production of RIP-Specific Antiserum

1. Prepare 4 mL of a solution of RIP at a concentration of 0.2 mg/mL in PBSA. Sterilize by passing the solution through a 0.22-μm filtration unit in a sterile hood.
2. Mix 2 mL of the RIP solution with 2 mL of Freund's complete adjuvant and emulsify, using a high-speed mixer.
3. Inject the rabbit intramuscularly in the two hind-legs with 0.5 mL of the RIP emulsion per site, i.e., 50 μg of RIP per site (*see* Notes 1–3).
4. Five weeks later, administer four subcutaneous injections of 0.25 mL of the RIP solution in PBSA prepared in step 1, i.e., 50 μg of RIP per site, to boost the antibody response of the animal.
5. One week later, bleed out the rabbit (*see* Note 4).
6. Allow the blood to clot for 1 h at room temperature in a glass container and then leave to stand overnight at 4°C to allow the clot to shrink in size.
7. Dislodge the clot from the sides of the tube and transfer the supernatant to a centrifuge tube.
8. Centrifuge the clot at 2500g for 30 min at 4°C. Remove any liquid carefully and combine with the supernatant from step 7.
9. Centrifuge the pooled supernatants at 1500g for 15 min at 4°C to remove intact blood cells.
10. Treat the serum for 30 min at 56°C to inactivate complement and pass through 0.45- and 0.22-μm filtration units in succession. Dispense 5-mL aliquots into suitable containers, freeze rapidly, and store at −70°C in the presence of 0.02% (w/v) NaN$_3$.

3.2. Affinity Purification of Anti-RIP Antibody

1. Prepare a solution containing between 10 and 20 mg of RIP in about 10 mL of bicarbonate buffer. Pass the solution through a 0.22-μm filtration unit to ensure that it is free of particulate matter.
2. Swell 2 g of CNBr-activated Sepharose 4B (equivalent to about 6–7 mL of swollen gel) in 1 mM HCl and wash with a further 500 mL of 1 mM HCl on a glass sinter, removing the liquid under vacuum from a water pump.
3. Mix the acid-washed gel directly with the RIP solution prepared in step 1 and incubate for 2 h at room temperature with gentle inversion (*see* Notes 5 and 6).
4. Remove the solution from the gel by careful filtration on a glass sinter, followed by washing of the gel with a small volume of bicarbonate buffer. Measure the optical density of the pooled filtrate at 280 nm to determine the amount of protein that has not coupled to the gel (*see* Note 7).
5. Mix the gel immediately with ethanolamine solution to block remaining active groups on the gel and incubate for 2 h at room temperature with gentle inversion.
6. Remove the ethanolamine solution by careful filtration on the glass sinter.

7. Wash the gel alternately with at least three cycles of the acetate/saline and borate/saline buffers to remove noncovalently adsorbed protein.
8. Pour the gel into a glass chromatography column and equilibrate with phosphate/saline buffer.
9. Prewash the column by pumping through one column volume of saline solution, followed by the eluting solution to remove any noncovalently adsorbed protein.
10. Reequilibrate the column with phosphate/saline buffer.
11. Apply the antiserum (*see* Note 8) to the column and elute with phosphate/saline buffer.
12. Monitor fractions from the column by measuring the optical density at 280 nm.
13. Continue eluting until the nonbinding material has passed through the column, i.e., when the optical density readings have returned to the baseline value.
14. Apply one column volume of saline solution, followed by 10 mL of eluting solution to remove the adsorbed antibody. Then reequilibrate the column with phosphate/saline buffer (*see* Note 9).
15. Dialyze the affinity-purified antibody against two changes of 2 L of phosphate/saline buffer, pass through a 0.22-μm filter, and store at 4°C in the presence of 0.02% (w/v) NaN₃.

3.3. High Performance Immunoaffinity Chromatography

1. Prepare a solution containing affinity purified rabbit anti-RIP antibody at a concentration of approx 1 mg/mL of loading buffer and pass through a 0.22-μm filtration unit.
2. Load the antibody solution onto the HPLC column at a flow rate of 0.5 mL/min for 5 min. Then recycle the solution through the column at a flow rate of 0.2 mL/min for 20 h at room temperature (*see* Notes 10–12).
3. Wash the column with 5 mL of the loading buffer and measure the optical density of the pooled cycling and washing solutions at 280 nm to determine the amount of antibody that has not coupled to the column.
4. Equilibrate the column with the running buffer.
5. Expose the column to several cycles of the low pH elution procedure (*see* step 10 *below*) to remove any noncovalently adsorbed antibody.
6. Before using the column to purify antibody–toxin conjugate, apply a solution of the RIP at a concentration of 1 mg/mL to block any high affinity binding sites. Remove the RIP using the elution procedure (*see* Note 13).
7. Load the sample (1 mL) of the antibody–toxin conjugate preparation (at a concentration up to 1 mg/mL in running buffer) and elute with the running buffer at a flow rate of 0.5 mL/min.
8. Monitor fractions from the column by measuring the optical density at 280 nm.
9. Continue eluting with the running buffer until the nonbinding material has passed through the column, i.e., when the optical density readings have returned to the baseline value.
10. Apply a pulse of eluting buffer (2.0 mL) by means of the sample loop at a reduced flow rate of 0.2 mL/min to prevent trailing of the eluted conjugate peak. Collect

fractions into tubes containing neutralizing buffer to minimize the exposure of the conjugate to the low pH elution conditions (*see* Note 14).

11. Dialyze the affinity-purified antibody–toxin conjugate into PBSA, filter-sterilize in a sterile hood, and store at 4°C or, freeze rapidly and store at –70°C (*see* Notes 15 and 16).

3.4. ELISA

1. Prepare a solution of affinity-purified anti-RIP antibody at a concentration between 2 and 4 µg antibody/mL in carbonate/bicarbonate buffer. Add 100 µL to each well of a microtiter plate. This step requires at least 10 mL of the solution per plate (*see* Note 17).
2. Incubate the plate overnight at 4°C in a humidified chamber to minimize evaporation.
3. Perform all subsequent steps at room temperature. Keep plates in the humidified box during incubation steps.
4. Prepare dilutions of the antibody–toxin conjugate samples with casein buffer to give an approximate concentration of between 0.5 and 5 ng of conjugated RIP/mL of buffer in each case. At least 300 µL of each dilution is required for step 7 (*see* Note 18).
5. Wash the plate four times with casein buffer (*see* Note 19).
6. Fill the wells with casein buffer and incubate the plate for 30 min.
7. Remove the casein buffer. Add 100 µL of each diluted antibody–toxin conjugate sample (prepared in step 4) to the plates in triplicate.
8. Incubate the plates for 2 h. Wash the plates four times with casein buffer.
9. Add 100 µL of SAMIg–HRP solution, freshly prepared by diluting the stock solution by 1 in 4000 to 1 in 10,000 with casein buffer. This step requires at least 10 mL of the solution per plate (*see* Note 20).
10. Incubate the plate for 1 h. Wash the plate four times with casein buffer, then twice with PBSA (*see* Note 21).
11. Add 100 µL of the substrate solution to each well. This step requires at least 10 mL of the solution per plate.
12. Incubate the plate for 10 min and stop the reaction by adding 50 µL of H_2SO_4 solution. This step requires at least 5 mL of the acid solution per plate (*see* Note 22).
13. Read the optical density of the dark orange/brown solution in the wells at 492 nm (*see* Note 23).
14. Calculate the concentration of antibody–toxin conjugate in sample wells by comparison with a standard curve (*see* Note 23).

4. Notes
4.1. Production of RIP-Specific Antiserum

1. Animals must only be handled by properly trained personnel in accordance with the pertinent regulations.
2. RIPs of plant origin elicit a strong antibody response in the rabbit. It is advisable to immunize two rabbits at the same time, because the antibody responses of individual animals can differ.

3. The titer of anti-RIP antibody can be determined before bleeding out the rabbit, by comparison with a sample of serum taken from the animal before immunization.
4. A single rabbit can be expected to yield about 50 mL of antiserum, which should contain at least 10 mg of RIP-specific antibody.

4.2. Affinity Purification of Anti-RIP Antibody

5. Ricin A chain in solution is prone to precipitate with even mild agitation. It is recommended that the gel-coupling procedure be performed without constant inversion.
6. For the purification of antibody raised against ricin and abrin A chains, a useful alternative to affinity chromatography on columns made with the isolated A chains is the use of immobilized *Ricinus* and *Abrus* agglutinins, which crossreact immunologically with the corresponding toxins but are much less toxic.
7. The amount of RIP coupled to CNBr-activated Sepharose 4B, calculated as the difference between the amount applied and the measured amount of RIP that has failed to couple to the gel, is generally in excess of 95%.
8. The immobilized RIP columns bind at least 2 mg of RIP-specific antibody. The precise volume of antiserum that can be applied without exceeding the binding capacity of the column must be determined by experiment in each case.
9. RIP affinity columns can be stored at 4°C in the presence of 0.02% (w/v) NaN$_3$ for several years with little loss of performance.

4.3. High Performance Immunoaffinity Chromatography

10. Using the coupling procedure described, 3–4 mg of affinity-purified anti-RIP antibody can be coupled to the HPLC column matrix. The procedure requires a minimum of 6 mL of anti-RIP antibody solution to allow cycling of the solution via the liquid reservoir, prepump solvent filter, pump, precolumn filter, the column itself, and all the connecting tubing.
11. The entire loading and pulsing cycle as described takes approx 30 min. Using an increased flow rate of 1 mL/min and a single elution pulse, at least 20 mg of antibody–toxin conjugate can be purified within a day on this size of HPLC column.
12. The capacity of immunoaffinity HPLC columns prepared using affinity-purified antibody against ricin A chain, abrin A chain, gelonin, and momordin varies between 400 and 600 µg/mL of bed vol for the appropriate RIP. In the case of the antibody–toxin conjugates made with these RIPs, the capacity is at least 2 mg/mL of bed vol.
13. The ricin and abrin A chains used to block high affinity binding sites on the column should be alkylated to remove the free sulfhydryl group that could interfere with conjugate purification.
14. The elution procedure using the low pH buffer removes 85–95% of the affinity-bound conjugate. The remaining bound conjugate can be removed by a second pulse with the elution buffer (*see* Fig. 1).
15. All the antibody–toxin conjugates bind in their entirety to the appropriate immunoaffinity HPLC column and are completely separated from free antibody. There is no adverse affect on the integrity of the conjugates as judged by gel electrophoresis, size exclusion HPLC, and assays of cytotoxic potency *(5)*.

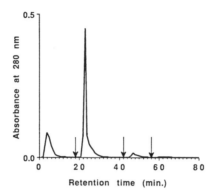

Fig. 1. High performance liquid immunoaffinity chromatography of an antibody–toxin conjugate preparation. An abrin A chain conjugate preparation obtained following Sephacryl S–200 (SF) chromatography was applied to an immunoaffinity HPLC column bearing immobilized affinity-purified rabbit anti-abrin A chain. Each arrow indicates the injection of a pulse of low pH eluting buffer. The first peak that emerges from the column in running buffer consists of unconjugated antibody only. The first elution pulse removes the majority of the bound conjugate from the column. The remainder of the bound conjugate is removed by the second pulse.

16. The anti-RIP antibody HPLC columns can be stored at 4°C in the presence of 0.02% (w/v) NaN₃ for several years with little loss of performance.

4.4. ELISA

17. The quality of microtiter plates varies according to the supplier and the batch. It is advisable to check individual batches for their suitability and consistency in use.
18. Casein buffer is used during steps 4–10 in Section 3.4., as a blocking agent to prevent the nonspecific adsorption of reagents to the plate, which otherwise gives rise to high background values of optical density *(6)*.
19. During washing (Section 3.4., steps 5, 8, and 10), the best results are obtained by completely filling the wells of the microtiter plate with casein buffer. A plate-washing machine is recommended. It is important to flush the tubing of the machine immediately after each batch of washes with casein buffer to prevent the liquid dispensing system from becoming blocked. At the end of the washing steps, the plates should be inverted and slapped vigorously onto a pad of tissue to remove any remaining liquid from the wells.
20. The use of SAMIg–HRP that has been adsorbed against rabbit Ig to prevent crossreactivity with the rabbit anti-RIP antibody immobilized on the plate is recommended to prevent high background absorbance.
21. The final washes with PBSA (Section 3.4., step 10) are important to remove traces of casein that can cause turbidity on the addition of H_2SO_4 to the substrate solution.

22. The time for color development should be carefully controlled. Plates should be read soon after the color has developed. If this is impossible, store the plates in the dark to minimize the fading of color.
23. The ELISA method for measuring the concentration of antibody–toxin conjugates works successfully with conjugates containing several different types of ricin A chain, with abrin A chain, gelonin, and momordin. A sample of conjugate at a concentration of 5 ng/mL gives an optical density of about 0.5 at 492 nm using between 2 and 4 µg/mL of affinity-purified anti-RIP antibody and dilutions of SAMIg–HRP of 1 in 4000 to 1 in 10,000. The optimal concentrations of these reagents must be established experimentally in each case.
24. The concentration of antibody–toxin conjugate in samples is determined from the optical density values at 492 nm, given by a standard curve. The standard curve is obtained by the same procedure using dilutions of the stock antibody–toxin solution having final concentrations between 0.125 and 20 ng/mL in casein buffer.

References

1. Cumber, A. J., Forrester, J. A., Foxwell, B. M. J., Ross, W. C. J., and Thorpe, P. E. (1985) Preparation of antibody–toxin conjugates. *Methods Enzymol.* **112**, 207–225.
2. Wawrzynczak, E. J. and Thorpe, P. E. (1987) Methods for preparing immunotoxins: effect of the linkage on activity and stability, in *Immunoconjugates: Antibody Conjugates in Radioimaging and Therapy of Cancer* (Vogel, C.-W., ed.), Oxford University Press, New York and Oxford, pp. 28–55.
3. Lambert, J. M. and Blattler, W. A. (1988) Purification and biochemical characterization of immunotoxins, in *Immunotoxins* (Frankel, A. E., ed.), Kluwer Academic Publishers, Boston, MA, pp. 323–348.
4. Knowles, P. P. and Thorpe, P. E. (1987) Purification of immunotoxins containing ricin A chain and abrin A chain using Blue Sepharose CL-6B. *Anal. Biochem.* **160**, 440–443.
5. Cumber, A. J., Henry, R. V., Parnell, G. D., and Wawrzynczak, E. J. (1990) Purification of immunotoxins containing the ribosome-inactivating proteins gelonin and momordin using high performance liquid immunoaffinity chromatography compared with Blue Sepharose CL-6B affinity chromatography. *J. Immunol. Methods* **135**, 15–24.
6. Kenna, J. G., Major, G. N., and Williams, R. S. (1985) Methods for reducing nonspecific antibody binding in enzyme-linked immunosorbent assays. *J. Immunol. Methods* **85**, 409–419.

15

Competitive ELISA

Kittima Makarananda, Lucinda R. Weir, and Gordon E. Neal

1. Introduction

Enzyme-linked immunosorbent assay (ELISA) is a very useful technique for the specific and sensitive assay of certain compounds, in which suitable antibodies, monoclonal or polyclonal, to the compounds are available. The technique has found particular application in the monitoring of environmental contaminants and toxins, either studying the primarily contaminated materials, e.g., foodstuffs, or body fluids of potentially exposed humans. The technique has been increasingly applied to monitoring the carcinogenic mycotoxins, the aflatoxins.

The principle of the direct ELISA system is a double-antibody sandwich technique, which is illustrated in Fig. 1. The binding of the primary antibody to the antigen, which is immobilized on the bottom of the wells in multiwell ELISA plates, is followed by the addition of the secondary antibody, which has an affinity for the primary antibody. The secondary antibody is linked to an enzyme that is then reacted with a chromogenic substrate. The color formed is proportional to the amounts of both of the antibodies, and hence, to the amount of antigen. The use of the secondary antibody can amplify the signal from the antigen-bound primary antibody. In the competitive ELISA, two antigens are involved: one, the sample antigen to be assayed and the other, a constant level of "binding" antigen immobilized in the multiwell plate. The primary antibody is allowed to react in solution with the sample antigen it is required to assay, before applying to the ELISA plates. The amount of binding antigen with which the wells are coated, necessary to give quantitative competition curves over a useful range, is determined in preliminary assays. Since only unbound primary antibody, i.e., that which has not undergone reaction with the sample antigen, is now available to bind to the immobilized, constant level of antigen coating

From: *Methods in Molecular Biology, Vol. 80: Immunochemical Protocols, 2nd ed.*
Edited by: J. D. Pound © Humana Press Inc., Totowa, NJ

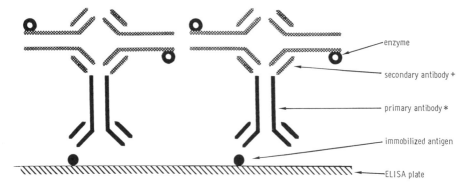

Fig. 1. Diagrammatic representation of the double-antibody-labeling technique used in the ELISA.

the wells, there is an inverse relationship between the level of enzymically formed color and the amount of antigen in the sample. Calibration curves are constructed using a range of concentrations of antigen in the competition reaction. This method of assaying antigens can be widely used. It is illustrated here as an assay for aflatoxins (*see* Note 1), in which case it is usually carried out using aflatoxin B_1 (AFB$_1$) as the standard. Polyclonal and monoclonal antibodies raised against aflatoxins usually detect a wide spectrum of aflatoxin metabolites, but with differing sensitivities. If the nature of the aflatoxin under investigation is known, a suitable calibration curve can be constructed. If it is not known or if it is a mixture of aflatoxins, the results can be expressed as AFB$_1$ equivalents.

2. Materials

1. Rabbit anti-AFB$_1$ serum.
2. Antirabbit IgG–peroxidase conjugate.
3. Bovine serum albumin–AFB$_1$ conjugate (BSA–AFB$_1$).
4. Phosphate-buffered saline (PBS), pH 7.3: 8 g of NaCl, 0.2 g of KCl, 1.15 g of Na$_2$HPO$_4$ · 2H$_2$O, and 0.2 g of KH$_2$PO$_4$ made up to 1 L with distilled water.
5. Standard concentrations of AFB$_1$ ranging from 0.01 to 100 ng/mL in PBS (*see* Note 1).
6. 3% BSA in PBS (PBS-BSA).
7. Washing buffer (PBS, pH 7.4, 1.5 mM MgCl$_2$, 0.05% Tween-20).
8. Dilution buffer (10 mM K$_2$HPO$_4$/150 mM NaCl, 1% BSA, 0.1% Tween-20, pH 7.2).
9. 3,3',5,5'-Tetramethylbenzidine (*see* Note 2).
10. Dimethyl sulfoxide (DMSO) (Spectrosol-grade).
11. 0.1M Sodium acetate buffer, pH 6.0.
12. 100 vol Hydrogen peroxide.
13. 2M H$_2$SO$_4$.

14. Microtiter plates, model M129E (Dynatech Laboratories Inc., VA).
15. Plate sealing tapes.
16. Microtiter plate shaker.
17. Microtiter plate reader.

3. Method

1. Determine the protein content of BSA–AFB$_1$ prepared as described by Sizaret et al. *(1)*, using Lowry's method *(2,3)*. The molar ratio of BSA:AFB$_1$ usually obtained is on the order of 1:7.
2. Dilute the BSA–AFB$_1$ to 5 ng of protein/50 μL of PBS.
3. Coat the microtiter plates with the diluted BSA–AFB$_1$ by adding 50 μL to each well.
4. Leave the plates to dry overnight at 37°C (*see* Note 3).
5. The plates can be stored at –20°C until required.
6. Wash the plates four times with washing buffer, using the immersion technique. This is carried out by totally immersing each plate in approx 800 mL of the washing buffer solution in a plastic box. Care must be taken to avoid air locks causing some wells not to be washed. This can be achieved by passing a small roller over the submersed plates (*see* Note 4).
7. Dry the plates by vigorously banging the inverted plate on several layers of absorbent paper (*see* Note 5).
8. Incubate each well with 200 μL of PBS–BSA (to block the nonspecific sites) for 60 min at room temperature (*see* Note 6).
9. Prepare a concentration range of AFB$_1$ standards (0.01–100 ng/mL) and pipet 200 μL of each into small thoroughly clean glass test tubes (2-mL capacity). One tube is also prepared using PBS to serve as a noninhibited standard.
10. Dilute "unknown" samples appropriately (all assays are carried out using a 200 μL sample volume).
11. Dilute rabbit anti-AFB$_1$ serum 1:10,000 using 2 μL of antibody in 20 mL of dilution buffer. Optimal dilution of rabbit serum is determined in a preliminary experiment using a range of serum dilutions against a range of AFB$_1$ concentrations (*see* Notes 7 and 8).
12. Add the diluted antibody to the AFB$_1$ concentration standards or "unknown" samples, using a 1:1 ratio of antibody to sample. Then incubate the tubes at 37°C with continuous shaking for 60 min. The tubes should be covered to prevent evaporation.
13. After the incubation to block nonspecific sites on the plate (step 8), discard the solution, and wash the plates twice with washing buffer. Then dry the plates (as in steps 6 and 7).
14. Load each well with 50 μL of the mixture obtained from step 12, cover the plates with plate-sealing tape, and incubate, with continuous shaking using a microtiter plate shaker, for 90 min at room temperature.
15. Dilute rabbit anti-IgG–peroxidase conjugate 1:5000, using 4 μL of antibody in 20 mL of dilution buffer, approx 5 min before use, and leave it in ice (*see* Note 9).

16. Stop the plate shaker after 90 min (step 14), remove the sealing tape, and discard the solution into a waste bucket containing 0.5% sodium hypochlorite to destroy the toxin. Wash the plates five times with washing buffer and dry them as in steps 6 and 7.

17. Add 50 µL of diluted antirabbit IgG–peroxidase conjugate (from step 15) into each well, and then seal the plates, and incubate at room temperature for another 90 min with continuous shaking.

18. Prepare the substrate by warming (approx 40°C) 24.75 mL of $0.1M$ sodium acetate buffer, pH 6.0, for 30 min, then adding 250 µL of tetramethylbenzidine solution (10 mg in 1 mL of DMSO), and warming it for another 30 min (*see* Note 10).

19. Stop the plate shaker after the 90-min incubation (in step 17), remove the tape, and discard the solution. Wash the plates five times with washing buffer, followed by a single distilled water wash, and dry the plates as in step 7.

20. Add 10 µL of 100 vol hydrogen peroxide to the substrate solution (from step 18) *immediately* before use, and thoroughly mix by shaking (*see* Note 11).

21. Dispense 50 µL of substrate solution into each well. Incubate at room temperature for 30 min. A blue color will develop.

22. Stop the reaction by adding 50 µL of $2M$ H_2SO_4 to each well. The color will change to yellow. Leave the plates for 15 min.

23. Read the absorbance at 450 nm using a microtiter plate reader (*see* Notes 11 and 12).

24. Calculate the percentage inhibition using the non-AFB$_1$-containing PBS standard as the uninhibited control absorbance. Absorbance of the PBS standard is routinely in the range 1.4–1.6. Inhibition of 50% is usually achieved using concentrations in the order of 0.25 ng of AFB$_1$/mL.

4. Notes

1. The aflatoxins are extremely potent hepatotoxins and hepatocarcinogens, exerting their biological effect at the microgram level in animal model systems. Extreme caution is therefore necessary when using these materials to avoid contact with them. Decontamination of contaminated glassware using 0.5% sodium hypochlorite, followed by extensive rinsing in water, should be routinely carried out. All combustible contaminated materials should be sealed in plastic bags and incinerated. Solutions of aflatoxins to be discarded should also be exposed to a final concentration of 0.5% sodium hypochlorite for several hours, followed by extensive rinsing of the container in running tap water.

2. Tetramethylbenzidine is used because of its noncarcinogenic property.

3. When the plates are coated with BSA–AFB$_1$ and dried overnight, ensure that they are **completely** dry. Otherwise, binding antigen will be lost from the plates during subsequent procedures.

4. **All** the plate washings are carried out using the immersion technique. Care must be taken to ensure that all wells are filled with the washing solution.

5. The plates are dried by inverting, followed by vigorous banging on absorbent paper to ensure that washing buffer is completely removed. Otherwise, it may interfere with the subsequent binding of the antibodies or the substrate.

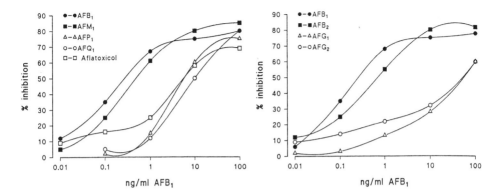

Fig. 2. Competitive ELISA curves obtained using primary aflatoxins **(left)** and some aflatoxin metabolites **(right)**.

6. In each incubation step, the plates should be properly sealed to prevent evaporation. Otherwise varying concentration of the reactants will lead to lack of constant results between wells.

7. All the dilutions of the antibodies required should be prepared shortly before use, and they should be kept cool in ice.

8. The appropriate dilutions of the antibodies giving suitable curves in the competitive ELISA should be determined in preliminary experiments. Suitable antiserum for use in ELISA has been found to have working dilutions of between 1 in 10,000 and 1 in 20,000.

9. Peroxidase is routinely used because it is sufficiently sensitive to permit the detection of small quantities of antigen. Other enzymes linked to the second antibody, e.g., alkaline phosphatase, have been examined, but have generally been less satisfactory than peroxidase *(4)*.

10. Sodium acetate buffer has to be warmed to 40°C before the tetramethylbenzidine is added to avoid precipitation.

11. Hydrogen peroxide should be added to the substrate solution **immediately** before use.

12. Standard curves should be included in every batch of assays. Figure 2 shows typical competition curves obtained using a range of aflatoxins.

13. Use replicate wells (usually six) for each concentration assayed.

References

1. Sizaret, P., Malaveille, C., Montesano, R., and Frayssinet, C. (1982) Detection of aflatoxins and related metabolites by radioimmunoassay. *J. Natl. Cancer Inst.* **69,** 1375–1381.

2. Lowry, O. H., Rosebrough, N. J., Farr, A. L., and Randall, L. J. (1961) Protein measurement with the Folin phenol reagent. *J. Biol. Chem.* **193,** 265–275.

3. Waterborg, J. H. and Matthews, H. R. (1984) The Lowry method for protein quantitation, in *Methods in Molecular Biology,* vol. 1 (Walker, J., ed.), Humana, Clifton, NJ, pp. 1–3.

4. Martin, C. N., Garner, R. C., Tursi, F., Garner, J. V., Whittle, H. C., Ryder, R. W., Sizaret, P., and Montesano, R. (1984) An enzyme linked immunosorbent procedure for assaying aflatoxin B_1, in *Monitoring Human Exposure to Carcinogenic and Mutagenic Agents* (Berlin, A., Draper, M., Hemminki, K., and Vainio, H., eds.), IARC Scientific Publication No. 59, IARC, Lyon, France, pp. 313–321.

16

Epitope Mapping

Glenn E. Morris

1. Introduction

The aim of epitope mapping is to find out which part of its antigen a given antibody binds to, and mapping methods are most widely applied to protein antigens. It is possible to think of epitope mapping as a "simple" biochemical problem of finding out how one well-defined protein (a monoclonal antibody [MAb]) binds to another (the antigen). The term "epitope mapping" is also used to describe the attempt to determine all the major sites on a protein surface that can elicit an antibody response, at the end of which one might claim to have produced an "epitope map" of the protein antigen. This information might be very useful, for example, to someone wishing to produce antiviral vaccines. However, it is questionable how far one can go down this road, since the final map will depend on the individual immune response (although immuno-dominant regions undoubtedly exist) and on how MAbs are selected, and may depend also on the mapping method used. Epitope mapping is usually done with MAbs, though it can be done with polyclonal antisera in a rather less rigorous way, bearing in mind that antisera behave as a mixture of MAbs of variable complexity. Some authors have extended the epitope concept to the inter-action between peptide hormones and their receptors (1); however one feels about this, it does make the point that in mapping epitopes, we are studying a biological process of fundamental importance, that of protein–protein interaction.

At their most elaborate, epitope mapping techniques can provide detailed information on the amino acid residues in a protein antigen, which are in direct contact with the antibody binding site. X-ray crystallography of antibody–anti-gen complexes can identify contact residues directly and unequivocally, though not surprisingly in view of the effort required, this method is not in routine use. At the other extreme, demonstration by competition enzyme-linked immuno-sorbent assay (ELISA) methods that two antibodies bind to different sites on

From: *Methods in Molecular Biology, Vol. 80: Immunochemical Protocols, 2nd ed.*
Edited by: J. D. Pound © Humana Press Inc., Totowa, NJ

the same antigen is also epitope mapping of a kind, experimentally simple, but producing results that lack molecular detail. There are many different reasons for wanting to identify epitopes; you may want to use an antibody as a very specific research tool at the molecular level, use the antibody–antigen system as a model for understanding protein–protein interactions, learn about the immune response that an organism mounts against the antigen, understand better the specificity of a commercially important immunoassay, and so on. The degree of precision required in mapping and, hence, the choice of method, may depend on the application envisaged for the mapped antibodies.

To understand epitopes, both from a theoretical and practical point of view, the problem of antigen conformation must be tackled from the outset. Most native proteins are formed of highly convoluted peptide chains, so that residues that lie close together on the protein surface are often far apart in the amino acid sequence. Consequently, most epitopes on native, globular proteins are conformation-dependent or "assembled," and they disappear if the protein is denatured or fragmented. Sometimes, by accident or design, antibodies are produced against "local" (linear, sequential) epitopes, which survive denaturation, though such antibodies usually fail to recognize the native protein. The simplest way to find out whether an epitope is conformational is by Western blotting after sodium dodecyl sulfate-polyacrylamide gel electrophoresis (SDS-PAGE). If the antibody still binds after the protein has been boiled in SDS and 2-mercaptoethanol (2-ME), the epitope is unlikely to be highly conformational. Many, though not all, conformational epitopes are destroyed when the antigen binds to plastic in an ELISA test. Antibodies against assembled epitopes often display the high avidities and specificities required for immunoassays, but they are difficult to map. Mapping methods are either rather vague (e.g., competition ELISA), incomplete (e.g., antibody protection of antigen from chemical modification), or long and involved (e.g., X-ray studies or construction of recombinant chimeric antigens). Antibodies against local epitopes, on the other hand, can be mapped by fragmentation methods, which lend themselves to library approaches in which powerful screening methods (λ libraries) or even more powerful selection methods (phage display libraries) can be applied to complex mixtures of antigenic fragments or random peptides (*see* Chapter 47). MAbs produced as tools for cell and molecular biology research are often against local epitopes, since ability to work on Western blots is a very desirable property. Screening hybridoma supernatants against both denatured (Western blot) and native (e.g., immunohistochemistry or sandwich ELISA) antigen often produces the most useful MAb for research, though they may be quite unrepresentative of the overall immune response to the antigen. Table 1 lists and compares some of the mapping methods that have been used. Full details of these methods can be found in *Epitope Mapping Protocols,* another volume in this series *(2)*.

Table 1
A Selection of Epitope Mapping Methods[a]

X-ray analysis of Ab–Ag complexes	A, P, H, E	*(14)*
NMR of Ab–peptide complexes	S, P, H, E	*(15)*
Neutralization escape mutants of viruses	A, H	*(16)*
Competition ELISA	A, S, L, C	*(17)*
Surface plasmon resonance of Ab–Ag interaction	A, S, L	*(18)*
Protection by antibody		
Protection of Ag from proteolysis	A, S, P, M	*(19)*
Protection of Ag from chemical modification	A, S, P, H (limited)	*(20)*
Fragmentation of Ag		
Chemical fragmentation	S, P, M, C	*(8)*
Proteolytic fragmentation	S, P, M, C	*(21)*
Mass spectrometry of Ab-bound fragments	S, M, E	*(22)*
Synthetic peptides	S, H	
On pins		*(23)*
As SPOTS		*(24)*
As "positional scanning" libraries		*(25)*
Recombinant DNA methods		
Peptide libraries in filamentous phage	S, R, H	*(26)*
DNase fragment expression libraries	S, R, M	*(27,28)*
Expression of PCR-generated subfragments	S, R, M	
In bacterial plasmids		*(29)*
By in vitro translation		*(30)*
Deletion mutagenesis	S, R, M	*(31)*
Transposon mutagenesis	S, R, M, C	*(32)*
Early termination of in vitro translation	S, R, M, C	*(33)*
Random PCR mutagenesis	S, R, M	*(34)*
Site-directed mutagenesis	A, S, R, H	*(35)*
Construction of chimeric antigens	A, R, M	*(36)*

[a]Most methods are mainly suited to either assembled (A) or sequential (S) epitopes. Some methods are applicable only to Ags expressed from cloned cDNA (R; recombinant), whereas others need purified protein (P). Resolution of mapping may be low (L; sequences not defined), medium (M, sequence defined to within 10–100 amino acids), or high (H; individual amino acids defined). Some methods are particularly expensive (E) or cheap (C) in terms of the equipment and/or skilled labor required. Finally (not shown in the table), some methods may not be useful for your particular Ab–Ag combination.

It is now possible to identify T-cell epitopes, which are recognized by receptor complexes on the T-lymphocyte surface, in addition to the B-cell epitopes recognized by antibodies (which are also the B-lymphocyte receptors). T-cells are stimulated by small peptide fragments of antigens produced by intracellular proteolytic processing, so problems of conformation do not arise, and synthetic peptides are a popular and valid approach. At present, T-cell epitopes are usually recognized by their ability to stimulate T-lymphocyte division, rather than by direct receptor binding, and this limits the number of mapping methods that can be used.

I shall describe a relatively simple "library" approach for MAb mapping in which overlapping antigen fragments, generated by chemical or proteolytic digestion, are screened with antibody on Western blots. It is widely applicable insofar as it is not restricted to recombinant antigens only, though it cannot be used for highly assembled epitopes and the amino acid sequence of the antigen must be known. Chemicals that cut proteins at uncommon amino acids are used to produce fragments; cyanogen bromide (CNBr) cuts at Met *(3)*, nitro-thiocyanobenzoic acid (NTCB) at Cys *(4)*, iodosobenzoic acid (IBA) at Trp *(5)*, and formic acid between Asp–Pro bonds *(6)*. The fragments on Western blots can often be recognized unequivocally using M_rs predicted from the sequence. Proteases tend to cut at common amino acid residues; trypsin at basic residues, especially Arg and Lys; chymotrypsin at large hydrophobic residues, especially Tyr and Phe; endoproteinase Glu-C (V8) at Glu, and so forth. However, the digestion is carried out under native or only partially denaturing conditions under which most sites are protected by protein folding and a restricted range of fragments is obtained. To identify proteolytic fragments, it is necessary to sequence each of them. N-terminal sequence can be obtained directly from stained bands on Western blots using automated microsequencers. Automated methods for C-terminal sequencing are being developed.

Assembly of the Western blot data into a map is illustrated by chemical cleavage results with creatine kinase *(7–11)*. Figure 1A shows the amino acid sequence of chick muscle creatine kinase (M_r 43,000) with Met, Cys, and Trp residues in bold type (except the CNBr-resistant Met–Thr bonds *[3]*). Figure 1B shows the limiting fragments expected for each digestion. These fragments are separated by SDS-PAGE, and the fragment reacting with any given MAb can be identified by Western blotting. The epitopes can be defined more precisely from the overlaps between the different fragments, and this is illustrated in Fig. 1B for two MAbs, CK-2A7 and CK-JAC. The third MAb, CK-ART, illustrates several interesting points about this method. The smallest fragment it will recognize is the 10.6-kDa C-terminal NTCB fragment E. It will also recognize the slightly larger 12-kDa C-terminal IBA fragment Z, but only after prolonged reduction of the Met-sulfone produced by IBA back to Met, suggesting that a Met is involved in the ART epitope. Consistent with this, CK-ART will not recognize any CNBr fragments cleaved at Met residues. Other experiments, however, suggest that CK-ART recognizes a conformational epitope, although one that is resistant to permanent denaturation by SDS *(8)*. This being so, the Met-sulfones might be causing a conformational change in

MPFSSTHNKHKLKFSAEEEFPDLSKHNNH**M**AKVLTPELYKR
LRDKETPSGFTLDDVIQTGVDNPGHPFIMTVG**C**VAGDEESY
EVFKDLFDPVIQDRHGGYKPTDKHRTDLNHENLKGGDDLDP
KYVLSSRVRTGRSIKGYSLPPH**C**SRGERRAVEKLSVEALNS
LEGEFKGRYYPLKAMTEQEQQQLIDDHFLFDKPVSPLLLAS
GMARD**W**PDARGI**W**HNDNKTFLV**W**VNEEDHLRVIS**M**EKGGN**M**
KEVFRR**FC**VGLKKIEEIFKKAGHPF**MW**TEHLGYILTCPSNL
GTGLRGGVHVKLPKLSQHPKFEEILHRLRLQKRGTGGVDTA
AVGAVFDISNADRLGFSEVEQVQMVVDGVKLMVEMEKKLEQ
NQPIDD**M**IPAQK

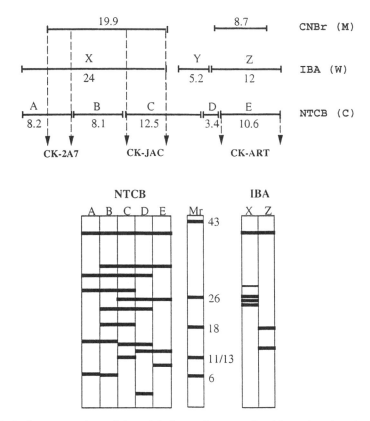

Fig. 1. Epitope mapping of three MAbs against creatine kinase by chemical cleavage at methionine, tryptophan, or cysteine residues.

the C-terminal region, which prevents CK-ART binding, and removal of the last 30 amino acids by CNBr might also affect conformation. Thus, Met may not be a "contact" residue in the epitope after all. This shows that effects of conformation still have to be kept in mind even when using methods that normally are only useful for "sequential" determinants. In practice, chemical cleavage is rarely complete, and the usual result is a more complex pattern of partial digestion products on the Western blot. However, a "fingerprint," or ladder, of bands on a Western blot can often be more informative than a single product of complete digestion.

Figure 1C shows all five NTCB "fingerprints" for MAbs recognizing regions A–E in Fig. 1B and three of these (A–E) match the patterns obtained with CK-2A7, CK-JAC, and CK-ART, respectively. Two MAbs binding to regions A and B, respectively, would be difficult to distinguish if only the smallest NTCB fragments were detectable on the Western blot (8.2 and 8.1 kDa, respectively), but the two "fingerprints" (lanes A and B in Fig. 1C) are quite distinctive. IBA cleavage is more complete and not every possible fragment is observed. In Fig. 1C, lanes X and Z show the actual patterns obtained with CK-JAC and CK-ART MAbs, respectively. There are three tryptophans near the X–Y junction in Fig. 1B, and a triplet of bands (24, 25, and 26 kDa) is seen with CK-JAC instead of the 2-kDa band only. Similarly, CK-ART detects both fragments Z (12 kDa) and YZ (17.2 kDa).

Creatine kinase sequences are known for many different species and isoforms, so species-specificity of MAbs can often be used for refining the details of epitope mapping. Natural variants that prevent MAb binding are likely to involve "contact" residues, because the overall protein structures (and enzyme activity) are likely to be retained. The CK-2A7 MAb in Fig. 1B binds between Met-29 and Cys-73. It recognizes rabbit and *Torpedo* CKs, as well as chick CK, but it fails to bind to either rat muscle CK or rabbit brain CK. This suggests that Lys-39 is required for CK-2A7 binding, since it is replaced by Asn in rat muscle CK and by Ala in rabbit brain CK *(7)*, and is the only amino acid change consistent with the observed CK-2A7 specificity.

2. Materials

2.1. Digestions

1. CNBr (toxic and may produce toxic gas; carry out all steps in an efficient fume hood): Dissolve the whole bottle to make a 100 mg/mL stock in distilled water, and store in a well-sealed bottle at –20°C.
2. NTCB (toxic): Prepare a fresh 25 mg/mL solution in water each time. Add 5*M* NaOH in microliter amounts until the NTCB is dissolved (goes completely clear).
3. IBA (toxic): Prepare a fresh 5 mg/mL solution in IBA buffer each time.
4. Dithioerythritol (DTE): a 100 m*M* solution in water should be freshly prepared.
5. SDS: 20% (w/v) stock solution in water.

6. 2-ME.
7. Sucrose.
8. Bromophenol blue.
9. Formic, acetic, and hydrochloric acids (analytical-grade).
10. *p*-Cresol (toxic and volatile: Handle it, and all solutions containing it, in a fume hood).
11. Sephadex G-15 (Pharmacia, Uppsala, Sweden).
12. Sephadex buffer (prepare freshly): $8M$ urea (ultra-pure) in 125 mM Tris-HCl, pH 6.8.
13. NTCB buffer 1: $5M$ guanidine HCl (analytical-grade) in 200 mM Tris-acetate, pH 8.0 (pH is critical).
14. NTCB buffer 2: $8M$ urea in 200 mM Tris-acetate, pH 9.0 (pH is critical).
15. IBA buffer: $4M$ guanidine HCl/80% acetic acid/2% *p*-cresol. The *p*-cresol prevents IBA cleavage at tyrosine residues.
16. Protease buffer: 50 mM Tris-HCl, pH 6.8.
17. Phenylmethyl sulfonyl fluoride (PMSF): **Highly toxic**. Handle powder and stock solutions in a fume hood. Prepare a 100-mM stock solution in 95% ethanol, and store at –20°C. Warm to redissolve crystals before use.
18. TPCK-treated trypsin, TLCK-treated chymotrypsin, and endoproteinase-Glu-C (Staphlococcal V8 protease) are all obtainable from Sigma (Poole, UK).
19. For gel filtration: Glass columns (12 × 1 cm, approximately with 10-cm gel height) with glass sinters at the bottom and no "dead volume" below the sinter.

2.2. SDS-PAGE and Western Blotting

Materials are described in detail in Chapter 20.

1. Laemmli buffers *(12)* for SDS-PAGE are only satisfactory for fragments of 6 kDa or greater, and a Tris-Tricine system *(13)* is recommended if resolution of smaller peptides is necessary.
2. Low-M_r range prestained protein markers are essential for identification of cleavage fragments on blots. These are available from Life Technologies (Gaithersburg, MD) or Novex (SeeBlue and Multimark, San Diego, CA)
3. Nitrocellulose (e.g., Schleicher and Schull [Keene, NH] BA85) is a relatively inexpensive, if rather fragile, medium for blots, but PVDF membranes (e.g., Problott, Applied Biosystems-Perkin Elmer, Foster City, CA) are needed for automated microsequencing of proteolytic fragments.

3. Methods

3.1. Digestions

The protocols are for 0.5 mg of antigen in a 0.5-mL reaction volume, but if the antigen is in short supply, it may be possible to scale down both weight and volume by using a smaller Sephadex column or replacing it with a microspin column (check to ensure that the same separation is obtained).

3.1.1. CNBr for Met

All steps are performed in a fume hood.

1. Take 0.5 mg of protein antigen in 125 µL or less of distilled water (or buffer) in a glass vial, and add 350 µL of formic acid.
2. Add 5 µL of CNBr stock solution, and make up to 0.5 mL with distilled water (*see* Note 1). Mix, and leave for 18 h at 20°C (*see* Note 2)
3. Load onto the column of Sephadex G-15 swollen and pre-equilibrated in Sephadex buffer and precalibrated to identify the "excluded volume" fractions (*see* Note 3). Elute with Sephadex buffer, and collect 1-mL fractions.
4. To each "excluded volume" fraction, add 50 µL of 20% SDS, 50 µL of 2-ME, and 10 µL of bromophenol blue, and boil for 2 min for SDS-PAGE.

3.1.2. NTCB for Cys

1. Dissolve 0.5 mg of antigen in 0.5 mL of NTCB buffer 1, pH 8.0 (*see* Note 4).
2. Add 5 µL of 100 mM DTE, and leave for 30 min at 20–25°C.
3. Add 30 µL of 25 mg/mL NTCB, and incubate at 37°C for 15 min.
4. Load immediately onto a Sephadex G-15 column equilibrated with NTCB buffer 2, pH 9.0, and elute with the same buffer collecting 1 mL fractions (*see* Note 5).
5. Incubate "excluded volume" column fractions (*see* Note 3) at 37°C for 16 h (*see* Note 6).
6. Adjust fractions to pH 6.8 using a predetermined amount of 5M HCl. Add 50 µL of 20% SDS, 50 µL of 2-ME, 10 µL of bromophenol blue, 100 mg of sucrose, and boil for 2 min for SDS-PAGE.

3.1.3. IBA for Trp

1. Dissolve 0.5 mg of antigen in 450 µL of IBA buffer, and add 50 µL of 5 mg/mL IBA in the same buffer. Mix, and leave at 20–25°C for 24 h.
2. Follow steps 3 and 4 of the CNBr method.
3. Optional: Add solid DTE (700 mM final conc.) to each column fraction, and incubate at 37°C for 24 h or longer (*see* Note 7). If this option is followed, the 2-ME may be omitted from the previous step.

3.1.4. Formic Acid for Asp–Pro bonds

1. Dissolve 1 mg of antigen in 0.5 mL of 75% formic acid, and incubate for 24–48 h at 37°C (*see* Note 8).
2. Follow steps 3 and 4 of the CNBr method.

3.1.5. Proteolysis

Proteolysis occurs at much more common residues than chemical cleavage, but protein folding usually ensures that some regions are much more sensitive to proteolysis (i.e., more unfolded) than others, so that fragments are not too small or too numerous to be resolved. Native proteins may be very resistant to proteolysis, in which case a brief pretreatment of the antigen with 0.1% SDS or 0.6M guanidinium chloride will usually give a good pattern of fragments *(37)* (*see* Note 9).

1. To a tube containing 1 mg of antigen in 0.5 mL protease buffer at 0°C, add 10 μL of 1 mg/mL trypsin, chymotrypsin, or V8, and mix.
2. Place in a 37°C water bath, and remove 100 μL samples into 1.5-mL Eppendorf tubes containing 2 μL of 100 mM PMSF at room temperature after 0.5, 2, 5, 15, and 45 min (*see* Note 10).
3. Add 5 μL of 20% SDS, 5 μL of 2-ME, 1 μL of bromophenol blue, and 5–10 mg of sucrose, and boil for 2 min for SDS-PAGE.

3.2. SDS-PAGE and Western Blotting

Acrylamide (20%) with 0.5% bisacrylamide is appropriate for the separating gel. PVDF blots are stained with amido black, and all clearly visible bands are excised for direct microsequencing on the membrane, using an Applied Biosystems 476A or 494 sequencer *(37)*.

4. Notes

1. The CNBr should be in 30-fold molar excess over the Met residues in the antigen; this works out at about 1:1 (w/w) for a typical protein with 1 Met/30–40 residues.
2. CNBr cleavage is usually almost complete under these conditions, except that Met-Thr bonds are not noticeably cleaved at all.
3. The gel-filtration step removes formic acid and excess CNBr, and gets the antigen fragments into a buffer compatible with SDS-PAGE. An important safety feature is that CNBr never leaves the fume hood and can be destroyed later by elution into bleach. The buffer described is for the Laemmli PAGE system *(12)* and should be replaced if other PAGE systems are used. The urea prevents any possible precipitation on the column. G-15 allows fragments of $M_r > 2000$ to pass unretarded in the excluded volume; the column should be precalibrated with blue dextran to identify the excluded volume fractions (usually one or two main fractions). Since the column takes only a few minutes to run, elution buffer can be applied and fractions collected manually.
4. pH is critical in this procedure. If your antigen sample contains buffer salts, make sure the final pH is unaffected.
5. The gel-filtration step has a twofold purpose: first, to replace GdnHCl (which is not compatible with SDS-PAGE) with urea and, second, to raise the pH to 9.0 for the subsequent cleavage step.
6. Cleavage is usually incomplete with NTCB, and a complete spectrum of partial digestion products is produced. It is necessary to work out a theoretical "fingerprint" for each epitope location and compare them with the experimental result (*see* Fig. 1).

7. IBA oxidizes Met side chains to the sulfoxide, and this makes it difficult to map epitopes that require Met by this method. The problem can be solved by the prolonged incubation with DTE described here.
8. Although rather similar conditions are used for CNBr cleavage (70% formic acid instead of 75%), relatively little Asp–Pro cleavage appears to occur at the lower temperature (20°C instead of 37°C).
9. Urea should not be used because its effects on amino groups interfere with the Edman degradation in subsequent microsequencing. For similar reasons, microsequencing can rarely be applied to chemical cleavage fragments.
10. V8 protease is not inhibited by PMSF, so the aliquots should be boiled with SDS as soon as possible and kept at 0°C in the meantime. Di-isopropyl fluorophosphate (DFP) does inhibit, but its hazards are best avoided if inhibition is not essential. PefaBloc (Boehringer Mannheim) is a possible nontoxic alternative.

Acknowledgments

This work was supported by grants from the Muscular Dystrophy Group of Great Britain and Northern Ireland and from HEFC (Wales) DevR.

References

1. Wells, J. A. (1995) Structural and functional epitopes in the growth hormone receptor complex. *Biotechnology* **13**, 647–651.
2. Morris, G. E. (ed.) (1996) *Methods in Molecular Biology, vol. 66: Epitope Mapping Protocols*, Humana, Totowa, NJ.
3. Croft, L. R. (1980) *Handbook of Protein Sequence Analysis.* Wiley-Interscience, Chichester, UK.
4. Fontana, A., Dalzoppo, D., Grandi, C., and Zamboni, M. (1983) Cleavage at tryptophan with ortho–iodosobenzoic acid. *Methods Enzymol.* **91**, 311–318.
5. Stark, G. A. (1977) Cleavage at cysteine by nitro-thio-cyano-benzoic acid. *Methods Enzymol.* **47**, 129–132.
6. Sonderegger, P., Jaussi, R., Gehring, H., Brunschweiler, K., and Christen, P. (1982) Peptide mapping of protein bands from polyacrylamide gel electrophoresis by chemical cleavage in gel pieces and re-electrophoresis. *Anal. Biochem.* **122**, 298–301.
7. Morris, G. E., Frost, L. C., Newport, P. A., and Hudson, N. (1987) Monoclonal antibody studies of creatine kinase. Antibody-binding sites in the N-terminal region of creatine kinase and effects of antibody on enzyme refolding. *Biochem. J.* **248**, 53–59.
8. Morris, G. E. (1989) Monoclonal antibody studies of creatine kinase. The ART epitope: evidence for an intermediate in protein folding. *Biochem. J.* **257**, 461–469.
9. Morris, G. E. and Cartwright, A. J. (1990) Monoclonal antibody studies suggest a catalytic site at the interface between domains in creatine kinase. *Biochim. Biophys. Acta* **1039**, 318–322
10. Nguyen thi Man, Cartwright, A. J., Osborne, M., and Morris, G. E. (1991) Structural changes in the C-terminal region of human brain creatine kinase studied with monoclonal antibodies. *Biochim. Biophys. Acta* **1076**, 245–251.

11. Morris, G. E. and Nguyen thi Man (1992) Changes at the N-terminus of human brain creatine kinase during a transition between inactive folding intermediate and active enzyme. *Biochim. Biophys. Acta* **1120,** 233–238.
12. Laemmli, U. K. (1970) Cleavage of structural protein during the assembly of the head of bacteriophage T4. *Nature* **227,** 680–685.
13. Shagger, H. and von Jaggow, G. (1987) Tricine-sodium dodecyl sulfate polyacrylamide gel electrophoresis for the separation of proteins in the range 1 to 100 kDa. *Anal. Biochem.* **166,** 368–379.
14. Amit, P., Mariuzza, R., Phillips, S., and Poljak, R. (1986) Three-dimensional structure of an antigen–antibody complex. *Science* **233,** 747–753.
15. Zvi, A., Kustanovich, I., Feigelson, D., Levy, R., Eisenstein, M., Matsushita, S., Richalet-Secordel, P., Regenmortel, M. H. V., and Anglister, J. (1995) NMR mapping of the antigenic determinant recognized by an anti-gp120, human immunodeficiency virus neutralizing antibody. *Eur. J. Biochem.* **229,** 178–187.
16. Ping, L. H. and Lemon, S. M. (1992) Antigenic structure of human hepatitis-A virus defined by analysis of escape mutants selected against murine monoclonal antibodies. *J. Virol.* **66,** 2208–2216.
17. Tzartos, S. J., Rand, D. E., Einarson, B. L., and Lindstrom, J. M. (1981) Mapping of surface structures of Electrophorus acetylcholine receptor using monoclonal antibodies. *J. Biol. Chem.* **256,** 8635–8645.
18. Johne, B., Gadnell, M., and Hansen, K. (1993) Epitope mapping and binding kinetics of monoclonal antibodies studied by real time Biospecific Interaction Analysis using surface plasmon resonance. *J. Immunol. Methods* **160,** 191–198.
19. Jemmerson, R. and Paterson, Y. (1986) Mapping antigenic sites on a protein antigen by the proteolysis of antigen–antibody complexes. *Science* **232,** 1001–1004.
20. Burnens, A., Demotz, S., Corradin, G., Binz, H., and Bosshard, H. R. (1987) Epitope mapping by differential chemical modification of free and antibody-bound antigen. *Science* **235,** 780–783.
21. Mazzoni, M. R., Malinski, J. A., and Hamm, H. E. (1991) Structural analysis of rod GTP-binding protein, Gt-limited proteolytic digestion pattern of Gt with four proteases defines monoclonal antibodies epitope. *J. Biol. Chem.* **266,** 14,072–14,081.
22. Zhao, Y. and Chait, B. T. (1995) Protein epitope mapping by mass spectrometry. *Anal. Chem.* **66,** 3723–3726.
23. Geysen, H. M., Meleon, R. H., and Barteling, S. J. (1984) Use of peptide synthesis to probe viral antigens for epitopes to a resolution of a single amino acid. *Proc. Natl. Acad. Sci. USA* **81,** 3998–4002.
24. Frank, R., Kiess, M., Lahmann, H., Behn, Ch., and Gausepohl, H. (1995) Combinatorial synthesis on membrane supports by the SPOT technique, in *Peptides 1994* (Maia, H. L. S., ed.), ESCOM, Leiden, pp. 479,480.
25. Houghten, R. A., Pinilla, C., Blondelle, S. E., Appel, J. R., Dooley, C. T., and Cuervo, J. H. (1991) Generation and use of synthetic peptide combinatorial libraries for basic research and drug discovery. *Nature* **354,** 84–86.
26. Scott, J. K. and Smith, G. P. (1990) Searching for peptide ligands with an epitope library. *Science* **249,** 386–390.

27. Stanley, K. K. (1988) Epitope mapping using pEX. *Methods Mol. Biol.* **4,** 351–361.
28. Nguyen thi Man and Morris, G. E. (1993) Use of epitope libraries to identify exon-specific monoclonal antibodies for characterization of altered dystrophins in muscular dystrophy. *Am. J. Hum. Genet.* **52,** 1057–1066.
29. Thanh, L. T., Nguyen thi Man, Hori, S., Sewry, C. A., Dubowitz V., and Morris, G. E. (1995) Characterization of genetic deletions in Becker Muscular Dystrophy using monoclonal antibodies against a deletion-prone region of dystrophin. *Am. J. Med. Genet.* **58,** 177–186.
30. Burch, H. B., Nagy, E. V., Kain, K. C., Lanar, D. E., Carr, F. E., Wartofsky, L., and Burman, K. D. (1993) Expression polymerase chain reaction for the in vitro synthesis and epitope mapping of autoantigen. Application to the human thyrotropin receptor. *J. Immunol. Methods* **158,** 123–130.
31. Gross, C. H. and Rohrmann, G. F. (1990) Mapping unprocessed epitopes using deletion mutagenesis of gene fusions. *Biotechniques* **8,** 196–202.
32. Sedgwick, S. G., Nguyen thi Man, Ellis, J. M., Crowne, H., and Morris, G. E. (1991) Rapid mapping by transposon mutagenesis of epitopes on the muscular dystrophy protein, dystrophin. *Nucleic Acids Res.* **19,** 5889–5894.
33. Friguet, B., Fedorov, A. N., and Djavadi-Ohaniance, L. (1993) In vitro gene expression for the localization of antigenic determinants—application to the *E. coli* tryptophan synthase beta2 subunit. *J. Immunol. Methods* **158,** 243–249.
34. Ikeda, M., Hamano, K., and Shibata, T. (1992) Epitope mapping of anti-recA protein IgGs by region specified polymerase chain reaction mutagenesis. *J. Biol. Chem.* **267,** 6291–6296.
35. Alexander, H., Alexander, S., Getzoff, E. D., Tainer, J. A., Geysen, H. M., and Lerner, R. A. (1992) Altering the antigenicity of proteins. *Proc. Natl. Acad. Sci. USA* **89,** 3352–3356.
36. Wang, L. F., Hertzog, P. J., Galanis, M., Overall, M. L., Waine, G. J., and Linnane, A. W. (1994) Structure–function analysis of human IFN-alpha—Mapping of a conformational epitope by homologue scanning. *J. Immunol.* **152,** 705–715.
37. Webb, T., Jackson, P. J., and Morris, G. E. (1997) Protease digestion studies of an equilibrium intermediate in the unfolding of creative kinase. *Biochem J.* **321,** 83–88.

17

Coupling of Antibodies with Biotin

Rosaria P. Haugland and Wendy W. You

1. Introduction

The avidin–biotin bond is the strongest known biological interaction between a ligand and a protein (K_d = 1.3 × $10^{-15}M$ at pH 5.0) *(1)*. The affinity is so high that the avidin–biotin complex is extremely resistant to any type of denaturing agent *(2)*. Biotin (Fig. 1) is a small, hydrophobic molecule that functions as a coenzyme of carboxylases *(3)*. It is present in all living cells. Avidin is a tetrameric glycoprotein of 66,000–68,000 molecular weight, found in egg albumin and in avian tissues. The interaction between avidin and biotin occurs rapidly, and the stability of the complex has prompted its use for *in situ* attachment of labels in a broad variety of applications, including immunoassays, DNA hybridization *(4–6)*, and localization of antigens in cells and tissues *(7)*. Avidin has an isoelectric point of 10.5. Because of its positively charged residues and its oligosaccharide component, consisting mostly of mannose and glucosamine *(8)*, avidin can interact nonspecifically with negative charges on cell surfaces and nucleic acids, or with membrane sugar receptors. At times, this causes background problems in histochemical and cytochemical applications. Streptavidin, a near-neutral, biotin-binding protein *(9)* isolated from the culture medium of *Streptomyces avidinii,* is a tetrameric nonglycosylated analog of avidin with a molecular weight of about 60,000. Like avidin, each molecule of streptavidin binds four molecules of biotin, with a similar dissociation constant. The two proteins have about 33% sequence homology, and tryptophan residues seem to be involved in their biotin binding sites *(10,11)*. In general, streptavidin gives less background problems than avidin. This protein, however, contains a tripeptide sequence Arg-Tyr-Asp (RYD) that apparently mimics the binding sequence of fibronectin Arg-Gly-Asp (RGD), a universal recognition domain of the extracellular matrix that specifically promotes cell adhesion. Consequently,

From: *Methods in Molecular Biology, Vol. 80: Immunochemical Protocols, 2nd ed.*
Edited by: J. D. Pound © Humana Press Inc., Totowa, NJ

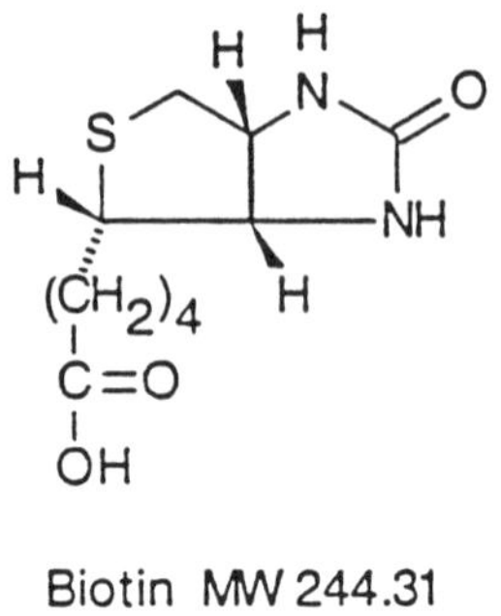

Biotin MW 244.31

Fig. 1. Structure of biotin.

the streptavidin–cell-surface interaction causes high background in certain applications *(12)*.

As an alternative to both avidin and streptavidin, a chemically modified avidin, NeutraLite™ avidin (NeutraLite is a trademark of Belovo Chemicals, Bastogne, Belgium), has recently become available. NeutraLite avidin consists of chemically deglycosylated avidin, which has been modified to reduce the isoelectric point to a neutral value, without loss of its biotin binding properties and without significant change in the lysines available for derivatization *(13)*. (Fluorescent derivatives and enzyme conjugates of NeutraLite avidin, as well as the unlabeled protein, are available from Molecular Probes, Eugene, OR.)

As shown in Fig. 1, biotin is a relatively small and hydrophobic molecule. The addition to the carboxyl group of biotin of one (*X*) or two (*XX*) amino-hexanoic acid "spacers" greatly enhances the efficiency of formation of the complex between the biotinylated antibody (or other biotinylated protein) and the avidin–probe conjugate, where the probe can be a fluorochrome or an enzyme *(14,15)*. Each of these 7- or 14-atom spacer arms has been shown to improve the ability of biotin derivatives to interact with the binding cleft of avidin. The comparison between streptavidin binding activity of proteins biotinylated with biotin-*X* or biotin-*XX* (labeled with same number of moles of biotin/mol of protein) has been performed in our laboratory (Fig. 2). No difference was found between the avidin or streptavidin–horseradish peroxidase conjugates in their ability to bind biotin-*X* or biotin-*XX*. However, biotin-*XX* gave consistently higher titers in enzyme-linked immunosorbent assays (ELISAs), using biotinylated goat antimouse Ig (GAM), bovine serum albumin (BSA), or protein A (results with avidin and with protein A are not presented here). Even nonroutine conjugations performed in our laboratory have consistently yielded excellent results using biotin-*XX*.

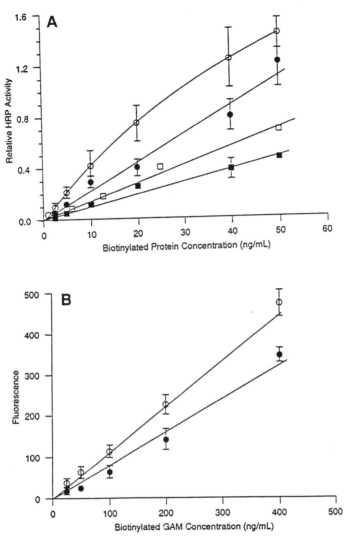

Fig. 2. (A) ELISA-type assay comparing the binding capacity of BSA and GAM biotinylated with biotin-*X* or biotin-*XX*. The assay was developed using streptavidin-HRP conjugate (0.2 μg/mL) and *o*-phenylenediamine dihydro-chloride (OPD). The number of biotin/mol was: 4.0 biotin-*X*/GAM (●), 4.4 biotin-*XX*/GAM (○), 6.7 biotin-*X*/BSA (■), and 6.2 biotin-*XX*/BSA (□). Error bars on some data points have been omitted for clarity. **(B)** Similar assay using GAM biotinylated with biotin-*X* (●) or biotin-*XX* (○). The assay was developed with streptavidin–R-phycoerythrin conjugate (25 μg/mL using a Perceptive Biosystems CytoFluor™ fluorescence microplate reader).

Biotin, biotin-*X,* and biotin-*XX* have all been derivatized for conjugation to amines or thiols of proteins and aldehyde groups of glycoproteins or other polymers. The simplest and most popular biotinylation method is to label the ε-amino groups of lysine residues with a succinimidyl ester of biotin. Easy-to-use biotinylation kits that facilitate the biotinylation of 1–2 mg of protein or oligonucleotides are commercially available *(16)*. One kit for biotinylating smaller amounts of protein (0.1–3 mg) utilizes biotin-*XX* sulfosuccinimidyl ester *(17)*. This compound is water-soluble and allows for the efficient labeling of dilute protein samples. Another kit uses biotin-*X* 2,4-dinitrophenyl-X-lysine succinimidyl ester (DNP-biocytin) as the biotinylating reagent. DNP-biocytin was developed by Molecular Devices (Menlo Park, CA) for their patented Threshold-Immunoligand System *(18)*. DNP-biocytin permits the direct measurement of the degree of biotinylation of the reaction product by using the molar extinction coefficient of DNP (15,000/cm at 364 nm). Conjugates of DNP-biocytin can be probed separately or simultaneously using either anti-DNP antibodies or avidin/streptavidin; this flexibility is useful when combining techniques, such as fluorescence and electron microscopy. Biotin iodoacetamide or maleimide, which could biotinylate the reduced sulfhydryls located at the hinge region of antibodies, is not usually used for this purpose. More examples in the literature describe biotinylation of antibodies with biotin hydrazide at the carbohydrate prosthetic group, located in the Fc portion of the molecule, relatively removed from the binding site. Conjugation of carbohydrates with hydrazides requires the oxidation of two adjacent hydroxyls to aldehydes and optional stabilization of the reaction with cyanoborohydride *(19)*.

Because of its strength, the interaction between avidin and biotin cannot be used for preparing matrices for affinity column purification, unless columns prepared with avidin monomers are used *(20)*. The biotin analog, iminobiotin, which has a lower affinity for avidin, can be used for this purpose *(21,22)*. Iminobiotin in reactive form is commercially available, and the procedure for its conjugation is identical to that used for biotin. Detailed, practical protocols for biotinylating antibodies at the lysine or at the carbohydrate site, and a method to determine the degree of biotinylation are described in detail in this chapter (*see* Notes 1–10 for review of factors that affect optimal conjugation and yield of biotinylated antibodies).

2. Materials
2.1. Conjugation with Amine-Reactive Biotin

1. Reaction buffer: 1*M* sodium bicarbonate, stable for about 2 wk when refrigerated. Dissolve 8.3 g of NaHCO$_3$ in 100 mL of distilled water. The pH will be about 8.3. Dilute 1:10 before using to obtain a 0.1*M* solution. Alternate reaction buffer: 0.1*M* sodium phosphate, pH 7.8. Dissolve 12.7 g Na$_2$HPO$_4$ and 1.43 g NaH$_2$PO$_4$

in 800 mL of distilled water. Adjust pH to 7.8 if necessary. Bring the volume to 1000 mL. This buffer is stable for 2 mo when refrigerated.

2. Anhydrous dimethylformamide (DMF) or dimethyl sulfoxide (DMSO).
3. Phosphate-buffered saline (PBS): Dissolve 1.19 g of K_2HPO_4, 0.43 g of $KH_2PO_4 \cdot H_2O$, and 8.8 g NaCl in 800 mL of distilled water, adjust the pH to 7.2 if necessary or to the desired pH, and bring the volume to 1000 mL with distilled water.
4. Disposable desalting columns or a gel-filtration column: Amicon GH-25 and Sephadex G-25 or the equivalent, equilibrated with PBS or buffer of choice.
5. Good-quality dialysis tubing as an alternative to the gel-filtration column when derivatizing small quantities of antibody.
6. Biotin, biotin-*X*, or biotin-*XX* succinimidyl ester: As with all succinimidyl esters, these compounds should be stored well desiccated in the freezer.

2.2. Conjugation with Biotin Hydrazide at the Carbohydrate Site

1. Reaction buffer: $0.1M$ acetate buffer, pH 6.0. Dilute 5.8 mL acetic acid in 800 mL distilled water. Bring the pH to 6.0 with $5M$ NaOH and the volume to 1000 mL. The buffer is stable for several months when refrigerated.
2. 20 mM Sodium metaperiodate: Dissolve 43 mg of $NaIO_4$ in 10 mL of reaction buffer, protecting from light. Use fresh.
3. Biotin-*X* hydrazide or biotin-*XX* hydrazide.
4. DMSO.
5. Optional: 100 mM sodium cyanoborohydride, freshly prepared. Dissolve 6.3 mg of $NaBH_3CN$ in 10 mL of 0.1 mM NaOH.

2.3. Determination of the Degree of Biotinylation

1. 10 mM 4' Hydroxyazobenzene-2-carboxylic acid (HABA) in 10 mM NaOH.
2. 50 mM Sodium phosphate and 150 mM NaCl, pH 6.0. Dissolve 0.85 g of Na_2HPO_4 and 6.07 g of NaH_2PO_4 in 800 mL of distilled water. Add 88 g of NaCl. Bring the pH to 6.0 if necessary and the volume to 1000 mL.
3. 0.5 mg/mL Avidin in 50 mM sodium phosphate and 150 mM NaCl, pH 6.0.
4. 0.25 mM Biotin in 50 mM sodium phosphate, and 150 mM NaCl, pH 6.0.

3. Methods

3.1. Conjugation with Amine-Reactive Biotin

1. Dissolve the antibody, if lyophilized, at approx 5–15 mg/mL in either of the two reaction buffers described in Section 2.1. If the antibody to be conjugated is already in solution in 10–20 mM PBS, without azide, the pH necessary for the reaction can be obtained by adding 1/10 vol of $1M$ sodium bicarbonate. IgM should be conjugated in PBS, pH 7.2 (*see* Note 3).
2. Calculate the amount of a 10 mg/mL biotin succinimidyl ester solution (biotin-SE) needed to conjugate the desired quantity of antibody at the chosen biotin/antibody molar ratio, according to the following formula:

$$(\text{mL of 10 mg/mL biotin-SE}) = \{[(\text{mg antibody} \times 0.1)/\text{mol wt}$$
$$\text{of antibody}] \times R \times \text{mol wt of biotin-SE})\} \qquad (1)$$

where R = molar incubation ratio of biotin/protein. For example, using 5 mg of IgG and a 10:1 molar incubation ratio of biotin-XX-SE, Eq. (1) yields:

$$(\text{mL of 10 mg/mL biotin-}XX\text{-SE}) =$$
$$\{[(5 \times 0.1)/145,000] \times (10 \times 568)\} = 0.02 \text{ mL} \qquad (2)$$

3. Weigh 3 mg or more of the biotin-SE of choice, and dissolve it in 0.3 mL or more of DMF or DMSO to obtain a 10 mg/mL solution. **It is essential that this solution be prepared immediately before starting the reaction,** since the succinimidyl esters or any amine-reactive reagents hydrolyze quickly in solution. Any remaining solution should be discarded.
4. While stirring, slowly add the amount of 10 mg/mL solution, calculated in step 2, to the antibody prepared in step 1, mixing thoroughly.
5. Incubate this reaction mixture at room temperature for 1 h with gentle stirring or shaking.
6. The antibody conjugate can be purified on a gel-filtration column or by dialysis. When working with a few milligrams of dilute antibody solution, care should be taken not to dilute the antibody further. In this case, dialysis is a very simple and effective method to eliminate unreacted biotin. A few milliliters of antibody solution can be effectively dialyzed in the cold against 1 L of buffer with three to four changes. Small amounts of concentrated antibody can be purified on a pre-packaged desalting column equilibrated with the preferred buffer, following the manufacturer's directions. Five or more milligrams of antibody can be purified on a gel-filtration column. The dimensions of the column will have to be proportional to the volume and concentration of the antibody. For example, for 5–10 mg of antibody in 1 mL solution, a column with a bed volume of 10×300 mm will be adequate. To avoid denaturation, dilute solutions of biotinylated antibodies should be stabilized by adding BSA at a final concentration of 0.1–1%.

3.2. Conjugation with Biotin Hydrazide at the Carbohydrate Site

1. It is essential that the entire following procedure be carried out with the sample completely protected from light (*see* Note 9).
2. Dissolve antibody (if lyophilized) or dialyze solution of antibody to obtain a 2–10 mg/mL solution in the reaction buffer described in Section 2.1., item 1. Keep at 4°C.
3. Add an equal volume of cold metaperiodate solution. Incubate the reaction mixture at 4°C for 2 h in the dark.
4. Dialyze overnight against the same buffer protecting from light, or, if the antibody is concentrated, desalt on a column equilibrated with the same buffer. This step removes the iodate and formaldehyde produced during oxidation.
5. Dissolve 10 mg of the biotin hydrazide of choice in 0.25 mL of DMSO to obtain a 40 mg/mL solution, warming if needed. This will yield a 107 mM solution of

biotin-*X* hydrazide or an 80 m*M* solution of biotin-*XX* hydrazide. These solutions are stable for a few weeks.

6. Calculate the amount of biotin hydrazide solution needed to obtain a final concentration of approx 5 m*M,* and add it to the oxidized antibody. When using biotin-*X* hydrazide, 1 vol of hydrazide should be added to 20 vol of antibody solution. When using biotin-*XX* hydrazide, 1 vol of hydrazide should be added to 15 vol of antibody solution.

7. Incubate for 2 h at room temperature with gentle stirring.

8. This step is optional. The biotin hydrazone–antibody conjugate formed in this reaction (steps 6 and 7) is considered by some researchers to be relatively unstable. To reduce the conjugate to a more stable, substituted hydrazide, treat the conjugate with sodium cyanoborohydride at a final concentration of 5 m*M* by adding a 1/20 vol of a 100-m*M* stock solution. Incubate for 2 h at 4°C (*see* Note 5).

9. Purify the conjugate by any of the methods described for biotinylating antibodies at the amine site (*see* Section 3.1., step 6).

3.3. Determination of the Degree of Biotinylation

The dye HABA interacts with avidin yielding a complex with an absorption maximum at 500 nm. Biotin, because of its higher affinity, displaces HABA, causing a decrease in absorbance at 500 nm proportional to the amount of biotin present in the assay.

1. To prepare a standard curve, add 0.25 mL of HABA reagent to 10 mL of avidin solution. Incubate 10 min at room temperature and record the absorbance at 500 nm of 1 mL avidin–HABA complex with 0.1 mL buffer, pH 6.0. Distribute 1 mL of the avidin–HABA complex into six test tubes. Add to each the biotin solution in a range of 0.005–0.10 mL. Bring the final volume to 1.10 mL with pH 6.0 buffer, and record the absorbance at 500 nm of each concentration point. Plot a standard curve with the nanomoles of biotin vs the decrease in absorbance at 500 nm. An example of a standard curve is illustrated in Fig. 3.

2. To measure the degree of biotinylation of the sample, add an aliquot of biotinylated antibody of known concentration to 1 mL of avidin–HABA complex. For example, add 0.05–0.1 mL of biotinylated antibody at 1 mg/mL to 1 mL of avidin–HABA mixture. Bring the volume to 1.10 mL, if necessary, incubate for 10 min, and measure the decrease in absorbance at 500 nm.

3. Deduct from the standard curve the nanomoles of biotin corresponding to the observed change in absorbance. The ratio between nanomoles of biotin and nanomoles of antibody used to displace HABA represents the degree of biotinylation, as seen from the following equation:

$$[(\text{nmol biotin} \times 145{,}000 \times 10^{-6})/(\text{mg/mL antibody} \times 0.1 \text{ mL})] = (\text{mol of biotin/mol of antibody}) \tag{3}$$

where 145,000 represents the mol wt of the antibody and 0.1 mL is the volume of 1 mg/mL of biotinylated antibody sample.

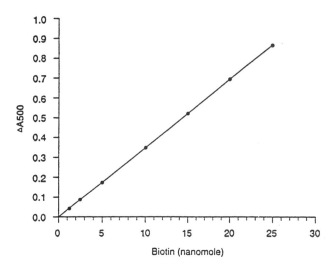

Fig. 3. Examples of standard curve for biotin assay with avidin-HABA reagent, obtained as described in Section 3.3.

4. Notes

4.1. Factors that Influence the Biotinylation Reaction

1. Protein concentration: As in any chemical reaction, the concentration of the reagents is a major factor in determining the rate and the efficiency of the coupling. Antibodies at a concentration of 5–20 mg/mL will give better results; however, it is often difficult to have such concentrations or even such quantities available for conjugation. Nevertheless, the antibody should be as concentrated as possible. In the case of solutions of antibody <2–3 mg/mL, the molar ratio of biotinylating reagent (or of both the oxidizing and biotinylating reagent, in the case of labeling the carbohydrate region) should be increased. It is also essential that the antibody solutions do not contain gelatin or BSA, which are often added to stabilize dilute solutions of antibodies. These proteins, generally present at a 1% concentration, will also react with biotinylating reagents.

2. pH: The reactivity of amines increases at basic pH. Unfortunately, so does the rate of hydrolysis of succinimidyl esters. We have found that the best pH for biotinylation of the ε-amino groups of lysines is 7.5–8.3. IgM antibodies, which denature at basic pH, can be biotinylated at pH 7.2 by increasing the molar ratio of the biotinylating reagent to antibody to at least 20. The optimum pH for oxidation and conjugation with hydrazides is 5.5–6.0.

3. Buffer: Bicarbonate or phosphate buffers are suitable for biotinylation. Organic buffers, such as Tris, which contain amines, should be avoided, because they react with amino-labeling reagents or interfere with the reaction between aldehydes and hydrazides. However, HEPES and EPPS, which contain tertiary amines, are suit-

able. Antibodies dissolved in 10–20 mM PBS can be readily prepared for conjugation at the lysine site by adding 1/10–1/5 of the volume of 1M sodium bicarbonate. As noted, because IgM antibodies are unstable in basic solution, biotinylation at the ε-amino group of lysines should be attempted in PBS or equivalent buffer at pH 7.2. Reactions of antibodies with periodate and biotin hydrazide can be performed in PBS at pH 7.0 or in acetate buffer, pH 6.0 (*see* Section 2.2.).

4. Temperature: Biotinylations at the amino group sites are run at room temperature, at the carbohydrate site at 0–4°C.
5. Time: Succinimidyl ester derivatives will react with a protein within 1 h. Periodate oxidation will require 2 h at pH 6.0. Reaction with biotin hydrazide can be performed in a few hours. Stabilization with cyanoboro-hydride requires <2 h.
6. Desired degree of biotinylation and stability of the conjugate: Reaction of an antibody with biotin does not significantly alter the size or charge of the molecule. However, because of the size of avidin or its analogs (molecular weight = 60,000–68,000), an increase in the number of biotins per antibody will not necessarily increase the number of avidins capable of reacting with one antibody molecule. Because biotin, biotin-*X*, and biotin-*XX* are very hydrophobic molecules, a high degree of biotinylation might increase the background or might destabilize the antibody. To obtain a degree of biotinylation of about 3–7 biotins/IgG, generally a molar ratio of 15 mol of amino biotinylating reagent/mol of protein is used. When the concentration of the antibody is <3 mg/mL, this ratio should be increased. The amount of increase should be determined experimentally, because the reactivity of the lysines available for conjugation varies for each antibody. This could become a significant factor, especially at low antibody concentrations.

The succinimidyl esters or hydrazides of biotin, biotin-*X*, and biotin-*XX* exhibit similar degrees of reactivity, and the choice is up to the researcher. In general, the longer spacer arm in biotin-*XX* should be advantageous (Fig. 2). The overall stability of biotinylated monoclonal antibodies derivatized with a moderate number of biotin should be similar to the stability of the native antibody, and the storage conditions also should be the same.

4.2. Factors that Affect Antibodies

7. Most antibodies can withstand biotinylation with minimal change in activity and stability, especially if the degree of biotinylation is about 3–6 biotins/mol.
8. Biotin or any of its longer chain derivatives do not contribute to the absorbance of the antibody at 280 nm. Consequently, the concentration of the antibody can be measured by using A $^{1\%}_{1cm}$ = 14 at 280 nm.
9. It is essential that the entire procedure for biotinylation of antibodies at the carbohydrate site (Section 3.2.) be performed in the dark, protected from light.
10. It should be noted that dry milk, serum, and other biological fluids contain biotin and, consequently, they should not be used as blocking agents in systems where blocking is required.

References

1. Green, N. M. (1963) Avidin. 3. The nature of the biotin binding site. *Biochem. J.* **89,** 599–609.
2. Green, N. M. (1963) Avidin. 4. Stability at extremes of pH and dissociation into subunits by guanidine hydrochloride. *Biochem. J.* **89,** 609–620.
3. Knappe, J. (1970) Mechanism of biotin action. *Annu. Rev. Biochem.* **39,** 757–776.
4. Wilchek, M. and Bayer, E. A. (1988) The avidin–biotin complex in bioanalytical applications. *Anal. Biochem.* **171,** 1–32.
5. Wilchek, M. and Bayer, E. A. (1990) Avidin–biotin technology, in *Methods in Enzymology,* vol. 184, Academic, New York, pp. 213–217.
6. Levi, M., Sparvoli, E., Sgorbati, S., and Chiantante, D. (1990) Biotin–streptavidin immunofluorescent detection of DNA replication in root meristems through Brd Urd incorporation: cytological and microfluorimetric applications. *Physiol. Plantarum* **79,** 231–235.
7. Armstrong, R., Friedrich, V. L., Jr., Holmes, K. V., and Dubois-Dalcq, M. (1990) *In vitro* analysis of the oligodendrocyte lineage in mice during demyelination and remyelination. *J. Cell Biol.* **111,** 1183–1195.
8. Bruch, R. C. and White, H. B., III (1982) Compositional and structural heterogeneity of avidin glycopeptides. *Biochemistry* **21,** 5334–5341.
9. Hiller, Y., Gershoni, J. M., Bayer, E. A., and Wilchek, M. (1987) Biotin binding to avidin: oligosaccharide side chain not required for ligand association. *Biochem. J.* **248,** 167–171.
10. Green, N. M. (1975) Avidin, in *Advances in Protein Chemistry,* vol. 29 (Anfinsen, C. B., Edsall, J. T., and Richards, F. M., eds.), Academic, New York, pp. 85–133.
11. Chaiet, L. and Wolf, F. J. (1964) The properties of streptavidin, a biotin-binding protein produced by *Streptomyces. Arch. Biochem. Biophys.* **106,** 1–5.
12. Alon, R., Bayer, E. A., and Wilcheck, M. (1990) Streptavidin contains an Ryd sequence which mimics the RGD receptor domain of fibronectin. *Biochem. Biophys. Res. Commun.* **170,** 1236–1241.
13. Wilchek, M. and Bayer, E. A. (1993) Avidin–biotin immobilization systems, in *Immobilized Macromolecules: Application Potentials* (Sleytr, U. B., ed.), Springer-Verlag, New York, pp. 51–60.
14. Gretch, D. R., Suter, M., and Stinski, M. F. (1987) The use of biotinylated monoclonal antibodies and streptavidin affinity chomatography to isolate Herpes virus hydrophobic proteins or glycoproteins. *Anal. Biochem.* **163,** 270–277.
15. Hnatowich, D. J., Virzi, F., and Rusckowski, M. (1987) Investigations of avidin and biotin for imaging applications. *J. Nucleic Med.* **28,** 1294–1302.
16. Haugland, R. P. (1996) Biotin and Haptens, in *Handbook of Fluorescent Probes and Research Chemicals,* 6th ed. (Spence, M., ed.), Molecular Probes, Inc., Eugene, OR, Chapter 4.
17. LaRochelle, W. J. and Froehner, S. C. (1986) Determination of the tissue distributions and relative concentrations of the postsynaptic 43-kDa protein and the acetylcholine receptor in *Torpedo. J. Biol. Chem.* **261,** 5270–5274.

18. Briggs, J. and Panfili, P. R. (1991) Quantitation of DNA and protein impurities in biopharmaceuticals. *Anal. Chem.* **63,** 850–859.

19. Wong, S. S. (1991) Reactive groups of proteins and their modifying agents, in *Chemistry of Protein Conjugation and Crosslinking,* CRC, Boston, MA, pp. 27–29.

20. Kohanski, R. A. and Lane, M. D. (1985) Receptor affinity chomatography. *Ann. NY Acad. Sci.* **447,** 373–385.

21. Orr, G. A. (1981) The use of the 2-iminobiotin–avidin interaction for the selective retrieval of labeled plasma membrane components. *J. Biol. Chem.* **256,** 761–766.

22. Hoffmann, K., Wood, S. W., Brinton, C. C., Montibeller, J. A., and Finn, F. M. (1980) Iminobiotin affinity columns and their application to retrieval of streptavidin. *Proc. Natl. Acad. Sci. USA* **77,** 4666–4668.

18

Preparation of Avidin Conjugates

Rosaria P. Haugland and Mahesh K. Bhalgat

1. Introduction

The high-affinity avidin–biotin system has found applications in different fields of biotechnology, including immunoassays, histochemistry, affinity chromatography, and drug delivery, to name a few. A brief description of avidin and avidin-like molecules, streptavidin, deglycosylated avidin, and NeutraLite avidin is presented in the previous chapter (Chapter 17). With four biotin binding sites per molecule, the avidin family of proteins is capable of forming tight complexes with one or more biotinylated compounds (1). Typically, the avidin–biotin system is used to prepare signal-amplifying "sandwich" complexes between specificity reagents (e.g., antibodies) and detection reagents (e.g., fluorophores, enzymes, and so on). The specificity and detection reagents are independently conjugated, one with avidin and the other with biotin, or both with biotin, providing synthetic flexibility (2).

Avidin conjugates of a wide range of fluorophores, phycobiliproteins, secondary antibodies, microspheres, ferritin, and enzymes commonly used in immunochemistry are available at reasonable prices, making their small scale preparation impractical and not cost effective (see Note 1). However, conjugations of avidin to specific antibodies, to uncommon enzymes, and to other proteins and peptides are often performed on-site. A general protocol for the conjugation of avidin to enzymes, antibodies, and other proteins is described in this chapter.

Avidin conjugates of oligodeoxynucleotides are hybrid molecules that not only provide multiple biotin binding sites, but can also be targeted to complimentary DNA or RNA sequences, by annealing interactions. Such conjugates are useful for the construction of macromolecular assemblies with a wide vari-

From: *Methods in Molecular Biology, Vol. 80: Immunochemical Protocols, 2nd ed.*
Edited by: J. D. Pound © Humana Press Inc., Totowa, NJ

ety of constituents *(3)*. The protocol outlined in Section 3.1. can be modified (*see* Note 2) for the conjugation of oligonucleotides to avidin.

Streptavidin conjugates are also being evaluated for use in drug delivery systems. A two-step imaging and treatment protocol has been developed that involves injection of a suitably prepared tumor-specific monoclonal antibody (MAb), followed by a second reagent that carries an imaging or therapeutic agent, capable of binding to the tumor-targeted antibody *(4)*. Owing to complications associated with the injection of radiolabeled biotin *(5)*, conjugation of the imaging or therapeutic agent to streptavidin is being considered instead. A protocol for radioiodination of streptavidin using IODO-BEADS *(6)* is described in Section 3.2. Some other methods that have been developed include the iodogen method *(7,8)*, the Bolton-Hunter reagent method *(9)*, and a few that do not involve direct iodination of tyrosine residues *(10–13)*. Streptavidin-drug conjugates are also candidates for therapeutic agents. Synthesis of a streptavidin-drug conjugate involves making a chemically reactive form of the drug followed by its conjugation to streptavidin. The synthetic methodology thus depends on the structure of the specific drug to be conjugated *(14–16)*.

The avidin–biotin interaction can also be exploited for affinity chromatography; however, there are limitations to this application. For example, a biotinylated protein captured on an avidin affinity matrix would likely be denatured by the severe conditions required to separate the high affinity avidin–biotin complex. On the other hand, an avidin affinity matrix may find utility in the removal of undesired biotinylated moieties from a mixture or for the purification of compounds derivatized with 2-iminobiotin. The biotin derivative 2-iminobiotin has reduced affinity for avidin, and its moderate binding to avidin at pH 9.0 is greatly diminished at pH 4.5 *(17)*. Another approach to reducing the affinity of the interaction is to denature avidin to its monomeric subunits. The monomeric subunits have greatly reduced affinity for biotin *(18)*. We describe here a protocol for preparing native *(19)* and monomeric avidin matrices *(20)*. Recently, modified streptavidins, hybrids of native and engineered subunits with lower binding constants, have been prepared that may also be suitable for affinity matrices *(21)*.

2. Materials
2.1. Conjugation with Antibodies and Enzymes

1. Avidin.
2. Antibody, enzyme, peptide, protein, or thiolated oligonucleotide to be conjugated to avidin.
3. Succinimidyl 3-(2-pyridyldithio)propionate (SPDP) (*see* Note 3).
4. Succinimidyl *trans*-4-(*N*-maleimidylmethyl)cyclohexane-1-carboxylate (SMCC).
5. Dithiothreitol (DTT).

6. *Tris* (2-carboxyethyl)phosphine (TCEP).
7. *N*-ethylmaleimide (NEM).
8. Anhydrous dimethyl sulfoxide (DMSO) or anhydrous dimethylformamide (DMF).
9. $0.1M$ Phosphate buffer: $0.1M$ sodium phosphate, $0.1M$ NaCl at pH 7.5. Dissolve 92 g of Na_2HPO_4, 21 g of $NaH_2PO_4 \cdot H_2O$, and 46.7 g of NaCl in approx 3.5 L of distilled water and adjust the pH to 7.5 with $5M$ NaOH. Dilute to 8 L. Store refrigerated.
10. $1M$ Sodium bicarbonate (*see* Note 4): Dissolve 8.4 g in 90 mL of distilled water and adjust the volume to 100 mL. A freshly prepared solution has a pH of 8.3–8.5.
11. Molecular exclusion matrix with properties suitable for purification of the specific conjugate. Sephadex G-200 (Pharmacia Biotech, Uppsala, Sweden), Bio-Gel A-0.5 m or Bio-Gel A-1.5 m (Bio-Rad Laboratories, Hercules, CA) are useful for relatively small to large conjugates, respectively.
12. Sephadex G-25 (Pharmacia Biotech) or other equivalent matrix.

2.2. Radioiodination Using IODO-BEADS

1. Streptavidin.
2. $Na^{131}I$ or $Na^{125}I$, as desired.
3. IODO-BEADS (Pierce Chemical, Rockford, IL).
4. Phosphate-buffered saline (PBS), pH 7.2: Dissolve 1.19 g of K_2HPO_4, 0.43 g of KH_2PO_4, and 9 g of NaCl in 900 mL of distilled water. Adjust the pH to 7.2 and dilute to 1 L with distilled water.
5. Saline solution: 9 g of NaCl dissolved in 1 L of distilled water.
6. 0.1% Bovine serum albumin (BSA) solution in saline: 0.1 g of BSA dissolved in 100 mL of saline solution.
7. Trichloroacetic acid (TCA), 10% (w/v) solution in saline: Dissolve 1 g TCA in 10 mL of saline solution.
8. Bio-Gel P-6DG Gel (Bio-Rad).

2.3. Avidin Affinity Matrix

1. 50–100 mg of avidin.
2. Sodium borohydride.
3. 1,4-Butanediol-diglycidylether.
4. Succinic anhydride.
5. $6M$ Guanidine $\cdot$ HCl in $0.2M$ KCl/HCl, pH 1.5: Dissolve 1.5 g of KCl in 50 mL of distilled water. Add 57.3 g of guanidine $\cdot$ HCl with stirring. Adjust the pH to 1.5 with $1M$ HCl. Adjust the volume to 100 mL with distilled water.
6. $0.2M$ Glycine $\cdot$ HCl pH 2.0: Dissolve 22.3 g of glycine $\cdot$ HCl in 900 mL of distilled water. Adjust the pH to 2.0 with $6M$ HCl and the volume to 1 L with distilled water.
7. PBS: *see* Section 2.2., item 4.
8. $0.2M$ Sodium carbonate, pH 9.5: Dissolve 1.7 g of sodium bicarbonate in 80 mL of distilled water. Adjust the pH to 9.5 with $1M$ NaOH and the volume to 100 mL with distilled water.

9. $0.2M$ Sodium phosphate, pH 7.5: Weigh 12 g of Na_2HPO_4 and 2.5 g of NaH_2PO_4 H_2O and dissolve in 900 mL of distilled water. Adjust the pH to 7.5 with $5M$ NaOH and the volume to 1 L with distilled water.
10. 20 mM Sodium phosphate, $0.5M$ NaCl, 0.02% sodium azide, pH 7.5: Dilute 100 mL of the buffer described in item 9 to 900 mL with distilled water. Add 28 g of NaCl and 200 mg of sodium azide. Adjust pH if necessary, and dilute to 1 L with distilled water.
11. Sepharose 6B (Pharmacia Biotech) or other 6% crosslinked agarose gel.

3. Methods

3.1. Conjugation with Antibodies and Enzymes

3.1.1. Avidin Thiolation

An easy-to-use, protein-to-protein crosslinking kit is now commercially available (Molecular Probes, Eugene, OR). This kit allows predominantly 1:1 conjugate formation between two proteins (0.2–3.0 mg) through the formation of a stable thioether bond *(22)*, with minimal generation of aggregates. A similar protocol is described here for conjugation of 5 mg avidin to antibodies or enzymes. Modifications of the procedure for conjugation of avidin to thiolated oligonucleotides and peptides are described in Notes 2 and 5, respectively. Although the protocol described in this section uses avidin for conjugation, it can be applied for the preparation of conjugates using either avidin, streptavidin, deglycosylated avidin, or NeutraLite avidin.

1. Dissolve 5 mg of avidin (76 nmol) in 0.5 mL of $0.1M$ phosphate buffer to obtain a concentration of 10 mg/mL.
2. Weigh 3 mg of SPDP and dissolve in 0.3 mL of DMSO to obtain a 10 mg/mL solution. This solution must be prepared **fresh** immediately before using. Vortex or sonicate to ensure that the reagent is completely dissolved.
3. Slowly add 12 μL (380 nmol) of the SPDP solution (*see* Note 3) to the stirred solution of avidin. Stir for 1 h at room temperature.
4. Purify the thiolated avidin on a 7 × 250 mm size exclusion column, such as Sephadex G-25 equilibrated in $0.1M$ phosphate buffer.
5. Determine the degree of thiolation (optional):
    a. Prepare a 100-mM solution of DTT by dissolving 7.7 mg of the reagent in 0.5 mL of distilled water.
    b. Transfer the equivalent of 0.3–0.4 mg of thiolated avidin (absorbance at 280 nm of a 1.0 mg/mL avidin solution = 1.54) and dilute to 1.0 mL using $0.1M$ phosphate buffer. Record the absorbance at 280 and 343 nm.
    c. Add 50 μL of DTT solution. Mix well, incubate for 3–5 min at room temperature, and record the absorbance at 343 nm.
    d. Using the extinction coefficient at 343 nm of 8.08×10^3/cm/M *(23)*, calculate the amount of pyridine-2-thione liberated during the reduction, which

Table 1
Molar Extinction Coefficients at 280 nm
and Molecular Weights of Avidin and Avidin-Like Proteins

Protein	Molecular weight	$E_{avidin}^M/cm/M$
Avidin	66,000	101,640
Deglycosylated avidin/neutraLite avidin	60,000	101,640
Streptavidin	60,000	180,000

is equivalent to the number of thiols introduced on avidin, using the following equation along with the appropriate extinction coefficient shown in Table 1:

$$\text{Number of thiols/avidin} = [\Delta A_{343}/(8.08 \times 10^3)] \times [E_{avidin}^M/(A_{280} - 0.63\Delta A_{343})] \tag{1}$$

where ΔA_{343} = change in absorbance at 343 nm; E_{avidin}^M = molar extinction coefficient; and $0.63\Delta A_{343}$ = correction for the absorbance of pyridyldithiopropionate at 280 nm *(23)*.

6. Equation (1) allows the determination of the average number of moles of enzyme or antibody that can be conjugated with each of avidin (*see* Note 6). For a 1:1 protein–avidin conjugate, avidin should be modified with 1.2–1.5 thiols/mol. Thiolated avidin prepared by the above procedure can be stored in the presence of 2 mM sodium azide at 4°C for 4–6 wk.

3.1.2. Maleimide Derivatization of the Antibody or Enzyme

In this step, which should be completed prior to the deprotection of thiolated avidin, some of the amino groups from the antibody or enzyme are transformed into maleimide groups by reacting with a bifunctional crosslinker, SMCC (*see* Note 7).

1. Dissolve or, if already in solution, dialyze the protein in 0.1M phosphate buffer to obtain a concentration of 2–10 mg/mL. If the protein is an antibody, 11 mg are required to obtain an amount equimolar to 5 mg of avidin (*see* Note 6).
2. Prepare a **fresh** solution of SMCC by dissolving 5 mg in 500 µL of dry DMSO to obtain a 10 mg/mL solution. Vortex or sonicate to ensure that the reagent is completely dissolved.
3. While stirring, add an appropriate amount of SMCC solution to the protein solution to obtain a molar ratio of SMCC-to-protein of approx 10. (If 11 mg of an antibody is the protein used, 30 µL of SMCC solution are required.)
4. Continue stirring at room temperature for 1 h.
5. Dialyze the solution in 2 L of 0.1M phosphate buffer at 4°C for 24 h, with four buffer changes using a membrane with a suitable molecular weight cut-off.

3.1.3. Deprotection of the Avidin Thiol Groups

This procedure is carried out immediately before reacting thiolated avidin with the maleimide derivative of the antibody or enzyme prepared in Section 3.1.2.

1. Dissolve 3 mg of TCEP in 0.3 mL of $0.1M$ phosphate buffer.
2. Add 11 µL of TCEP solution to the thiolated avidin solution. Incubate for 15 min at room temperature.

3.1.4. Formation and Purification of the Conjugate

1. Add the thiolated avidin-TCEP mixture dropwise to the dialyzed maleimide-derivatized protein solution with stirring. Continue stirring for 1 h at room temperature, followed by stirring overnight at 4°C.
2. Stop the conjugation reaction by capping residual sulfhydryls with the addition of NEM at a final concentration of 50 µM. Dissolve 6 mg of NEM in 1 mL DMSO and dilute 1:1000 in the conjugate reaction mixture. Incubate for 30 min at room temperature or overnight at 4°C (*see* Note 8). The conjugate is now ready for final purification.
3. Concentrate the avidin–protein conjugate mixture to 1–2 mL in a Centricon-30 (Amicon, Beverly, MA) or equivalent centrifuge tube concentrator.
4. Pack appropriate size columns (e.g., 10 × 600 mm for approx 15 mg of final conjugate) with a degassed matrix suitable for the isolation of the conjugate from unconjugated reagents. If the protein conjugated is an antibody, a matrix such as Bio-Gel A-0.5 m is suitable. For other proteins, Sephadex G-200 or a similar column support may be appropriate, depending on the size of the protein–avidin conjugate.
5. Collect 0.5–1 mL fractions. The first protein peak to elute contains the conjugate; however, the first or second fraction may contain some aggregates. Analyze each fraction absorbing at 280 nm for biotin binding and assay it for the antibody or enzyme activity. HPLC may also be performed for further purification, if necessary.

3.2. Radioiodination Using IODO-BEADS

The radioiodination procedure (*see* Note 9) described here uses IODO-BEADS, which contain the sodium salt of *N*-chloro-benzenesulfonamide immobilized on nonporous, polystyrene beads. Immobilization of the oxidizing agent allows for easy separation of the latter from the reaction mixture. This method also prevents the use of reducing agents.

1. Wash 6–8 IODO-BEADS twice with 5 mL of PBS. Dry the beads by rolling them on a clean filter paper.
2. Add 500 µL of PBS to the supplier's vial containing 8–10 mCi of carrier free Na^{125}I or Na^{131}I. Place the beads in the same vial and gently mix the contents by swirling. Allow the mixture to sit for 5 min at room temperature with the vial capped.
3. Dissolve or dilute streptavidin in PBS to obtain a final concentration of 1 mg/mL. Add 500 µL of streptavidin solution to the vial containing sodium iodide. Cap the

vial immediately and mix the contents thoroughly. Incubate for 20–25 min at room temperature, with occasional swirling (*see* Note 10).

4. Carefully remove and save the liquid from the reaction vessel; this is the radioiodinated streptavidin solution. Wash the beads by adding 500 µL of PBS to the reaction vial. Remove the wash solution and add it to the radioiodinated streptavidin.

5. For purification, load the reaction mixture onto a 9 × 200 mm Bio-Gel P-6DG column packed in PBS (0.1% BSA may be added as a carrier to the PBS to reduce loss of streptavidin by adsorption to the column). Elute the column with PBS and collect 0.5-mL fractions. The first set of radioactive fractions (as determined by counting in a γ-ray counter) contains radioiodinated streptavidin, while the unreacted radioiodine elutes in the later fractions. Pool the radioiodinated streptavidin fractions.

6. Assessment of protein-associated activity with trichloroacetic acid precipitation:
   a. Dilute a small volume of the pooled radiolabeled streptavidin with saline solution such that 50 µL of the diluted solution has 10^4–10^6 cpm.
   b. Add 50 µL of the diluted streptavidin solution to a 12 × 75-mm glass tube, followed by 500 µL of a 0.1% BSA solution in saline.
   c. For precipitating the proteins, add 500 µL of 10% (w/v) TCA solution in saline.
   d. Incubate the solution for 30 min at room temperature and count the radioactivity of the solution for 10 min ("total counts").
   e. Centrifuge the tube at 500 g for 10 min and carefully discard the supernatant in a radioactive waste container.
   f. Resuspend the pellet in 1 mL of saline and count its radioactivity for 10 min ("bound counts").
   g. The percentage of radioactivity bound to streptavidin is determined using the following equation:

$$[(\text{Bound counts})/(\text{Total counts})] \times 100 = \% \text{ of radioactivity bound to streptavidin} \qquad (2)$$

3.3. Avidin Affinity Matrices
3.3.1. Native Avidin Affinity Matrix

1. Wash 10 mL of sedimented 6% crosslinked agarose with distilled water on a glass or Buchner filter and remove excess water by suction.

2. Dissolve 14 mg of NaBH$_4$ in 7 mL of 1*M* NaOH. Add this solution along with 7 mL of 1,4-butanediol-diglycidylether to the washed agarose, with mixing. Allow the reaction to proceed for 10 h or more at room temperature with gentle stirring.

3. Extensively wash the activated gel with distilled water on a supporting filter. The washed gel can be stored in water at 4°C, for up to 10 d.

4. Dissolve 50–100 mg of avidin in 10–20 mL of 0.2*M* sodium carbonate, pH 9.5, and suspend the sedimented activated agarose gel in the same buffer to obtain a workable slurry.

5. Slowly drip the agarose slurry into the stirred protein solution and allow the binding to take place at room temperature for 2 d with continuous gentle mixing.
6. Wash the avidin–agarose mixture in PBS until the filtrate shows no absorbance at 280 nm. Store at 4°C in the presence of 0.02% sodium azide.

3.3.2. Monomeric Avidin Affinity Matrix

1. Filter the avidin–agarose matrix (from Section 3.3.1., step 6) on a glass or Buchner filter (or pack in a column) and wash four times with 2 vol of $6M$ guanidine · HCl in $0.2M$ KCl, pH 1.5, to dissociate the tetrameric avidin.
2. Thoroughly wash the gel with $0.2M$ potassium phosphate, pH 7.5, and suspend in 10 mL of the same buffer.
3. Add 3 mg of solid succinic anhydride to succinylate the monomeric avidin and incubate for 1 h at room temperature with gentle stirring.
4. Wash the gel with $0.2M$ potassium phosphate, pH 7.5, pack in a column, and saturate the binding sites by running through three volumes of 1 mM biotin dissolved in the same buffer.
5. Remove biotin from the low affinity binding sites by washing the column with $0.2M$ glycine · HCl, pH 2.0.
6. Store the column equilibrated in 20 mM sodium phosphate, $0.5M$ NaCl, 0.02% sodium azide, pH 7.5. The column is now ready to use.
7. Load the column with the mixture to be purified. Elute any unbound protein by adding 20 mM sodium phosphate, $0.5M$ NaCl, pH 7.5. Add biotin to the same buffer to obtain a final concentration of 0.8 mM to elute the biotinylated compound.
8. Regenerate the column after each run by washing with $0.2M$ glycine · HCl, pH 2.0.

4. Notes

1. A detailed procedure for the conjugation of fluorophores to antibodies has been recently published *(24)*. This protocol can be modified for conjugation of fluorophores to avidin or avidin-related proteins by using a dye-to-avidin molar ratio of 5–8:1.
2. The conjugation reaction for oligonucleotides synthesized with a disulfide containing a protecting group should be performed under nitrogen or argon. Deprotect the disulfide of the oligonucleotide using DTT. Add 1 mg of DTT to 140 µL of a 6 µM oligonucleotide (21–33 mer) solution in $0.1M$ phosphate buffer containing 5 mM ethylenediaminetetra-acetic acid. Stir the solution at 37°C for 0.5 h. Purify the reaction mixture using a disposable desalting column. Combine the oligonucleotide-containing fractions with thiolated avidin prepared as described in Section 3.1.1. It should be noted that, in this case, conjugation occurs through the formation of a disulfide bond instead of a thioether bond. Disulfides are sensitive to reducing agents; however, they make reasonably stable conjugates, useful in most applications *(25)*. Purify the conjugate as outlined in Section 3.1.4.

3. Using a molar ratio of SPDP to avidin of 5 yields 1–2 protected sulfhydryls per molecule of avidin. This range of thiols per mole is found to produce the best yield of a 1:1 conjugate.

4. Buffer and pH: The entire procedure for preparation of conjugates through thioether bonds can be performed at pH 7.5. (**Note:** Organic buffers containing amines, such as Tris, are unsuitable.) Antibodies or enzymes in PBS can be prepared for reaction with SMCC by adding 1/10 vol of $1M$ sodium bicarbonate solution. This step eliminates dialysis and consequent dilution of the protein. Presence of azide at concentrations above 0.1% may interfere with the reaction of the protein with SMCC or of avidin with SPDP. IgM antibodies denature above pH 7.2. They can, however, be conjugated in PBS at pH 7.0 by increasing the molar ratio of maleimide to antibody.

5. Peptides (20–25 amino acids) containing a single cysteine can also be conjugated to thiolated avidin by modifying the procedure described in Section 3.1. and performing the reaction under argon or nitrogen *(26)*. Peptide–avidin conjugate formation described here also involves the formation of a disulfide bond. For conjugation with 5 mg avidin, dissolve 1.6 mg of a lyophilized cysteine-containing peptide in 900 μL water/methanol (2:1 v/v) using 50 mM NaOH (a few microliters at a time) to improve solubility. Immediately prior to use, cleave any cystine-bridged homodimer that may be present by the addition of TCEP solution (10 mg/mL in 0.1M phosphate buffer) to obtain a TCEP-to-peptide ratio of 3. Incubate for 15 min at room temperature. Purify the peptide-TCEP mixture using a disposable desalting column. Combine the peptide-containing fractions with thiolated avidin prepared as described in Section 3.1.1. Purify the conjugate as described in Section 3.1.4.

6. Avidin and antibody or enzyme concentration: The concentration of avidin as well as that of the protein to be conjugated should be 2–10 mg/mL. The crosslinking efficiency and, consequently, the yield of the conjugate decreases at lower concentrations of the thiolated avidin and maleimide-derivatized protein. To obtain 1:1 conjugates, equimolar concentrations of avidin and the protein are desirable. However, most methods of conjugation will generate conjugates of different sizes, following the Poisson distribution. The size range obtained with the method described here is much narrower because the number of proteins reacting with each mole of avidin can be regulated by the degree of thiolation of avidin.

7. It is essential that the procedure described in Section 3.1.2. be performed approx 24 h before the procedure described in Section 3.1.3., because the deprotected thiolated avidin and the maleimide derivative of the protein are unstable. Purification of the maleimide-derivatized protein by size exclusion chromatography can be performed more rapidly than dialysis; however, the former leads to dilution of the protein and a decrease in the yield of the conjugate.

8. If the molecule being conjugated to avidin is β-galactosidase or other free thiol-containing oligonucleotide or protein, NEM treatment is not performed.

9. Radioiodination of streptavidin uses procedures similar to those used for stable nuclides. However, some distinct differences remain, since radioiodinations are

performed in dilute solutions. Also, the radioiodination mixture contains minor impurities formed during the preparation and purification of the radionuclide. Thus, optimization of reaction parameters is essential for performing radio-iodination. This reaction is carried out in small volumes; it is therefore essential to ensure adequate mixing at the outset of the reaction. Inadequate mixing is often responsible for poor radioiodination yield.

10. Specific activity using the method described in Section 3.2. is usually in the range of 10–50 mCi/mg and the protein-bound radioactivity obtained is >95%. Higher specific activity can be achieved by increasing the reaction time of step 3 in Section 3.2. by using more beads, or by increasing the amount of radioiodine. However, one must bear in mind that at longer incubation times, the risk of damage to streptavidin is greater.

11. Storage and stability of avidin conjugates: Most avidin conjugates can be stored at 4 or –20°C after lyophilization. Because of the variation in antibody structure, there is no general rule on the best method to store avidin–antibody conjugates, and the best conditions are determined experimentally. Aliquoting in small amounts and freezing is generally satisfactory. Radiolabeled streptavidin is aliquoted (~100 mL/tube) and stored at 4 or –20°C until use.

References

1. Green, N. M. (1975) Avidin, in *Advances in Protein Chemistry*, vol. 29 (Anfinsen, C. M., Edsall, J. T., and Richards, F. M., eds.), Academic, New York, pp. 85–133.
2. Bayer, E. A. and Wilchek, M. (1980) The use of the avidin–biotin complex as a tool in molecular biology. *Meth. Biochem. Anal.* **26**, 1–45.
3. Niemeyer, C. M., Sano, T., Smith, C. L., and Cantor, C. R. (1994) Oligo-nucleotide-directed self-assembly of proteins: semisynthetic DNA–strepta-vidin hybrid molecules as connectors for the generation of macroscopic arrays and the construction of supramolecular bioconjugates. *Nucleic Acids Res.* **22**, 5330–5339.
4. Paganelli, G., Belloni, C., Magnani, P., Zito, F., Pasini, A., Sassi, I., Meroni, M., Mariani, M., Vignali, M., Siccardi, A. G., and Fazio, F. (1992) Two-step tumor targetting in ovarian cancer patients using biotinylated monoclonal antibodies and radioactive streptavidin. *Eur. J. Nucl. Med.* **19**, 322–329.
5. van Osdol, W. W., Sung, C., Dedrick, R. L., and Weinstein, J. N. (1993) A distrib-uted pharmacokinetic model of two-step imaging and treatment protocols: appli-cation to streptavidin-conjugated monoclonal antibodies and radiolabeled biotin. *J. Nucl. Med.* **34**, 1552–1564.
6. Markwell, M. A. K. (1982) A new solid-state reagent to iodinate proteins. I. Con-ditions for the efficient labeling of antiserum. *Anal. Biochem.* **125**, 427–432.
7. Salacinski, P. R. P., McLean, C., Sykes, J. E. C., Clement-Jones, V. V., and Lowry, P. J. (1981) Iodination of proteins, glycoproteins, and peptides using a solid-phase oxidizing agent, 1,3,4,6-tetrachloro-3α,6α-diphenyl glycoluril (iodogen). *Anal. Biochem.* **117**, 136–146.

8. Mock, D. M. (1990) Sequential solid-phase assay for biotin based on ^{125}I-labeled avidin. *Methods Enzymol.* **184,** 224–233.
9. Bolton, A. E. and Hunter, W. M. (1973) The labeling of proteins to high specific radioactivity by conjugation to an ^{125}I-containing acylating agent. Applications to the radioimmunoassay. *Biochem. J.* **133,** 529–539.
10. Vaidyanathan, G., Affleck, D. J., and Zalutsky, M. R. (1993) Radioiodination of proteins using N-succinimidyl 4-hydroxy-3-iodobenzoate. *Bioconjugate Chem.* **4,** 78–84.
11. Vaidyanathan, G. and Zalutsky, M. R. (1990) Radioiodination of antibodies via N-succinimidyl 2,4-dimethoxy-3-(trialkylstannyl)benzoates. *Bioconjugate Chem.* **1,** 387–393.
12. Hylarides, M. D., Wilbur, D. S., Reed, M. W., Hadley, S. W., Schroeder, J. R., and Grant, L. M. (1991) Preparation and *in vivo* evaluation of an N-(p-^{125}I]iodophenethyl)maleimide-antibody conjugate. *Bioconjugate Chem.* **2,** 435–440.
13. Arano, Y., Wakisaka, K., Ohmomo, Y., Uezono, T., Mukai, T., Motonari, H., Shiono, H., Sakahara, H., Konishi, J., Tanaka, C., and Yokoyama, A. (1994) Maleimidoethyl 3-(tri-*n*-butylstannyl)hippurate: A useful radioiodination reagent for protein radiopharmaceuticals to enhance target selective radioactivity localization. *J. Med. Chem.* **37,** 2609–2618.
14. Willner, D., Trail, P. A., Hofstead, S. J., Dalton King, H., Lasch, S. J., Braslawsky, G. R., Greenfield, R. S., Kaneko, T., and Firestone, R. A. (1993) (6-Maleimidocaproyl)hydrazone of doxorubicin—A new derivative for the preparation of immunoconjugates of doxorubicin. *Bioconjugate Chem.* **4,** 521–527.
15. Arnold Jr., L. J. (1985) Polylysine-drug conjugates. *Methods Enzymol.* **112,** 270–285.
16. Pietersz, G. A. and McKenzie, I. F. (1992) Antibody conjugates for the treatment of cancer. *Immunol. Rev.* **129,** 57–80.
17. Orr, G. A. (1981) The use of the 2-iminobiotin–avidin interaction for the selective retrieval of labeled plasma membrane components. *J. Biol. Chem.* **256,** 761–766.
18. Dimroth, P. (1986) Preparation, characterization, and reconstitution of oxaloacetate decarboxylase from *Klebsiella aerogenes*, a sodium pump. *Methods Enzymol.* **125,** 530–540.
19. Dean, P. D. G., Johnson, W. S., and Middle, F. S. (1985) Activation procedures, in *Affinity Chromatography. A Practical Approach,* IRL, Washington, DC, pp. 34,35.
20. Kohanski, R. A. and Lane, D. (1990) Monovalent avidin affinity columns. *Methods Enzymol.* **184,** 194–220.
21. Chilkoti, A., Schwartz, B. L., Smith, R. D., Long, C. J., and Stayton, P. S. (1995) Engineered chimeric streptavidin tetramers as novel tools for bioseparations and drug delivery. *Bio/Technology* **13,** 1198–1204.
22. Wong, S. S. (1991) Reactive groups of proteins and their modifying agents, in *Chemistry of Protein Conjugation and Crosslinking,* CRC, Boston, MA, pp. 7–48.
23. Carlsson, J., Drevin, H., and Axen, R. (1978) Protein thiolation and reversible protein–protein conjugation. N-Succinimidyl 3-(2-pyridyldithio)propionate, a new heterobifunctional reagent. *Biochem. J.* **173,** 723–737.

24. Haugland, R. P. (1995) Coupling of monoclonal antibodies with fluorophores, in *Methods in Molecular Biology*, vol. 45 (Davis, W. C., ed.), Humana, Totowa, NJ, pp. 205–221.

25. Kronick, M. N. and Grossman, P. D. (1983) Immunoassay techniques with fluorescent phycobiliprotein conjugates. *Clin. Chem.* **29,** 1582–1586.

26. Bongartz, J.-P., Aubertin, A.-M., Milhaud, P. G., and Lebleu, B. (1994) Improved biological activity of antisense oligonucleotides conjugated to a fusogenic peptide. *Nucleic Acids Res.* **22,** 4681–4688.

19

Enhanced Chemiluminescence Immunoassay

Richard A. W. Stott

1. Introduction

Chemiluminescence results from reactions with a very high energy yield, which produce a potentially fluorescent product molecule; reaction energy passed to the product may result in an excited state and subsequent production of a single photon of light. The light yield is usually low, but can approach one photon per molecule in bioluminescent reactions catalyzed by dedicated enzymes.

A wide variety of immunoassay systems that use chemiluminescence or bioluminescence have been developed with the aim of detecting low concentrations of biologically active molecules. Even when emission efficiencies are <1%, chemiluminescence is a sensitive label detection method compared with isotopic methods in which very large numbers of molecules must be present for each detected disintegration (e.g., about 1×10^7 atoms of ^{125}I give 1 count/s). The production of light against a low background permits detection of small numbers of reacting molecules by measuring total light output. Luminescent emissions can be measured over a range of at least six orders of magnitude by all but the simplest luminometers. This is in marked contrast to fluorescent or spectrophotometric detection of reaction products, where sensitivity and instrument linear range are limited by the stability of light sources and wavelength selection. For example, a good spectrophotometer may achieve a linear range slightly greater than three orders of magnitude.

Directly labeled chemiluminescent systems produce <1 photon/label and require complex chemical synthesis to produce each new labeled molecule *(1,2)*. In contrast, chemiluminescent detection of enzyme labels combines the advantages of a high specific activity label with the convenience of relatively simple coupling chemistries, which use commercial reagents. A number of enzyme labels can be detected via chemiluminescent or bioluminescent reac-

From: *Methods in Molecular Biology, Vol. 80: Immunochemical Protocols, 2nd ed.*
Edited by: J. D. Pound © Humana Press Inc., Totowa, NJ

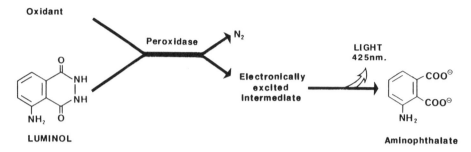

Fig. 1. Chemiluminescent oxidation of luminol by peroxidase.

tions, including β-galactosidase *(3)*, alkaline phosphatase *(4)*, peroxidase, luciferin and a variety of enzymes indirectly linked via production of ATP or NADH *(5)*. Systems that use alkaline phosphatase and peroxidase have the additional advantage of commercial availability of a wide range of labeled molecules and complete assay kits suitable for adaptation to luminescent detection.

Enhanced chemiluminescence is based on the reaction of luminol (3-aminophthalhydrazide) with an oxidizing agent, such as hydrogen peroxide or sodium perborate. This reaction is catalyzed by metal ions at high pH, resulting in emission of blue light (emission peak about 425 nm). At lower pH, the reaction is catalyzed by heme-containing enzymes, such as horseradish peroxidase, catalase, cytochrome C, and hemoglobin (Fig. 1). However, the light output is low with a half-life of a few seconds. The presence of any one of a series of "enhancer molecules" increases the light emission from horseradish peroxidase by 1000-fold or more, and alters the kinetics so that a steady glow is produced lasting several hours *(6,7)*. Microparticles, plastic beads, plastic tubes, microtiter plates, membranes, and plastic pins have all been used successfully as solid supports in a wide range of enhanced chemiluminescence assays, including competitive immunoassays, immunometric assays, and RNA and DNA binding assays *(6,8,9)*.

In common with all other sensitive detection systems, maintenance of the label enzyme in its active state is important. The precautions detailed in Notes 1–3 should be observed to maximize the sensitivity achieved. Reagents for enhanced chemiluminescence can be prepared in the laboratory or are available commercially (*see* Note 4). The purity of the substrate solution is important in achieving maximum sensitivity. Therefore, the precautions detailed in Notes 5–7 should be followed if preparing substrate solutions. The free base form of luminol undergoes rearrangement to a mixture of luminol and a series of contaminants. Therefore, luminol should be purified by recrystallization as the sodium salt before use (*see* Note 8).

1.1. Light Measurement Instruments (Luminometers)

Commercial luminometers range from low-cost manual single tube instruments to fully automated high-capacity machines and have been reviewed previously *(10)*. However, application-specific requirements are rarely discussed, and the first-time user will require some guidance in matching an instrument to the chemistry or chemistries to be used.

There is normally no requirement for wavelength selection, because very few reactions produce significant light output. Therefore, a simple luminometer can consist of a detector and some means of presenting a sample or samples in a light-tight compartment. There may also be a system for adding reagents to the sample while in the chamber. The detector is usually a photomultiplier tube for sensitive instruments, but can be a photodiode in a portable instrument *(7,11)* or photographic film, if a semiquantitative result is sufficient *(2,12)*.

Luminometers designed for use with short-lived reactions have complex high-precision reagent injection systems. There may also be a short measurement prior to reagent injection to correct for background owing to light leaks, phosphorescence, and scintillation from sample tubes. Photon-counting and cooled detectors may also be used to achieve maximal light-detection sensitivity. None of these features is essential for use with enhanced chemiluminescence.

Relatively high light intensities and prolonged emission are produced by enhanced chemiluminescence detection of peroxidase and the substituted dioxetane-based detection reactions for alkaline phosphatase or β-galactosidase *(3,4)*. These reactions require a short stabilizing time before reading and are conveniently performed by adding the reagents before the sample reaches the measuring position. This can only be done if any preinjection blank measurement can be disabled. It is also practical to handle large numbers of samples using a timed reagent addition outside the instrument, completely eliminating the need for automatic reagent handling. High light output can lead to "pulse pileup" in photon-counting electronics, resulting in nonlinearity and eventually zero apparent signal *(13)*. Linearity can be improved via mathematical correction for the dead time or insertion of a neutral density filter.

Although light output from individual transparent microtiter wells can be measured in a luminometer designed for tubes, it is more convenient to use opaque microtiter plate wells and one of the purpose-designed readers. Prolonged light output makes it possible to start the reaction outside the instrument in the same pattern as the light emission is read. However, the presence of other glowing wells introduces the possibility of light carryover into the well being read. Carryover is important if the dynamic range of light emissions from a plate is expected to be higher than three orders of magnitude; in this case,

Table 1
Carryover from a Single Glowing Well in a Rigid[a]
Black Microtiter Plate Measured Using a Prototype Luminometer

0.02%	0.01%	0.007%	ND	ND
0.04%	0.035%	0.018%	0.005%	ND
0.71%	0.075%	0.034%	0.007%	ND
Source	0.1%	0.03%	0.007%	ND
0.045%	0.034%	0.025%	0.006%	ND
0.03%	0.025%	0.013%	0.005%	ND
0.009%	0.009%	0.006%	ND	ND

[a]Data represent the mean of several readings obtained for empty wells expressed as a percentage of the mean light output of the source well. Positions marked ND gave readings that were not significantly different from the photomultiplier background.

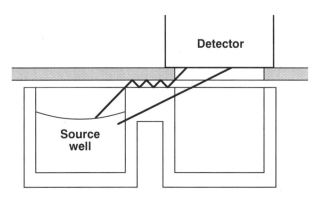

Fig. 2. Origin of light carryover between wells of an "opaque" microtiter plate.

there is a risk of false-positive results owing to a fraction of a percent of the emission from a very high sample being transmitted to a low one as much as three positions away (Table 1).

Both white and black microtiter plates are available in single-well, strip, and plate formats. The plastic is made opaque by incorporating colored particles into transparent plastic. Therefore, some light can pass through the plastic. The light transmission differs considerably between formats and individual manufacturers. However the greatest carryover occurs via external reflection from the shiny top surface (Fig. 2). Carryover is least for black plastic, although the loss of reflection within the well also reduces the signal available to the detector. Multiwell strips have higher carryover along the strip than between adjacent strips owing to the plastic web that links the wells. Similarly, individual wells have lower carryover than joined ones.

Carryover varies considerably between instruments, but it is particularly low if the instrument has an antireflection mask between the plate and detector. Individual instruments should be assessed for carryover using the type of plates that will be used with it. The pattern of carryover should be determined by reading light output from all wells of a plate containing a single glowing well with a light output, which represents the highest expected from the assay. The location of this well may affect the results, and carryover should be assessed using each corner well and one close to the center of the plate.

2. Materials

1. High-quality deionized water (*see* Note 3).
2. Luminol stock solution: 1.25 mM luminol in 0.1M Tris-HCl buffer, pH 8.6. Store at 4°C in the dark. Make up fresh each week. Luminol should be recrystallized as the sodium salt before use (*see* Note 8).
3. Hydrogen peroxide: 30% (w/v). Store at 4°C.
4. *p*-Iodophenol stock solution: *p*-iodophenol, 1 mg/mL in dimethyl sulfoxide (DMSO). Make up fresh each day.
5. Microfluor "B" microtiter plates (Dynatech Laboratories, Chantilly, VA).
6. Coating buffer: 0.1M glycine, pH 8.8. Adjust pH using NaOH. Store at 4°C, and make up fresh each week.
7. Rabbit anti-α fetoprotein (AFP) (Dako [Glostrup, Denmark] cat. no. A0008).
8. Phosphate-buffered saline (PBS), pH 7.2: 0.14M NaCl, 2.7 mM KCl, 1.5 mM KH_2PO_4, and 8.1 mM Na_2HPO_4. Store at 4°C, and make fresh each week.
9. Blocking solution: PBS containing bovine serum albumin (BSA) 0.1% (w/v). Make up fresh each day.
10. PBS-Tween: PBS containing Tween-20, 0.05% (v/v). Make an additional batch using high-quality deionized water (*see* Note 3). Store at 4°C, and make fresh each week.
11. Assay diluent: PBS-Tween containing BSA 0.5% (w/v). Make up fresh each day.
12. Working standards concentration range 0–800 ng/mL made fresh for each assay batch by serial dilution of stock standard using normal human serum. Stock standard (1600 ng/mL) is made by diluting AFP standard serum (Dako cat. no. X900 or Boehring Diagnostics [Westwood, MA] cat. no. OTOD 02/03) in human serum containing 0.05% (w/v) sodium azide. Store frozen as 1-mL aliquots.
13. Peroxidase-conjugated anti-AFP (Dako cat. no. P128) diluted 1/1000 in assay diluent. Make up fresh for each assay batch.
14. Working enhanced chemiluminescence substrate solution (*see* Note 9)—either:
    a. *p*-iodophenol-enhanced substrate: luminol 1.25 mM, *p*-iodophenol 4 μM, H_2O_2 2.7 mM). Add 15 μL of stock hydrogen peroxide and 40 mL of *p*-iodophenol stock solution to 50 mL of stock substrate solution,, and mix well. Make up daily using high-quality deionized water (*see* Note 3), and store in the dark when not in use, or
    b. *p*-Hydroxycinnamic acid-enhanced substrate (luminol 1.25 mM, *p*-hydroxycinnamic acid 30 μM, H_2O_2 2.7 mM). Add 15 mL of stock hydrogen peroxide

and 1 mg of *p*-hydroxycinnamic acid (alternative names: *p*-coumaric acid or 4-hydroxycinnamic acid, e.g., Aldrich [Gillingham, UK] cat. no. 2,320-7) to 50 mL of stock substrate solution. Mix for 30 min before using. Make up daily using high-quality deionized water (*see* Note 3), and store in the dark when not in use.

3. Method

1. Coat the wells of a microtiter plate with 100 mL of anti-AFP (1/1000 in coating buffer). Allow the protein to bind for either 2 h at room temperature or overnight at 4°C (*see* Note 10).
2. Empty the wells, and wash off any unbound antibody by filling each well with PBS and shaking the plate to re-empty. Repeat the wash and block unbound sites by incubating with 200 mL/well of blocking solution for 30 min at room temperature.
3. Empty the wells, and wash the plate twice (as described in step 2) with PBS-Tween to remove any unbound albumin.
4. Prepare 1/20 dilutions of samples, standards, and quality control specimens using assay diluent, and add 150 µL to each of the microtiter plate wells. Cover the plate with plastic film, and incubate at 37°C for 1 h.
5. Empty the wells, and wash the plate three times with PBS-Tween. Shake the plate over a sink to ensure complete removal of wash solution. Add 150 µL of working conjugate to each well, cover, and incubate at 37°C for 1 h.
6. Empty the wells, and wash the plate three times with PBS-Tween made using high-quality deionized water (*see* Note 3).
7. Add 150 µL of enhanced chemiluminescent substrate to each well in the same order and preferably with the same timing as used by the plate reader. Allow at least 2 min for the light output to stabilize before reading the plate.
8. Obtain unknown specimen results either by reading off a plotted calibration curve or use a computer program to calculate from a fitted curve.

4. Notes

1. Peroxidase is inactivated by anions and certain antimicrobial agents, including azide, cyanide, and thiomersal. Antimicrobial agents may be present in concentrated enzyme label solutions and assay buffers at typically active concentrations, but must not be present in wash solutions or substrate. The latter reagents must be freshly made each day from concentrated stocks.
2. Powerful oxidizing or reducing agents may interfere with any peroxidase detection reaction by inactivating peroxidase, oxidizing the substrates or reducing the oxidants in the reagents. There are potentially many of these in the laboratory environment, including chlorine in water, disinfectants, paper dust, laboratory coats, skin, and so forth. Care should be taken to avoid contamination of individual assay wells or equipment.
3. For best possible sensitivity, the final assay wash (step 6) and all substrate reagents should be made up in water of the highest possible purity. Trace contamination with bacteria, algae, organic compounds, and chlorine is a particular problem.

Laboratory-grade distilled or reverse osmosis water should be further treated using a deionization cartridge. The water plant must be well maintained to avoid bacterial growth in deionization columns, plumbing, and storage tanks. Alternatively, commercial HPLC-grade water has been found to be satisfactory.

4. Amerlite signal reagent (Johnson and Johnson Clinical Diagnostics) is supplied as separate bottles of buffer and substrate tablets. One "A" and one "B" substrate tablet (cat. no. LAN.4401) are dissolved in each bottle of substrate buffer (cat. no. LAN. 4402) prior to use. This reagent is stable for a day at room temperature providing it is kept in the dark glass bottle.

5. In order to ensure stable concentrations, the anhydrous form of sodium luminol is preferred molecular weight 199.1. This should be stored over silica gel in the dark. Luminol solutions should be stored in the dark at 4°C. Stock solutions must be made up at least weekly and working substrate daily.

6. DMSO is a colorless, odorless compound. However, it is hygroscopic and acquires an onion-like smell. DMSO in this state has been found to be inhibitory in the enhanced chemiluminescent reaction. Therefore, the highest available grade should be purchased in small amounts and carefully stored to minimize water uptake.

7. Hydrogen peroxide is a powerful oxidant, but gradually loses activity. The highest available grade should be purchased in small amounts, and stored at 4°C.

8. Luminol is available as the free base under alternative chemical names from several chemical suppliers, including:
   a. 5-Amino-2,3-dihydro-1,4-phthalazinedione (Sigma [St. Louis, MO], cat. no. A 8511P).
   b. 3-Aminophthalhydrazide (Aldrich cat. no. 12,307-2).
   There is considerable batch to batch variability in commercial luminol. The purity of the original material is only important in determining how many recrystallization steps are required. Recrystallization gives a consistently high activity product and may be performed as follows (for further details, *see* ref. *7*):
   a. Dissolve luminol in 5% (w/v) sodium hydroxide at room temperature until close to saturation (about 200 g/L). The color of this solution will depend on the original luminol. Cool the solution in an ice bath and allow to crystallize for 4 h. Recover the sodium luminol crystals using suction filtration on a glass fiber filter disk (Whatman GFA or similar), and wash using a small volume of ice-cold 5% sodium hydroxide. The crystals should be white or only slightly discolored. Sodium luminol should be recrystallized at least twice after a white product is obtained.
   b. Dissolve the sodium luminol in a minimum volume of 5% sodium hydroxide at room temperature. Allow to crystallize on an ice bath for 18 h. A refrigerator can be used as an alternative, although crystallization may be slower and yield may be low. Recover the crystals by filtration as above.
   The initial crystalline form is the hexa-hydrate, which converts to an anhydrous powder on drying over silica gel. Sodium luminol is stable to heat (melting point >400°C), but undergoes photochemical reactions and should be stored in the dark.

Sodium luminol has recently become available from Sigma (cat. no. A 4685). The author has no experience with this product.

9. The substrate solutions detailed here (Section 2., item 14) are essentially interchangeable with no sensitivity advantage for either. Both systems are optimized for a reasonably steady light output at a peroxidase concentrations typically encountered in immunoassays. Use of final peroxidase activities that are markedly higher will result in declining light output owing to substrate exhaustion. This cannot be avoided by alteration of the reaction conditions. Slight reduction in enhancer concentration may give more stable light output for assays with atypically low peroxidase activity.

10. For best results, plates should be coated with the IgG fraction of an antiserum, this can be conveniently prepared using caprylic acid precipitation (*see* Chapter 10 and ref. *15*). Where this is not possible, indirect capture may be used, such as antispecies antibody on the plate, or the streptavidin–biotin system. Any indirect capture system must be compatible with the final label, e.g., labeled antigen or different species antisera with no crossreaction with the indirect coating antibody.

11. Safety data (from ref. *16*):
    a. Luminol (commercial-grade): Irritating to eyes, respiratory system, and skin. No specific information is available for pure luminol or for the sodium salt.
    b. Hydrogen peroxide: Contact with combustible materials may cause fire. Causes burns. Keep in a cool place. After contact with skin, wash immediately with plenty of water.
    c. DMSO: Irritant to eyes, skin, and respiratory system. Harmful by inhalation, skin contact, and if swallowed. May cause sensitization by inhalation or skin contact.
    d. *p*-Iodophenol: Irritant to eyes, skin, and respiratory system.
    e. *p*-Hydroxycinnamic acid: Irritant to eyes, skin, and respiratory system.

References

1. Zomer, G., Stavenuiter, J. F. C., Van Den Berg, R. H., and Jansen, E. H. J. M. (1991) Synthesis, chemiluminescence and stability of acridinium ester labeled compounds, in *Luminescence Techniques in Chemical and Biochemical Analysis* (Bayens, W. R. G., De Kekeleire, D., and Korkidis, K., eds.), Dekker, New York, pp. 505–521.
2. Jansen, E. H. J. M., Zomer, G., and Van Peteghem, C. H. (1991) Chemiluminescence immunoassays in vetinary and food analysis, in *Luminescence Techniques in Chemical and Biochemical Analysis* (Bayens, W. R. G., De Kekeleire, D., and Korkidis, K., eds.), Dekker, New York, pp. 477–504.
3. Bronstein, I. and McGrath, P. (1989) Chemiluminescence lights up. *Nature* **333,** 599,600.
4. Bronstein, I., Voyta, J. C., Thorpe, G. H. G., Kricka, L. J., and Armstrong, G. (1989) Chemiluminescent assay of alkaline phosphatase applied in an ultrasensitive enzyme immunoassay of thyrotropin. *Clin. Chem.* **35,** 1441–1446.
5. Bronstein, I. and Kricka, L. J. (1989) Clinical applications of luminescent assays for enzymes and enzyme labels. *J. Clin. Lab. Anal.* **3,** 316–322.

6. Thorpe, G. H. G. and Kricka, L. J. (1986) Enhanced chemiluminescent reactions catalyzed by horseradish peroxidase. *Methods Enzymol.* **133,** 331–354.

7. Kricka, L. J., Stott, R. A. W., and Thorpe, G. H. G. (1991) Enhanced chemiluminescent detection of horseradish peroxidase labels in ligand binder assays, in *Luminescence Techniques in Chemical and Biochemical Analysis* (Bayens, W. R. G., De Kekeleire, D., and Korkidis, K., eds.), Dekker, New York, pp. 599–635.

8. Thorpe, G. H. G., Stott, R. A. W., Sankolli, G. M., Catty, D., Raykundalia, C., Roda, A. and Kricka, L. J. (1987) Solid supports and photodetectors in enhanced chemiluminescent immunoassays, in *Bioluminescence and Chemiluminescence. New Perspectives* (Scholmerich, J., Andreesen, R., Kapp, M., and Woods, W. G., eds.), Wiley, Chichester, UK, pp. 209–213.

9. Matthews, J. A., Batki, A., Hynds, C., and Kricka, L. J. (1985) Enhanced chemiluminescent method for the detection of DNA dot-hybridization assays. *Analytical Biochem.* **151,** 205–209.

10. Stanley, P. E. (1992) A survey of more than 90 commercially available luminometers and imaging devices for low light measurements of chemiluminescence and bioluminescence, including instruments for manual, automatic and specialized operation, for HPLC, LC, GLC, and microtiter plates. Part 1 Descriptions. *J. Bioluminescence Chemiluminescence* **7,** 77–108.

11. Marks, K., Killeen, P. R., Goundry, J., Gibbons, J. E. C., and Bunce, R. A. (1987) A portable silicon photodiode luminometer. *J. Bioluminescence Chemiluminescence* **1,** 173–179.

12. Kricka, L. J. and Thorpe, G. H. G. (1986) Photographic detection of chemiluminescent and bioluminescent reactions. *Methods Enzymol.* **133,** 404–420.

13. Stott, R. A. W., Moseley, S. B., Williams, L. A., Thorpe, G. H. G. and Kricka, L. J. (1987) Enhanced chemiluminescent quantitation of horseradish peroxidase labels in commercial EIA kits using a modified Berthold LB950T, in *Bioluminescence and Chemiluminescence. New Perspectives* (Scholmerich, J., Andreesen, R., Kapp, M., and Woods, W. G., eds.), Wiley, Chichester, UK, pp. 249–252.

14. Stott, R. A. W. and Kricka, L. J. (1987) Purification of luminol for use in enhanced chemiluminescence immunoassay, in *Bioluminescence and Chemiluminescence. New Perspectives* (Scholmerich, J., Andreesen, R., Kapp, M., and Woods, W. G., eds.), Wiley, Chichester, UK, pp. 237–240.

15. Steinbuch, M. and Audran, R. (1969) The isolation of IgG from mammalian sera with the aid of caprylic acid. *Arch. Biochem. Biophys.* **134,** 279–284.

16. Lenga, R. E. and Votoupal, K. L. (eds.) (1993) *The Sigma-Aldrich Library of Regulatory and Safety Data.* Sigma-Aldrich Corporation.

20

Nonradioactive Methods
for Visualization of Protein Blots

Michael Finney

1. Introduction

The ability to detect specific proteins that have been immobilized on nitrocellulose or polyvinylidene difluoride (PVDF) membranes has become an invaluable technique in all areas of the biological sciences. In the past, visualization of low-abundance proteins required the use of radioactive markers, such as [125]Iodine, but with the advent of enhanced chemiluminescent technology and amplified colorimetric detection, this is no longer the case *(1–3)*. This chapter details two of the more popular nonradioactive methods for immobilized protein detection, both of which rely on the indirect labeling of specific proteins with enzyme-linked antibodies. The location and abundance of these enzyme markers are then realized in a reaction producing a colored end product or by the generation of light in a chemiluminescent reaction. These techniques can identify <20 pg of protein.

Transfer of proteins onto nitrocellulose or PVDF membranes is usually performed after separation of complex protein mixtures by polyacrylamide gel electrophoresis (PAGE). Proteins can be separated on the basis of their molecular weight or isoelectric point, under reducing or nonreducing conditions, and it is therefore for the investigator to establish the most appropriate separation conditions for particular samples. Full details of PAGE can be found in refs. *4* and *5*, and the reader is encouraged to use these as sources of further details.

The transfer of proteins from the gel to the membrane is achieved by laying a sheet of nitrocellulose or PVDF on the side of the gel and applying an electrical current across the two surfaces *(6)*. Proteins migrate toward the anode and move onto the membrane where they irreversibly bind to its surface. The spatial separation achieved during electrophoresis is therefore retained in an immo-

From: *Methods in Molecular Biology, Vol. 80: Immunochemical Protocols, 2nd ed.*
Edited by: J. D. Pound © Humana Press Inc., Totowa, NJ

bilized and accessible form. The method of choice for this transfer uses a semidry blotter that allows rapid transfer with the use of only a small amount of buffer (*7,8; see* Note 1). Once transfer is complete, the blot can be processed immediately or can be dried and stored dry for up to 3 mo at 4°C before being analyzed (*see* Note 2).

The visualization of specific proteins on such blots typically involves four stages:

1. Blocking any surplus binding capacity on the membrane.
2. Incubation with a specific primary antibody.
3. Incubation with an enzyme-linked secondary antibody.
4. Treatment with a chemical substrate to reveal the location of the enzyme marker.

The first visualization procedure detailed here indirectly labels the immobilized protein with alkaline phosphatase. The location of this enzyme is then revealed by treatment with a chromogenic substrate containing 5-bromo-4-chloro-3-indolylphosphate (BCIP) and nitroblue tetrazolium (NBT), which produces a purple insoluble end product *(3)*. The second uses horseradish peroxidase (HRP) as the enzyme marker that is subsequently visualized by treating the membrane with a commercially available solution (Amersham's ECL™ system [Amersham, Bucks, UK]) containing luminol, hydrogen peroxide, and phenol-based enhancers, and results in the generation of light *(2,9)*. The position and intensity of this light are then measured using photographic film.

2. Materials

2.1. Semidry Transfer

1. Membranes: Two types of membrane can be used (*see* Note 3).
    a. Nitrocellulose: Nitrocellulose membranes have been traditionally used in protein blotting procedures but suffer from being brittle and difficult to handle. A suitable alternative is supported nitrocellulose (such as Hybond™C-extra or Hybond C-super, Amersham International [Amersham]), which contains an inert matrix that makes the membrane more robust. Many suppliers also provide nitrocellulose that has been optimized for use with chemiluminescent visualization procedures (such as Hybond-ECL, Amersham); this type tends not to be of this supported type. Nitrocellulose membranes need to be soaked in buffer (transfer or TST, whichever is appropriate) for 5 min to wet the surface before being used.
    b. PVDF: PVDF (such as Immobilon™-P, Millipore [Bedford, MA]) is the material of choice for protein blotting owing to its strength and protein binding characteristics. PVDF suffers from being extremely hydrophobic and, therefore, requires prewetting with 100% methanol for a few seconds before being washed in four changes of distilled water (20 s/wash). These water washes replace the methanol within the membrane and allow aqueous solu-

tions access to the membrane surface. PVDF membranes must be treated in this way before proteins are transferred to its surface, and it is recommended that the blot not be allowed to dry out before visualization is complete. If drying does occur (e.g., for storage after transfer; *see* Note 2) the membrane must be wet once more with 100% methanol for a few seconds, and the methanol then washed out with distilled water before proceeding with the visualization process *(10)*.

2. Transfer buffer: 25 mM Tris, 150 mM glycine, 20% (v/v) methanol. The pH of this solution will be around 8.5 and does not need to be adjusted. Approx 200 mL of buffer are required for each transfer. The solution is stable for 2–4 wk at room temperature in a sealed container. Alternatively, the buffer can be made up without methanol (i.e., as 31.2 mM Tris, 187.5 mM glycine) and the methanol added to 20% just before use. This solution is stable for 6 mo at room temperature.

2.2. General Blotting Procedure

1. Tris/saline/Tween™ (TST): 0.1 M NaCl, 10 mM Tris, pH 7.5, 0.05% Tween-20 (polyoxyethylenesorbitan monolaurate). Dissolve NaCl and Tris in 4/5 of the final volume of distilled water and adjust pH to 7.5 with HCl. Add Tween-20, mix, and make up to the final volume with distilled water. Approximately 1 L is required/blot. The solution is stable for 3 mo at room temperature.

2. Blocking buffer: 5% (w/v) freeze-dried nonfat milk (e.g., "Marvel," Premier Beverages, Stafford, UK) in TST. Make up fresh as required. The quality of the dried milk is important, since some brands contain significant amounts of fat (*see* Note 4).

3. Primary and secondary antibodies: The choice of primary antibody depends on what specific antisera are available for the protein of interest; both monoclonal antibodies (MAbs) and polyclonal antibodies are suitable. Choice of secondary antibody is more important: this must be matched for the primary reagent in terms of species recognition. If, for example, the primary antibody is a mouse monoclonal IgG1, the secondary antibody must be from another species (such as rabbit) and raised against murine IgG1. Secondary antibodies are usually available as a variety of conjugates, linked either to marker enzymes or to biotin. Biotinylated antibodies are subsequently visualized using enzyme-linked streptavidin. Most commercial suppliers of primary antibodies can provide suitable matched secondary antibodies (*see* Note 5).

4. Additional equipment: rocking table, plastic bag sealer, and a number of plastic containers in which to perform the membrane washes (*see* Note 6).

2.3. Colorimetric Visualization of Alkaline Phosphatase (AP) Labels

1. AP staining buffer: 0.1M NaCl, 0.1M Tris, pH 9.5, 50 mM MgCl$_2$. Dissolve Tris and NaCl in distilled water (4/5 final volume), adjust pH to 9.5 with HCl. Make up a small stock solution of 4M MgCl$_2$ in distilled water (e.g., 50 mL), and add the appropriate amount to the staining buffer (12.5 mL/L). Make up to the final volume with distilled water and store at room temperature. Stable for 6 mo.

2. NBT stock solution: 75 mg/mL in 70% dimethylformamide (DMF). Stable if stored at 4°C in a dark container.

3. BCIP stock solution: 50 mg/mL in 100% DMF. Stable if stored at 4°C in a dark container. Solubility of BCIP in DMF is minimal, but a white slurry is produced.

2.4. Chemiluminescent Visualization
of Horseradish Peroxidase (HRP) Labels

1. A number of kits are available that provide the various reagents required for chemiluminescent visualization. The most popular of these, the ECL™ kit from Amersham (cat. No. RPN 2109), is the one described here, but others, designed for use with AP labels, are also available (Aurora™ from ICN [Thame, UK] and Immun-lite™ from Bio-Rad [Hemel Hempstead, UK]). All of these come with comprehensive instructions.

2. Additional materials: "Cling-film" (*see* Note 7), an autoradiography cassette and autoradiography film (*see* Note 8). Access to a darkroom is also required along with film-processing facilities (*see* Note 9).

3. Methods

The following procedures are summarized in Fig. 1.

3.1. Semidry Transfer

N.B. Always wear gloves when handling blotting membranes to prevent the transfer of protein from fingers onto the membrane surface.

1. Remove the gel from the electrophoresis apparatus, and remove any stacking gel that may be present. Measure the size of the gel, and transfer it to a container for incubation with transfer buffer for 15 min. This incubation is to equilibrate the gel in the new buffer and to reduce the level of SDS, since this reduces the binding of protein to the membrane. Gels >1-mm thick will require a 30-min incubation in transfer buffer for this equilibration to take place.

2. Cut six sheets of Whatman 3MM filter paper to the same dimensions as the gel, and soak them in transfer buffer.

3. Cut a sheet of nitrocellulose or PVDF membrane to the same dimensions as the gel and prewet the membrane (*see* Section 2.1.). Equilibrate in transfer buffer.

4. Assemble the transfer sandwich as in Fig. 2. It is important to exclude any air bubbles from the various layers, since these can reduce transfer efficiency.

    Place three soaked sheets of filter paper on the anode, one on top of the other. The sheets should be saturated, but not dripping with excess buffer. Place the sheet of wet membrane on top of the filter paper stack and cover with the gel. Roll a glass rod (or similar) over the surface of the gel to push out any air bubbles, and to ensure good contact between the gel and the membrane. Finally, place the three remaining sheets of soaked filter paper on top of the gel.

5. Rest the cathode plate on top of the sandwich, making sure it is sitting flat, and connect the assembly to the power supply.

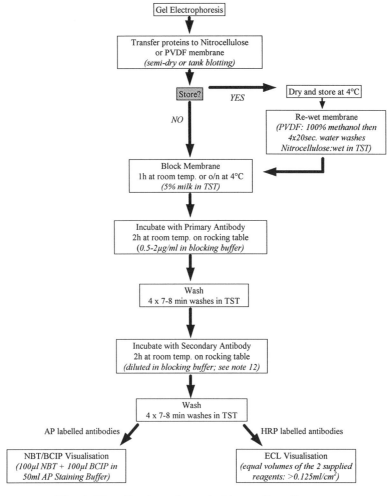

Fig. 1. Visualization of protein blots—flow diagram.

Set the supply to deliver 0.75–1.0 mA/cm^2 membrane constant current for 1 h, and turn the supply on. The voltage will start between 5 and 10 V but will gradually rise throughout the course of the run.

6. Turn off the power after 1 h, and remove the cathode plate. Remove the membrane from the sandwich.
7. Rinse the membrane briefly in transfer buffer or distilled water. The membrane can be reversibly stained with Ponceau S to confirm the transfer of protein (*see* Note 10).
8. If the membrane is to be stored at this stage place it between 2 sheets of filter paper (Whatman 3MM) to dry and store at 4°C (*see* Note 2). If not stored, continue straight on to the next stage (Section 3.2., step 2): Do not allow the blot to dry out.

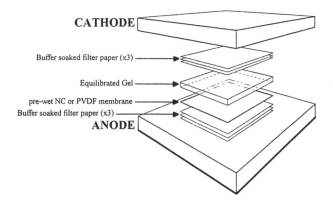

Fig. 2. Semidry blotting assembly.

3.2. General Blotting Procedure

1. If the membrane is dry, prewet it as appropriate (*see* Section 2.1.).
2. Place the blot in blocking buffer (>1 mL/cm² membrane), and incubate on a rocking table for 1 h at room temperature or overnight at 4°C, whichever is more convenient.
3. Dilute the primary antibody in blocking buffer to give a final concentration between 0.5 and 2 μg/mL (*see* Note 11).
4. Incubate the blot in the primary antibody solution for 2 h at room temperature with continuous agitation provided by a rocking table.
5. Decant the primary antibody solution and wash the membrane for 30 min in four changes of TST (i.e., 4 × 7–8 min washes; *see* Note 12). Do not economize on the volume of TST used—the membrane must be thoroughly washed.
6. Dilute the enzyme-conjugated secondary antibody in blocking buffer. Follow any recommendations that may be provided by the supplier regarding antibody dilution (*see* Note 13).
7. Incubate the blot in the secondary antibody solution for 2 h at room temperature with continuous agitation provided by a rocking table.
8. Decant and discard the secondary antibody solution and wash the membrane for 30 min in four changes of TST (i.e., 4 × 7–8 min washes). Again, washing must be thorough. The blot is then ready for visualization. Do not store the blot at this stage.

3.3. Colorimetric Visualization
of Alkaline Phosphatase (AP) Labels

1. Vortex mix the NBT and BCIP stock solutions, and add 100 μL of each to 50 mL AP staining buffer. When pipeting BCIP, it is useful to snip off the end of the pipet tip to widen its bore.
2. Rinse the blot briefly in staining buffer (15 s) before submerging it in the staining solution. Cover the container in aluminum foil to block out any light. AP reactions can develop quite slowly, and it may take an hour or more before an acceptable

level of staining is reached. If the staining solution turns from yellow to purple, replace it with some fresh staining solution.

3. Stop the reaction by pouring off and discarding the staining solution, and rinse the membrane briefly in two changes of distilled water. The membrane can then be dried between filter paper and, once dry, can be photographed for a permanent record. The image will remain on the blot if it is stored in the dark, but otherwise will fade with time.

3.4. Chemiluminescent Visualization of HRP Labels

1. Mix equal volumes of the two supplied solutions to give a final volume of at least 0.125 mL/cm² of membrane, and place the solution in a tray roughly the same size as the membrane. There must be sufficient detection reagent to cover the bottom of the container; add more reagent if necessary.

    N.B. Perform the following operations in a darkroom (lights can be on for the following three steps).

2. Drain off any excess wash buffer from the membrane, and place it in the detection reagent for 1 min. It is important that the membrane be completely covered by the reagent.

3. Lift the membrane out of the detection reagent, and drain off any excess. Place protein face down on a flat piece of cling-film, and gently wrap over the edges of the cling-film sheet to enclose the membrane.

4. Turn the wrapped membrane over (protein side up), place in an autoradiography cassette, and gently smooth out any air bubbles that may be between the membrane and the cling-film.

5. Turn off the lights (red safe lights can be on), and place a sheet of autoradiography film over the wrapped membrane for 10 s.

6. Remove the film and process immediately as usual (*see* Note 9).

7. Examine the resulting image and assess how long to expose a subsequent piece of film (*see* Note 14).

4. Notes

1. Semidry blotting has a number of advantages over the traditional tank blotting procedure. First, the length of time required to perform the transfer is greatly reduced (approx 1 h), and the electrical current required is much smaller (<1 mA/cm² membrane). These currents can be supplied by a standard electrophoresis power supply, thus avoiding the requirement for a dedicated supply. Also, because of this reduced current requirement, the temperature of transfer is low; there is no need to have special cooling arrangements. A number of suppliers provide semidry blotting equipment (Sigma [Poole, UK], Millipore, Bio-Rad, Hoefer [Pharmacia, Milton Keynes, UK]), all of which come with full instructions.

    If tank blotting equipment is the only option available, then perfectly acceptable results can be obtained. Recommended conditions for tank blotting are overnight transfer (>8 h) at 0.2 A (50 V) with water cooling in Tris/glycine/20% methanol transfer buffer (*see* Section 2.1.).

2. The length of time that blots can be stored dry depends on the nature of the antigens of interest. Some proteins can degrade slowly even when stored at 4°C, and this is particularly evident with proteins losing posttranslational modifications (such as phosphorylation). This may or may not be important depending on whether the modified motif is within the antigenic site, but of course is crucial if probing for phosphoproteins with an antiphospho-amino acid antibody (such as antiphosphotyrosine). It is advisable to use fresh blots wherever possible.

3. Nylon membranes are not recommended for protein blotting, since they almost always suffer from high background staining.

4. Membrane blocking: This is an essential step to prevent the nonspecific binding of antibodies to the membrane surface. Other proteins can be used as the basis of this solution, such as 1–10% bovine serum albumin (BSA) in TST or 0.5–3% gelatin in TST if preferred, although the time, concentration, and temperature of the blocking step would need to be optimized. Increasing the temperature of the blocking step to 37°C decreases the time required for effective blocking.

5. Some suppliers provide enzyme-linked primary antibodies that can be used in these protocols, thus avoiding the necessity for a secondary antibody incubation. This does reduce the length of time required for the procedure, but does have some disadvantages with regard to sensitivity. The treatment with a secondary antibody does provide a degree of amplification in the system that allows detection of smaller amounts of protein. Also, the choice of visualization procedure is limited to the enzyme type conjugated to the primary antibody.

6. Plastic sandwich boxes make good containers for blot washing, but often have a much larger base area than the size of the membrane. It is useful to have a few containers that have a base of similar dimensions to the membrane, so that incubations can be carried out in as small a volume as possible. Incubations with antibody solutions can be performed in heat-sealed plastic bags (*see* Note 11), but this is not practical for other steps, particularly incubations with visualization solutions. Lids from pipet tip holders make suitable containers for small blots from minigels.

7. Most brands of laboratory cling-film are satisfactory for use in the ECL procedure, although Amersham particularly recommends SaranWrap™. Some brands can quench the light-generating reaction, so if a weak signal is consistently obtained, it may be worth checking other brands of cling-film.

8. Standard autoradiography film can be used to visualize ECL reactions, although Amersham does provide a number of products that have been optimized for use in this procedure. Hyperfilm™-ECL and Hyperpaper™-ECL are both recommended. Please note that Hyperpaper-ECL has photographic emulsion on only one side, so the appropriate side must be exposed to the membrane (the emulsion side has a glossy appearance).

Membranes can be labeled with phosphorescent tape (Sigma, cat. no. L5149), which can be written on with a permanent black marker. This produces a negative image of the writing on the film.

9. Exposed film can be developed manually or using an automated processor. With automated processors, it is advisable to transfer the exposed film to an empty autoradiography cassette for transport to the machine. Manual processing can be achieved with standard chemicals (e.g., Kodak GBX developer and fixer for film, Kodak Dektol developer and fixer for paper; available from Sigma).

10. Blots can be reversibly stained with Ponceau S to confirm transfer has taken place. This must be done before the blocking stage, since after this, the membrane is saturated with protein. This is not a highly sensitive stain—only major bands are revealed.

   Make up a staining solution of 0.1% (w/v) Ponceau S (Sigma, cat. no. P3504) in 5% acetic acid and a destain solution of 0.1M NaOH.

   After transfer is complete, wash the membrane in the stain solution for 3–5 min. Pour off the stain (it can be reused until no longer effective), and wash the membrane in four to five changes of distilled water (2 min/wash). The red background will wash away leaving red-stained bands visible. The position of any molecular weight markers can be noted (N.B.: Not all the markers may be revealed).

   To destain the blot, cover with 0.1M NaOH. As soon as the bands disappear (after turning purple), tip off the alkali and wash the membrane thoroughly in four changes of distilled water. This treatment may result in a slight loss of protein from the membrane but losses are not usually significant if the procedure is carried out rapidly.

11. The volume of antibody solution required depends on the size of the blot and the container in which the incubation will occur. Incubation in heat-sealed plastic bags can significantly reduce the required volume, with a blot from a minigel (8.5 × 5.5 cm) needing only 5 mL of primary antibody solution when incubated in this way. If you are unsure of what volume is required, then seal the membrane (or one of the same size) in a plastic bag with a volume of TST, and check that there is enough fluid to cover the membrane.

   For sealing membranes into bags it is easiest to cut two sheets of plastic and place one underneath and one on top of the membrane. Heat seal around three sides to make a bag, add the incubation solution, remove any air bubbles and seal the fourth side.

12. The primary antibody solution can be saved and reused two to three times within the following 2 wk if stored at 4°C, and no bacterial growth is evident. It is not advisable to use sodium azide as an antimicrobial agent, particularly when using HRP-labeled antibodies: azide inhibits peroxidase reactions.

13. The appropriate dilution required for a particular secondary antibody needs to be established empirically, but usually falls in the range of 1/2000–1/20,000. Higher concentrations often lead to unacceptable background staining. It is advisable to run a gel of some control samples so that the appropriate dilution can be established. Run a number of lanes of a control sample interspersed with prestained molecular weight markers on a gel, and then transfer the protein to a membrane. The membrane can then be cut into strips along the prestained marker lanes, and the strips blocked and treated with primary antibody. After washing, the strips

can be incubated with different concentrations of secondary antibody (suggested dilutions: 1/1000, 1/2500, 1/5000, 1/10000, 1/20,000) and then visualized in the appropriate way. Select the dilution that gives the maximum signal with the minimum background. Even higher dilutions may be optimal for HRP/ECL visualization.

14. If the image is very faint (or absent), it may be necessary to expose another piece of film for up to an hour. If the image is overexposed, it may be necessary to wait for 5–10 min before exposing another piece of film to allow the light intensity to reduce.

    If the background is high, even with a short exposure, then it may be necessary to wash the membrane a few more times. Remove the membrane from its cling-film wrapper, and wash it in three changes of TST (3 × 5 min washes). Drain off excess wash buffer, and submerge the blot in the detection reagent for 1 min. Wrap in a fresh piece of cling-film, and expose another sheet of film. Higher dilutions of secondary antibody may be required if the background is still high (*see* Note 13).

References

1. Whitehead, T. P., Thorpe, G. H. G, Carter, T. J. N., Groucutt, C., and Kricka, L. J. (1983) Enhanced luminescence procedure for sensitive determination of peroxidase-labeled conjugates in immunoassay. *Nature* **305,** 158,159.
2. Thorpe, G. H. G. and Kricka, L. J. (1986) Enhanced chemiluminescent reactions catalysed by horseradish peroxidase. *Methods Enzymol.* **133,** 331–353.
3. Pluzek, K.-J. and Ramlau, J. (1988) Alkaline phosphatase labeled reagents, in *CRC Handbook of Immunoblotting of Proteins,* vol. 1, *Technical Descriptions* (Bjerrum, O. J. and Heegaard N. H. H., eds.), CRC, Boca Ration, FL, pp. 177–188.
4. Laemmli, U. K. (1970) Cleavage of structural proteins during the assembly of the head of bacteriophage T4. *Nature* **227,** 680–685.
5. Hames, B. D. and Rickwood, D. (eds.) (1990) *Gel Electrophoresis of Proteins,* 2nd ed., IRL, Oxford, UK.
6. Towbin, H., Staehelin, T., and Gordon, J. (1979) Electrophoretic transfer of proteins from polyacrylamide gels to nitrocellulose sheets: procedure and some applications. *Proc. Natl. Acad. Sci. USA* **76,** 4350–4354.
7. Kyhse-Anderson, J. (1984) Electroblotting of multiple gels: a simple apparatus without buffer tank for rapid transfer of proteins from polyacrylamide to nitrocellulose. *J. Biochem. Biophys. Methods* **10,** 203–209.
8. Lauriere, M. (1993) A semidry electroblotting system efficiently transfers both high-molecular-weight and low-molecular-weight proteins separated by SDS-PAGE. *Anal. Biochem.* **212,** 206–211.
9. "ECL™ western blotting protocols" Amersham International plc. Bucks, UK.
10. Millipore Technical Protocols 006/007 (1987) Millipore Corporation, Bedford, MA.

21

Colloidal Gold Staining and Immunoprobing on the Same Western Blot

Denise Egger and Kurt Bienz

1. Introduction

Proteins, blotted from polyacrylamide gels onto nitrocellulose sheets (Western blots) can be stained nonspecifically with a variety of dyes, or they can be identified individually by probing with appropriate antibodies. These procedures may be performed on duplicate blots, staining the total protein pattern on one blot and using the second blot for the immune reaction *(1,2)*. This chapter describes how to combine both methods on one blot, i.e., staining the blot first for total protein, followed by an indirect immune reaction *(3)*.

Possible applications of this method include:

1. Viewing the blot for artifacts, resolution, and so on, before probing with a (precious) antibody;
2. Cutting out the desired region for immunoprobing (e.g., in screening monoclonal antibodies);
3. Locating immunoreactive proteins or protein A-containing fusion proteins on the blot in relation to the total protein pattern of a given sample;
4. Testing the degree of purity obtained during purification of a protein. Examples are shown in Fig. 1.

The simultaneous demonstration of the whole protein pattern and the individual immunoreactive proteins on one single blot can be achieved in two different ways: Either the immune reaction is performed first and the total protein stain is applied afterward. This method, using "AuroDye" (formerly obtainable from Janssen, Belgium, now from Amersham, UK, or Aurion, Wageningen, Holland) as a protein stain, is described in detail in *Methods in Molecular Biology*, Volume 3, Chapter 34. Or, as presented here, the blot is first stained for total protein, using colloidal gold (referred to as "citrate gold"

From: *Methods in Molecular Biology, Vol. 80: Immunochemical Protocols, 2nd ed.*
Edited by: J. D. Pound © Humana Press Inc., Totowa, NJ

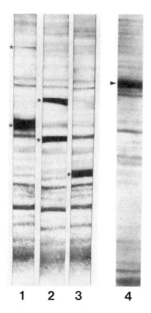

Fig. 1. Examples of Western blots stained with colloidal gold for total protein followed by immunostaining of individual antigens. Lanes 1–3: Proteins on a Western blot from a cytoplasmic extract of poliovirus-infected HEp-2 cells were stained with colloidal gold. The probing monoclonal antibodies, recognizing the viral proteins VP1 and precursor, VPO and VP2, and VP3, respectively, are detected by peroxidase-coupled rabbit-antimouse antibody (asterisks). Lane 4: Western blot of an *E. coli* lysate, containing a fusion protein composed of protein A and the poliovirus protein 2B. The fusion protein (arrowhead) is detected on the gold-stained blot by peroxidase-coupled IgG that binds to the protein A moiety.

because of the method of preparation) and then, after blocking free protein binding sites on the nitrocellulose as usual, the immune reaction is performed.

In deciding which method to use, the following differences should be considered: in contrast to the "AuroDye" method, in which only Tween-20 can be used to block free binding sites on the nitrocellulose, the citrate gold method allows for optimal blocking with one of a variety of proteins (gelatin, ovalbumin, milk powder, and so on) or Tween-20. This often results in a much lower background and preserves the highest possible immunoreactivity. Even more important is that the two gold preparations differ at least 30-fold in their sensitivity for protein staining. This should be kept in mind when the relative amount of immunoreactive antigen in the protein mixture under study is small and, therefore, a large amount of total protein has to be loaded on the gel to obtain enough antigen on the blot for immunological detection. In this case, the lower sensitivity of the citrate gold is preferable over "AuroDye" in order not to overstain the blot and to obtain clear staining of the protein bands. The immunoreactivity of the blotted proteins after staining with citrate gold is qualitatively and quantitatively the same as in unstained blots. Using peroxidase-labeled antibody for the immune reaction, a blue reaction product is obtained that contrasts well with the red stained protein pattern, and allows an easy documentation, even by black and white photography.

2. Materials

1. Colloidal gold: This can be prepared by the citrate method ("citrate gold") (*see also* Chapter 29) using gold chloride and sodium citrate. $H(AuCl_4)$: 2% stock solution in water, stable for 1–2 yr at 4°C. Dilute to 0.01% in water just before use. Sodium citrate: 1% in water, freshly prepared. All solutions are made up in double-distilled water of highest purity. Glassware has to be extremely clean (*see* Note 1).
2. Filters: To filter the working solutions from above, use 0.45-μm nitrocellulose filters (e.g., Millex-HA, Millipore).
3. Siliconized Erlenmeyer flask: A 200 mL flask is siliconized by rinsing it with silicone solution (e.g., SERVA) and curing the silicone film for 1 h at 100–150°C.
4. Nitrocellulose for blotting: Nitrocellulose sheets with 0.45-μm pore size are available from several suppliers.
5. Blotting buffer: 25 mM Tris, 192 mM glycine, pH 8.4, 20% methanol, and 0.02% SDS.
6. Wash after blotting: 100 mM Tris-HCl, pH 7.4 or 100 mM Tris-HCl, pH 7.4 in 150 mM NaCl (*see* Table 1).
7. Blocking solutions: The following blocking solutions have been successfully used (*see* Table 1): 0.25% gelatin and 3% ovalbumin; 5% skimmed milk (commercial milk powder, dissolved in the appropriate buffer); 0.3% Tween-20. Other solutions may work equally well, depending on the nature of the proteins under study.
8. The primary antibody is diluted according to the blocking solution employed (*see* Table 1). The dilution factor has to be found empirically. We use hybridoma supernatant diluted to 1:10.
9. The secondary, peroxidase-coupled antispecies antibody is diluted 1:200–1:2000 in the buffer indicated in Table 1.
10. Washing solutions: After primary and secondary antibody stages, washes are done in the solutions given in Table 1. PBS: 8 g of NaCl, 0.2 g of KCl, 1.44 g of $Na_2HPO_4 \cdot 2H_2O$, 0.2 g of KH_2PO_4, 1000 mL of distilled water, final pH 7.4.
11. 4-Chloro-1-naphthol: This substrate for the peroxidase is prepared as stock solution of 0.3% in methanol. Add 0.6 mL of the stock solution and 2 μL of H_2O_2 (30%) to 9.4 mL of distilled water just before use.
12. Kodak TP-Film (Technical Pan).
13. Yellow or orange filter (e.g., OG1 barrier filter from I.F.-microscope).
14. Kodak D19-developer.

Table 1
Immunoprobing with Different Blocking Agents

Blocking agent	Ovalbumin/gelatin	Skimmed milk	Tween-20
Wash after blotting	100 mM Tris, pH 7.4 room temperature (R.T.), 5 min	100 mM Tris, pH 7.4, 150 mM NaCl, R.T., 5 min	100 mM Tris, pH 7.4, R.T., 5 min
Blocking solution	100 mM Tris, pH 7.4, 3% ovalbumin, 0.25% gelatin, 40°C, 60 min	100 mM Tris, pH 7.4, 150 mM NaCl, 5% (w/v) skimmed milk, R.T., 30 min	PBS, 0.3% Tween-20, 37°C, 30 min
Wash	—	100 mM Tris, pH 7.4, 150 mM NaCl, 0.1% NP40, R.T., 3 × 5 min, rinse in 100 mM Tris, 150 mM NaCl	—
Primary antibody	Diluted in blocking solution, R.T., overnight	Diluted in 100 mM Tris, pH 7.4, 150 mM NaCl, R.T., overnight	Diluted in PBS, 0.05% Tween-20, R.T., overnight
Wash	50 mM Tris, pH 7.4, 5 mM EDTA, 150 mM NaCl, 0.25% gelatin, 0.5% NP40, R.T., 5 × 10 min	100 mM Tris, pH 7.4, 150 mM NaCl, 0.1% NP40, R.T., 3 × 5 min, rinse in 100 mM Tris, 150 mM NaCl	PBS, 0.05% Tween-20, R.T., 3 × 10 min
Labeled secondary antibody	Diluted in blocking solution, R.T., 2.5 h	Diluted in 100 mM Tris, pH 7.4, 150 mM NaCl, R.T., 20 min–2.5 h	Diluted in PBS, 0.05% Tween-20, R.T., 2.5 h
Wash	50 mM Tris, pH 7.4, 5 mM EDTA, 450 mM NaCl, 0.4% Sarkosyl, R.T., 5 × 10 min	As after primary antibody, R.T., 3 × 5 min	PBS, 0.05% Tween-20, R.T., 3 × 10 min

3. Methods

3.1. Preparation of Colloidal Gold (see Note 1)

1. Filter the 0.01% gold chloride and the 1% sodium citrate solutions through 0.45-μm nitrocellulose filters.
2. Bring 100 mL of the gold chloride solution to a vigorous boil in a siliconized 200 mL Erlenmeyer flask.
3. Add 4 mL of the sodium citrate solution at once while shaking the flask. Keep the mixture boiling constantly. Don't worry if some of the fluid evaporates; reflux cooling is not necessary. The solution will stay colorless for 2–3 min, then turn purple for 9 min, and change to bright red thereafter. Keep boiling for a total of 12–15 min until the *bright* red color is obtained. Let it cool. This is the final staining solution. It consists of 20 nm gold grains with an OD_{515} of 1–1.1 and a pH of 6. If kept at 4°C, the shelf-life is at least 1 yr.

3.2. Blotting

1. Prepare SDS-polyacrylamide gels or 2D-gels (*see Methods in Molecular Biology*, Volume 1, Chapter 6 and Volume 3, Chapters 16 and 17).
2. Blot the gels onto nitrocellulose by standard procedures (*see* Chapter 20). An additional nitrocellulose sheet on the cathodic side of the gel might be helpful to absorb impurities. We blot routinely at 48 V with cooling during 1–1.5 h.
3. Wash the blots briefly with 100 m*M* Tris-HCl pH 7.4, for 5 min.
4. Air-dry the blots and store at 4°C or process for gold staining.

3.3. Gold Staining of Protein Bands (see Note 2)

1. Wash the blot in double-distilled water before gold staining.
2. Stain the blots with the gold solution at room temperature on a shaker for 10–45 min until the protein bands are visible. Use sufficient gold solution to cover the blot easily.
3. After staining, rinse the blot in double-distilled water.

3.4. Blocking and Immune Reaction

1. To block free binding sites on the nitrocellulose, use the blocking solution that gives the most intense immunostaining of the antigen and the lowest background for the other proteins. This has to be found empirically; Table 1 may be used as a guide.
2. After blocking, incubate the blots in a suitable dilution of antibody (Table 1) overnight in an airtight container at room temperature on a shaker.
3. Wash and incubate the blots in peroxidase-labeled antispecies antibody at room temperature, as indicated in Table 1.
4. Wash again, rinse in distilled water, and incubate in freshly prepared substrate for 5–30 min until the immunoreactive bands are clearly visible.
5. Rinse with distilled water and air-dry.

3.5. Photography (see Note 3)

1. Take black-and-white photographs of the blots on Technical Pan film (Kodak), setting 125/22°. If an OG1 filter is used to enhance contrast further, the setting is 75/19°.
2. Develop for 3–4 min in undiluted (or in a 1:2 dilution) of D19 developer. This developer yields especially high contrast.

4. Notes

1. Colloidal gold: For preparation of the citrate gold, highly purified water and cleanliness of the glassware is essential. Adjusting the pH of the citrate gold in the range between 3.7 and 8.0 does not change its staining properties for the blots, but may impair its stability. It is best to use it without any addition or pH adjustment.
2. Gold staining of blot: Blots that are to be stained with colloidal gold have to be handled with extreme care, since they are very sensitive to mechanical damage (scratches, impression marks) and dirt, such as grease from the seal of the glass plates in the gel apparatus or impurities from the blotting buffer. Handle the blots at the edge only with clean forceps.

    As outlined above, the gold stain should be matched in sensitivity to the amount of protein loaded on the gel. This can be estimated as follows: if a strip of the gel from which the blot is to be made can be adequately stained with Coomassie blue, citrate gold will yield a good stain of the blot, whereas "AuroDye" will heavily overstain it. If the gel contains so little protein that it has to be detected by silver staining, "AuroDye" and the corresponding method (*see Methods in Molecular Biology*, Volume 3, Chapter 34) should be used.
3. Photography: On black and white photographs, the contrast can be enhanced by using an orange or yellow filter, i.e., a filter similar in color to the gold stain and complementary to the (blue) immunoreactive bands. This renders the immune reaction bands on the final print intensely black and the red gold-stained proteins contrastingly gray.

    Faint immunoreactive bands tend to fade during drying. They are easier to recognize and photograph on wet blots laid on a clean glass plate.

References

1. Rohringer, R. and Holden, D. W. (1985) Protein blotting: detection of protein with colloidal gold, and of glycoproteins and lectins with biotin-conjugated and enzyme probes. *Anal. Biochem.* **144,** 118–127.
2. Hancock, K. and Tsang, V. C. W. (1983) India ink staining of proteins on nitrocellulose paper. *Anal. Biochem.* **133,** 157–162.
3. Egger, D. and Bienz, K. (1987) Colloidal gold staining and immunoprobing of proteins on the same nitrocellulose blot. *Anal. Biochem.* **166,** 413–417.

22

Erasure of Western Blots After Autoradiographic or Chemiluminescent Detection

Scott H. Kaufmann and Udo Kellner

1. Introduction

Western blotting (reviewed in refs. *1–3*) refers to formation and detection of an antibody–antigen complex between an antibody and a polypeptide that is immobilized on derivatized paper. Most commonly, polypeptides in a complex mixture are separated by electrophoresis through polyacrylamide gels in the presence of sodium dodecyl sulfate (SDS), electrophoretically transferred to thin sheets of nitrocellulose or nylon, and reacted sequentially with one or more antibody-containing solutions. This sequence of manipulations can be utilized to determine whether a polypeptide recognized by a specific antiserum is present in a particular biological sample (cell type, subcellular fraction, or biological fluid), to follow the purification of the polypeptide, or to assess the location of epitopes within the polypeptide after chemical or enzymatic degradation. If suitable antibodies are available, this same approach can be utilized to search for proteins that bear a particular physiological or pathological posttranslational modification (e.g., refs. *4–6*). Alternatively, the same procedure can be utilized to determine whether antibodies that recognize a particular polypeptide are detectable in a sample of biological fluid. Because Western blotting takes advantage of the power of electrophoresis for separating complex mixtures of polypeptides, it is possible to derive large amounts of information from this technique without necessarily purifying the antigen being studied.

There are certain circumstances in which it is convenient to be able to dissociate the antibodies from a Western blot after detection of antibody–antigen complexes. If, for example, the experiment gives an unexpected

From: *Methods in Molecular Biology, Vol. 80: Immunochemical Protocols, 2nd ed.*
Edited by: J. D. Pound © Humana Press Inc., Totowa, NJ

result regarding the subcellular distribution of a polypeptide, it is convenient to be able to reprobe the blot with an antibody that recognizes a second polypeptide in order to confirm that the samples have been properly prepared, loaded, and transferred. Likewise, if the polypeptides being analyzed are derived from a precious source (e.g., biological fluid, tissue, or organism that is not readily available), it is convenient to dissociate the antibody–antigen complexes and reutilize the blots.

Several methods for removing antibodies from Western blots have been previously described. In early experiments, proteins were covalently bound to diazotized paper. Antibodies that were subsequently (noncovalently) bound to the paper were removed by treating the paper at 60°C with $10M$ urea *(7)* or 2% (w/v) SDS *(8)* under reducing conditions. Because of several undesirable properties (reviewed in refs. *1–3*), diazotized paper has been largely replaced by nitrocellulose or polyvinylidene fluoride (PVDF), solid supports to which proteins are presumably noncovalently bound. It has been reported that treatment of nitrocellulose blots with glycine at pH 2.2 *(9)* or with $8M$ urea at 60°C *(10)* will remove antibodies and permit reuse of blots. Although these techniques are effective at disrupting low-affinity interactions between antigens and antibodies, they appear to be ineffective at disrupting interactions between immobilized antigens and high-affinity antibodies *(9,11)*.

Two subsequent observations have allowed the development of a more widely applicable technique for the removal of antibodies from Western blots. First, it was observed that treatment of nitrocellulose with acidic solutions of methanol would "fix" transferred polypeptides to the nitrocellulose (reviewed in ref. *3; see also* refs. *12* and *13*). Polypeptides treated in this fashion remained bound to the nitrocellulose even during treatment with SDS at 70–100°C under reducing conditions *(11,12)*. Second, it was observed that removal of antibodies from nitrocellulose after Western blotting could be facilitated by reincubation of the blot with a large excess of irrelevant protein immediately prior to drying and autoradiography *(11)*. Based on these observations, a technique that allows the reutilization of Western blots after reaction with a wide variety of antibodies or with lectins was developed. In brief, polypeptides immobilized on nitrocellulose are stained with dye dissolved in an acidic solution of methanol. After unoccupied binding sites have been saturated with irrelevant protein, the nitrocellulose is treated sequentially with unlabeled primary antibodies and radiolabeled secondary antibodies. Prior to drying, the blot is briefly incubated in a protein-containing buffer. After subsequent drying and autoradiography, the antibodies are removed by treating the nitrocellulose with SDS at 70°C under reducing conditions. A similar erasure procedure removes peroxidase-coupled antibodies after detection of antigens by enhanced chemiluminescence.

2. Materials

1. Apparatus for transferring polypeptides from gel to solid support (design principles are reviewed in refs. *2* and *3*).
   a. TE52 reservoir-type electrophoretic transfer apparatus (Hoefer Scientific, San Francisco, CA) or equivalent.
   b. Polyblot semidry blotter (Pharmacia, Piscataway, NJ) or equivalent.
2. Paper support for binding transferred polypeptides.
   a. Nitrocellulose.
   b. Nylon (e.g., Genescreen from New England Nuclear, Boston, MA, or Nytran from Schleicher and Schuell, Keene, NH).
   c. PVDF (e.g., Immobilon from Millipore, Bedford, MA).
3. Fast green FCF for staining polypeptides after transfer to solid support.
4. 10,000 U/mL Penicillin and 10 mg/mL streptomycin.
5. Reagents for electrophoresis (acrylamide, bis-acrylamide, 2-mercaptoethanol, SDS) should be electrophoresis grade.
6. All other reagents (Tris, glycine, urea, methanol) are reagent grade.
7. Transfer buffer: 0.02% (w/v) SDS, 20% (v/v) methanol, 192 mM glycine-HCl, and 25 mM Tris base. Prepare enough buffer to fill the chamber of the transfer apparatus and a container for assembling cassette.
8. TS buffer: 150 mM NaCl, 10 mM Tris-HCl, pH 7.4. This can be conveniently prepared as a 10X stock (1.5M NaCl, 100 mM Tris-HCl, pH 7.4). The 10X stock can be stored indefinitely at 4°C and then used to prepare 1X TS buffer, TSM buffer, and the other buffers described below.
9. TSM buffer: TS buffer containing 5% (w/v) powdered milk, 100 U/mL penicillin, 100 µg/mL streptomycin, and 1 mM sodium azide. This buffer can be stored for several days at 4°C. Note that sodium azide is poisonous and can form explosive copper salts in drain pipes if not handled properly.
10. TS buffer containing 2M urea and 0.05% (w/v) Nonidet P-40: Prepare 300 mL/blot by combining 0.15 g of Nonidet P-40, 30 mL of 10X TS buffer, 75 mL of 8M urea (freshly deionized over Bio-Rad AG1X-8 mixed-bed resin to remove traces of cyanate), and 195 mL of water.
11. TS buffer containing 0.05% (w/v) Nonidet P-40. Prepare 300 mL/blot.
12. Fast green stain: 0.1% (w/v) Fast green FCF in 20% (v/v) methanol–5% (v/v) acetic acid. This stain is reusable. Prepare 50–100 mL/blot.
13. Fast green destain: 20% (v/v) Methanol in 5% (v/v) acetic acid.
14. Blot erasure buffer: 2% (w/v) SDS, 62.5 mM Tris-HCl, pH 6.8, and 100 mM 2-mercaptoethanol. The SDS/Tris-HCl solution is stable indefinitely at 4°C. Immediately prior to use, 2-mercaptoethanol is added to a final concentration of 6 µL/mL.
15. Primary antibody.
16. ^{125}I-labeled secondary antibody. Secondary antibodies can be labeled as previously described *(11)* or purchased commercially. Radiolabeled antibodies should only be used by personnel trained to properly handle radioisotopes properly.
17. In lieu of radiolabeled secondary antibody, reagents for detection by chemiluminescence: This approach requires enzyme-coupled secondary antibody and a substrate

that becomes chemiluminescent as a consequence of enzymatic modification, e.g., peroxidase-coupled secondary antibody and luminol (Amersham [Arlington Heights, IL]) ECL enhanced chemiluminescence kit or equivalent (*see* Chapter 20).

3. Methods

3.1. Transfer of Polypeptides to Nitrocellulose

The following description is appropriate for transfer in a transfer reservoir. If a semidry transfer apparatus is to be used, follow the manufacturer's instructions (*see* Note 1).

1. Perform SDS-polyacrylamide gel electrophoresis (SDS-PAGE) using standard techniques (*see* ref. *14* for description of this method).
2. Wear disposable gloves while handling the gel and nitrocellulose at all steps. This avoids cytokeratin-containing fingerprints.
3. Cut nitrocellulose sheets to a size slightly larger than the polyacrylamide gel (*see* Note 2).
4. Fill the transfer apparatus with transfer buffer (*see* Note 3).
5. Fill a container large enough to accommodate the transfer cassettes with transfer buffer. Assemble the cassette under the buffer in the following order:
   a. Back of the cassette.
   b. Two layers of filter paper.
   c. The gel.
   d. One piece of nitrocellulose—gently work bubbles out from between the nitrocellulose and gel by rubbing a gloved finger or glass stirring rod over the surface of the nitrocellulose.
   e. Two layers of filter paper—again, gently remove bubbles.
   f. Sponge or flexible absorbent pad.
   g. Front of the cassette.
6. Place the cassette in the transfer apparatus so that the front is oriented toward the positive pole.
7. Transfer at 4°C in a cold room with the transfer apparatus partially immersed in an ice-water bath. Power settings: 90 V for 5–6 h or 60 V overnight.
8. Place the Fast green stain in a container with a surface area slightly larger than one piece of nitrocellulose (*see* Note 4). After the transfer is complete, place all the pieces of nitrocellulose in the stain, and incubate for 2–3 min with gentle agitation. Decant the stain solution, which can be reused (*see* Note 5).
9. Destain the nitrocellulose by rinsing it for 3–5 min in Fast green destain solution with gentle agitation. Decant the destain, which can also be reused. Rinse the nitrocellulose four times (5 min each) with TS buffer (200 mL/rinse).
10. Mark the locations of lanes, standards, and any other identifying features by writing on the blot with a standard ballpoint pen.
11. Coat the remaining protein binding sites on the nitrocellulose by incubating the blot in TSM buffer (50–100 mL/blot) for 6–12 h at room temperature (*see* Note 6). Remove the blot from the TSM buffer. Wash the blot four times in quick

succession with TS buffer (25–50 mL/wash), and dry the blot on fresh paper towels. Either before or after coating of the unoccupied protein binding sites, blots can be dried, and stored indefinitely in an appropriate container, e.g., Ziplock disposable food storage bags (1–2 blots/bag).

3.2. Detection of Antibody–Antigen Complexes Using Radiolabeled Secondary Antibody

1. Place the nitrocellulose blot in an appropriate container for reaction with the antibody. A 15- or 20-lane sheet can be reacted with 15–20 mL of antibody solution in a Ziplock bag. A 1- or 2-lane strip can be reacted with 2–5 mL of antibody solution in a disposable 15-mL conical test tube.
2. If the nitrocellulose has been dried, rehydrate it by incubation for a few minutes in an appropriate volume of TSM buffer (*see* previous step).
3. Add an appropriate dilution of antibody to the TSM buffer, and incubate overnight (10–15 h) at room temperature with gentle agitation (*see* Notes 7 and 8).
4. Remove the antibody solution and save for reuse (*see* Note 9).
5. Wash the nitrocellulose (100 mL/wash for each large blot or 15–50 mL/wash for each individual strip) with TS buffer containing $2M$ urea and 0.05% NP-40 (three washes for 15 min each) followed by TS buffer (one wash for 5 min) (*see* Note 10).
6. Add fresh TSM buffer to the nitrocellulose sheets or strips. For nitrocellulose sheets (or pooled strips) in Ziplock bags, it is convenient to use 50 mL of TSM buffer. Add 5–10 µCi ^{125}I-labeled secondary antibody (*see* Note 11). Incubate for 90 min at room temperature with gentle agitation.
7. Remove the radiolabeled antibody and discard appropriately.
8. Wash the sheets (100 mL/wash for each large blot or each group of pooled strips) with TS buffer containing 0.05% NP-40 (three or more washes for 15 min each) followed by TS buffer (one wash for 5 min).
9. Before drying blots, incubate them for 5 min with TSM buffer. This incubation step facilitates subsequent removal of antibody and reuse of the blot (*see* Note 12 and Fig. 1).
10. After incubating the blot with TSM buffer, immediately dry it between several layers of paper towels. After 5 min, move the blot to fresh paper towels to prevent the nitrocellulose from sticking to the paper towels. Allow the blot to dry thoroughly.
11. Mount the dried blot on heavy paper, cover it with clear plastic wrap, and subject it to autoradiography (*see* ref. *17* for details).

3.3. Dissociation of Antibodies from Western Blots

1. After the blot has been subjected to autoradiography for the desired length of time, remove it from its mounting, and place it in a Ziplock bag.
2. Add 50 mL of erasure buffer, seal the bag, and incubate in a water bath at 70°C for 30 min with gentle agitation every 5–10 min (*see* Notes 13 and 14).
3. Decant and discard the erasure buffer. Wash the blot twice (5 min each) with 50–100 mL of TS buffer to remove SDS.

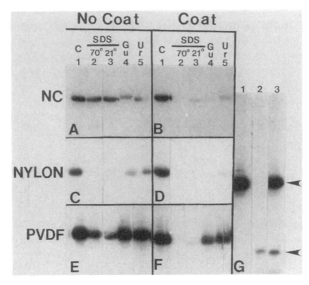

Fig. 1. Conditions for dissociating radiolabeled antibodies from Western blots after immobilization of polypeptides on various solid supports. Replicate samples containing 2×10^6 rat liver nuclei were subjected to PAGE in the presence of SDS as previously described *(15)*. The separated polypeptides were transferred to nitrocellulose paper **(A,B)**, Nytran nylon sheets **(C,D)**, or Immobilon PVDF paper **(E–G)** *(see* Note 2). Unoccupied binding sites were blocked by incubation with milk-containing buffer (Section 3.1., step 11). Blots were incubated with chicken polyclonal antiserum, which reacts with the nuclear envelope polypeptide lamin B *(15)* followed by ^{125}I-labeled rabbit antichicken IgG (Section 3.2., steps 1–8). Half of each blot (B,D,F,G) was coated with milk-containing buffer for 5 min prior to drying (Section 3.2., step 9); the other half of each blot was dried without being recoated with protein (A,C,E). Autoradiography (not shown) confirmed that the signal in all lanes of a given panel was identical prior to subsequent manipulation. (A–F) To investigate the efficacy of various conditions for dissociating antibodies, samples were incubated at 70°C for 30 min with SDS erasure buffer (lane 2), with $6M$ guanidine hydrochloride in 50 mM Tris-HCl (pH 6.8) containing 100 mM 2-mercaptoethanol (lane 4), or with $8M$ urea in 50 mM Tris-HCl (pH 6.8) containing 100 mM 2-mercaptoethanol (lane 5). Alternatively, samples were incubated at 21°C for 30 min with SDS erasure buffer (lane 3). Strips were then washed twice with TS buffer and dried for autoradiography. Untreated strips (lane 1) served as controls. In each pair of panels, nonadjacent wells from a single autoradiograph have been juxtaposed to compose the figure. It is important to note that coating with milk prior to drying (Section 3.2., step 9) does not affect the amount of radiolabeled antibody initially bound to the blots (cf. lane 1 in A and B, C and D, E and F). The efficacy of various treatments in removing antibodies varies depending on the solid support. For nitrocellulose or PVDF, coating of the blots with protein prior to drying (B,F) greatly facilitates the dissociation of antibodies. In both cases, SDS-containing buffer (lanes 2 and 3) is more effective than guanidine hydrochloride (lane 4), or urea (lane

4. To ensure that nonspecific binding sites on the blot are well coated, incubate with TSM buffer for 6–8 h at room temperature with gentle agitation.

5. The blot is ready to be stored (Section 3.1., step 11) or to be incubated with a new antibody as described in the previous section.

4. Notes

4.1. Transfer of Polypeptides to Nitrocellulose

1. The method described is for transferring polypeptides after electrophoresis in SDS-containing polyacrylamide gels. Alternative methods have been described for transferring polypeptides after acid-urea gels and after isoelectric focusing (reviewed in refs. *2* and *3*).

2. Choice of solid support for polypeptides: Figure 1 shows the results obtained when various solid supports (nitrocellulose, nylon, PVDF) are used for Western blotting, stripped of antibodies, and reused. Nitrocellulose (Fig. 1A,B) has the advantage of ease of use. It is compatible with a wide variety of staining procedures. With multiple cycles of blotting and erasing, however, nitrocellulose becomes brittle. Derivatized nylon (Fig. 1C,D) has the advantage of greater protein binding capacity and greater durability, but avidly binds many nonspecific protein stains (reviewed in refs. *1–3*). The higher binding capacity of nylon is said to contribute to higher background binding despite the use of blocking solutions containing large amounts of protein (reviewed in ref. *3*). Antibodies can be more easily dissociated from nylon than from nitrocellulose (cf. Fig. 1C,A). PVDF membranes (Fig. 1E–G) are durable, are compatible with a variety of nonspecific protein stains, and are capable of being stripped of antibody (Fig. 1F) and reutilized (Fig. 1G).

---

5) at dissociating the antibodies. For nylon, SDS-containing buffer is again more effective at dissociating the antibodies (cf. lanes 2–5 in C). When SDS-containing erasure buffer is used, it is not necessary to recoat nylon with protein prior to drying for autoradiography (cf. lanes 2 or 3 in C and D). On the other hand, when guanidine hydrochloride-containing buffer is used to dissociate antibodies, it is necessary to recoat the nylon (cf. lane 4 in C and D). (G) Reutilization of blots after dissociation of antibodies. Nuclear polypeptides were immobilized on PVDF, reacted with antibodies, and treated with milk-containing buffer (Section 3.2., step 9) prior to drying. Autoradiography (not shown) confirmed that all three lanes initially had indistinguishable signals for the 66-kDa lamin B polypeptide. After lane 2 was treated with SDS erasure buffer and recoated with milk (Section 3.3., steps 2–5), lanes 2 and 3 (a lane that was not erased) were reacted sequentially with chicken antiserum that recognizes the 38-kDa nucleolar polypeptide B23 *(16)* and ^{125}I-labeled rabbit antichicken IgG. The signal for B23 (lower arrow) was readily detectable on the strip that had previously been erased (lane 2) as well as the strip that had not been erased (lane 3), indicating that treatment with SDS erasure buffer did not remove the nuclear polypeptides from the PVDF paper or substantially alter their reactivity with polyclonal antibodies. The absence of a signal for lamin B after erasure (upper arrow, lane 2) indicates that the erasure buffer efficiently dissociated the antilamin B primary antibodies as well as the radiolabeled secondary antibodies from the PVDF-immobilized polypeptides.

3. Various compositions of transfer buffer have been described (reviewed in refs. *1–3*). Methanol is said to facilitate the binding of polypeptides to nitrocellulose, but to retard the electrophoretic migration of polypeptides out of the gel. In the absence of SDS, polypeptides with molecular weights above 116 kDa do not transfer efficiently. Low concentrations of SDS (0.01–0.1%) facilitate the transfer of larger polypeptides, but simultaneously increase the current generated during electrophoretic transfer, necessitating the use of vigorous cooling to prevent damage to the transfer apparatus.

4. Alternative staining procedures (reviewed in refs. *1–3*) utilize Coomassie blue, Ponceau S, Amido black, India drawing ink, colloidal gold, or silver. A highly sensitive technique utilizing eosin Y has also been described *(18)*.

5. A washing step in acidified alcohol is probably essential to immobilize the polypeptides on the nitrocellulose *(3,12,13)*. The Fast green staining procedure satisfies this requirement. Polypeptides are observed to elute from nitrocellulose under mild conditions if a wash in acidified alcohol is omitted *(13,19)*.

6. Various proteins have been utilized to block unoccupied binding sites on nitrocellulose (reviewed in refs. *2* and *3*). These include 5% (w/v) powdered dry milk, 3% bovine serum albumin, 1% hemoglobin, and 0.1% gelatin. Although the choice of protein can affect antibody binding (e.g., Fig. 3D), blots of polypeptides immobilized on nitrocellulose have been successfully stripped of antibody and reutilized after coating of unoccupied binding sites with any of these protein solutions *(11)* if the blot is recoated with the protein solution immediately prior drying (Section 3.2., step 9).

4.2. Formation of Antigen–Antibody Complexes

7. No guidelines can be provided regarding the appropriate dilution of antibody to use. Some antisera are useful for blotting at a dilution of >1:20,000. Other antisera are useful at a dilution of 1:5 or 1:10. When attempting to blot with an antiserum for the first time, it is reasonable to try one or more arbitrary concentrations in the range of 1:10–1:500. If a strong signal is obtained at 1:500, further dilutions can be performed in subsequent experiments.

8. Different investigators incubate blots with primary antibodies for different lengths of time (reviewed in ref. *3*). Preliminary studies with some of our antibodies have revealed that the signal intensity on Western blots is greater when blots are incubated with antibody overnight rather than 1–2 h at room temperature (G. Humphrey and S. H. K., unpublished observations).

9. Diluted antibody solutions can be reused multiple times. They should be stored at 4°C after additional aliquots of penicillin/streptomycin and sodium azide have been added. Some workers believe that the amount of nonspecific (background) staining on Western blots diminishes as antibody solutions are reutilized. Antibody solutions are discarded or supplemented with additional antibody when the intensity of the specific signal begins to diminish.

10. Choice of wash buffer after incubation with primary antibody: $2M$ urea is included in the suggested wash buffer to diminish nonspecific binding. Alternatively, some

investigators include a mixture of SDS and nonionic detergent (e.g., 0.1% [w/v] SDS and 1% [w/v] Triton X-100) in the wash buffers. For antibodies with low avidity (especially monoclonal antibodies and antipeptide antibodies), the inclusion of $2M$ urea or SDS might diminish the signal intensity. These agents are, therefore, optional depending on the properties of the primary antibody used for blotting.

11. ^{125}I-labeled protein A can be substituted for radiolabeled secondary antibody. Protein A, however, can bind to the immunoglobulins present in milk, causing a high background on the blot. Therefore, when ^{125}I-labeled protein A is to be used, milk should not be utilized to block unoccupied binding sites (Section 3.1., step 11), nor as a diluent for antibodies (Section 3.2., steps 2, 3, and 6). Instead, bovine serum albumin, hemoglobin, or gelatin should be considered (*see* Note 6).

4.3. Dissociation of Antibodies After Autoradiography

12. Reincubation of blots with protein-containing buffer prior to drying has been found to be essential for efficient dissociation of antibodies from nitrocellulose (cf. Fig. 1A,B) or PVDF paper (cf Fig. 1E,F). Recoating the blots is not required in order to dissociate antibodies from Western blots performed on certain types of nylon (Fig. 1C).

13. Choice of erasure buffer: Preliminary experiments have shown that the SDS/2-mercaptoethanol erasure buffer is more effective than urea, guanidine hydrochloride, or acidic glycine at dissociating polyclonal antibodies from Western blots on nitrocellulose (ref. *11; see also* Fig. 1B) or PVDF (Fig. 1F). On the other hand, $6M$ guanidine hydrochloride is effective under certain conditions at removing antibodies from nylon (ref. *11* and Fig. 1D).

14. Incubation:
   a. Temperature of incubation: When blotting is performed after immobilization of polypeptides on nitrocellulose, complete removal of antibodies requires heating of erasure buffer to $\geq 50°C$ for 30 min (ref. *11; see also* Fig. 1B, lanes 2 and 3). On the other hand, after immobilization of polypeptides on nylon, antibodies are efficiently dissociated by erasure buffer at room temperature (lane 3 in Fig. 1C,D).
   b. Length of incubation: When blotting is performed on nitrocellulose, complete dissociation of antibodies at 70°C requires a minimum of 20 min of incubation with erasure buffer *(11)*. Incubation times for removal of antibodies from nylon and PVDF have not been investigated.

4.4. Removal of Antibodies After Chemiluminescent Detection

15. The technique described above is not useful for removing colored peroxidase reaction products (e.g., diaminobenzidine oxidation products) from blots. Thus, we avoid detection methods based on these reactions. On the other hand, peroxidase-based luminescent assays *(20)* do not deposit a chemical reaction product on the blot and are compatible with this erasure method *(21)*. An example of the use of this erasure method (Section 3.3., steps 1–5) after chemiluminescent detection is shown in Fig. 2.

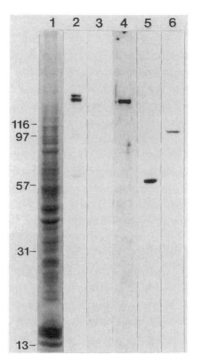

Fig. 2. Removal of antibodies after antigen detection by enhanced chemiluminescence. Replicate gel lanes containing protein from 3×10^5 HL-60 human leukemia cells were stained with Coomassie blue (lane 1) or transferred to nitrocellulose. After unoccupied binding sites on the nitrocellulose were blocked by incubation with milk-containing buffer (Section 3.1., step 11), multiple identical strips (lanes 2–6) were reacted with antiserum directed against both isoforms of the nuclear enzyme topoisomerase II (ref. 22), and washed with TS buffer containing $2M$ urea and 0.05% (w/v) NP-40 (Section 3.2., steps 1–5). The strips were then incubated for 60 min with peroxidase-coupled goat antirabbit IgG, washed with phosphate-buffered saline containing 0.05% (w/v) Tween-20, incubated with luminol, and covered with plastic wrap as described in ref. 21. After detection of the chemiluminescence (lane 2), nitrocellulose strips were stored overnight. The blots were treated as described in Section 3.3., steps 1–5 to dissociate the antibodies and recoat any unoccupied binding sites. The strips were then incubated in TSM buffer without primary antibody (lane 3), or with rabbit antisera raised against the 170-kDa isoform of topoisomerase II (lane 4), the c-*myc* protein (lane 5, kindly provided by Chi Dang, Johns Hopkins University School of Medicine), or human topoisomerase I (lane 6, kindly provided by Leroy F. Liu, Robert Wood Johnson School of Medicine). Washing and chemiluminescent detection were performed as described above. The absence of a signal at 180 kDa in lanes 3–6 confirms that the primary antibody used in the first detection step (lane 2) has been successfully removed.

In the case of blots subjected to chemiluminescent detection, the antibody removal technique is successful even though the strips were not recoated with protein-containing solution immediately prior to the detection step (Section 3.2., step 9). The need for recoating the blots (Section 3.2., step 9 and Note 12) is apparently obviated by covering the strips with plastic wrap and preventing drying during the detection and storage steps.

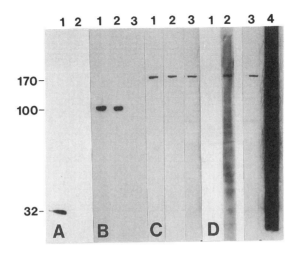

Fig. 3. Effect of various treatments on antigen recognition during Western blotting. **(A)** Replicate aliquots containing polypeptides from 2×10^5 K562 human leukemia cells were separated by SDS-PAGE, transferred to nitrocellulose, and stained with Fast green FCF (Section 3.1., steps 1–9). Strip 2 was then treated as described in Section 3.3., steps 1–5 to simulate an erasure procedure. Strips were blocked with 10% (w/v) milk in TS buffer and blotted with the earliest released version of a mouse monoclonal IgG recognizing the CPP32 cysteine protease (Transduction Laboratories, Lexington, KY). The epitope recognized by this antibody is destroyed by erasure (lane 2). **(B,C)** Replicate gel lanes containing identical amounts of protein from a single batch of HL-60 lysate were transferred to nitrocellulose 1 wk (strips 1 and 2), or 3 yr (strip 3) prior to blotting. Strip 2 was treated as described in Section 3.3., steps 1–5 to simulate an erasure procedure. After unoccupied binding sites were blocked by incubation with TS buffer containing 10% (w/v) milk, the strips were incubated with MAb C-21 recognizing DNA topoisomerase I (B) (kindly provided by Y-C. Cheng, Yale University Cancer Center) or MAb Ki-S1 to DNA topoisomerase IIα (C). Washing and chemiluminescent detection were performed as described in the legend to Fig. 2. In B, the absence of a signal in lane 3 and presence in lane 2 indicate that the epitope recognized by antibody C-21 has been damaged by prolonged storage (lane 3) but not by the erasure procedure (lane 2). In contrast, the epitope recognized by antibody Ki-S1 (C) is resistant to the erasure procedure (lane 2) and to storage of blots (lane 3). **(D)** Effect of blocking solution on reactivity. Replicate gel lanes containing protein from 3×10^5 HL-60 cells were blocked with TS buffer containing 10% milk (strip 1), or 3% albumin (strip 2), and then reacted with antibody Ki-S1 diluted 1:1000 in the corresponding protein solution. After reaction with peroxidase-coupled antimouse IgG diluted in the corresponding protein solution, the strips were treated with luminol and exposed to Kodak XAR-5 film for 20 s (lanes 1 and 2) or 60 min (lanes 3 and 4). The signal was much stronger when albumin was used as a blocking reagent (cf. lanes 1 and 2), but the background was much cleaner using milk as a blocking reagent (cf. lanes 2 and 3).

4.5. General Notes

16. The techniques described above can be applied to the detection of glycoproteins by radiolabeled lectins. For this application, blots would be coated with albumin or gelatin, reacted with radiolabeled lectin (Section 3.2., steps 6–8), and recoated with albumin or gelatin (Section 3.2., steps 9 and 10) prior to drying. After autoradiography, the radiolabeled lectin would be solubilized in warm SDS under reducing conditions (Section 3.3., steps 1–5).

17. Although most epitopes are resistant to the erasure procedure (Figs. 1 and 2; *see also* refs. *10* and *11*), epitopes recognized by an occasional MAb are destroyed by erasure (Fig. 3A *[previous page]*, lane 2). Observations from our laboratory also indicate that certain epitopes are lost on prolonged storage of blots (Fig. 3B, lane 3). There does not appear to be any relationship between the loss of epitopes on blot storage and the damage of epitopes during the erasure procedure.

References

1. Gershoni, J. M. and Palade, G. E. (1983) Protein blotting: principles and applications. *Anal. Biochem.* **131,** 1–15.
2. Beisiegel, U. (1986) Protein blotting. *Electrophoresis* **7,** 1–18.
3. Stott, D. I. (1989) Immunoblotting and dot blotting. *J. Immunol. Methods* **119,** 153–187.
4. Evans, J. P., Wickremasinghe, R. G., and Hoffbrand, A. V. (1987) Detection of tyrosine protein kinase substrates in fresh leukemia cells and normal blood cells using an immunoblotting technique. *Leukemia* **1,** 782–785.
5. Guther, M. L. S., de Almeida, M. L. C., Rosenberry, T. L., and Ferguson M. A. J. (1994) The detection of phospholipase-resistant and -sensitive glycosyl-phosphatidylinositol membrane anchors by Western blotting. *Anal. Biochem.* **219,** 249–255.
6. Laycock, C. A., Phelan M. J. I. Bucknall, R. C., and Coleman J. W. (1994) A western blot approach to detection of human plasma protein conjugates derived from D-penicillamine. *Ann. Rheum. Dis.* **53,** 256–260.
7. Renart, J., Reizer, J., and Stark, G. R. (1979) Transfer of proteins from gels to diazobenzyloxymethyl-paper and detection with antisera: a method for studying antibody specificity and antigen structure. *Proc. Natl. Acad. Sci. USA* **76,** 3116–3120.
8. Gullick, W. J. and Lindstrom, J. M. (1982) Structural similarities between acetylcholine receptors from fish electric organs and mammalian muscle. *Biochemistry* **21,** 4563–4569.
9. Legocki, R. P. and Verma, D. P. S. (1981) Multiple immunoreplica technique: screening for specific proteins with a series of different antibodies using one polyacrylamide gel. *Anal. Biochem.* **111,** 385–392.
10. Erickson, P. F., Minier, L. N., and Lasher, R. S. (1982) Quantitative electrophoretic transfer of polypeptides from SDS polyacrylamide gels to nitrocellulose sheets: a method for their reuse in immunoautoradiographic detection of antigens. *J. Immunol. Methods* **51,** 241–249.

11. Kaufmann, S. H., Ewing, C. M., and Shaper, J. H. (1987) The erasable Western blot. *Anal. Biochem.* **161,** 81–95.

12. Parekh, B. S., Mehta, H. B., West, M. D., and Montelaro, R. C. (1985) Preparative elution of proteins from nitrocellulose membranes after separation by sodium dodecylsulfate-polyacrylamide gel electrophoresis. *Anal. Biochem.* **148,** 87–92.

13. Salinovich, O. and Montelaro, R. C. (1986) Reversible staining and peptide mapping of proteins transferred to nitrocellulose after separations by sodium dodceylsulfate-polyacrylamide gel electrophoresis. *Anal. Biochem.* **156,** 341–347.

14. Gallagher, S. R. and Smith, J. A. (1991) Electrophoretic separation of proteins, in *Current Protocols in Molecular Biology* (Ausubel, F. M., Brent, R., Kingston, R. E., Moore, D. D., Seidman, J. G., Smith, J. A., and Struhl, K., eds.), Wiley, New York.

15. Kaufmann, S. H. (1989) Additional members of the rat liver lamin polypeptide family: structural and immunological characterization. *J. Biol. Chem.* **264,** 13,946–13,955.

16. Fields, A. P., Kaufmann, S. H., and Shaper, J. H. (1986) Analysis of the internal nuclear matrix: oligomers of a 38 kD nucleolar polypeptide stabilized by disulfide bonds. *Exp. Cell Res.* **164,** 139–153.

17. Laskey, R. A. and Mills, A. D. (1977) Enhanced autoradiographic detection of ^{32}P and ^{125}I using intensifying screens and hypersensitized film. *FEBS Lett.* **82,** 314–316.

18. Lin, F., Fan, W., and Wise G. E. (1991) Eosin Y staining of proteins in polyacrylamide gels. *Anal. Biochem.* **196,** 279–283.

19. Lin, W. and Kasamatsu, H. (1983) On the electrotransfer of polypeptides from gels to nitrocellulose membranes. *Anal. Biochem.* **128,** 302–311.

20. Leong, M. M. L., Fox, G. R., and Hayward, J. S. (1988) A photodetection devise for luminol-based immunodot and western blotting assays. *Anal. Biochem.* **168,** 107–114.

21. ECL Western Blotting Protocols (1991) Amersham International plc, Amersham, UK.

22. Kaufmann, S. H., McLaughlin, S. J, Kastan, M. B., Liu, L. F., Karp, J. E., and Burke, P. E. (1991) *Cancer Res.* **51,** 3534–3543.

23

Colloidal Gold Staining and Immunodetection in 2D Protein Mapping

Anthony H. V. Schapira

1. Introduction

This chapter extends the use of the technique described in Chapter 21 to two-dimensional (2D) protein gels, as well as containing some alternatives and modifications to the method.

Two-dimensional sodium dodecyl sulfate-polyacrylamide gel electrophoresis (SDS-PAGE) provides a rapid and reproducible method for the separation and analysis of complex mixtures of proteins. Proteins may be separated in the first dimension either by isoelectric focusing (IEF) *(1)* or nonequilibrium pH gradient electrophoresis (NEPHGE) *(2),* and by SDS-PAGE in the second dimension. Such gels have the capacity to resolve over 1000 individual polypeptides. The identification and characterization of individual polypeptides separated by these techniques is the natural extension of the study of proteins by electrophoresis. A protein may be identified directly from the gel by cutting out the specific gel segment in which it is contained, and then eluting and sequencing the protein. Alternatively, a protein may be identified by specific antibody binding and detected with enzyme-linked or radiolabeled second antibodies. Detection by these methods is generally performed after the proteins in the gel have been transferred to a solid matrix, such as nitrocellulose. The mapping of individual proteins is then dependent on the identification of the protein(s) of interest within the whole protein map. This chapter describes a colloidal gold method of staining all proteins transferred to nitrocellulose followed by antibody binding, which allows the precise mapping of an individual protein within the whole 2D gel picture.

From: *Methods in Molecular Biology, Vol. 80: Immunochemical Protocols, 2nd ed.*
Edited by: J. D. Pound © Humana Press Inc., Totowa, NJ

2. Materials

1. Tube gel and slab gel electrophoresis equipment.
2. Electroblotting equipment.
3. Nitrocellulose (*see* Note 1).
4. 1% Milk powder or 1% bovine serum albumin (BSA) in phosphate-buffered saline (PBS), pH 7.4.
5. 1% (w/v) Analar grade gold chloride. This can be made up in a solution of 100 mL and stored at 4°C in a dark bottle.
6. 20% (v/v) Tween-20 in distilled water.
7. Stannous chloride solution: Dissolve 250 mg of stannous chloride in 1.25 mL of 1*M* HCl and make up to 25 mL with distilled water. Prepare fresh.
8. Citric acid solution: Dissolve 2.42 g of anhydrous citric acid in 250 mL of distilled water.
9. Photographic facilities for high resolution photography.
10. Specific primary antibodies for individual polypeptides.
11. Appropriate antispecies second antibodies linked to horseradish peroxidase (*see* Note 2).
12. 4-Chloro-1-naphthol (*see* Note 2).
13. PBS, pH 7.4.

3. Method

The techniques of 1D and 2D SDS-PAGE (*see Methods in Molecular Biology*, Volumes 1 and 3), electroblotting (*see Methods in Molecular Biology*, Volume 3), and immunoblotting (*see* Chapter 20) are described elsewhere.

First dimension gels may be run either by IEF or NEPHGE. Following the electrophoretic separation of proteins, the gel may be equilibrated for 10–15 min in Tris-glycine-methanol before electroblotting to nitrocellulose. This reduces any distortion from swelling or contraction of the gel relative to nitrocellulose sheet. Prolonged equilibration beyond this time-period may lead to loss of protein from the gel. Electroblotting is now most conveniently performed by the semidry method. This reduces transfer time considerably, utilizes very small amounts of buffer, and the uniform field strength produces consistent transfer of protein over the whole gel.

For consistent results, the gold stain should be prepared fresh for each batch of nitrocellulose filters. The gold stain is prepared essentially as described by Righetti et al. *(3),* with some modifications *(4)* (*see also*, Chapter 29).

1. To a clean 2-L glass flask or beaker, add 750 mL of distilled water. Place on a magnetic stirrer and begin stirring—this will be continued throughout (*see* Note 3).
2. Add dropwise 10 mL of the 1% gold chloride solution. Leave to stir for 5 min.
3. Slowly add 100 mL of 20% (v/v) Tween-20 (*see* Note 4). Leave to stir for 15 min.
4. Add dropwise 4 mL of freshly prepared stannous chloride solution to the gold/Tween mixture (*see* Note 5). The color of the solution will change from gold to burgundy. Leave to stir for 5 min.

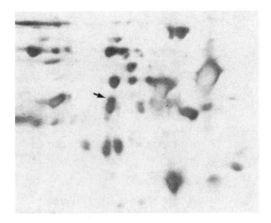

Fig. 1. Gold stain of 2D separation of proteins from beef heart mitochondria. Arrow indicates the 49-kDa protein of NADH CoQ reductase (*see* Figs. 2 and 3).

5. Slowly add 250 mL of citric acid solution to the gold solution. Leave to stir for 20–30 min. The color of the solution should develop into red (*see* Note 6).
6. Following transfer of proteins from the gel, quickly rinse the nitrocellulose in two changes of distilled water. Pour 150–200 mL of the gold stain into a clean glass or plastic container and lay the nitrocellulose face up on top of the gold stain. Shake gently, allowing the stain to cover the filter. Proteins will begin to stain within 15 min, often appearing as a "ghost" before fully developing. A good fresh gold stain will give a pink color to the proteins.
7. Filters should be photographed before blocking overnight with a solution of 1% milk powder or 1% BSA in PBS. Immunoblotting may then be performed as described in Chapter 21 (*see* Notes 7 and 8).

3.1. Example of Technique

Figure 1 shows the gold stain of a section of a 2D gel of beef heart mitochondria proteins separated by isoelectric focusing and then by SDS-PAGE, and transferred to nitrocellulose. The filter was then probed with antibody specific to the 49-kDa iron sulfur protein of NADH CoQ reductase. The blot was photographed with (Fig. 2) and without (Fig. 3) a red filter following development with 4-chloro-1-naphthol. The position of the 49-kDa protein can then be determined by back reference to Fig. 1 (*see* arrow).

4. Notes

1. The nitrocellulose should always be handled with gloves. Otherwise, the gold stain will bring out fingerprints.
2. It is best to use horseradish peroxidase-linked compounds and to develop with 4-chloro-1-naphthol, as this blue-black stain provides a good contrast to the pink of the gold stain.

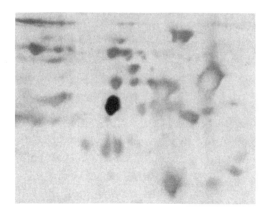

Fig. 2. Immunoblotting with antibody to the 49-kDa protein demonstrates its position on the 2D separation. Photographed with red filter.

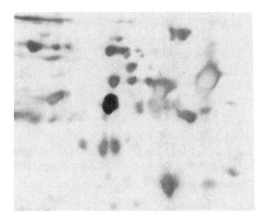

Fig. 3. As for Fig. 2, but photographed without a filter.

3. The volumes of solutions used can be adjusted to the number of filters to be stained. The method described provides sufficient stain for six filters of 14 × 14-cm nitrocellulose.
4. The addition of the Tween-20 before the stannous chloride enhances the stability of the gold colloid and leads to more reproducible results.
5. The slow, dropwise addition of the stannous chloride is also important in establishing a stable stain. The Tween-20 and citric acid solutions can be added at a slow pour. Constant stirring is mandatory.
6. The color of the final solution after 20–30 min of stirring is a good guide to stain quality: A burgundy color is good; a darker purple hue indicates an unstable gel. The longer the stain is left before use, the more purple the stained proteins will

be, and this will contrast less well with the 4-chloro-1-naphthol-developed immunoblot.

7. For greatest sensitivity, the biotin–streptavidin system should be used in antibody detection, especially since proteins separated in 2D are often more difficult to detect than when separated in 1D.

8. The best, most unequivocal results are obtained by immunoblotting a 2D separation with an antibody to a single protein. This can then be developed and photographed. Further antibodies can then be used in sequence on the same filter, with developing and photography recording the position of each protein as the respective antibody is used. There is no need to requench filters between each blot. Washing for 30 min in three changes of PBS–0.1% Tween-20 is sufficient to clean the filter before the next overlay.

References

1. O'Farrell, P. H. (1975) High resolution two dimensional electrophoresis of proteins. *J. Biol. Chem.* **250,** 4007–4021.
2. O'Farrell, P. Z., Goodman, H. M., and O'Farrell, P. H. (1977) High resolution two dimensional electrophoresis of basic as well as acidic proteins. *Cell* **12,** 1133–1142.
3. Righetti, P. G., Casero, P., and Del Campo, G. B. (1986) Gold staining in cellulose acetate membranes. *Clin. Chem. Acta* **157,** 167–174.
4. Schapira, A. H. V. and Keir, G. (1988) Two dimensional protein mapping by gold stain and immunoblotting. *Analyt. Biochem.* **169,** 167–171.

24

Enzyme–Antienzyme Method for Immunohistochemistry

Michael G. Ormerod, Elizabeth Philp, and Susanne F. Imrie

1. Introduction

Immunohistochemical stains use antibodies to identify specific constituents in tissue sections. In order to detect the site of reaction, the antibody is labeled with an enzyme that can be reacted with a suitable substrate to give a colored product. The alternative is to use a fluorescent label. The advantage of an enzyme label is that the nuclei can be counter stained thereby revealing the tissue architecture, and that the stain fades slowly, if at all, allowing the slides to be stored.

In the original method, the section was incubated with the primary antibody followed by a secondary antibody to which a suitable enzyme had been attached. For example, if the primary antibody was a mouse monoclonal, the secondary antibody could be a goat antimouse immunoglobulin. It was later found that the number of enzyme molecules/molecule of primary antibody could be increased by using an enzyme–antienzyme method, thereby increasing the sensitivity of the method.

The basic enzyme–antienzyme method is outlined in Fig. 1. The primary antibody is bound to the antigen of interest, followed by incubation with an appropriate anti-immunoglobulin antibody, and finally with a complex of enzyme–antienzyme antibodies. The primary antibody and the antienzyme antibodies are raised in the same species, so that the anti-immunoglobulin will link the two together. The enzyme used is usually either horseradish peroxidase, in which case the method is called peroxidase–antiperoxidase (PAP), or alkaline phosphatase, where the method is referred to as APAAP. These enzymes are chosen because they have a high turnover number (giving a high yield of product) and have substrates that can give an insoluble, colored product.

From: *Methods in Molecular Biology, Vol. 80: Immunochemical Protocols, 2nd ed.*
Edited by: J. D. Pound © Humana Press Inc., Totowa, NJ

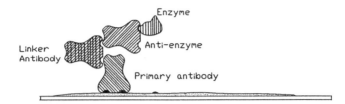

Fig. 1. The enzyme–antienzyme method. The primary antibody and the antienzyme antibody must have been raised in the same species. Because there are several epitopes on the enzyme and the immunoglobulins are divalent, a large complex of enzyme–antienzyme molecules builds up. This increases the number of enzyme molecules linked to each primary antibody molecule. This effect is not shown in the figure, because it would make the diagram too complicated.

For further general reading about immunohistochemistry, *see* refs. *1–3*. For a more detailed discussion of the methods involved in immunohistochemistry, *see* ref. *4*.

2. Materials

1. Xylene or Histoclear (BDH, Atherstone, UK).
2. Ethanol.
3. Phosphate-buffered saline (PBS): 8.5 g of sodium chloride, 1.07 g of disodium hydrogen *ortho*-phosphate (or 2.7 g of $Na_2HPO_4 \cdot 12H_2O$), 0.39 g of sodium dihydrogen *ortho*-phosphate (or 0.51 g of $NaH_2PO_4 \cdot 2H_2O$). Make up to 1 L with distilled water.
4. Bovine serum albumin (BSA).
5. Detergent—BRIJ or Tween-80.
6. Primary antibody (*see* Notes 3 and 4).
7. Anti-immunoglobulin (linking) antibody raised against the species used to produce the primary antibody (*see* Section 1. and Note 4).
8. Enzyme–antienzyme complexes: The antienzyme antibody must have been raised in the species used to produce the primary antibody (*see* Section 1. and Note 4).
9. Diaminobenzidine (DAB) solution: Dissolve 9 mg of DAB in 9 mL of $0.1M$ Tris buffer, pH 7.2. Add 9 mL of distilled water containing 6 µL of 30% H_2O_2.
10. Mayer's hemalum: 1 g of hematoxylin, 50 g of aluminum potassium sulfate, 0.2 g of sodium iodate, 1 g of citric acid, 50 g of chloral hydrate, and 1 L distilled water. Dissolve the hematoxylin in distilled water using gentle heat, if necessary. Add the aluminum potassium sulfate, heat if necessary. Add the sodium iodate, mix well, and leave overnight. Then add citric acid, mix well, and add the chloral hydrate.
11. Hanker Yates Reagent (HYR): Dissolve 7.5 mg of HYR in 5 mL of $0.1M$ Tris-HCl buffer, pH 7.6, and add 6 µL of 30% H_2O_2. (HYR contains *para*-phenylene-diamine plus pyrocatechol.)

12. Carbazole: Dissolve 2 mg of 3-amino, 9-ethyl carbazole in 0.5 mL of dimethyl formamide (DMF) in a glass tube. Add 9.5 mL of 0.2M acetate buffer, pH 5. Just before use, add 5 µL of 30% H_2O_2.
13. DPX—mountant for cover slips (as supplied by manufacturer).
14. Glycerin jelly (alternative mountant): 10 g of gelatin, 70 mL of glycerin, 0.25 g of phenol, and 60 mL of distilled water. Dissolve the gelatin in distilled water using gentle heat. Add glycerin and phenol, and mix well. Aliquot into 10 mL batches and store in the refrigerator. For use, melt in a water bath at 60°C—avoid shaking since this creates air bubbles.
15. Chloronaphthol: Dissolve 20 mg of 4 chloro-1-naphthol in 40 mL of 20% methanol in 0.05M Tris saline, pH 7.6 (0.6 g of Trizma base plus 3 g of NaCl in 100 mL of distilled water, adjust the pH to 7.6 with HCl). Add 13.5 µL of 30% H_2O_2 and heat gently to 50°C before use.
16. Tetramethyl benzidine: Dissolve 5 mg of tetramethyl benzidine in 2 mL of DMSO. Add to 50 mL of 0.02M acetate buffer, pH 3.3, containing 20 µL of 30% H_2O_2 immediately before use.
17. Methyl green.
18. Veronal acetate buffer: 0.97 g of sodium acetate (trihydrate), 1.47 g of sodium barbitone, 250 mL of fresh distilled water (CO_2 free), and 2.5 mL of 0.1M hydrochloric acid, pH 9.2.
19. Fast red salt: Dissolve 5 mg of naphthol AS BI phosphoric acid sodium salt in 1 drop of DMF in a glass tube. Dissolve 5 mg of Fast red TR salt in 10 mL of veronal acetate buffer, pH 9.2. Mix the two solutions together and filter.
20. Fast blue salt: Dissolve 5 mg of naphthol AS BI in DMF in a glass tube, and add to 5 mg of Fast blue BB salt in 10 mL of 0.1M Tris-HCl buffer, pH 9.0.
21. New Fuchsin: Mix 250 µL of a 4% solution of New Fuchsin in 2M HCl with 250 µL of 4% sodium nitrite. Leave the mixture to stand in the cold for 5 min, and then add it to 40 mL of 0.2M Tris-HCl buffer, pH 9.0, and add 10 mg of naphthol AS TR phosphoric acid dissolved in 0.2 mL of DMF in a glass tube.
22. Periodic acid.
23. Potassium borohydride.
24. Acetic acid: a 20% solution in distilled water.
25. Pronase solution: 50 µg of pronase/mL of PBS.
26. 3-Amino propyl triethoxysilane (APTS).
27. Citrate buffer (pH 6.0): Dissolve 21.0 g citric acid in 10 L distilled water; add 265 mL 1M NaOH. Adjust pH.
28. A domestic microwave oven fitted with a temperature probe.
29. Levamisole.

3. Methods

3.1. The Basic Method

1. If the section has been cut from a paraffin block, take it through xylene (or Histoclear) and ethanol to water (*see* Note 2).

2. Block endogenous enzyme as appropriate (*see* Section 3.3.). Wash the section in water.

3. Use treatment with a proteolytic enzyme or in a microwave oven if appropriate (*see* Section 3.4.). Wash the section in water.

4. Rinse the section in PBS, and then wipe any excess from the slide, so that the antiserum is not diluted too much on the slide.

5. Incubate for 1 h at room temperature in a moist chamber with 100 µL of primary antibody appropriately diluted in either PBS, 0.5% BSA, or (preferably) PBS, 5% serum, the serum being obtained from the species in which the second antibody was raised (*see* Notes 3–6).

6. Wash the section with PBS, 0.5% BSA followed twice by PBS containing 0.01% detergent (BRIJ or Tween-80).

7. Repeat step 4.

8. Incubate for 1 h at room temperature in a moist chamber with 100 µL of second, anti-immunoglobulin, antibody appropriately diluted (*see* Note 4).

9. Repeat steps 6 and 7.

10. Incubate for 1 h at room temperature in a moist chamber with 100 µL of the enzyme–antienzyme complex appropriately diluted.

11. Repeat steps 6 and 7. Wash in distilled water.

12. Develop the color and counterstain, and mount as appropriate (*see* Notes 7 and 8 and Section 3.2.).

3.2. Developing the Colored Product

These procedures relate to step 12 in Section 3.1. For all the methods listed below, the substrate solutions should be prepared fresh and the sections should be at room temperature.

3.2.1. Peroxidase Substrates (see Note 9)

1. DAB: Cover the section with this substrate, and incubate the slide for 5 min. The product is brown, and is stable in alcohols and in xylene. Counterstain with Mayer's hemalum for 5 min. Wash in tap water. Dip the slide in saturated lithium carbonate for a few seconds; this makes the nuclear stain blue. Wash in tap water. Dehydrate through ethanol and xylene (or Histoclear), and mount in a permanent mountant, e.g., DPX.

2. HYR: Incubate the slides for 15 min. The product is blackish-brown, and is stable in xylene and alcohols. Counterstain with hemalum, and mount in DPX.

3. Carbazole: Incubate the slides for 15 min. The product is red and insoluble in water, but dissolves in organic solvents. Counterstain with hemalum, and mount in a water-based mountant, e.g., glycerin jelly.

4. Chloronaphthol: Incubate the slides for 8 min. The product is blue and soluble in xylene. We do not know a suitable counterstain; hemalum being blue is unsuitable, and methyl green is water-soluble. Mount in glycerin jelly.

5. Tetramethyl benzidine: Incubate for 15 min. The product is blue, and stable in xylene and alcohols. Counterstain with methyl green, and mount in DPX.

3.2.2. Alkaline Phosphatase Substrates

1. Fast red salt: Cover the section with this substrate, and incubate for 45–60 min. The product is red and is soluble in organic solvents. Counterstain with hemalum, and mount in glycerin jelly.
2. Fast blue salt: Use two or three 5-min incubations each in fresh substrate. The product is blue and soluble in organic solvents. There is no satisfactory counterstain. Mount in glycerin jelly.
3. New Fuchsin: Incubate the slides for 10 min. The product is red, and stable in xylene and alcohols. Counterstain with hemalum, and mount in DPX.

3.3. Blocking Endogenous Enzymes

The tissue under study may contain endogenous enzyme, which is the same as that used in the enzyme–antienzyme stain. It is desirable that this should be destroyed. Otherwise, interpretation of the stained slide is difficult.

1. For peroxidase, incubate the section in one of the following solutions for the time indicated, and then wash in tap water before starting the method in Section 3.1.
   a. 2.3% Periodic acid in distilled water for 5 min;
   b. 0.03% Potassium borohydride in distilled water (freshly prepared) for 2 min; or
   c. 0.1% Phenylhydrazine in PBS for 5 min.
   The last treatment is the most gentle and should be used for labile antigens.
2. For alkaline phosphatase, incubate the section in 20% acetic acid for 5 min, and then wash it in tap water. This treatment may destroy the antigen. An alternative for tissues other than the intestine is to make the substrate solution (Section 3.2.2.) in 1 mM levamisole (increase to 2 mM for tissues rich in alkaline phosphatase, e.g., kidney or placenta) (*see* Note 10).

3.4. Revealing "Hidden" Antigens

In fixed tissue, some antigens can be revealed by treatment with a proteolytic enzyme or by heating the section in a microwave oven *(5)*.

3.4.1. Treatment with a Proteolytic Enzyme

This protocol uses pronase.

1. Dewax the section in xylene or Histoclear, and take it through ethanol to water.
2. Incubate the section in PBS at 37°C for 5 min, and then in pronase solution at 37°C for 20 min.
3. Wash the section in running tap water for 5 min, and then wash twice in PBS.

After enzyme treatment the sections are very fragile and must be handled with care.

3.4.2. Treatment in a Microwave Oven

1. Cut 5-μm sections from a paraffin block, and mount them on slides coated with APTS.

2. Dewax sections, take them down to water, and place the sections in a plastic holder.
3. Put 500 mL citrate buffer in a plastic container with a lid that has a hole cut to take the temperature probe in the microwave oven (*see* Note 11). Heat the buffer to 90°C.
4. Place slides in the citrate buffer, and heat in the microwave oven at 90°C for 10 min.
5. Remove slides from oven, and leave to cool in the citrate buffer for 15 min.
6. Wash sections in running tap water. Block endogenous phosphatase by treatment of choice (*see* Section 3.3., step 2). Wash in PBS.
7. Continue as for the basic method.

4. Notes

1. DAB is a suspected carcinogen and must be treated with care. Use in a fume hood.
2. For routine histopathology, tissues are usually fixed in formalin and embedded in paraffin wax. Sections cut from this material must be dewaxed in xylene and taken through ethanol to water. This gives sections of high quality but, unfortunately, many antigens are destroyed by this process. Some will survive fixation in ethanol based fixatives, such as Methacarn (60% methanol, 30% chloroform, 10% glacial acetic acid). Some antigens can be revealed by treating either with a proteolytic enzyme or by brief heating in a microwave oven (*see* Section 3.4.). Others will not survive embedding in paraffin and must be studied in sections cut from unfixed, frozen tissue. These sections are often briefly fixed before use. The correct fixative has to be determined empirically for each antigen under study.
3. The primary antibody can be in the form of a polyclonal antiserum or a monoclonal antibody produced either in a culture supernatant or in an ascitic fluid. The concentration of the antibody in an ascitic fluid will be an order of magnitude greater than that in the culture supernatant, but the latter will be free of other immunoglobulins.
4. The appropriate concentration of the primary antibody must be determined by using serial dilutions on a set of sections cut from a tissue known to carry the antigen of interest. The linking antibody and the enzyme–antienzyme complex are best used at the concentration recommended by the manufacturer. If desired, this can be checked using serial dilutions.
5. For incubations in antibody, the slides are usually placed in a suitable box in which they can be kept horizontally in a humid atmosphere. This is important because the solutions must not be allowed to dry out during incubation.
6. In the methods described, incubation at room temperature is recommended. However, room temperature can vary considerably and if the final product is to be quantified (for example, by image cytometry), the temperature of incubation should be carefully controlled.
7. The substrate chosen for color development depends on the enzyme used and the final color required by the investigator. For routine work, DAB is normally used with peroxidase, and Fast red with alkaline phosphatase.

8. The choice of mountant depends on the solubility characteristics of the colored product. Permanent mountants, such as DPX, are based on organic solvents. If the colored product is soluble in such solvents, then a water-based mountant must be used. Guidance is given for each substrate described.

9. When using peroxidase and DAB, it is sometimes necessary to bleach the brown pigment found in fixed tissue sections, e.g., in formol saline fixed red blood cells. Bleach with 7.5% hydrogen peroxide in distilled water for 5 min. Wash well in tap water.

10. Different tissues contain different isoenzymes of alkaline phosphatase, and the intestinal isoenzyme is not inhibited by levamisole. The enzyme used in immunohistochemistry is extracted from calf intestine, so that levamisole can be used as an inhibitor without affecting the desired reaction. For labile antigens in the intestine, it is better to switch to the peroxidase method.

11. It is important that the sections be immersed in a large volume of buffer to ensure an even distribution of heat.

12. Control sections should be included with each set of stained slides. A positive control from a tissue known to contain the antigen should be included for each primary antibody used. The negative control is normally a section stained with the omission of the primary antibody.

13. The negative control should be quite clean. If a reaction is observed, check for the presence of endogenous enzyme or pigment. In their absence, try to reduce the background by more careful washing and increasing the protein in the washing solution. Finally, try fresh secondary reagents purchased from a different source.

14. If no staining is observed in the positive control, check whether a reagent has been inadvertently omitted or whether the wrong reagent has been used (for example, antimouse Ig on a rat monoclonal). This is easy to do if several different antibodies from different species are being used.

15. If staining is weak, one of the reagents may have deteriorated. For example, stock solutions of H_2O_2 should be renewed regularly.

References

1. Sternberger, S. S. and De Lellis, R. A. (eds.) (1982) *Diagnostic Immunohistochemistry.* Masson Publishing, New York.
2. Bullock, G. R. and Petrusz., P. (eds.) (1982 and 1983) *Techniques in Immunocytochemistry,* vols. 1 and 2, Academic, London.
3. Polak, J. M. and van Noorden, S. (eds.) (1983) *Immunocytochemistry.* John Wright and Sons, Bristol, UK.
4. Ormerod, M. G., and Imrie, S. F. (1989) Immunohistochemistry in *Light Microscopy in Biology. A Practical Approach* (Lacey, A. J., ed.), Oxford University Press, Oxford, UK.
5. Cuevas, E. C., Bateman, A. C., Wilkins, B. S., Johnson, P. A., Williams, J. H., Lee, A. H. S., Jones, D. B., and Wright, D. H. (1994) Microwave antigen retrieval in immunocytochemistry: a study of 80 antibodies. *J. Clin. Pathol.* **47,** 448–452.

25

Immunohistochemical Detection of Bromodeoxyuridine-Labeled Nuclei for In Vivo Cell Kinetic Studies

Jonathan A. Green, Richard E. Edwards, and Margaret M. Manson

1. Introduction

The classical technique for identifying cells engaged in DNA synthesis is by their uptake of [^{3}H]-thymidine, detected using autoradiography. However, this method can be inconvenient, as specialized darkroom and radioisotope facilities are required, with the potential health hazard that handling isotopes entails. Bromodeoxyuridine (BrdU), the halogenated 5-substituted derivative of deoxyuridine, is a thymidine analog specifically incorporated into the DNA of proliferating cells during S phase. This is now a well-established alternative to [^{3}H] thymidine, since it has been shown that labeling indices for the two molecules are the same *(1,2)*. The development of a monoclonal antibody *(3)* that recognizes BrdU incorporated into single-stranded DNA has resulted in several techniques using immunocytochemical staining to detect incorporated BrdU in frozen, paraffin- and plastic-embedded sections of tissue by light microscopy. It has also proved extremely valuable for studies in conjunction with flow cytometry and even, for in vivo studies of human tumor cell kinetics (*see* Chapter 26). We describe here a method to detect DNA synthesis by in vivo labeling of nuclei with BrdU, followed by indirect immunological detection in paraffin-embedded tissue *(4)*.

2. Materials

1. Bromodeoxyuridine: 50 μg/g body weight dissolved in 1 mL of sterile 0.9% saline. Prepare fresh.
2. Carnoys fixative: 60% absolute alcohol, 30% chloroform, and 10% glacial acetic acid.

From: *Methods in Molecular Biology, Vol. 80: Immunochemical Protocols, 2nd ed.*
Edited by: J. D. Pound © Humana Press Inc., Totowa, NJ

3. Glass microscope slides that have been coated with 3-amino-propyltriethoxysilane (APES) (*see* Note 1).
4. Xylene.
5. 100, 90, and 70% ethanol series.
6. Phosphate-buffered saline (PBS), pH 7.4: 8 g of NaCl, 0.2 g of KH_2PO_4, 2.8 g of $Na_2HPO_4 \cdot 12H_2O$, 0.2 g of KCl dissolved and made up to 1 L in distilled water.
7. 0.3% H_2O_2 in distilled water.
8. 1M HCl.
9. Monoclonal antibody to BrdU: A rat monoclonal obtained from Sera-Lab (Crawley Down, Sussex, UK).
10. Rabbit antirat peroxidase-conjugated secondary antibody.
11. Substrate solution: A stock solution of diaminoazobenzidine (DAB) is made up at 5 mg/mL in PBS, aliquoted into 0.5 mL amounts, and stored frozen. For use, add 4.5 mL of PBS to 0.5 mL of DAB stock and add 50 μL of freshly prepared 1% H_2O_2 immediately before use.
12. Hematoxylin.
13. Mountant: DPX.

3. Method

3.1. Preparation of Tissue Sections

1. Dissolve the required amount of BrdU in 1 mL of sterile saline immediately prior to use and protect the solution from light to prevent photo-decomposition.
2. Inject the solution ip and sacrifice the animal 1 h later (*see* Notes 2 and 3).
3. Dissect out the liver and gently wipe excess blood from the outside of the organ (*see* Note 4).
4. Using a single edge razor blade, cut thin (2–3 mm) slices of liver and place them immediately into Carnoys fixative.
5. Leave the tissues in the fixative for a minimum of 2 h to a maximum of 18 h and then transfer them to 95% ethanol (*see* Note 5).
6. Embed the tissues in paraffin wax by routine histological procedures as soon as possible to avoid excessive hardening.
7. Cut sections 5-μm thick and mount on coated glass slides. Dewax the slides in xylene for 3 × 20 min and then rehydrate in 100% ethanol (2 × 2 min), then 95% and 70% ethanol and water for 2 min each.

3.2. Immunohistochemistry

1. Wash the sections in PBS for 2 min. It is convenient to place the slides on a rack over the sink to carry out all washing steps.
2. Inhibit endogenous peroxidase activity in the tissue sections by incubating in 0.3% H_2O_2 for 20 min.
3. Wash the sections in running tap water for 10 min, then rinse in distilled water at 60°C.
4. Incubate the sections in 1M HCl at 60°C for exactly 8 min (*see* Notes 6 and 7). This step denatures the DNA just sufficiently to allow access of the anti-BrdU antibody.

5. Wash briefly in tap water, then distilled water, and finally, PBS.
6. Dry around the section with a tissue (*see* Note 8) and incubate in monoclonal antibody against BrdU, diluted 1:100 in PBS, for 30 min at room temperature in a humid box to prevent the sections from drying out. One hundred microliters of solution should be enough to cover the tissue.
7. Wash 3 × 5 min in PBS.
8. Dry around the sections again and apply rabbit antirat IgG peroxidase conjugate diluted 1:100 in PBS and incubate as in step 6.
9. Wash 3 × 5 min in PBS.
10. Incubate the sections in freshly prepared DAB substrate solution for 10 min (*see* Note 9). A brown product will be deposited at the site of BrdU incorporation.
11. Wash the sections in PBS.
12. Counterstain lightly with hematoxylin.
13. Dehydrate the sections in increasing concentrations of ethanol (70, 90, 100%), clear with xylene, and mount in DPX (*see also* Chapter 24).

4. Notes

1. Clean the slides in 5% DECON 90 or an equivalent detergent overnight. Rinse in hot water for 30 min, then twice in deionized water. Dry at 60°C. Dip the slides in a 4% solution of APES in acetone for 2 min, then rinse twice in acetone. Dry the slides in an oven at 60°C. They can then be stored at room temperature indefinitely.
2. It is vital that the BrdU is injected into the peritoneal cavity and not the gut. Injection of BrdU into the gut is the most common reason for failure to see any stained nuclei.
3. After injection of the BrdU, the time before sacrifice may be extended to give a higher degree of incorporation into the dividing nuclei. However, a single injection of BrdU will be undetectable after three cell divisions.
4. This method can be applied to other tissues in the animal where active DNA synthesis is occurring, for instance, the small intestine. In fact, it is good practice to prepare a composite block containing the tissue of interest and a piece of small intestine as a positive control (*see* Fig. 1).
5. We have also used this method on acetone-fixed paraffin-embedded material with equal success. Slices of fresh liver are fixed in ice-cold acetone for at least 4 h. Material can then be transferred to a –20°C freezer prior to routine embedding and sectioning. In this case, uncoated glass slides were used.
6. This is the most important step in the procedure. The exact time (usually between 2 and 10 min) must be determined empirically, if other fixatives such as acetone are used.
7. Some workers neutralize the HCl with 0.1*M* borax buffer, pH 8.5 for 5 min.
8. A pen for drawing a hydrophobic ring around the tissue section is marketed by Dako. It obviates the need to wipe around the sections after each step and reduces the amounts of antibody solution required.

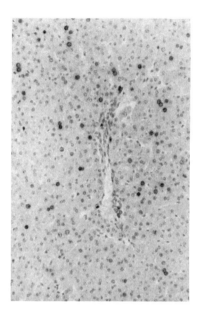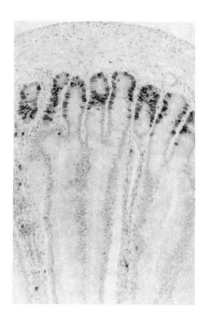

Fig. 1. Nuclei in liver (**left**), and small intestine (**right**) that have incorporated BrdU during DNA synthesis are stained more darkly.

9. The rabbit antirat antibody may alternatively be conjugated with alkaline phosphatase and detected with naphthol AS-BI and fast red. In this case, incorporation will be indicated by a red color. *See also* Chapter 24 for alternative conjugates and substrates.

References

1. Schutte, B., Reynders, M. M. J., Bosman, F. T., and Blijham, G. H. (1987) Studies with antibromodeoxyuridine antibodies: II simultaneous immunocytochemical detection of antigen expression and DNA synthesis by *in vivo* labelling of intestinal mucosa. *J. Histochem. Cytochem.* **35,** 371–374.
2. Lanier, T. L., Berger, E. K., and Eacho, P. I. (1989) Comparison of 5-bromo-2-deoxyuridine and [^{3}H]thymidine for studies of hepatocellular proliferation in rodents. *Carcinogenesis* **10,** 1341–1343.
3. Gratzner, H. G. (1982) Monoclonal antibody to 5-bromo and 5-iododeoxyuridine: a new reagent for detection of DNA replication. *Science* **218,** 474,475.
4. Wynford-Thomas, D. and Williams, E. D. (1986) Use of bromodeoxyuridine for cell kinetic studies in intact animals. *Cell Tissue Kinetics* **19,** 179–182.

26

Cell Kinetic Studies Using a Monoclonal Antibody to Bromodeoxyuridine

George D. Wilson

1. Introduction

Cell kinetics is defined as the measurement of time parameters in biological systems. Traditionally, this has involved the use of radioactive precursors of DNA, such as tritiated thymidine (^{3}HTdR), and autoradiography to detect their incorporation into DNA. This technique has provided detailed knowledge of cell kinetics in both in vitro and in vivo experimental systems. The technique, however, is time consuming and arduous and is not readily applicable to human tumor research because of ethical problems involved in incorporation of a radioisotope into DNA.

The development of monoclonal antibodies which recognize halogenated pyrimidines such as 5-bromo-2-deoxyuridine (BrdU) incorporated into DNA *(1)* and of flow cytometric (FCM) techniques to simultaneously measure BrdU uptake and total DNA content *(2)* have led to a renaissance in cell kinetic studies. The speed and quantitative power of the flow cytometer, in conjunction with the specificity and sensitivity of monoclonal antibody techniques, provide the basis for the adoption and success of the BrdU technique in experimental and clinical investigations.

The BrdU/FCM technique offers several advantages over ^{3}HTdR/autoradiography method in many cell kinetic studies.

1. The simultaneous measurement of BrdU incorporation and DNA content confers sensitivity and versatility in detection of cell cycle perturbations in response drugs or radiation and tracing the lineage of a cell within the cell cycle. The use of computer-generated windows facilitates the analysis of any population of cells within any phase of the cell cycle and is not restricted to the "mitotic window," as is the case with ^{3}HTdR/autoradiography.

From: *Methods in Molecular Biology, Vol. 80: Immunochemical Protocols, 2nd ed.*
Edited by: J. D. Pound © Humana Press Inc., Totowa, NJ

2. The results from a cell kinetic study can be obtained, literally, within 1 d using BrdU/FCM, whereas ^{3}HTdR/autoradiography may take several weeks to obtain an answer.
3. It is now possible to study routinely human tumor cell kinetic studies in vivo, because BrdU does not have to be a radioisotope as it is detected by a monoclonal antibody. BrdU shows no toxicity in the doses required for cell kinetic studies in humans.

BrdU/DNA flow cytometry offers flexibility and diversity in the study of cell kinetics from cells in culture to human tumors in vivo. The essence of the procedure is to pulse label with BrdU by a short-term incubation in vitro or by a single injection in vivo; samples are then taken at time intervals thereafter and stained after fixation in ethanol. The cells are then stained with a monoclonal antibody against BrdU that can be either directly conjugated to a fluorochrome (usually fluorescein isothiocyanate [FITC]) or, alternatively, bound to a second antibody conjugated with FITC. The cells are then counterstained with propidium iodide (PI) to measure the DNA content and analyzed on the flow cytometer. The results are displayed as linear-red fluorescence on the x-axis vs linear or log-green fluorescence on the y-axis.

2. Materials

1. BrdU: This can be obtained from Sigma (Poole, UK) for experimental purposes. A preparation suitable for human use can be obtained from the Investigational Drugs Branch of the National Cancer Institute (Bethesda, MD). Alternatively individual Hospital Pharmacies can formulate their own preparation.
2. 70% Ethanol for fixation.
3. $2M$ Hydrochloric acid.
4. Phosphate-buffered saline (PBS), pH 7.4.
5. 0.4 mg/mL Pepsin in $0.1M$ HCl, pH 1.5 or 0.2 mg/mL pepsin in $2M$ HCl. The pepsin is dissolved in a small volume of PBS or water before addition of HCl.
6. Antibody incubation buffer: 0.5% normal goat serum (NGS) and 0.5% Tween-20 in PBS.
7. Monoclonal antibody against BrdU: Many are available from various manufacturers. Some have differing specificities for different halogenated pyrimidines (*see* later). The antibodies used routinely by our group are a rat IgG$_{2a}$ (BUI/75 ICR) available from Sera-Lab (Crawley Down, Sussex, UK) and a mouse IgG (BU20a) from Dako (High Wycombe, Bucks, UK).
8. Goat antirat or antimouse IgG (whole molecule) FITC (Sigma).
9. 35-μM Pore nylon filter.
10. 12-mL Conical bottom tube.
11. Swinnex holders.
12. 10 mL Syringe.
13. Propidium iodide (PI) (Sigma).
14. A flow cytometer.

3. Methods

A prerequisite for FCM is a single cell or nuclei suspension. In vivo studies in solid tumors and tissues require disaggregation of the material into single cells or nuclei. The staining method described here includes a method for obtaining nuclei from solid tumors. However, it is not appropriate to describe detailed methods for obtaining cell suspensions from solid tumors in this chapter. Readers are directed to ref. *3* for a review on methods for obtaining single cell suspensions for FCM studies.

3.1. BrdU Incorporation

1. To incorporate BrdU in vitro into monolayers or cell suspensions, the cells are incubated with 10–20 μM BrdU for 10–20 min. Concentrations as small as 1 μM can be detected, whereas concentrations >50 μM may cause cell cycle perturbations. The BrdU is thoroughly washed out by two washes in PBS or medium. It is important to keep everything at 37°C for cell kinetic studies to avoid any perturbations caused by lowering the temperature.
2. To incorporate BrdU in vitro into 1–2 mm^3 solid pieces of tissue in explant culture, use concentrations of 50 μM or greater in the culture medium for 1 h under high pressure oxygen to ensure maximum diffusion of the DNA precursor into the core of the tissue *(4)*.
3. For in vivo incorporation of BrdU in experimental animals, inject 10–100 mg/kg of BrdU in 0.9% saline by the ip route. A concentration of 10 mg/mL is routinely used. The animal is sacrificed after 1 h for labeling index studies or at 1–2 hourly time intervals for cell cycle progression studies. In vivo incorporation of BrdU into humans at Mount Vernon Hospital involves iv injection of 200 mg of BrdU in 20 mL of normal saline as a single bolus over 3–5 min.

3.2. Fixation

Prior to the staining procedures, fix cells in 70% ethanol. Best results are obtained by resuspending the cell pellet in 1 mL of PBS and adding 9 mL of ice-cold 70% ethanol while vortexing to prevent agglutination. Solid pieces of tissue can be fixed as 5 mm^3 pieces directly in ice-cold 70% ethanol. Cells and tissues are usually left at least 1 h prior to staining. Fixed cells or tissues should be stored at 4°C and, in the author's experience, will remain suitable for BrdU staining studies for at least 3 yr.

3.3. Staining Procedure

1. Cut solid tumors or tissues, removed from the fixative, into 1–2 mm^3 pieces and incubate in 5–10 mL of 0.1 M HCl containing 0.4 mg/mL pepsin, pH 1.5, for 30–60 min at 37°C with constant agitation. The period of incubation varies from one tumor or normal tissue to another (*see* Notes 1 and 2).
2. When the tissue starts to break up, ensure complete dissociation into individual nuclei by pipeting using a 5-mL automatic pipet.

3. Filter the suspension of nuclei into a 12-mL conical-bottomed tube through 35-µ*M* pore nylon filter, in a Swinnex holder and 10 mL syringe, to remove large debris and dumped nuclei.
4. Centrifuge the suspension at 2000 rpm for 5 min.
5. If cell suspensions are used as starting material, then omit steps 1–4. Centrifuge the suspension from cultures or dissociated from solid tissues at 1000 rpm for 5 min and decant the fixative.
6. The pellets from nuclei obtained from solid tumors are resuspended in 2 mL of 2*M* HCl and incubated for 10–15 min at room temperature. This can also be done with the whole cell suspension, although 20–30 min in 2*M* HCl is required. In the author's experience, optimal staining of cell suspensions is achieved resuspending the pellet in 2.5 mL of 0.2 mg/mL pepsin in 2*M* HCl for 20 min (*see* Note 3). All of these variations are carried out at room temperature with occasional mixing (*see* Note 3). The step achieves partial unwinding of the DNA into single strands to allow monoclonal antibody access to the binding sites.
7. Add 5 mL of PBS to the HCl and centrifuge the tubes at 2000 rpm for nuclei, or 1000 for cells, for 5 min.
8. Add 5 mL of PBS to the pellets and repeat the centrifugation. The washes with PBS are sufficient to remove all the acid (*see* Note 4).
9. Resuspend the pellet in 0.5 mL of antibody incubation buffer and 25 µL of monoclonal antibody. The dilution of monoclonal antibody will vary according to the preparation (*see* Notes 5 and 6). The monoclonal antibody used in the author's studies is derived directly from the supernatant from the antibody producing cell line. Incubate the tubes for 1 h at room temperature with occasional mixing (*see* Note 7).
10. Add 5 mL of PBS and centrifuge the tubes at 2000 rpm for nuclei, or 1000 rpm for cells, for 5 min.
11. Resuspend the pellets in 0.5 mL of antibody incubation buffer containing 25 µL of goat antirat or antirat IgG (whole molecule) FITC conjugate. Allow binding of the second antibody to proceed for 30–60 min at room temperature with occasional mixing.
12. Repeat step 10 (*see* Note 8).
13. Resuspend the resulting pellet in 1–3 mL of PBS containing 10 µg/mL PI.
14. Analyze on a flow cytometer (*see* Notes 9 and 10). This type of staining can be analyzed on any of the modern flow cytometers with the proviso that the machine is equipped with a pulse processing facility to enable the discrimination of cell doublets. The most commonly used flow cytometer is the Becton Dickinson FACScan. In this machine, PI should be collected into FL3 rather than FL2 to overcome any crossover of the FITC into the FL2 channel. The FL3 detector should be routinely set around 400, whereas FL1 is usually set at around 500 in linear amplification. Controls, without either BrdU or the monoclonal antibody, should be included whenever possible to determine the lower limits of detection of the DNA precursor. At least 10,000 events should be analyzed, but more might be required in the case of slowly proliferating (low BrdU incorporation) tissues or tumors.

3.4. Examples of Data and Data Analysis

Cell kinetic data can be generated from a wide range of experimental conditions using BrdU/FCM. Figure 1 shows bivariate distributions obtained from a "pulse chase" experiment of V79 cells cultivated in vitro. The basic cell populations can be separated from each other by considering both their BrdU uptake and DNA content. Two populations show little BrdU uptake, those at channel 270 are G1 cells and those at channel 550 are G2 + M cells. The S-phase cells lie between these two populations in terms of DNA content, but are separated from them by virtue of their BrdU uptake. Early S-phase cells can be seen arising from the G1 populations, as can mid- and late-S-phase cells, owing to their increasing DNA content. The progression of cells through the cell cycle can be easily detected in the subsequent profiles at hourly intervals. BrdU-labeled cells increase their DNA as they move through S-phase. They spend a short time in G2 before dividing and entering G1. Thus, at 3 h, the original BrdU-labeled population is clearly separated into two subpopulations. One cohort of BrdU-labeled cells is progressing through mid- and late-S-phase and G2, whereas the other comprises cells that have divided (indicated by an arrow in Fig. 1) and now reside in G1. With time, this latter compartment increases as more of the original S-phase cells divide, whereas the former diminishes as the early S-phase cells reach late S and G2. At 7 h, virtually all the original S-phase cells have either divided or are in G2. In addition, some of these cells (those that were in late S-phase at time zero) have progressed through G1 and entered early and mid-S-phase. By 9 h, the population has almost regained the 1 h profile as the cell cycle is almost complete. The unlabeled cells can also be tracked around their cell cycle. The arrow in the 4-h profile shows the movement of G1 cells into early S-phase.

Analysis of this type of data is handled by the computer facilities of the flow cytometer. Basically, regions of interest or windows can be set in any phase of the cell cycle looking at both BrdU and non-BrdU-labeled cells. Figure 2 shows an example of analysis regions set on the 4-h profile from Fig. 1. The left-hand panel shows the bivariate distribution in which a region (R1) has been set to discriminate the BrdU-labeled cells. Two single parameter histograms have been generated; the middle panel displays the DNA profile (PI-FL3) of all cells and the right-hand panel displays the DNA profile of BrdU-labeled cells gated from R1. Within each of these DNA profiles, three regions have been set. R2 describes the cells resident in G1, R3 delineates the cells in G2, and R4 analyses a narrow window in mid-S. These basic regions can give information on all cell cycle parameters and in most experimental conditions.

Region 4 in the gated and ungated DNA profile can generate a curve analogous to a "pulse-labeled mitosis" analysis from ^{3}HTdR/autoradiography. A plot

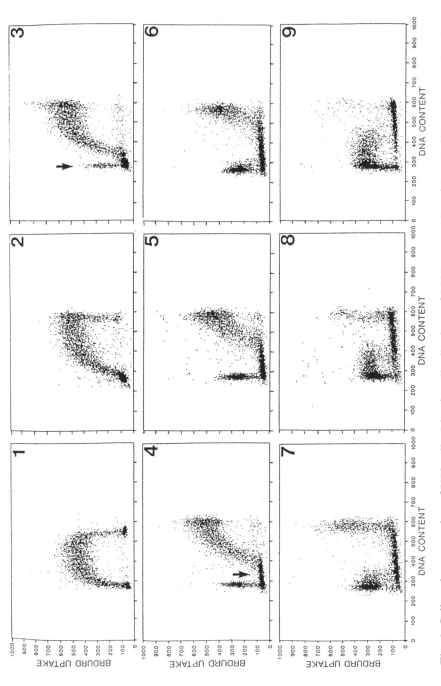

Fig. 1. Cell cycle progression of V79 cells. Bivariate distributions of DNA content (x-axis) vs BrdU uptake (y-axis) of V79 cells removed at hourly intervals after pulse labeling with BrdU. Cells in exponential growth, were pulse labeled with 10 μM BrdU for 20 min. After washing out the BrdU, the cells were resuspended in fresh medium and harvested at 1-h intervals.

260

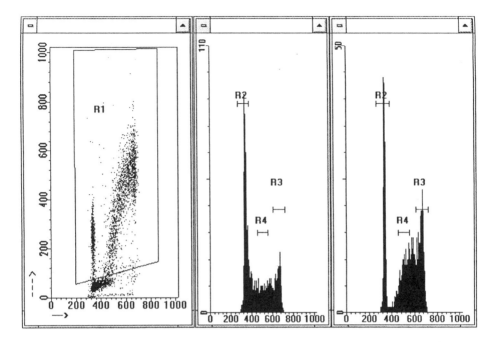

Fig. 2. FCM profiles of V79 cells 4 h after pulse labeling with BrdU. The left-hand panel shows the bivariate distribution, the middle panel shows the DNA profile of the total cell population, while the right-hand panel consists of the DNA profile of BrdU-labeled cells only (gated on R1).

of time vs the ratio of cells in the mid-S window of the BrdU-labeled DNA profile as a fraction of the total number of cells in this window from the ungated DNA profile produces the curve seen in Fig. 3. From this analysis, the mid-S ratio should stay at its maximum (theoretically 1.0) for a time equal to half T_S (duration of S-phase). The ratio then falls to a value which should approach zero and remain low for a period equal to the cell cycle time (T_C) minus T_S; this can be read off from the midpoint of the maximum and minimum mid-S ratio values. The ratio will then rise again and the T_C can be read off from the midpoint of the second peak. The duration of G2 + M (T_{G2+M}) can be estimated by plotting the entry of BrdU-labeled cells into G1; this can be generated by plotting the number of cells in R2 of the gated DNA profile (right panel) as a function of time. Extrapolation of the data, over the first 4–6 h, back to 0 equates to T_{G2+M}.

In human tumors, both the labeling index (LI) and T_S can be calculated from a single observation *(5)*. These two parameters can be used to calculate the potential doubling time (T_{pot}), which describes the shortest possible time a cell

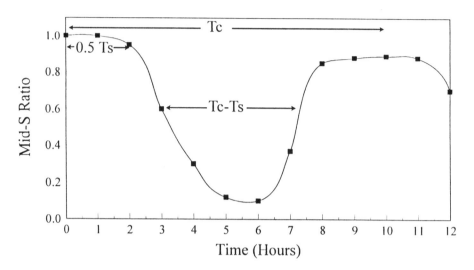

Fig. 3. Cell cycle analysis of BrdU/DNA profiles. The curve is generated from narrow regions set in mid-S phase. One region is set around the BrdU-labeled cells and the other encompasses all cells in mid-S. The y-axis is calculated from the ratio of cells in the BrdU-labeled compartment divided by that in the total mid-S region (R4 in the gated and ungated DNA profiles in Fig. 2).

population can double its number in the absence of cell loss. This procedure is based on the measurement of the mean DNA content of the BrdU-labeled cohort of cells.

Immediately after labeling, as in the 1-h profile from Fig. 1, the mean DNA of the BrdU-labeled cells will be halfway between that of G1 and G2 cells, because there is a uniform distribution throughout S-phase. If this were expressed as a function of the difference in DNA content between G1 and G2 cells (i.e., by subtracting the G1 mean DNA content from the mean S DNA content, and dividing by the G1 subtracted from the G2), then the starting value would be 0.5. As the BrdU-labeled cells progress through S-phase, then this value will increase (ignoring the cells that divide) until the only cells which are BrdU-labeled, and have not divided, are in G2. The value or relative movement will be 1.0. Assuming linearity of T_S then, the progression of 0.5–1.0 will describe the movement of early S-phase cells to G2 (i.e., T_S). Thus, by taking a biopsy several hours after an injection of BrdU, T_S can be calculated.

An example of a human tumor analyzed by this method is shown in Fig. 4. This was an adenocarcinoma of the colon removed 6 h after injection. The profile shows the complex nature of many human tumors that possess abnormal DNA content. The first major peak, in the DNA profile, is diploid G1 cells, followed by a peak of aneuploid G1 cells that have 1.5 times more DNA than

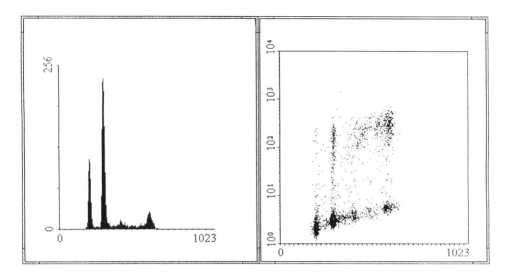

Fig. 4. BrdU/DNA profile of a human colonic adenocarcinoma. Bivariate BrdU/DNA distribution **(right)** and DNA profile **(left)** of a human colonic adenocarcinoma. These profiles were obtained 6 h after injection of 200 mg of BrdU.

the diploid cells. The bivariate distribution clearly shows the redistribution of BrdU-labeled cells through the cell cycle after 6 h. One population has divided and resides in G1, whereas the other is still progressing through mid- and late-S and G2 + M. It is also clear from this profile that virtually all proliferation is associated with the cells with aneuploid DNA content. From the profile, the T_S was calculated to 14.5 h and the LI of the aneuploid cells was 13.8%. The LI has to be corrected for those cells that have divided and shared their BrdU between the two daughter cells. This is simply done by measuring the number of G1 cells with BrdU uptake, halving that number and recalculating a corrected LI by subtracting it from the total BrdU-labeled and total cell number. These values of LI and T_S compute a T_{pot} of 3.5 d. This technique has permitted routine analysis of proliferative characteristics of human solid tumors on a time scale useful for prognostic or diagnostic purposes *(6)*.

4. Notes

1. The concentration of cells or nuclei is important. The procedure outlined in this chapter is designed for a starting density of 2–3 million cells. The volume of HCl should be increased and the antibody dilution decreased if more cells are used. A cell or nuclei count is usually performed prior to step 6 in Section 3.3.
2. The procedure described in this chapter has been kept simple, with as few steps as possible. However, many variations exist that may have benefit in certain systems. For cell suspensions, digestion into nuclei prior to staining,

with 0.4 mg/mL pepsin in 0.1*M* HCl for up to 30 min at room temperature, may improve results *(7)*. This step may be particularly useful if cells have a tendency to clump or have a large cytoplasm:nucleus ratio that may cause problems with nonspecific staining. The incubation time of cells or tissues in pepsin varies from one cell type to another. Solid tissues should be monitored throughout the incubation and the digestion stopped when the large pieces disappear. Thirty-minutes digestion is usually the optimum incubation period, but this can be as long as 1 h.

3. The denaturation step is perhaps the most crucial of the assay. Enough unwinding of DNA is required to ensure sufficient antibody binding, but not enough to disrupt the stoichiometry of PI binding, which requires double-stranded DNA. The denaturing agent, HCl, has proved the most reliable method, with little loss of material. The incubation time in HCl varies according to the material being stained. Normal tissues require much less denaturation than tumors (10 min vs 15–20 min). Cells require much longer denaturation than nuclei (20–30 min vs 10–15 min). The optimum denaturation period should be characterized for each particular experimental system. The use of HCl, however, is relatively mild and does not result in extensive denaturation of DNA. If increased sensitivity of BrdU detection is required, an alternative method involving incubation of cells in 0.1*M* HCl containing 0.7% Triton X-100 at 0°C for 10 min, followed by boiling in 2 mL of distilled water for 10 min *(8)*, will increase sensitivity by a factor of 20–30. This procedure, and several like it, suffer the drawback that cell loss is a major problem; in the case of hematopoietic cells, up to 90% of the staining material may be lost during the process. Procedures have been developed to combine denaturation with digestion *(9)* using 0.2 mg/mL pepsin in 2*M* HCl for 30 min at room temperature. This technique has proved particularly useful for epidermal cells and the author has adapted this to his own staining procedure. One other potentially useful method for denaturing DNA is the use of restriction endonucleases and exonuclease III *(10)*. In these procedures, nuclear protein is extracted with 0.1*M* HCl, *Dde*I, *Eco*RI or *Hin*dIII, followed by digestion with exonuclease III. This procedure may achieve the sensitivity of heat denaturation without severe cell loss, morphology change, or protein loss.

4. Many procedures employ 0.1*M* sodium tetraborate, pH 8.5, to neutralize after the acid denaturation. This does not appear to be necessary when large volumes of PBS are used as a washing medium.

5. Many monoclonal antibodies are commercially available to detect halogenated pyrimidines. Most antibodies will detect both BrdU and iododeoxyuridine. However, Br3 shows extremely high specificity for BrdU *(11)*, whereas IU4 (both available from Caltag) shows much higher specificity for IUdR *(12)*. These antibodies have opened the pathway for double labeling experiments on the FCM. The dilution of the monoclonal will depend on its specificity and whether it is a purified, ascitic or supernatant preparation; for instance, we routinely use IU4 at a dilution of 1:2000 compared to 1:20 for the Sera-Lab antibody.

6. Some workers prefer to carry out the antibody incubations at 4°C because some monoclonal preparations were found to have DNase activity from mycoplasma contaminants. This should not be a problem with commercial preparations.

7. There is no need to perform the assay in dark conditions. BrdU is photosensitive, but there is no advantage when incubations are carried out in the dark.
8. It has been reported that incubation of cells in 0.1% sodium borohydride in 1 mL PBS for 30 min at room temperature, after the antibody incubations, reduces autofluorescence and nonspecific staining. This has not proved to be advantageous in the author's hands.
9. The author found that stained preparations can be kept for up to at least 1 mo at 4°C with little loss of fluorescence.
10. If the staining procedure fails to detect BrdU incorporation, it is always worth repeating the antibody incubations. One of the most common reasons for failure is an excess of cellular or nuclear material.

References

1. Gratzner, H. (1982) Monoclonal antibody against 5-bromo and 5-iodo-deoxyuridine: a new reagent for detection of DNA replication. *Science* **218,** 474,475.
2. Dolbeare, F., Gratzner, H., Pallavicini, M., and Gray, J. W. (1983) Flow cytometric measurement of total DNA content and incorporated bromo-deoxyuridine. *Proc. Natl. Acad. Sci. USA* **80,** 5573–5577.
3. Pallavicini, M. G. (1987) Solid tissue dispersal for cytokinetic analyses, in *Techniques in Cell Cycle Analysis* (Gray, J. W. and Darzynewicz, Z., eds.), Humana, Clifton, NJ, pp. 139–162.
4. Wilson, G. D., McNally, N. J., Dunphy, E., Karcher, H., and Pfragner, R. (1985) The labelling index of human and mouse tumours assessed by bromo-deoxyuridine staining *in vitro* and *in vivo* and flow cytometry. *Cytometry* **6,** 641–647.
5. Begg, A. C., McNally, N. J., Shrieve, D. C., and Karcher, H. (1985) A method to measure the duration of DNA synthesis and the potential doubling from a single sample. *Cytometry* **6,** 620–626.
6. Wilson, G. D., McNally, N. J., Dische, S., Saunders, M. I., des Rochers, C., Lewis, A. A., and Bennett, M. H. (1988) Measurement of cell kinetics in human tumours in vivo using bromodeoxyuridine incorporation and flow cytometry. *Br. J. Cancer* **58,** 423–431.
7. Schutte, B., Reynders, M. M. J., van Assche, C. L. M. V. J., Hupperets, P. S. G. J., Bosman, F. T., and Blijham, G. H. (1987) An improved method for the immuno-cytochemical detection of bromodeoxyuridine labelled nuclei using flow cytometry. *Cytometry* **8,** 372–376.
8. Beisker, W., Dolbeare, F., and Gray, J. W. (1987) An improved immunocyto-chemical procedure for high sensitivity detection of incorporated bromo-deoxyuridine. *Cytometry* **8,** 235–239.
9. van Erp, P. E. J., Brons, P. P. T., Boezeman, J. B. M., de Jongh, G. J., and Bauer, F. W. (1988) A rapid flow cytometric method for bivariate bromodeoxyuridine/ DNA analysis using simultaneous proteolytic enzyme digestion and acid denaturation. *Cytometry* **9,** 627–630.

10. Dolbeare, F. and Gray, J. W. (1988) Use of restriction endonuclease and exonuclease III to expose halogenated pyrimidines for immunochemical staining. *Cytometry* **9,** 631–635.
11. Dolbeare, F., Kuo, W. L., Vanderlaan, M., and Gray, J. W. (1988) Cell cycle analysis by flow cytometric analysis of the incorporation of iododeoxyuridine (IdUrd) and bromodeoxyuridine (BrdUrd). *Proc. Am. Assoc. Cancer Res.* **29,** 1896–1901.
12. Vanderlaan, M., Watkins, B., Thomas, C., Dolbeare, F., and Stanker, L. (1986) Improved high-affinity monoclonal antibody to iododeoxyuridine. *Cytometry* **7,** 499–507.

27

Immunohistochemical Detection of Cells in the Division Cycle Using Antibodies to Proliferating Cell Nuclear Antigen (PCNA)

Richard E. Edwards and Jerry Styles

1. Introduction

The detection and quantification of cells undergoing proliferation have centered on methods that identify specific stages of the cell cycle. Thus, the replication of DNA or S-phase (the labeling index) is detected by the use of [³H]-thymidine and autoradiography, or by bromodeoxyuridine and immunohistochemical labeling. The other stage of the cell cycle that is frequently examined is mitosis, or M-phase (the mitotic index), via the use of spindle inhibitors, such as colchicine. These techniques detect only phases of the cell cycle and require that the animal or cell culture be dosed with [³H]-thymidine or bromodeoxyuridine, or with colchicine. These parts of the cell cycle are of differing durations and do not give a direct measure of the growth fraction. Proliferating cell nuclear antigen (PCNA) is an endogenous nuclear protein that functions as an accessory protein to DNA polymerase (pol) δ *(1)*. Since PCNA is present in all cycling cells, the entire proportion of dividing cells present at any instant in a population can be detected *(2,3)*.

This chapter describes a simple immunoperoxidase method for detection of PCNA in tissue sections. A flow cytometric method for demonstrating PCNA in single cells is given in Chapter 36.

2. Materials

1. Carnoy's fixative: 60% absolute ethanol, 30% chloroform, and 10% glacial acetic acid.
2. Glass microscope slides that have been coated with 3-aminopropyl-triethoxy-silane (APES) (*see* Note 1).
3. Xylene.

From: *Methods in Molecular Biology, Vol. 80: Immunochemical Protocols, 2nd ed.*
Edited by: J. D. Pound © Humana Press Inc., Totowa, NJ

4. 100, 90, and 70% Ethanols.
5. Dulbecco A phosphate-buffered saline (PBS) tablets made up to the appropriate volume.
6. 0.3% (v/v) Hydrogen peroxide in distilled water: Dilute just before use.
7. Monoclonal antibody (MAb) to PCNA: A suitable mouse MAb (cat. no. NCL-PCNA; IgG2a isotype) can be obtained from Euro-Path Ltd. (Stratton, Bude, UK) (*see* Note 2 for alternatives).
8. Rabbit antimouse IgG2a antibody peroxidase-conjugated second antibody (e.g., from Serotec, Kidlington, Oxford, UK).
9. Substrate solution: A stock solution of diaminobenzidine tetrachloride (DAB) (Sigma, St. Louis, MO) is made up at 5 mg/mL in PBS, aliquoted into 0.5-mL amounts, and stored at −20°C. For use, add 4.5 mL of PBS to 0.5 mL DAB stock, and add 50 μL of freshly prepared 1% hydrogen peroxide immediately before use.
10. Hematoxylin solution (Gill No. 2).
11. Microscope slide cover glasses.
12. Mounting medium: distrene, tricresyl phosphate, xylene (DPX).

3. Method
3.1. Preparation of Tissue Sections (see Note 3)

1. From a freshly killed animal, dissect out the organs of interest and gently wipe excess blood from the outside.
2. Using a sharp scalpel or razor blade, cut thin (2–3 mm) slices of the organ, and place them immediately in Carnoy's fixative (*see* Note 4).
3. Leave the tissues in the fixative for up to 48 h, and then transfer them to 95% ethanol to prevent excessive hardening.
4. Process the tissue as soon as possible using a routine paraffin wax processing schedule.
5. Cut sections 5-μm thick and mount on coated microscope slides. The drying temperature **must not exceed 37°C**, as higher temperatures cause denaturation of the antigen (*see* Note 5).

3.2. Immunohistochemistry

1. Dewax the sections in xylene for 3 × 20 min, and rehydrate in 100% ethanol (2 × 3 min) and then 95 and 70% ethanol and water for 3 min each.
2. Inhibit endogenous peroxidase activity in the tissue section by incubation in 0.3% hydrogen peroxide in distilled water for 10 min.
3. Wash the sections in running tap water for 10 min, then rinse in distilled water.
4. Dry around the section with a soft tissue and incubate in the freshly prepared primary antibody (diluted 1/25 with PBS) at room temperature in a moist chamber. Allow 100 μL of antibody for each section (*see* Notes 6 and 7).
5. Wash 3 × 5 min in PBS.
6. Dry around the section, and apply the freshly prepared rabbit antimouse IgG2a peroxidase-conjugate at a dilution of 1/50 in PBS. Incubate as in step 4.

7. Incubate the sections in freshly prepared DAB substrate solution for 10 min at room temperature. A brown reaction product will be deposited in the areas where the PCNA antigen is present.
8. Counterstain lightly with hematoxylin.
9. Dehydrate the sections in increasing concentrations of ethanol (70, 90, 100%), finally clear with xylene, and mount in DPX.

4. Notes

1. Coat slides with APES as follows:
   a. Soak in 5% Decon 90 or equivalent detergent overnight in staining racks.
   b. Rinse in hot water for 30 min and then twice in deionized water. Then dry at 60°C.
   c. Dip the slides in a 2% solution of APES in acetone, and rinse twice in acetone. This step should be carried out in a fume cupboard.
   d. Dry the slides at 60°C.
   The coated slides can be stored at room temperature indefinitely.
2. Other sources of mouse MAb anti-PCNA antibodies are given below:

Supplier	Clone	Isotype
Serotec	19A2	IgM
Serotec	Ki67	IgG1
Dako	PC10	IgG2a
Sigma	PC10	IgG2a

3. We have also used this method successfully on formalin-fixed paraffin-embedded material. For the technique to work under these conditions, the sections are microwaved in $0.01M$ citric acid, pH 6.0, for approx 14 min on full power (700 W). The exact time of incubation required varies depending on the tissue and must be determined by experimentation.
4. It is important that the fresh tissue, when placed in the Carnoy's fixative, is not allowed to drop to the bottom of the container and adhere to it, since this may result in uneven and unreliable fixation. The container should be inverted gently several times during the fixation period.
5. It is of vital importance that the sections, once cut and mounted on slides, are not exposed to temperatures in excess of 37°C, either on the drying hot plate or subsequently in the oven, since higher temperatures cause denaturation of the antigen.
6. As a guide, we have found that the following conditions give optimal results:

Tissue	Primary antibody		Secondary antibody	
	Dilution	Incubation time, h	Dilution	Incubation time, h
Rat	1/25	2	1/50	1
Mouse	1/20	3	1/50	1.5

Antibodies were diluted with PBS just before use.

7. A pen for drawing a hydrophobic ring around the tissue section is marketed by a number of companies, including Sigma and Dako (High Wycombe, UK). It obviates the necessity of wiping around the section after each washing step and reduces the amount of antibody solution required.

References

1. Bravo, R., Frank, R., Blundell, P. A., and MacDonald-Bravo, H. (1987) Cyclin/ PCNA is the auxiliary protein of DNA polymerase-δ. *Nature* **326,** 515–517.
2. Bravo, R. and MacDonald-Bravo, H. (1987) Changes in the nuclear distribution of cyclin (PCNA) but not its synthesis depend on DNA replication. *EMBO J.* **4,** 655–661.
3. Foley J., Ton T., Maronpot R., Butterworth B., and Goldsworthy T. L. (1993) Comparison of proliferating cell nuclear antigen to tritiated thymidine as a marker of proliferating hepatocytes in rats. *Environ. Health Persp.* **101(Suppl. 5),** 199–206.

28

Double Label Immunohistochemistry on Tissue Sections Using Alkaline Phosphatase and Peroxidase Conjugates

Jonathan A. Green and Margaret M. Manson

1. Introduction

One of the most common methods in immunohistochemistry involves the use of an antibody to the antigen of interest detected indirectly with an enzyme-labeled antispecies secondary antibody. The enzyme catalyzes the formation of a colored insoluble reaction product at the antigen site. It is possible, with careful choice of reagents, to label two antigens simultaneously, resulting in two different colored reaction products *(1)*. Cells or tissue sections can also be double labeled with two antispecies secondary antibodies carrying different fluorochromes (*see* Chapter 34), or by using suitable antibodies conjugated to different sizes of colloidal gold (*see* Chapter 32).

Described here is an indirect method for detecting two different cellular antigens in acetone-fixed tissue, using a rabbit polyclonal antibody, and a murine monoclonal antibody on the same section. One secondary antispecies antibody is conjugated with alkaline phosphatase, the other with peroxidase, thus resulting in two differently colored products showing the localization of the two antigens (Fig. 1).

2. Materials

1. Acetone-fixed, paraffin-embedded tissue sections (*see* Notes 1 and 2).
2. Xylene.
3. 70 and 100% Ethanol.
4. 15% Glacial acetic acid in water.
5. 0.3% Hydrogen peroxide in water.

From: *Methods in Molecular Biology, Vol. 80: Immunochemical Protocols, 2nd ed.*
Edited by: J. D. Pound © Humana Press Inc., Totowa, NJ

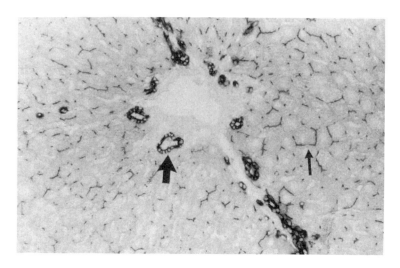

Fig. 1. Double label immunohistochemistry on rat liver. An acetone-fixed rat liver section was incubated with a polyclonal antiserum raised in rabbit to a hepatocyte cell surface protein (courtesy of Dr. S. Stamatoglou) and a mouse monoclonal antibody against a bile duct specific cytokeratin (courtesy of Dr. E. B. Lane). The hepatocyte protein was localized by use of a secondary peroxidase-conjugated antibody resulting in a red/brown product (thin arrow). The bile duct cytokeratin was identified by using an alkaline phosphatase-conjugated secondary antibody giving a blue color (thick arrow).

6. Phosphate-buffered saline (PBS), pH 7.4: 8 g of NaCl, 0.2 g of KH_2PO_4, 2.8 g of $Na_2HPO_4 \cdot 12H_2O$, and 0.2 g of KCl dissolved and made up to 1 L in distilled water.
7. PBS–BSA: PBS containing 1% bovine serum albumin.
8. PBS–Tween: PBS containing 0.05% (v/v) Tween-80.
9. Tris buffer: $0.1M$ Tris-HCl, pH 8.2.
10. Acetate buffer: $0.2M$ Sodium acetate, pH 5.0.
11. Primary antibody raised in rabbit against antigen 1 (*see* Note 3).
12. Peroxidase-conjugated antirabbit IgG raised in sheep (*see* Note 3).
13. Primary mouse monoclonal antibody against antigen 2.
14. Alkaline phosphatase-conjugated antimouse IgG raised in goat.
15. BCIP/NBT substrate: Dissolve 5-bromo-4-chloro-3-indolyl phosphate at 50 mg/mL in dimethyl formamide. Dissolve nitroblue tetrazolium at 75 mg/mL in 70% (v/v) dimethyl formamide. Add 30 μL of BCIP and 45 μL of NBT to 10 mL of Tris buffer, pH 8.2 immediately before use.
16. AEC substrate: Dissolve 2 mg of 3-amino, 9-ethyl carbazole, in 500 μL of dimethyl formamide. Add 9.5 mL of acetate buffer and 10 μL of 30% H_2O_2. Use immediately.
17. Aqueous mountant: Apathy's mountant.

3. Method

1. Place the sections (*see* Notes 2 and 3) in a slide rack, dewax in xylene for 20 min, followed by transfer to a fresh xylene bath for a further few minutes. Then rehydrate through an ethanol series, 2 × 100%, 1 × 70%, 1 × distilled water (*see* Note 4).
2. Rinse the sections in PBS–Tween. This helps to prevent nonspecific binding, and also makes subsequent solutions easier to apply to the slide.
3. Place the sections in the acetic acid solution for 15 min to block endogenous alkaline phosphatase activity (*see* Chapter 24).
4. Rinse as in step 2.
5. Place the sections in 0.3% hydrogen peroxide for 15 min to block endogenous peroxidase activity.
6. Rinse as in step 2.
7. Place the slides horizontally in a moist chamber and incubate for 30 min with 100 μL of PBS–BSA to block nonspecific binding sites.
8. Remove the solution from the slide and wipe the excess from around the section so that the antiserum is not diluted.
9. Incubate with both primary antibodies, suitably diluted in 100 μL of PBS–BSA (*see* Note 5), for 2 h in the moist chamber.
10. Rinse the slides three times with PBS–Tween, 2 min for each rinse.
11. Wipe around the sections as before and apply 100 μL of liquid containing both secondary antibodies diluted 1:100 in PBS–BSA and incubate in the humid chamber for 1 h.
12. Rinse the sections as in step 10.
13. Flood the sections with AEC substrate solution and incubate for 15 min (*see* Note 6).
14. Rinse the sections as in step 2.
15. Flood the sections with BCIP/NBT substrate solution and incubate for 15 min.
16. Wash as in step 2.
17. Dry around the sections and mount in Apathy's mountant (*see* Note 7).

Sites of positive reaction product are seen as a red/brown granular deposit where the peroxidase conjugated second antibody is bound, and a purple/blue deposit where the alkaline phosphatase-conjugated antibody is bound.

4. Notes

1. To prepare tissue, 2–3 mm slices are removed as quickly as possible into ice-cold acetone and left on ice for 4–6 h. (Less than 4 h can result in incomplete penetration of fixative and subsequent formation of ice crystals.) Samples are then stored in a −20°C freezer until they can be processed using routine paraffin embedding techniques.
2. Care should be taken not to allow the temperature of the paraffin bath to exceed 60°C, since most laboratories use embedding media containing plastics. Above 62°C, these will begin to form polymers, which are very difficult to remove, and may give rise to background staining. This will show up as a pale ring of staining extending beyond the tissue section.

3. One of the most likely reasons for failure with this technique is the wrong choice of antibodies. It is important that the two primary antibodies have been raised in different species and that the two secondary antibodies have been raised in species distinct from either of the primary antibody species.

4. Xylene should be changed frequently. Ideally, not more than 100 slides should be dewaxed per 400 mL. This helps to reduce background by removing the wax more efficiently. Xylene is toxic and should ideally be handled in a fume hood. Histoclear is a commercially available, safer alternative to xylene.

5. The dilution of the antibodies has to be determined empirically. Polyclonal antibodies can usually be diluted between 1:50 and 1:250. Monoclonal antibodies in tissue culture supernatant may need to be concentrated by centrifuging a frozen sample in a microfuge for 10 min and discarding the top third of the solution. This solution (100 μL) can then have the other primary antibody diluted into it in place of PBS–BSA. Monoclonal antibodies produced as ascites can usually be diluted between 1:200 and 1:1000.

6. It is important to carry out the reaction for peroxidase first since the H_2O_2 contained in this reaction mixture might bleach any color that was already deposited on the section.

7. No satisfactory counterstain is known. The blue of hematoxylin is too close to that of the alkaline phosphatase product to allow good photography.

Acknowledgments

The authors are grateful to Stamatis Stamatoglou, formerly of the National Institute for Medical Research, Mill Hill, London and Birgitte Lane, University of Dundee, UK for supplying antibodies.

Reference

1. Mason, D. Y. and Sammons, R. E. (1978) Alkaline phosphatase and peroxidase for double immunoenzymatic labelling of cellular constituents. *J. Clin. Pathol.* **31,** 454–460.

29

Preparation of Colloidal Gold Probes

David A. Hughes and Julian E. Beesley

1. Introduction

As long ago as 1857 *(1)*, Michael Faraday in an address to the Royal Society recognized the reactive properties of colloidal metal particles (in particular gold) with light. Since 1933 *(2)*, a range of methods have been devised for producing gold sols. It was not until 1971, however, that Faulk and Taylor *(3)* published a method for binding proteins to gold particles for use in immunocytochemistry at the electron microscope level. Nowadays, colloidal gold is incorporated into probes that are widely used in the biological sciences both for light and electron microscopy.

A gold probe is an electron-dense sphere of gold coated with an immunologically active protein. Making such a probe involves two major steps: production of the gold sol and binding of the gold to the probe molecule.

1.1. Production of Gold Sol

A suspension of gold spheres is produced by the chemical reduction of yellow gold chloride (chloroauric acid) in solution. This happens in a sequence of stages *(4)*. Initially, the reduction of Au^{3+} produces a supersaturated molecular Au solution. Nucleation is initiated when the concentration of Au increases, and the gold atoms cluster and form nuclei. Particle growth proceeds with the deposition of molecular gold on the nuclei. The theoretical size of the gold is inversely proportional to the cube root of the number of nuclei formed if it is assumed that the conversion of Au^{3+} to Au is complete and that the concentration of gold remains constant *(5)*.

The use of different reducing agents allows us to produce particles of a prechosen size range. The speed of reduction of the gold chloride determines how many gold nuclei are formed. In a closed system, this will determine the

From: *Methods in Molecular Biology, Vol. 80: Immunochemical Protocols, 2nd ed.*
Edited by: J. D. Pound © Humana Press Inc., Totowa, NJ

final size of the gold. The aim has always been to work toward monodisperse suspensions, avoiding particle aggregates, and to encourage as little variance as possible in the mean particle diameter of samples. Experience has shown that the desired routine sizes are 5, 10, and 15 nm. All these are useful for transmission electron microscope studies and the 5 nm gold are recommended for light microscopy. Gold spheres of 30 nm are occasionally used for scanning electron microscope immunocytochemistry. A 1-nm probe is now readily commercially available and is proving useful as a more efficient nucleus for silver-enhancement.

The following procedures have been described in the literature as being useful for colloidal gold production:

1. White phosphorus reduction: White phosphorus, and indeed sodium or potassium thiocyanate, are fast reducers. Chloroauric acid is boiled under reflux with white phosphorus *(6)* dissolved in diethylether. Boiling is continued until the solution turns from a brownish shade to red—this usually takes about 5 min. This method produces gold particles in the smaller size range (2–12 nm). Accurate production of the particle size range is not easy, and, since the procedure is potentially highly dangerous, it is not commonly used.
2. Ascorbate reduction: This method *(7)* entails the fairly rapid addition of sodium ascorbate to chloroauric acid while stirring. If the reaction is carried out on ice, the gold particle size range is between 6 and 8 nm. Higher temperatures tend to increase the particle size. The method is also really of academic interest nowadays, since it is not easy to control the final sphere diameter.
3. Citrate reduction: Chloroauric acid is boiled under reflux with sodium citrate *(5)* until the solution turns red. Particle sizes achieved are in the range of 15–150 nm, and a particular diameter is chosen for a batch by adjusting the amount of citrate added to the boiling flask. This method has been used, therefore, for producing probes in the larger particle size range.
4. Combined tannic acid-citrate reduction: In 1985, Slot and Geuze *(4)* described a method of using two reducing agents, tannic acid and sodium citrate, in combination to control accurately the diameter of gold particles yielded. Adjusting the amount of tannic acid in the mixture will control the sphere diameter very precisely at the point within the size range of 3–17 nm. The method produces sols with very little variance in mean particle diameter. Centrifugation to purify the end product is not usually needed, since gold particle aggregates are infrequently found.

1.2. Making Gold–Protein Complexes

To be of use as immunocytochemical markers, the gold spheres in the sol have to be bound to specific ligands, such as proteins (e.g., immunoglobulins) and lectins. The binding is by straightforward electrostatic absorption relying on the negative charge of the gold interacting with the positive charge of the protein, and the complex obtained is highly stable. Moreover, the molecules bound to the gold retain their biological properties, an indispensable feature for immunocytochemistry. Unbound gold sol is unstable and changes color from red to blue in the presence of salts (e.g., sodium chloride). This can be used as a test for finding the amount of protein required to saturate (i.e., stabilize) a given quantity of gold sol. The protein–gold complex is isolated from excess protein and gold particle aggregates by density centrifugation. The complexes thus retrieved are stable for at least a year when refrigerated. Samples may be stored for even longer periods in 50% glycerol at –20°C.

2. Materials

1. Gold chloride crystals.
2. 1% Aqueous trisodium citrate dihydrate.
3. 25 mM and 0.2M Potassium carbonate.
4. 0.1M Hydrochloric acid.
5. 10% Aqueous sodium chloride.
6. 1% Aqueous tannic acid.
7. Protein to be complexed with gold: It is essential that the isoelectric point of the protein is known.
8. Ultracentrifuge and 10-mL ultracentrifuge tubes.
9. Distilled water, double-distilled and filtered through a 0.45-μm Millipore filter.
10. All glassware should be thoroughly cleaned and siliconized (*see* Note 1).
11 Electron microscope facilities with Formvar/carbon-coated grids (*see* Note 2).
12. 1% Aqueous polyethylene glycol ([PEG], "Carbowax 20," Union Carbide).
13. Phosphate-buffered saline (PBS): 0.1M phosphate, 0.15M sodium chloride, pH 7.4.
14. PBS containing 0.2 mg/mL of PEG.
15. Sodium azide (**caution:** highly toxic).

3. Methods

There are three stages in the production of gold probes:

1. Production of gold spheres.
2. Estimation of the amount of protein to be added to the gold.
3. Making the required amount of probe.

3.1. Production of the Gold Spheres (ref. 4)

1. Freshly prepare a gold solution from an ampule of gold chloride crystals by adding 1 mL of a 1% aqueous gold chloride solution to 79 mL of distilled water.
2. Prepare the reducing mixture with 4 mL of 1% trisodium citrate dihydrate, 2 mL of 1% tannic acid, 2 mL of 25 mM potassium carbonate, and distilled water to make 20 mL.
3. Warm the solutions to 60°C and quickly add the reducing mixture to the gold solution while stirring. The temperature is critical at this stage. Evidence of sol formation is the red color of the mixture.

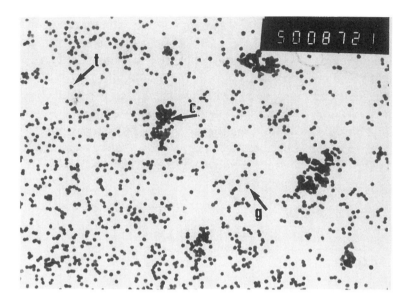

Fig. 1. Formvar grid coated with a colloidal suspension of 14-nm gold particles prepared using the method of Slot and Geuze *(4)*. Most gold particles are spherical singlets, duplets, or triplets (g). Occasionally, the particles are tetrahedral (t) or in clusters (c). Electron micrograph ×125,000.

4. After the sol has formed, heat the mixture to boiling, and then cool. According to Slot and Geuze *(4)*, the quantities stated here should produce 4-nm (±11.7%) particles. For 6-nm (±7.3%) particles, add 0.5 mL of potassium carbonate to the sodium citrate. The potassium carbonate counteracts the pH effect of the tannic acid. Below 0.5 mL, the tannic acid has no effect on the pH and may be omitted. Therefore, for 8.2-nm (±6.9%) particles, add 0.125 mL tannic acid to the sodium citrate, and for 11.5-nm (±6.3%) particles, add 0.03 mL tannic acid. The sol forms within seconds if a high amount of tannic acid has been added or will take up to 60 min if the tannic acid has been omitted. A calibration curve can be constructed to enable a rapid identification of the amounts of reducing agent required to produce a given gold particle size. The electron micrograph in Fig. 1 shows a Formvar grid preparation of 14-nm gold particles routinely prepared in the author's laboratory using the method of Slot and Geuze *(4)*.
5. Dry a small aliquot of the gold onto a Formvar/carbon-coated 400-mesh copper grid.
6. Wash away any salts in the preparation by floating the grid, specimen side down, on distilled water.
7. View the grid at ×125,000 with the transmission electron microscope. Electronmicrographs should be taken and scanned into either a monochrome or full-color image analyzer for morphometric analysis. It is also possible to attach the image analysis system directly to the electron microscope and so eliminate

the intermediary time-consuming photographic stage. Even the simplest of image analysis programs available now will be able to give a rapid evaluation of the gold particle size and shape distribution, and the level of aggregation. In a good preparation, at least 80–85% of gold particles should be unclustered singlets. If the size distribution is unacceptably high, the preparation can be purified by centrifugation over a continuous sucrose or glycerol density gradient *(4)*.

3.2. Titration to Determine the Minimum Amount of Protein to Stabilize the Gold Sol (ref. 7)

1. Adjust the pH of the gold sol to 0.5 pH units above the isoelectric point of the protein to be complexed. Care should be taken when adjusting the pH, since nonstabilized colloidal gold will plug the pore of the pH electrode. Take an aliquot of a few milliliters of the gold and add five drops of 1% aqueous polyethylene glycol, before measuring the pH. Make the necessary adjustments to the pH, and repeat until the required pH is obtained. Do not return these aliquots to the remaining colloidal gold sol. Add $0.1M$ HCl to lower the pH or add $0.2M$ potassium carbonate to raise the pH, each of these being carried out with vortexing.
2. Measure five aliquots of 0.5 mL of gold sol.
3. Prepare five aliquots of serially diluted protein in distilled water, and add one of these, while shaking, to each of the 0.5-mL gold sol aliquots.
4. After 1 min, add 0.1 mL of 10% aqueous sodium chloride to each tube. Where there is excess protein in the tubes, the sol will not change color, but in those tubes where there is insufficient protein to stabilize the gold, flocculation will have occurred and the liquid will be blue. The correct concentration of protein is the minimal amount that will inhibit flocculation. Horisberger *(8)* suggested that for accurate determination of color change, a spectrophotometric assay should be used.

3.3. Production of the Colloidal Gold Probe

Once the minimal amount of protein necessary to stabilize a given quantity of gold is known, any quantity of gold probe can be produced.

1. Dissolve the required amount of protein in 0.1–0.2 mL of distilled water in a centrifuge tube, and add 10 mL of the gold sol.
2. After 2 min, add 1 mL of 1% aqueous polyethylene glycol solution to stabilize the gold probe *(7)*.
3. Centrifuge the mixture at a speed depending on the size of the gold complex: 15 nm at 60,000*g* for 1 h at 4°C *(7)*, 12 nm at 50,000*g* for 45 min at 4°C *(4)*, 5–12 nm at 105,000*g* for 1.5 h at 4°C *(7)*, 5 nm at 125,000*g* for 45 min at 4°C *(4)*, and 2–3 nm at 105,000*g* for 1.5 h at 4°C *(7)*. The pellet formed consists of two phases *(7)*. There is a large loose part, which is the protein–gold complex. In addition, there is a tight, dense pellet on the side of the tube, which contains aggregated gold particles and gold particles that have not been fully stabilized.

4. Resuspend the loose part of the pellet in 1.5 mL of PBS containing 0.2 mg/mL of polyethylene glycol. This can be stored for up to 1 yr at 4°C. If necessary, 0.5 mg/mL of sodium azide may be added to prevent microorganisms from growing in the probe. It should then be suitably diluted before use. The technique described above is the basis for the preparation of colloidal gold probes, and the principles of probe production are identical for each type of probe. Those who are interested should refer to Slot and Geuze *(4)*, for preparation of protein A-gold probes, Roth *(7)* for production of antibody–gold complexes, Tolsen et al. *(9)* for production of the avidin–gold complex, Horisberger *(8)* for production of the lectin–gold complex, and Bendayan *(10)* for production of the enzyme–gold complex.

4. Notes

1. If these precautions are not taken, the gold spheres will adhere to the side vessel walls which is evidenced by a red coloration of the glass.
2. For complete quality control, access to a monochrome image analyzer is also required.
3. There are many ways of testing a gold probe, but the most convincing is by using a known positive sample. Therefore, this could be a histological section, an electron microscope specimen, or a dot-blot. Estimation of the concentration of the probe by optical density measurements is a good method to standardize the concentration of probes from one batch to another, but in addition, it is always preferable to test the performance of the probes on known positive samples.
4. It is reasonably easy to make good-quality probes in the laboratory, but the investigator has to consider nonscientific factors, such as time and cost. Many gold conjugates are available commercially, in particular the commonly used secondary antibodies used in indirect immunocytochemistry. A good compromise is to purchase the reagents that will be in constant demand and make the required quantity of those that are not readily available. When purchasing probes, it is important to seek information on the properties of the probe. Commercial gold probes are usually sold with certain variables closely controlled. The degree of particle aggregation is stated, and the optical density of the solution given as a guideline to the concentration of the probe. Particle size variance will have been calculated by one of two methods. A laser-diffraction particle sizer (Malvern Instruments, Malvern, Worcestershire, UK) might have been used or, alternatively, electron micrographs may have been made from Formvar grid preparations of the gold sol, particle sizes being measured by image analysis of the micrograph. In addition, especially when using double or triple labeling in transmission electron microscopy, the distribution of gold particle sizes and the variance should be noted—a 5-nm probe may comprise a particle size range of 3–6 nm, of which a large number of particles may potentially overlap with those from 1- or 10-nm samples with wide distributions.
5. Immunogold labeling is a well-established procedure in both transmission and scanning electron microscopy. The ability to bind a range of proteins to gold probes of different, but well-defined size offers great scope for single, double, or

even triple labeling at the electron microscope level (*see* Chapter 31). The different applications for gold probes in electron microscopy have been reviewed in detail *(11)*.

6. Using larger (e.g., 30-nm) gold labels, it is sometimes possible to build up enough gold label in frozen or paraffin sections to enable antigen localization at the light microscope level (*see* Chapter 30). This technique is no more sensitive, however, than immunoenzyme methods. Gold particles as small as 1 nm may be located by nanometer particle video microscopy (Nanovid) *(12)* but the ideal way to increase the sensitivity of immunogold labeling is by silver-enhancement (immunogold-silver staining or IGSS) *(13)*.

7. Because of the light-reflecting properties of gold *(14)* and silver *(15)* particles, it is possible to use either dark-ground or epipolarization microscopy *(16,17)* for the enhanced visualization of both types of labeling at the light microscope level. The technique is especially useful when used in conjunction with transmitted ordinary light, since other tissue structures may be examined at the same time. Epipolarization bright-field double illumination may also be used for image analysis of multilabeling immunocytochemistry *(18)*. More recently, immunogold visualization in highly sensitive capping experiments with leukocyte surface proteins has been demonstrated using confocal scanning microscopy *(19)*. Such methodology is starting to bridge the gap between light and electron microscopical studies.

8. It has been reported that some commercial preparations of colloidal gold–antibody complexes may contain free active antibody. Such free antibody will compete with antibody–colloidal gold particles for antigen binding sites and may reduce labeling intensity. The presence of free protein may be identified using a simple test procedure *(20)*.

9. The use of probes prepared by a covalent attachment procedure of gold particles and proteins has been recently described as offering a number of advantages over conventional gold probes, including better resolution, stability, uniformity, sensitivity, and complete absence of aggregation *(21)*.

References

1. Faraday, M. (1857) Experimental relations of gold (and other metals) to light. *Phil. Trans. Roy. Soc.* **147,** 145–181.
2. Weizer, H. B. (1933) *Inorganic Colloid Chemistry,* vol. 1. Wiley, New York.
3. Faulk, W. and Taylor, G. (1971) An immunogold method for the electron microscope. *Immunocytochemistry* **8,** 1081–1083.
4. Slot, J. W. and Geuze, H. J. (1985) A new method of preparing gold probes for multiple labelling cytochemistry. *Eur. J. Cell. Biol.* **90,** 533–536.
5. Frens, G. (1973) Preparation of gold dispersions of varying size: controlled nucleation for the regulation of the particle size in monodisperse gold suspensions. *Nature: Phys. Sci.* **241,** 20–22.
6. Slot, S. W. and Geuze, H. J. (1981) Sizing of protein A—colloidal gold probes for immunoelectron microscopy. *J. Cell. Biol.* **90,** 533–536.

7. Roth, J. (1982) The protein A gold (pAg) technique—a qualitative and quantitative approach for antigen localization on thin sections, in *Techniques in Immunocytochemistry*, vol. 1 (Bullock, G. R. and Petrusz. P., eds.), Academic, London, pp. 107–133.

8. Horisberger, M. (1985) The gold method as applied to lectin cytochemistry in transmission and scanning electron microscopy, in *Techniques in Immunocytochemistry*, vol. 3 (Bullock, G. R. and Petrusz. P., eds.), Academic, London, pp. 155–178.

9. Tolsen, N. D., Boothroyd, B., and Hopkins, C. R. (1981) Cell-surface labelling with gold colloidal particles: the use of avidin and staphylococcal protein A-coated gold in conjunction with biotin and Fc-bearing ligands. *J. Microsc.* **123**, 215–226.

10. Bendayan, M. (1985) The enzyme–gold technique: a new cytochemical approach for the ultrastructural localization of macromolecules, in *Techniques in Immunocytochemistry*, vol. 3 (Bullock, G. R. and Petrusz, P., eds.), Academic, London, pp. 179–201.

11. Beesley, J. E. (1985) Colloidal gold: a new revolution in marking immunocytochemistry. *Proc. R.M.S.* **20**, 187–196.

12. De Branbender, M., Nuydens, R., Geuens, G., Moeremans, M., and De Mey, J. (1986) The use of sub-microscopic gold particles combined with video contrast enhancement as a simple molecular probe for the living cell. *Cell Motil. Cytoskeleton* **6**, 105–113.

13. Holgate, C. S., Jackson, P., Cowen, P., and Bird, C. C. (1983) Immunogold-silver staining: a new method of immunostaining with enhanced sensitivity. *J. Histochem. Cytochem.* **31**, 938–944.

14. De Mey, J. (1983) Colloidal gold probes in immunocytochemistry, in *Immunocytochemistry: Practical Applications in Pathology and Biology* (Polak, J. M. and Van Noorden, S., eds.), Wright-SPG, Bristol, UK, pp. 82–112.

15. De Waele, M., De Mey, J., Renmans, W., Labeur, C., Jochmans, K., and Van Camp, B. (1986) Potential of immunogold-silver staining for the study of leucocyte sub-populations as defined by monoclonal antibodies. *J. Histochem. Cytochem.* **34**, 1257–1263.

16. Hughes, D. (1987) Developments in IGSS: A review. *Lab. Prac.* **36**, 62–69.

17. Ellis, I. O., Bell, J., and Bancroft, J. D. (1989) Polarized incident lightmicroscopical enhancement of immunogold and immunogold-silver preparations: its role in immunohistochemistry. *J. Pathol.* **159**, 13–16.

18. Hughes, D. (1990) *Immunocytochemistry*—selecting an approach to the identification of aspirated human renal allograft endothelium and epithelium. *Trans. R. M. S.* **1**, 701–706.

19. Shotton, D. M. (1989) Confocal scanning optical microscopy and its applications for biological specimens. *J. Cell. Sci.* **94**, 175–206.

20. Kramarcy, N. R. and Sealock, R. (1991) Commercial preparations of colloidal gold-antibody complexes frequently contain free active antibody. *J. Histochem. Cytochem.* **39**, 37–39.

21. Hainfield, J. F. and Furuya, F. R. (1992) A 1.4-nm gold cluster covalently attached to antibodies improves immunolabelling. *J. Histochem. Cytochem.* **40**, 177–184.

30

Immunogold Probes in Light Microscopy

David A. Hughes and Julian E. Beesley

1. Introduction

All immunocytochemical techniques are based on the same principle of incubating the target antigen with an appropriate antibody solution, but they may incorporate one from a range of different microscopically dense markers for visualizing, the sites of binding. Light microscope immunocytochemistry was initiated by the classical work of Coons and coworkers in 1950, who developed the immunofluorescence technique for antigen localization *(1,2)*. This was followed some time later in 1966 with the introduction by Nakane and Pierce of the immunoperoxidase procedure *(3)*, after which there have been various attempts to increase the sensitivity of techniques for localizing tissue antigens, including peroxidase antiperoxidase (PAP) *(4)*, avidin–biotin complex *(5)*, and alkaline phosphatase antialkaline phosphatase (APAAP) *(6)*. These techniques are all still routinely used for immunocytochemistry.

During the past decade, it has become possible to use colloidal gold probes for immunolabeling at the light microscope level. Gold spheres, usually between 1 and 15 nm in diameter and in colloidal suspension, are coated with an immunological protein. As in the immunoenzyme techniques, the immunological protein could be one of a wide range of proteins. It could be a primary antibody, for use in a one-step system, or a secondary or tertiary antibody, for indirect labeling. It could be protein A, protein G, or if an avidin–biotin system is used, streptavidin or an antibiotin monoclonal antibody (MAb) could be coupled to the gold. Immunolabeling is carried out by incubating the antigen with the primary antibody–gold complex in the direct technique, or primary antibody followed by the gold conjugate in the indirect technique. Strong immunogold labeling may sometimes be observed as its natural red/pink color under the light microscope, but frequently the labeling is too weak to detect unless a further enhancement stage is used.

From: *Methods in Molecular Biology, Vol. 80: Immunochemical Protocols, 2nd ed.*
Edited by: J. D. Pound © Humana Press Inc., Totowa, NJ

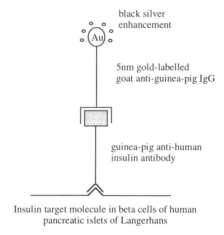

black silver
enhancement

5nm gold-labelled
goat anti-guinea-pig IgG

guinea-pig anti-human
insulin antibody

Insulin target molecule in beta cells of human
pancreatic islets of Langerhans

Fig. 1. Schematic representation of the indirect IGSS procedure as applied to the demonstration of insulin in human pancreatic islets of Langerhans.

Table 1
Historical Development of IGSS

Author	References	Development
Faraday (1857)	*9*	First mention of gold–protein complexing and interaction with light
Faulk and Taylor (1971)	*10*	EM gold probes established
Danscher (1981)	*7*	Silver probe for gold detection in tissue sections
Holgate et al. (1983)	*8*	Adaptation of the Danscher procedure for IGSS

Immunogold-silver staining (IGSS) is a technique that is applied in essentially the same manner as immunoenzyme staining but involves the use of colloidal gold-labeled antisera that are strongly visualized for light microscopy by silver-enhancement (Fig. 1). This method makes use of the Danscher physical developing solution *(7)* to create a layer of black, metallic silver over the gold-labeled binding sites. Table 1 describes the historical progression of the IGSS method. Danscher's reagent is a mixture of silver lactate (the silver ion source), hydroquinone (the silver reducer), and gum acacia (a colloid that prevents rapid, autoreduction of the silver lactate, which would lead to high background levels by a process known as "autonucleation"). A range of easy-to-use, commercial alternatives to this mixture are also now available.

2. Materials

1. An antibody of known specificity and species. It does not matter whether the antibody is monoclonal or polyclonal.
2. A gold probe, preferably 5-nm diameter or less, coated with an immunological protein specific to the primary antibody. In principle, small gold particles produce a higher labeling intensity of the target antigen owing to reduced steric hindrance. If the primary antibody is from a rabbit, gold coated with protein A or antirabbit antiserum may be used. If the primary antibody is from mouse, gold coated with protein G or an antibody raised against the correct isotype of IgG is used. If the antibody is biotinylated, gold complexed to either streptavidin or a MAb to biotin is used. These will be referred to as the gold probe. In the context of the final result, it does not matter which probe is used as long as it reacts with the primary antibody.
3. Lugol's iodine.
4. 5% Sodium thiosulfate.
5. Phosphate-buffered saline ([PBS]: $0.01M$ phosphate, $0.15M$ NaCl, pH 7.2, as suggested by Slot and Geuze *[11]*).
6. Heat-inactivated serum from the second antibody species (not for use with the protein A-gold technique).
7. 1% Bovine serum albumin (BSA) in PBS (BSA-PBS).
8. Commercial silver-enhancement kit.
9. Double-distilled water.
10. Gill's hematoxylin.
11. Industrial methylated spirit (IMS).
12. Xylene.
13. Gum acacia (500 g/L in distilled water).
14. Trisodium citrate dihydrate.
15. Citric acid.
16. Hydroquinone: 0.85 g/15 mL distilled water, freshly prepared.
17. Silver lactate: 0.11 g/15 mL distilled water, freshly prepared.
18. Tris-buffered saline (TBS): $0.05M$ Tris in isotonic (0.9%) NaCl, pH 7.6.
19. Trypsin: 0.1% in TBS.
20. Calcium chloride.
21. Neutral buffered formalin.
22. 1% Glutaraldehyde.
23. 1% Eosin in distilled water.

3. Methods

3.1. Paraffin Sections (Fig. 1)

1. Fix the specimen in neutral buffered formalin and embed in wax. Cut 3–5 μm sections.
2. Dewax the sections in xylene (two changes, 5 min each), and rehydrate through three changes of IMS to tap water.

3. Lugol's iodine/hypo sequence (in the author's experience, this is only required when using Danscher's reagent, and not if a commercial silver-enhancement kit is used). Immerse in Lugol's iodine (5 min), and remove the iodine by rinsing thoroughly in 5% sodium thiosulfate, followed by washing in PBS.

4. Wipe excess liquid from the area around the sections, and apply sufficient 5% heat-inactivated normal serum from the second antibody species to cover each entire section (15 min). If protein A-gold probes are used, flood the sections with BSA-PBS rather than normal serum. It is important to keep the sections covered and in a humid environment throughout all incubations, preferably using a purpose-made humidity chamber. Depending on the size of the section, about 50–200 µL of reagent is sufficient to cover each preparation.

5. Tip the slides, wipe away the normal serum from around the section, and replace, without rinsing, with specific primary antibody for 1 h. The appropriate dilution of the primary antibody should be decided previously either by following the manufacturer's recommendations or by titration assay—carrying out a series of dilutions and determining which gives the best signal-to-noise ratio.

6. Rinse the slides in BSA-PBS, three changes of 2 min each.

7. Cover the sections with gold probe, again suitably diluted in BSA-PBS following either the manufacturer's recommendations or by titration assay.

8. Rinse the slides in BSA-PBS, three changes of 2 min each.

9. If weak antibody–antigen binding is suspected, the binding may be stabilized by fixation in 1% glutaraldehyde in PBS for 10 min.

10. Rinse sections in high-quality distilled water to remove all traces of chloride ions and other impurities that might contaminate the silver-enhancing solution. Some commercial enhancement solutions are reported to be resistant to contamination; the user should evaluate this carefully, especially if high levels of nonspecific background are encountered.

11. If a commercial silver-enhancement kit is used, make up enhancer immediately before use according to the manufacturer's instructions, especially with respect to times, temperatures, and lighting conditions. Every 2 min, examine the progress of the enhancement using a bench microscope, but be aware that some of the more sensitive enhancers, in particular Danscher's reagent, may undergo spontaneous reduction when exposed to strong light. It may be useful to place a control slide continuously on the microscope stage; the lamp may then be turned on when required to examine the progress of enhancement.

12. When the reaction has developed sufficiently, according to the investigator's preference, wash the slides first in distilled water and then in running tap water.

13. To prevent the silver intensification from fading, fix the reaction product with 5% sodium thiosulfate for 5 min and wash with tap water.

14. Counterstain as required; either 1 min in Gill's hematoxylin alone, 1% eosin alone, or hematoxylin followed by eosin will give good contrast with the black silver deposition.

15. Wash well in tap water, dehydrate in IMS, clear in xylene, and mount in DPX.

16. Sites of antibody–antigen localization will appear black when viewed with transmitted white light (Fig. 2).

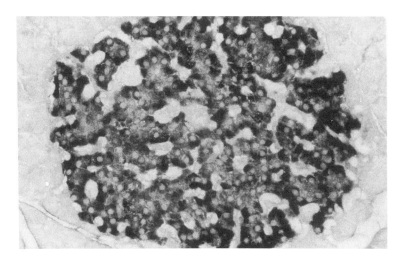

Fig. 2. Photomicrograph of β-cells in a pancreatic islet of Langerhans-IGSS labeling of insulin (magnification ×400).

3.2. Frozen Sections and Cytocentrifuge Preparations

Cryostat sections and cytocentrifuge preparations should be air-dried for at least 1 h, but preferably overnight before immunostaining. Before immunolabeling, cryostat sections should be fixed in cold acetone for 10 min and cytospin slides should be fixed for 90 s in a 1:1 mixture of acetone and methanol at room temperature. After fixation, follow the IGSS method for paraffin sections from step 3 in Section 3.1. Cytospin preparations are usually adequately covered by standard 25-μL aliquots of reagent. If immunolabeling is weak, the sections may be permeabilized for 5 min in 0.1% trypsin in TBS containing 0.1% calcium chloride at 37°C *(12)*.

3.3. Cell Suspensions

De Waele et al. *(13)* recommended immunolabeling isolated cells while in suspension. Following the final antibody incubation, cells are washed and cytocentrifuged, and then silver-enhanced and counterstained on the slide as usual. Although labeling may be stronger than in previously cytocentrifuged cells, the procedure involves centrifugation and resuspension of cell pellets after the labeling and washing stages, which may result in cell damage and depletion.

3.4. Preparation of Silver-Enhancement Solution

The silver solution for enhancing the gold probes is prepared by mixing the following reagents in the order given and using immediately. All solutions are made in distilled water.

1. 7.5 mL of gum acacia (500 g/L) prepared by stirring overnight and filtering through gauze. Stock solutions may be kept in frozen aliquots.
2. 10 mL of citrate buffer at pH 3.0 This consists of 23.5g trisodium citrate dihydrate and 2.5 g citric acid monohydrate dissolved in 100 mL distilled water.
3. 15 mL Freshly prepared hydroquinone.
4. 15 mL Freshly prepared silver lactate.

Keep the silver lactate and the final mixture containing the silver lactate dark by wrapping the containers within foil, and use in a darkroom. At the acid pH, silver lactate provides the source of silver ions necessary for deposition on the gold particles.

4. Notes

1. General notes: IGSS is still a fairly recent innovation in the fields of research and diagnostic histopathology, but the method is now making advances in some interesting applications, which are reviewed in ref. *14*. There have been reports describing labeling of leukocytes in hematology *(15)*, and also in transplantation pathology *(16)* and cytology *(17)*, the latter making use of Romanowsky counterstaining so that cells can be identified both morphologically and phenotypically at the same time. The IGSS method has been used in the MAb diagnosis of B-cell lymphomas using paraffin-embedded material *(18)*, and it has been suggested that cell-surface antigens can be better demonstrated with periodate-lysine-paraformaldhyde-dichromate (PLPD) fixed material *(19)*. IGSS has been found to give superior results with a whole range of antisera used in routine paraffin histopathology, including regulatory peptides, intermediate filaments, and S100 *(20)*. Using the procedures outlined in this chapter, it can be shown that IGSS offers a number of distinct advantages over other immunolabeling methods:
   a. Gold sols are easy and cheap to produce.
   b. Gold particle size can be closely regulated; smaller-size probes make a better nucleus for silver-enhancement.
   c. Antibody/gold conjugation is relatively straightforward, and the resulting probes remain stable for a long time if refrigerated.
   d. The method is economical, since greater sensitivity permits incubation with more highly diluted antisera.
   e. IGSS preparations are permanent and can be re-examined at later dates.
   f. Gold conjugates are nonhazardous, and the procedure does not involve the use of carcinogenic chromagens. No precautions are required for handling or disposal of materials.
2. Problems with labeling: Problems with immunolabeling have been discussed in detail elsewhere *(21,22)* and are usually either:
   a. Operator error.
   b. No antigen: The antigen may have been damaged during processing, or there may be no antigen in the sample.
   c. No antibody: The antibody may have been destroyed during preparation, or there may be no specific antibody in the serum.

Problems with IGSS labeling usually fall into two categories. Either there is no immunolabeling, or the labeling is so high that the accompanying background obscures the specific labeled sites. These problems are at first sight daunting, but usually the remedy is quite simple. When there is no immunolabeling, it is always advisable to run a positive control with each experiment to confirm that the reagents are functioning properly. If there is no immunolabeling on the experimental sections, the concentration of the antibody may be too low or indeed too high. In the latter case, there is no room for the antibody to bind, therefore reducing the signal *(21)*. It is possible that the antigen may be masked by the thickness of the section. Cut thinner sections or permeabilize the sections with a detergent, such as Triton X-100, or carry out proteolysis to unmask the antigen *(22)*. A common problem is the fixation regime. If the fixation is too harsh, the antigenicity of the specimen will be lost, whereas if the fixation regimen is too light, antigens and other material may leach from the tissue. Too much labeling is often accompanied by an unacceptably high background, and this may be caused by a very poor antibody. It is always wise to ascertain the titer and specificity of an antibody before immunolabeling and estimate the expected results. If a suitable antibody has been chosen, the concentration of immunological reagents may be too high, or there may be a nonspecific attachment of reagents to the tissue. The former is remedied by carrying out a series of dilutions of the reagents and silver development times and selecting concentrations that produce high signal-to-low noise. High background caused by the nonspecific attachment of reagents to the specimen is reduced by including 0.5% Triton X-100 in the buffers used for diluting the reagents. A preincubation of the specimen with 1% BSA and 1% gelatin in PBS *(22)* will block some of these nonspecific sites and will also, if necessary, block reactive electrostatic sites on the gold probes *(23)*. Beltz and Burd *(21)* recommend that the addition of up to 0.05 *M* sodium chloride should reduce nonspecific labeling by preventing ionic interactions between the sera and the tissue. They warn also that high salt concentration can interfere with low-affinity antigen–antibody binding, and this technique should be used with care. Beltz and Burd *(21)* also recommend that if there is trouble with background immunolabeling, the antiserum can be absorbed with fresh tissue from the same host that does not contain the antigen in question. If these fail, they suggest the selection of another antibody against the same antigen. Although immunocytochemistry is now a routine technique, care must still be taken to obtain optimum results. Pay particular attention to freshness of reagents, especially buffers, which will become contaminated with bacteria that may interfere with immunolabeling. During incubations, care should be taken to prevent the specimens from drying, since evaporation will concentrate the antibody solutions leading to increased background deposition.

3. Problems with nonspecific background silver deposition: Background silver deposition may be owing to the use of poor-quality antibodies, incorrectly diluted antibodies, old silver-enhancing solutions, poor-quality distilled water, or incorrect silver-enhancement times. The silver-enhancement procedure is tempera-

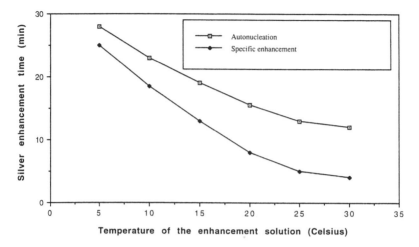

Fig. 3. Temperature-time curve for standardizing silver-enhancement. Silver-enhancement time in IGSS increases with lower operating temperature. The use of a calibration curve assists in optimizing the enhancement procedure.

ture-dependent, and where laboratory temperatures vary widely, especially at different times of the year, it is useful to construct a standardized temperature-enhancement time graph and keep it readily available at the bench (Fig. 3). As an example, adequate silver-enhancement may take only 5 min at 25°C, whereas the same result may take up to 15 min to obtain at 15°C. Enhancement times may be controlled more precisely by storing the enhancer components in the refrigerator at 4°C. Although autonucleation should not be a problem when using modern commercial enhancement kits, silver deposition may be avoided by performing the reaction in a darkroom with a Safelight 5902 or F904.

4. Epipolarization microscopy: An interesting extension of the IGSS techniques lies with some of the optical properties of silver grains. Sites of silver deposition are strikingly demonstrated under dark ground illumination, although it is not possible to *see* the surrounding tissue morphology at the same time. Most fluorescence microscopes may now be adapted to permit the study of IGSS under epipolarization, a procedure that has evolved from reflection contrast microscopy (*see* Table 2). Powerful episcopic illumination from a mercury vapor light source passes through interchangeable filters, an adjustable diaphragm, and into the special epipolarization block. This block contains a UV protection filter, a dichroic half-mirror, and an analyzer. The only light strong enough to pass through the polarizer and return from the sample in a correct plane to be passed by the analyzer is the intense, back-scattered light from silver labeling. The epipolarized light appears as a bright turquoise signal. The image is usually strong enough to allow ordinary diascopic light to be used at the same time for visualizing other tissue structures. Epipolarization is especially useful when silver-

Table 2
Historical Development of Epipolarization Microscopy

Author	References	Development
Jenkins and White (1950)	*24*	Reflection contrast microscopy
Ploem (1975)	*25*	Viewing of living cells attached to slides
De Mey (1983)	*26*	Epipolarization of immunogold alone
De Waele (1986)	*27*	
Ellis et al (1989)	*28*	Epipolarization of IGSS

enhancement is faint, in automated image analysis where the most clear, precise labeling is desirable, and also when a heavy counterstain has been used and the silver deposit is unclear. The use of water or oil medium-power objective lenses is recommended, since problems with glare may be encountered at low-power magnification when a dry objective is used. Also, since epipolarization microscopy greatly increases the sensitivity of IGSS detection, any background silver deposition will also be illuminated more sharply. Epipolarization will often still give a clear result with IGSS preparations that have either faded or turned brown following incomplete stabilization with sodium thiosulfate.

5. Image analysis and IGSS: Two aspects of IGSS make the technique highly suitable for subsequent study using image analysis. First, the intense, sharp, black reaction product is easily discriminated by either monochrome or full-color image analysis systems. Second, epipolarization may be used to provide even more discrimination between the IGSS signal and the background, which is particularly useful when a heavy counterstain has been employed for identifying other features of the preparation. A procedure has been described *(28)* whereby leukocyte subpopulations labeled with IGSS may be enumerated by examining the total, hematoxylin-counterstained leukocyte population under diascopic white light, and then changing to epipolarizing illumination to count the proportion of IGSS-labeled cells that are present (Fig. 4). Occasionally, caution is required with the interpretation of computer-analyzed IGSS data, for example, when other black tissue components are present, such as carbon particles within lung sections *(30)*.

6. Counterstaining IGSS preparations: Whereas most immunohistochemical procedures may only successfully employ a delicate nuclear counterstain, a wide variety of counterstains may be used following IGSS labeling, including trichromes and more selective techniques, such as those used in the identification of microorganisms. The Romanowsky procedure has been used as a counterstain for the morphological examination of leukocyte populations previously labeled with IGSS incorporating leukocyte subset markers *(17,27)*. Only silver impregnation procedures and techniques giving a black or near-black coloration should be avoided; epipolarsiation may be helpful in the latter situation, but silver impregnation preparations behave variably under epipolarized light.

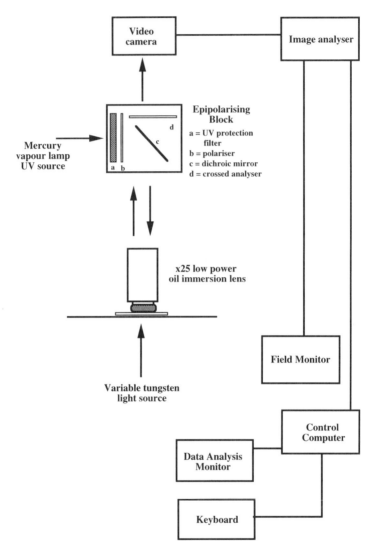

Fig. 4. Flow diagram illustrating the application of image analysis to IGSS using a conventional diascopic white light/episcopic polarized light double-illumination light microscope system. Adapted from ref. *28* with permission.

7. Color development of the IGSS signal: The color development of silver grains in IGSS has been used to convert the black silver signal to either red, yellow, or blue-green *(31)*. The method is a histochemical application of the chemical reactions more traditionally used in color photography.

8. Double labeling with IGSS and other immunocytochemical methods: The combination of IGSS with a variety of different immunoenzyme and immunofluores-

cence procedures has been evaluated *(32)*, and the application of IGSS followed by immunoalkaline phosphatase seems to provide the most successful results.

9. IGSS and *in situ* hybridization. IGSS is now being used for locating DNA probes with *in situ* hybridization, especially incorporating the new 1-nm gold labels *(33)*.

10. Microwave stimulation: Recent work has shown that IGSS labeling procedures can be performed more rapidly using microwave stimulation *(34)*.

11. IGSS may also be performed on cryostat sections, which may then be plastic embedded for semi-thin sectioning *(35)*.

12. Although the IGSS technique was originally introduced for use in light microscopy, the procedure has also found application in combined light microscope and electron microscope studies *(36)* as well as in the electron microscope field alone.

References

1. Coons, A. H., Creech, H. J., and Jones, R. N. (1941) Immunological properties of an antibody containing a fluorescent group. *Proc. Soc. Exp. Biol. Med.* **47,** 200–202.

2. Coons, A. H. and Kaplan, M. H. (1950) Localization of antigen in tissue cells. *J. Exp. Med.* **91,** 1–13.

3. Nakane, P. K. and Pierce, G. B. (1966) Enzyme-linked antibodies: preparation and application for localization of antigens. *J. Histochem. Cytochem.* **14,** 929–931.

4. Sternberger, L. A. (1970) The unlabelled antibody-enzyme method of histochemistry. Preparation and properties of soluble anigen–antibody complex (horseradish peroxidase-antihorseradish peroxidase) and its use in identification of spirochetes. *J. Histochem. Cytochem.* **18,** 315–333.

5. Hsu, S.-M., Raine, L., and Fanger, H. (1981) Use of avidin–biotin–peroxidase complex in immunoperoxidase techniques. *J. Histochem. Cytochem.* **29,** 577–580.

6. Cordell, J. L., Falini, B., Erber, W. N., Ghosh, A. K., Abdulaziz, Z., MacDonald, S., Pulford, K. A. F., Stein, H., and Mason, D. Y. (1984) Immunoenzymatic labelling of monoclonal antibodies using immune complexes of alkaline phosphatase and onoclonal anti-alkaline phosphatase (APAAP Complexes) *J. Histochem. Cytochem.* **32,** 219–229.

7. Danscher, G. (1981) Localization of gold in biological tissue. A photochemical method for light and electron microscopy. *Histochemistry* **71,** 81–88.

8. Holgate, C., Jackson, P., Cowen, P., and Bird, C. (1983) Immunogold-silver staining: a new method of immunostaining with enhanced sensitivity. *J. Histochem. Cytochem.* **31,** 938–944.

9. Faraday, M. (1857) Experimental relations of gold (and other metals) to light. *Phil. Trans. Roy. Soc.* **147,** 145–181.

10. Faulk, W. and Taylor, G. (1971) Immunogold method for the electron microscope. *Immunocytochemistry* **8,** 1081–1083.

11. Slot, J. W. and Geuze, H. J. (1985) A new method of preparing gold probes for multiple labelling cytochemistry. *Eur. J. Cell. Biol.* **90,** 533–536.

12. Finley, J. C. W. and Perutz, P. (1982) The use of proteolytic enzymes for improved localization of tissue antigens with immunocytochemistry, in *Techniques in Immunocytochemistry*, vol. 1 (Bullock, G. R. and Petrusz, P., eds.), Academic, New York, pp. 239–250.

13. De Waele, M., De Mey, K., Moeremans, M., De Brabender, M., and Van Camp, B. (1983) Immunogold staining for the light microscopic detection of leukocyte cell-surface antigens with monoclonal antibodies. *J. Histochem. Cytochem.* **31,** 938–944.

14. Hughes, D. (1987) Developments in IGSS: A review. *Lab. Prac.* **36,** 62–69.

15. Romasko, F., Rosenburg, J., and Wybran, J. (1985) An immunogold silver method for the light microscopic analysis of blood lymphocyte subsets with monoclonal antibodies. *Am. J. Clin. Pathol.* **84,** 307–316.

16. Sako, H., Nakane, Y., Okino, K., Nishihara, K., Kodama, M., Paku, K., Takayama, H., Tomoyoshi, T., Kawata, M., and Yamada, H. (1987) Immunocytochemical study of the cells infiltrating human renal allografts by the ABC and the IGSS methods using monoclonal antibodies. *Transplantation* **44,** 43–50.

17. Hughes, D. A., Kempson, M. G., Carter, N. P., and Morris, P. J. (1988) Immuno-gold-silver/Romanowsky staining: simultaneous immunocytochemical and morphological analysis of fine-needle aspirate biopsies. *Transplant. Proc.* **20,** 575,576.

18. Holgate, C. S., Jackson, P., Lauder, I., Cowen, P. N., and Bird, C. C. (1983) Surface membrane staining of immunoglobulins in paraffin sections of non-Hodgkins lymphomas using the immunogold-silver technique. *J. Clin. Pathol.* **36,** 742–746.

19. Holgate, C. S., Jackson, P., Pollard, K., Lunny, D., and Bird, C. C. (1986) Effects of fixation on T and B lymphocyte surface membrane antigen demonstration in paraffin-processed tissues. *J. Pathol.* **149,** 293–300.

20. Hacker, G. W., Springall, D. R., Van Noorden, S., Bishop, A. E., Grimelius, L., and Polak, J. M. (1985) The immunogold-silver technique: a powerful tool in histopathology. *Virchows Arch. (Pathol. Anat.)* **406,** 449–461.

21. Beltz, B. S. and Burd, G. D. (1989) *Immunocytochemical Techniques: Principles and Practice.* Blackwell, Oxford.

22. Beesley, J. E. (1989) Colloidal gold: a new perspective for cytochemical marking, in *Royal Microscopical Society Handbook,* vol. 17. Oxford Scientific Publications, Oxford, UK.

23. Behnke, O., Ammitzboll, T., Jessen, H., Klokker, M., Nilhausen, K., Tranum-Jensen, H., and Olsen, L. (1986) Nonspecific binding of protein-stabilized gold sols as a source of error in immunocytochemistry. *Eur. J. Cell. Biol.* **41,** 326–338.

24. Jenkins, E. W. and White, H. E. (1950) *Fundamentals in Optics.* McGraw-Hill, NY.

25. Ploem, J. S. (1975) Reflection contrast microscopy as a tool for the investigation of the attachment of living cells to glass surface, in *Mononuclear Phagocytes In Immunity, Infection And Pathology* (Von Furth, R., ed.), Blackwell, Oxford, UK, pp. 405–421.

26. De Mey, J. (1983) Colloidal gold probes in immunocytochemistry, in *Immunocytochemistry: Practical Applications in Pathology and Biology* (Polak, J. M. and Van Noorden, S., eds.), Wright-SPG, Bristol, UK, pp. 82–112.

27. De Waele, M., De Mey, J., Rewmans, W., Labeur, C., Rochmans, K., and Van Kamp, B. (1986) Potential of immunogold-silver staining for the study of leuko-cyte sub-populations as defined by monoclonal antibodies. *J. Histochem. Cytochem.* **34,** 1257–1263.

28. Ellis, I. O., Bell, J., and Bancroft, J. D. (1989) Polarized incident light microscopical enhancement of immunogold and immunogold-silver preparations: its role in immunohistology. *J. Pathol.* **159,** 13–16.
29. Hughes, D. A., Fowler, S., Chaplin, A. J., and Morris, P. J. (1991) Immunogold-silver staining of leukocyte populations in lung sections containing carbon particles requires cautious interpretation. *Histochem. J.* **23,** 196–199.
30. Fritz, P., Hoenes, J., Schenk, J., Mischelinski, A., Grau, A., Saal, J. G., Tuczek, H. V., Multhaupt, H., and Pfleiderer, G. (1986) Color development of immunogold-labelled antibodies for light microscopy. *Histochemistry* **85,** 209–214.
31. Gillitzer, R., Berger, R., and Moll, H. (1990) A reliable method for simultaneous demonstration of two antigens using a novel combination of immunogold-silver staining and immunoenzymatic labelling. *J. Histochem. Cytochem.* **38,** 307–313.
32. Jackson, P., Lalani, E. N., and Boutsen, J. (1988) Microwave stimulated immunogold-silver staining. *Histochem. J.* **20,** 353–358.
33. Jackson, P., Dockey, D. A. Lewis, F. A., and Wells, M. (1990) Applications of 1 nm gold probes on paraffin sections for *in situ* hybridization histochemistry. *J. Clin. Pathol.* **43,** 810–812.
34. Gao, K., Giffin, B. F., Morris, R. E., Cardell, E. L., and Cardell, R. R. (1994) Optimal visualization of immunogold-silver staining of hepatic PEPCK with epipolarized light microscopy. *J. Histochem. Cytochem.* **42,** 823–826.
35. Otsuki, Y., Maxwell, L. E., Magari, S., and Kubo, H. (1990) Immunogold-silver staining method for light and electron microscopic detection of lymphocyte cell-surface antigens with monoclonal antibodies. *J. Histochem. Cytochem.* **38,** 1215–1221.
36. Lackie, P. M., Hennessy, R. J., Hacker, G. W., and Polak, J. M. (1985) Investigation of immunogold-silver staining by electron microscopy. *Histochemistry* **83,** 545–550.

31

Immunogold Probes in Electron Microscopy

David J. P. Ferguson, David A. Hughes, and Julian E. Beesley

1. Introduction

Electron microscopy permits the detailed study of cell relationships within tissues and organelles within cells. Two ultrastructural techniques in which gold probes have proven invaluable are immunocytochemistry and *in situ* hybridization, and these will be described here. Until 1980, peroxidase was the marker of choice, but now colloidal gold is almost universally used. The advantages of colloidal gold are that:

1. It is particulate and very dense, therefore easily identified on biological sections;
2. It is small and will not obscure fine structural details;
3. It can be prepared in several different sizes for use in multiple labeling experiments and quantitation; and
4. It is easily conjugated to immunoglobulins or proteins A or G.

It is these features that make it the ideal label for the localization of antigens in immunocytochemistry and nucleic acid sequences by *in situ* hybridization.

1.1. Immunocytochemistry (see Note 1)

Immunoelectron microscopy is the use of immunocytochemical techniques to study subcellular location of antigens on and within cells. Unfortunately, immunoelectron microscopy involves two incompatible techniques in that the fixation required for good morphology damages the antigenic epitopes recognized by specific antibodies. Therefore, cell preparation for electron microscopy is a compromise between retaining sufficient antigenicity and preserving the cell ultrastructure.

In the basic technique, the specimen is prepared to expose antigens at the surface of the sample, and these samples are successively incubated with pri-

From: *Methods in Molecular Biology, Vol. 80: Immunochemical Protocols, 2nd ed.*
Edited by: J. D. Pound © Humana Press Inc., Totowa, NJ

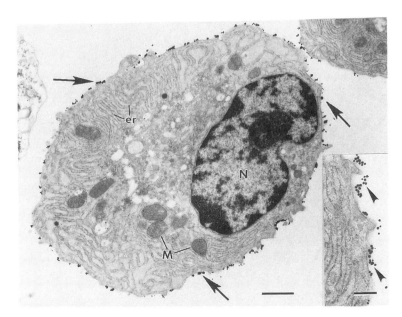

Fig. 1. Preembedding technique. A plasma cell from human bone marrow immunostained using a monoclonal antibody (E29) to epithelial membrane antigen prior to fixation and embedding showing the antigen is located along the plasmalemma (arrows). N, nucleus; M, mitochondrion; er, rough endoplasmic reticulum. Insert: Detail of the cell surface showing the numerous gold particles (arrowheads). Visualized using goat antimouse Ig conjugated to 20-nm gold. Bars are 1 and 0.2 μm, respectively (micrograph supplied by K. Zimmer, K. Gatter and D. Y. Mason).

mary antibody, a wash, and a secondary antibody that is complexed with an electron dense marker. Blocking steps are included to reduce nonspecific attachment of the reagents to either the sample or the background.

Some experiments require that antigenic information be obtained from the surface of the cell; others are interested in intramembrane antigens or intracellular antigens, or indeed the relationship of one antigen-bearing cell to another. The specimen can be prepared by one of several different methods to expose antigens and, thus, obtain the desired antigenic information from the sample *(1)*.

1. The preembedding technique allows external antigens to be localized. The sample, usually whole cells, is incubated with the immunological reagents before fixation, dehydration, embedding, and sectioning (Fig. 1).
2. In contrast, for the postembedding technique, the sample is embedded and sectioned before immunolabeling. This permits the localization of internal antigens (Fig. 2).

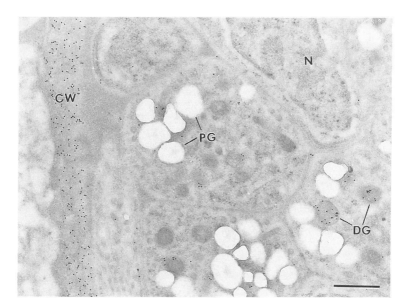

Fig. 2. Postembedding technique. Section through part of a tissue cyst of the protozoan parasite *Toxoplasma gondii* immunostained with a rat monoclonal antibody (CC2) which recognizes a molecule located in the cyst wall (CW) and in dense granules within the parasite (for details, *see* ref. *2*). N, nucleus; PG, polysaccharide granules. Three-step protocol: rat monoclonal followed by rabbit antirat Ig and visualized with goat antirabbit Ig conjugated to 10-nm gold. Bar is 0.5 μm.

3. The immunonegative stain technique is used for the localization of external antigens on viruses, bacterial pili, and any small objects that may be dried onto an electron microscope grid and immunolabeled *in situ* (Fig. 3).
4. When relationships between cells expressing particular surface antigens are of interest, specimens are immunolabeled before preparation for scanning electron microscopy. This allows the three-dimensional evaluation of immunolabeling on the surface of the cells.
5. The immunoreplica technique is a high-resolution technique for the localization of antigens on the plasma membrane of cultured cells. After immunolabeling, the cells are replicated with carbon and platinum to reveal immunolabeling on the cell surface.
6. The freeze-fracture immunolabeling technique can be used in two ways. In the first, the cells are immunolabeled and freeze-fractured. This shows immunolabeling of the outer surface of the cell membrane superimposed on a high-resolution replica of the inner surface of the membrane. In the second, the cells are fractured before immunolabeling. This permits immunolabeling to be correlated with large areas of the fractured faces.

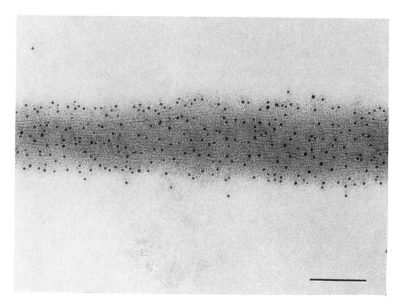

Fig. 3. Negative stain technique. Micrograph shows a bundle of pili from the bacterium *Neisseria meningitidis* immunostained with an antipilus rabbit polyclonal antibody visualized using Protein A conjugated to 5-nm gold followed by negative staining with 1% methyl tungstate. Bar is 0.1 μm.

The process of immunolabeling for each of these different methods is similar. The difference between the techniques is in preparation of the antigen and the contrasting method (*see* Note 3).

1.2. In Situ *Hybridization*

In situ hybridization has become a widely used method for the localization of nucleic acid sequences in chromosomes, single cells, and tissue sections at the light microscope level *(3)*. More recently, with the development of nonisotopic probe labeling techniques and immunogold detection methods, it has been possible to localize nucleic acid sequences at the ultrastructural level *(4,5)*. The technique has been applied to subcellular localization of RNA transcripts, analyses of intracellular viral life cycles (Fig. 4), and identification of the species of origin in xenograft tissue. The initial stage involves hybridization of the probe to the nucleic acid target, followed by localization of the probe using immunocytochemistry as described in Section 1.1.

The technical problems of maintaining morphology while exposing the target to the detection systems are similar to those described for immunoelectron

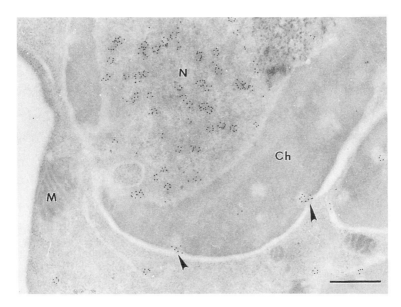

Fig. 4. *In situ* hybridization technique. Part of an erythroid precursor cell infected with the human parvovirus B19 and probed for viral DNA. The B19 nucleic acid is located within the central electron lucent area of the nucleus (N) and also at nuclear pores (arrowheads). Ch, chromatin; M, mitochondrion. A three-step detection protocol was used (*see* ref. *5* for details). Sheep antidigoxigenin followed by rabbit antisheep Ig and then goat antirabbit Ig conjugated to 10-nm gold. Bar is 0.5 μm.

microscopy *(6)*. As such, the three techniques that have been devised are similar to those described for immunoelectron microscopy (*see* Note 3).

1. Preembedding hybridization where permeabilized cells or vibratome sections are hybridized, and then postfixed and embedded as described in Section 3.1.2.
2. Hybridization to ultrathin cryosections.
3. Postembedding hybridization in which material is processed as described in Section 3.1.1., and the hybridization is carried out on thin sections.

1.3. Combined Immunocytochemistry and In Situ *Hybridization*

Using the techniques described in Sections 1.1. and 1.2., it is possible to label both nucleic acids sequences and proteins on the same section. This has been used to colocalize viral nucleic acids and proteins (Fig. 5) *(6,7)*.

The method is a combination of the techniques described in Sections 3.1. and 3.2. The *in situ* hybridization is carried out as described in Sections 3.2, steps 1–9, directly followed by immunolabeling as in Section 3.1.1.2., steps 4–10.

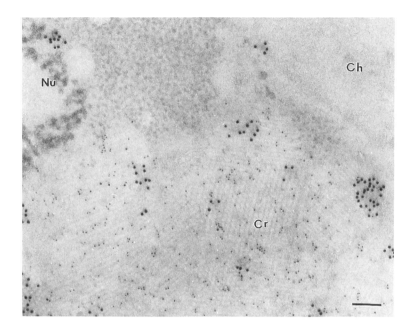

Fig. 5. Combined *in situ* hybridization and immunocytochemistry. Part of the nucleus of an erythroid precursor cell infected with parvovirus B19. There is colabeling of the viral DNA (10-nm gold) using *in situ* hybridization and the B19 capside protein (5-nm gold) by immunocytochemistry over an intranuclear crystalline array (Cr) of viral particles (*see* ref. *7* for details). Nu, nucleus; Ch, heterochromatin. Bar is 0.1 μm.

2. Materials

2.1. Immunocytochemistry

1. Antibody of known specificity.
2. Colloidal gold probe of the required size (10-nm diameter for routine use), which will react with the primary antibody (*see* Notes 2 and 5).
3. Phosphate-buffered saline (PBS): 0.01M phosphate, 0.15M NaCl, pH 7.2, as recommended by Slot and Geuze *(8)*.
4. 1% Gelatin in PBS.
5. 0.02M Glycine in PBS.
6. 1% Bovine serum albumin in PBS (BSA-PBS).
7. 1% Glutaraldehyde in PBS.
8. Distilled water.
9. Materials for embedding the samples in the pre- and postembedding techniques.
10. Contrasting reagents for samples (*see* individual techniques).
11. 4% Formaldehyde freshly prepared from paraformaldehyde powder, in 0.1M cacodylate buffer, pH 7.2, or 2% paraformaldehyde + 0.1% glutaraldehyde in 0.1M cacodylate buffer, pH 7.2.

12. Graded series of ethanol (70, 90, 100%).
13. 2.3M Sucrose.
14. 200-Mesh formvar/carbon-coated grids.
15. 1% Osmium tetroxide.
16. 2% Aqueous uranyl acetate.
17. 1% Uranyl acetate made up in 70% methanol.
18. Neutral uranyl acetate: To prepare neutral 2% uranyl acetate, mix equal quantities of 4% aqueous uranyl acetate and 0.3M oxalic acid, and adjust the pH to 7.2–7.4 with 10% ammonium hydroxide *(9)*.
19. Reynold's lead citrate stain *(10)*.
20. 1% Methyl tungstate.
21. Freon 22.
22. Liquid nitrogen.
23. Sodium hypochlorite.
24. 40% Chromic acid.
25. Parafilm or similar.

2.2. In Situ *Hybridization*

In addition to the materials listed in Section 2.1., the following are required:

1. Probes (oligonucleotides, cDNAs, or RNAs) labeled with biotin or digoxigenin.
2. SET buffer: 300 mM NaCl, 4 mM EDTA, 50 mM Tris, pH 7.0.
3. Hybridization buffer: 50% deionized formamide, 10% dextran sulfate, 250 µg/mL sheared herring sperm DNA, 0.01% polyvinyl pyrrolidone and 0.1% sodium dodecyl sulfate in 2X SET buffer.
4. 0.5M NaOH.
5. Tris-buffered saline/Triton: 50 mM Tris, 150 mM NaCl, pH 7.2, containing 0.5% Triton.
6. TBS/Triton/BSA: as in step 5, with 1% BSA added.
7. Antibodies to biotin or digoxigenin.

3. Methods
3.1. Immunocytochemistry

Some techniques require the specimen to be fixed. Fixation for electron microscopy depends very much on the antibody being used. If the antibody is a monoclonal, fixation is in 4% cacodylate-buffered formaldehyde. Keep the specimen in this fixative until further processing. The nature of polyclonal antibodies is such that the antigens may be able to withstand greater fixation, although very few can withstand routine glutaraldehyde fixation. Therefore, a reasonable compromise is 2% paraformaldehyde + 0.1% glutaraldehyde in cacodylate buffer. This preserves more ultrastructure than formaldehyde alone. The sample should be transferred to cacodylate buffer until further processing.

3.1.1. The Postembedding Technique (see Note 7)

This technique is the most popular of the immunolabeling techniques. All immunolabeling steps are carried out at room temperature, and the various reagents are placed dropwise on a piece of Parafilm in a Petri dish. If required, the chamber can be kept moist by inclusion of several pieces of damp filter paper.

3.1.1.1. SPECIMEN PREPARATION

1. Ascertain which primary antibody is to be used, and fix the specimen with either freshly prepared 4% formaldehyde or with 2% paraformaldehyde + 0.1% glutaraldehyde.
2. Dehydrate the specimen in a graded series of ethanol and embed in the resin of choice. This could be LR White *(1)*. If a more sensitive system is required, embedding in LR Gold or Lowicryl, at –20°C *(11)*, may retain antigenicity. For extremely sensitive antigens, cryoprotect the specimen in 2.3M sucrose for 1 h before freezing in liquid nitrogen, and cut ultrathin frozen sections that are collected and thawed on a droplet of 2.3M sucrose before mounting on 200-mesh formvar/carbon-coated grids and immunolabeling *(12,13)*.

3.1.1.2. IMMUNOLABELING

1. Float the grids, section side down, on 1% gelatin in PBS for 10 min. The gelatin adsorbs nonspecifically to nonimmunological sticky sites on the surface of the section. This prevents antibody attachment, thereby reducing nonspecific background.
2. Float the grid on 0.02M glycine in PBS for 3 min. This will block any free aldehyde groups in the tissue and prevent the antibodies from being fixed nonimmunologically on the tissue.
3. Rinse the sections with BSA-PBS for 2 min.
4. Incubate the sections with an appropriate dilution of specific antibody diluted with BSA-PBS for 1 h. The concentration of antibody is found by immunolabeling at different concentrations until a satisfactory signal:noise ratio is achieved. Suitable starting dilutions for monoclonal antibodies are 1:5, 1:10, and 1:20. For polyclonal antibodies, 1:10, 1:50, and 1:100 are recommended.
5. Rinse excess reagents from the section by floating the grid for 4 × 1 min washes on BSA-PBS.
6. Incubate the sections with a suitable dilution of colloidal gold probe, diluted with BSA-PBS. This dilution is found empirically by testing a number of dilutions. A good starting dilution is 1:20 for a 10 nm gold probe.
7. Wash excess reagents off the sections by floating the grid, 4 × 1 min, on PBS (no BSA).
8. Fix the reagents by floating the grid for 1 min on 2.5% glutaraldehyde in PBS (only necessary with frozen sections).
9. Wash the sections thoroughly with water, 4 × 1 min.
10. Stain resin sections with 1% methanolic uranyl acetate and lead citrate according to routine electron microscopy procedures. If ultrathin frozen sections are being

used, stain with 2% aqueous uranyl acetate, neutral uranyl acetate, and embed in methyl cellulose before examination *(13)*.

3.1.2. The Preembedding Technique

The preembedding technique is used to localize antigens on the surface of isolated cells, either prokaryotes or eukaryotes. If it is necessary to store the cells before immunolabeling, they must be fixed as in Section 3.1.1.1. If a very sensitive method is required, fixation may be omitted before immunolabeling.

1. Centrifuge the cells lightly into a pellet and resuspend this in the reagents, following the schedule from step 3 in Section 3.1.1.2. It is important to resuspend the cell suspensions thoroughly in each reagent. Otherwise, the cells in the center of the clump will not be immunolabeled because of poor penetration of reagents *(1)*.
2. After glutaraldehyde fixation (Section 3.1.1.2., step 8), fix the cells further with 1% osmium tetroxide, saturated uranyl acetate, dehydrate in an ascending series of ethanol (70, 90, 100%), and embed in epoxy resin. Ultrathin sections of the block, stained with 1% methanolic uranyl acetate and lead citrate, will reveal immunolabeling on the outer surface of the cells.

3.1.3. The Immunonegative Stain Technique

Carbon/formvar-coated grids are floated on suspensions of virus, bacteria, or even isolated cell organelles in buffer or distilled water, and immunolabeled as described in Section 3.1.1.2., steps 3–7. After immunolabeling (Section 3.1.1.2., step 7), the specimen is contrasted with a negative stain, such as 1% methyl tungstate. If a fixative is included (Section 3.1.1.2., step 8), the specimens are difficult to stain. For very small specimens, it is advisable to use the 5-nm gold probes. Care should be taken with highly pathogenic samples. If necessary, they should be killed with glutaraldehyde or formaldehyde, and tested for viability before immunolabeling.

3.1.4. The Immunoreplica Technique

The immunoreplica technique *(14)* is used when it is necessary to detect antigenic sites on the plasma membrane of cultured cells. The cells are cultured on coverslips, and are fixed as described above depending on the antibody in question, and immunolabeled *in situ* as described in Section 3.1.1.2., steps 3–9. After immunolabeling (Section 3.1.1.2., step 9), they are further fixed with 1% osmium tetroxide and are dehydrated in a graded series of ethanol (70, 90, 100%), critically point-dried, and replicated with a layer of carbon and platinum. The replicas are cleaned with sodium hypochlorite and chronic acid before examination with the transmission electron microscope. Large areas of the replicated plasma membrane remain intact for observation. Colloidal gold probes are probably the only probes of sufficient density that can be detected on these surfaces.

3.1.5. The Immunoscanning Electron Microscope Technique

Colloidal gold immunolabeling is suitable for scanning electron microscopy *(15)*. This yields a further useful dimension to the technique for observing external antigens. Specimens excised from the animal or cells grown in culture are suitably fixed in either 4% cacodylate buffered formaldehyde or 2% paraformaldehyde + 1% cacodylate-buffered glutaraldehyde, and immunolabeled as in Section 3.1.1.2., steps 3–8. After additional fixation with 2.5% glutaraldehyde. The samples are further fixed with 1% osmium tetroxide and prepared for scanning electron microscope observation by any of the routine techniques, such as the osmium tetroxide/thiocarbohydrazide technique *(16)*. Recent technical advances in the SEM (field emission guns and backscatter electron detectors) have increased the resolution and usefulness of this technique by allowing the direct visualization of 10-nm gold particles using the atomic number contrast of the gold. Thus, the three-dimensional distribution of antigens on the surface of cells can be identified.

3.1.6. The Immunofreeze-Fracture Techniques

These techniques were developed and have been pioneered by Pinto da Silva et al. *(17)*.

3.1.6.1. The Label-Fracture Technique *(18)*

Isolated cells, usually unfixed, may be immunolabeled with antibody and gold probe as in Section 3.1.1.2., steps 3–9, and freeze-fractured by routine techniques *(19)*. Briefly, the tissue is cryoprotected with a suitable agent, such as 30% glycerol, and rapidly frozen in Freon 22 cooled with liquid nitrogen. The specimen is fractured in a freeze-fracture plant, and the surfaces replicated. These replicas are thawed, and biological debris removed by cleaning with sodium hypochlorite and 40% chromic acid, followed by thorough washing in distilled water. After mounting on uncoated electron microscope grids, the replicated fracture faces can be observed simultaneously with immunolabeling on the outer surfaces of the cells.

3.1.6.2. The Fracture-Label Technique

Alternatively, the specimen may be fractured before immunolabeling *(17)*. The sample is fixed depending on which antibody is being used, cryoprotected, frozen rapidly, and ground into small pieces under liquid nitrogen in a homogenizer. The small pieces are thawed in glycerol and immunolabeled as in Section 3.1.1.2., steps 3–8. At this stage, they may be processed to resin for ultrathin sectioning to observe immunolabeling on the fractured faces (the thin section fracture-label technique), or they may be dehydrated, critical point-dried and replicated, before examination (the critical point-drying fracture-label technique) for observation of replicas of the labeled surface of fractured tissue.

3.2. In Situ *Hybridization*

Using the postembedding technique, sections prepared as described in Section 3.1.1.1. were floated face down on drops of the appropriate solution placed on fresh Parafilm starting at step 4.

Probe preparation:

1. Dissolve labeled probes in hybridization mixture at a final concentration of 1 µg/mL.
2. Denature probe mixture at 95°C for 15 min in Eppendorf tube.
3. Store probes on ice until used.

Section staining:

4. Denature sections on drops of 0.5M NaOH at room temperature for 5 min (if target is double-stranded DNA).
5. Wash sections in double-distilled water (dH$_2$O), 3 × 5 min, and then air-dry.
6. Incubate the sections on 15-µL drops of denatured probe mixture at 37°C in moist chamber for 4 h.
7. Wash in Tris/Triton/BSA, 3 × 5 min at 37°C.
8. Block nonspecific binding with Tris/Triton/BSA for 15 min at room temperature.
9. Incubate sections on antibodies to either biotin or digoxigenin conjugated to colloidal gold diluted 1:25 in Tris/Triton/BSA for 1 h.
10. Wash in Tris/Triton, 2 × 5 min.
11. Wash in dH$_2$O, 2 × 5 min.
12. Stain with 2% uranyl acetate.

Pretreatment of the grids prior to hybridization (step 4) with protease may improve the signal by further exposure of the nucleic acids. Also, pretreatments with RNase or DNase will allow differentiation between signals from DNA or RNA targets.

Owing to the low number of hybridization sites, better results may be obtained by amplifying the signal using a two- or three-step immunogold detection protocol *(5)*.

The major limiting factor in the technique is that there are usually few copies of the target, and since only those at the surface of the section can be hybridized, there is usually a low signal. Therefore, although the technique is very specific, it is relatively insensitive and is only useful where there is a large amount of target sequences present, as in virally infected cells (*see* Note 4).

4. Notes

1. Colloidal gold probes are the most popular of all the immunolabeling techniques for ultrastructural immunocytochemistry and *in situ* hybridization. Since individual gold probes can be easily identified with the electron microscope, there is

increased interest in multiple immunolabeling and quantitative studies. Unfortunately, there is no universally applicable technique, resulting in the development of a multitude of variations. The methods given in this chapter are very basic, but have proven to be satisfactory in this laboratory for certain antigens.

2. The choice of the size of gold to be used is often questioned. Small 5-nm gold particles are surrounded by fewer protein molecules than the 15-nm particles. Therefore, for a given number of closely spaced antigens, it can be assumed that there will be more 5-nm gold particles than 15-nm particles, since each 15-nm gold probe is able to saturate more antibodies than the 5-nm probe. There will also be less steric hindrance when using the 5-nm gold compared with the 15-nm probe. Therefore, it is advisable to use the smallest probe consistent with the magnification required to detect the structures of interest. For thin section studies (Sections 3.1.1., 3.1.2., and 3.1.5.), a gold probe of 10 nm is a useful size. When immunolabeling small virus particles, such as polio (Section 3.1.3.), the size of the probe could be reduced to 5 nm. For general work, the 15-nm probe is slightly large, and the level of immunolabeling is low.

3. Where there is a low signal in either immunocytochemistry or *in situ* hybridization, it is possible to amplify it by either using additional immunological steps in the visualization protocol or by using the small 1- or 5-nm gold followed by silver enhancement, where silver is deposited around the gold particle to increase its size. Both of these techniques increase the number of particles associated with the target.

4. It is possible to carry out double labeling using the *in situ* hybridization technique by attaching biotin to one probe and digoxigenin to another, which can then be visualized with antibiotin or digoxigenin antibodies. Care has to be taken with biotin, because many cells contain endogenous biotin, which can give false-positives results.

5. For multiple immunolabeling experiments, it is important that there be no overlap of sizes of the gold probe. It is advisable to use the 5-nm gold in conjunction with the 15-nm probe. There is no difficulty in differentiating these two-sized probes. The 5- and the 10-, or the 10- and the 15-nm probes could be used, if the size range of the probes were sufficiently small, but in triple immunolabeling with the 5-, 10-, and 15-nm probes, it is sometimes difficult to separate the 5- from the 10- and the 10- from the 15-nm probes. Care has to be taken to prevent crossreactions of the different probes, especially if multiple immunological amplification steps are used.

6. The postembedding technique (Section 3.1.1.) is the most popular of all the immunolabeling techniques. The preembedding technique (Section 3.1.2.), the immunonegative stain technique (Section 3.1.3.), and the immunoscanning electron microscope technique (Section 3.1.5.) are also reasonably popular. The remaining techniques are specialized, and although the information they provide is extremely useful, they are not widely used.

7. There is a continuing debate about which method of specimen preparation is optimum for the postembedding technique (Section 3.1.1.). There are reports

of the technique working with routinely fixed and embedded tissue, although these are exceptional. Methacrylate and LR White have been used for ambient temperature embedding, but there is now a great interest in the low-temperature techniques using LR gold and Lowicryl K4M. Advantages of these techniques are that at the low temperature, there is very little leaching of cell components, since, during dehydration at temperatures down to –40°C, proteins precipitate and are effectively stabilized within the tissue (PLT technique) *(20)*. There is also interest in techniques in which the unfixed sample is frozen before being dried and embedded in a resin *(21)*. Freeze (cryo) substitution is an alternative technique for formalin-fixed cryoprotected tissue. The sample is rapidly frozen with liquid nitrogen and the water substituted at –90°C with either acetone or methanol follow by embedding in Lowicryl HM20 at –45°C *(22,23)*. Another avenue is to freeze the sample and cut frozen sections, which are thawed at room temperature before immunolabeling *(12)*. The deciding factors in which technique to use are the abundance of the antigen, its distribution in the tissue, and its sensitivity to fixation. If the antigen is abundant and withstands fixation, sensitivity is not usually a problem.

8. Any of the gold probes may be conveniently used for immunolabeling provided they link with the primary antibody. Slight differences are seen between immunolabeling with the protein A-gold probes and the antibody–gold complexes. If the antibody–gold complex is used, up to 10 conjugated gold probes may attach to a single Fc component of the primary antibody, thereby producing labeling in clusters. Protein A possesses one binding site for the Fc region, and therefore, clumps of Protein A-gold probes are not observed. Protein A-gold may therefore be of more use in quantitative studies (although many other factors, such as steric hindrance and binding several antibodies with one probe, must be considered). Care is also required because the affinity of protein A to immunoglobulins of different species varies.

9. Immunolabeling for electron microscopy is theoretically identical to immunolabeling for light microscopy. The problems discussed in Chapter 30 describing light microscope immunolabeling are entirely relevant to electron immunocytochemistry.

10. Image analysis may be applied to gold labeling in electron microscopy in order to achieve improved localization and facilitate quantitative analysis of the gold particles *(24)*.

11. Gold chloride may be used to enhance the size of small gold particles where cell-surface and intraorganelle localization of particles is ambiguous *(25)*. Silver enhancement has also been used for improving the localization of antigens labeled using small gold particles *(26–29)*.

References

1. Beesley, J. (1989) Colloidal gold: a new perspective for cytochemical marking. *Royal Microscopical Society Handbook 17*. Oxford Science Publications, Oxford, UK.
2. Gross, U., Bormuth, H., Gaissmaier, C., Dittrich, C., Krenn, V., Bohne, W., and Ferguson, D. J. P. (1995) Monoclonal rat antibodies directed against Toxoplasma

gondii suitable for studying tackyzoite-bradyzoite interconversion in vivo. *Clin. Diag. Lab. Immunol.* **2,** 542–548.

3. Levy, E. R. and Herrington, C. S. (eds). (1995) *Nonisotopic Methods in Molecular Biology—A Practical Approach.* Oxford University Press, Oxford.

4. Morel, G. (ed). (1993) *Hybridization Techniques for Electron Microscopy.* CRC, Boca Raton, FL.

5. Morey, A. L., Ferguson, D. J. P., Leslie, K. O., Taatses, D. J., and Fleming, K. A. (1993) Detection of parvoviral and human DNA sequences at the ultrastructural level by *in situ* hybridization with digoxigenin-labeled probes. *Histochem. J.* **25,** 421–429.

6. Morey, A. L. (1995) Nonisotopic *in situ* hybridization at the ultrastructural level. *J. Pathol.* **176,** 113–121.

7. Morey, A. L., Ferguson, D. J. P., and Fleming, K. A. (1995) Combined immunocytochemistry and nonisotopic *in situ* hybridization for ultrastructural investigation of human parvovirus B19 infection. *Histochem. J.* **27,** 46–53.

8. Slot, J. W. and Geuze, H. J. (1984) Gold markers for single and double immuno-labeling of ultrathin cryosections, in *Immunolabeling for Electron Microscopy* (Polak, J. M. and Varndell, I. M., eds.), Elsevier, Amsterdam, pp. 129–142.

9. Tokuyasu, K. T. (1978) A study of positive staining of ultrathin frozen sections. *J. Ultrastruct. Res.* **63,** 287–307.

10. Reynolds, E. S. (1963) The use of lead citrate at high pH as an electron-opaque stain in electron microscopy. *J. Cell Biol.* **17,** 208–212.

11. Carlemalm, E., Garavito, R. M., and Villiger, W. (1982) Resin development for electron microscopy and an analysis of embedding at low temperature. *J. Microsc.* **126,** 123–143.

12. Griffiths, G., McDowall, A., Back, R., and Dubochet, J. (1984) On the preparation of cryosections for immunocytochemistry. *J. Ultrastruct. Res.* **89,** 68–78.

13. Tokuyasu, K. T. (1986) Immunocryoultramicrotomy. *J. Microsc.* **143,** 139–149.

14. Mannweiler, K., Hohenberg, H., Bohn, W., and Rutter, G. (1982) Protein A-gold particles as markers in replica immunocytochemistry: high resolution electron microscope investigations of plasma membrane surfaces. *J. Microsc.* **126,** 145–149.

15. Hodges, G. M., Southgate, J., and Toulson, E. C. (1987) Colloidal gold-a powerful tool in S. E. M. immunocytochemistry: an overview of bioapplications. *Scanning Electron Microscopy* **1,** 301–318.

16. Murphy, J. A. (1980) Noncoating techniques to render biological specimens conductive/1980 update. *Scanning Electron Microscopy* **1,** 209–220.

17. Pinto da Silva, P., Barbosa, M. L. F., and Aguas, A. P. (1986) A guide to fracture label: cytochemical labeling of freeze-fractured cells, in *Advanced Techniques in Biological Electron Microscopy* (Koehler, J. K., ed.), Springer-Verlag, Berlin, pp. 201–227.

18. Pinto da Silva, P. and Kan, F. W. (1984) Label-fracture: a method for high resolution labeling of cell surfaces. *J. Cell Biol.* **99,** 1156–1161.

19. Robards, A. W. and Sleytr, U. B. (1985) Low temperature methods in biological electron microscopy, in *Practical Methods in Electron Microscopy,* vol. 10 (Glauert, A. M., ed.), Elsevier, Amsterdam.

20. Robertson, D., Monaghan, P., Clark, C., and Atherton, A. J. (1992) An appraisal of low temperature embedding by progressive lowering of temperature into Lowicryl HM20 for immunocytochemical studies. *J. Microsc.* **168,** 85–100.

21. Dudek, R. W., Varndell, I. M., and Polak, J. M. (1984) Combined quick-freeze and freeze-drying techniques for improved electron immunocytochemistry, in *Immunolabeling for Electron Microscopy* (Polak, J. M. and Varndell, I. M., eds.), Elsevier, Amsterdam, pp. 235–248.

22. Oprins, A. D., Geuze, H. J., and Slot, J. W. (1994) Cryosubstitution dehydration of aldehyde-fixed tissue: a favourable approach to quantitative immunocytochemistry. *J. Histochem. Cytochem.* **42,** 497–503.

23. Monaghan, P. and Robertson, D. (1990) Freeze-substitution without aldehyde or osmium fixatives: ultrastructural and implication for immunocytochemistry. *J. Microsc.* **158,** 355–363.

24. Shimizu, H. and Nishikawa, T. (1993) Application of an image analyser to gold labeling in immunoelectron microscopy to achieve better demonstration and quantitative analysis. *J. Histochem. Cytochem.* **41,** 123–128.

25. Morris, R. E., Ciraolo, G. M., and Saelinger, C. B. (1991) Gold enhancement of gold-labeled probes: gold-intensified staining technique (GIST). *J. Histochem. Cytochem.* **39,** 1585–1591.

26. Lackie, P. M., Hennessy, R. J., Hacker, G. W., and Polak, J. M. (1985) Investigation of immunogold-silver staining using electron microscopy. *Histochemistry* **83,** 545–550.

27. Manara, G. C., Ferrari, C., Torresani, C., Sansoni, P., and De Panfilis, G. (1990) The immunogold-silver staining approach in the study of lymphocyte subpopulations in transmission electron microscopy. *J. Immunol. Methods* **128,** 59–63.

28. Otsuki, Y., Maxwell, L. E., Magari, S., and Kubo, H. (1990) Immunogold-silver staining method for light and electron microscopic detection of lymphocyte cell surface antigens with monoclonal antibodies. *J. Histochem. Cytochem.* **38,** 1215–1221.

29. Burry, R. W., Vandrè, D. D., and Hayes, D. M. (1992) Silver enhancement of gold antibody probes in preembedding electron microscopic immunocytochemistry. *J. Histochem. Cytochem.* **40,** 1849–1856.

32

Electron Microscopic-Silver Enhancement for Double Labeling with Antibodies Raised in the Same Species

Kurt Bienz and Denise Egger

1. Introduction

In immunoelectron microscopy (IEM), simultaneous labeling of two or more antigens on the same section is desirable for many applications. If the antibodies (Ab) to be used are raised in the same species, as is usually the case with monoclonal antibodies (MAb), the difficulty arises that the labeled secondary, antispecies Ab used in the first labeling step traps the primary Ab directed against the second antigen, thus leading to a nonspecific signal for the second antigen.

We describe here a method (electron microscopic [EM]-silver enhancement, ref. *1*) to overcome this problem. This procedure increases the size of the gold marker by a predetermined amount, thereby inactivating the antispecies Ab present on the gold grain, but fully retaining the immunoreactivity of the section. For IEM double labeling, therefore, the EM-silver enhancement (B in Fig. 1) has to be performed after the first labeling step (Fig. 1A) to render the section ready for a second immunocytochemical reaction (Fig. 1C) with primary Ab from the same species and with the same (small) gold marker as in the first labeling step.

The physical development employed in the silver enhancement procedure was originally used in photographic work, including EM autoradiography *(2,3)*, and is widely applied today in intensifying immunogold stains in light microscopic preparations or on Western blot (immunogold-silver stain, IGSS; refs. *4,5*). In essence, the method employs a photographic developer and dissolved silver ions. The photographic development reduces the silver ions to silver atoms on the surface of the gold particles in the immunocytochemical prepara-

From: *Methods in Molecular Biology, Vol. 80: Immunochemical Protocols, 2nd ed.*
Edited by: J. D. Pound © Humana Press Inc., Totowa, NJ

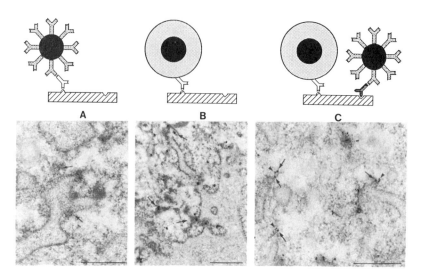

Fig. 1. Schematic representation and EM aspect of the IEM double-labeling method.
(A) The first antigen is labeled with the primary Ab (white) and a secondary antispecies
Ab (hatched), tagged with a small (e.g., 5–10 nm) gold grain (black). The EM picture
above shows a viral replication complex in a poliovirus-infected HEp-2 cell, labeled
(arrows) with a mouse MAb directed against the viral protein 2C and a goat-antimouse
(GAM) Ab tagged with 10 nm gold (Amersham Auroprobe EM-grade, GAM IgG G10).
Bar: 500 nm. **(B)** The EM-silver enhancement inactivates the antispecies Ab and enlarges
the gold grain by the deposition of a silver layer (shaded area) on its surface. EM-pic-
ture: same as (A), gold grains (arrows) enlarged approximately threefold by the silver
enhancement. Bar: 500 nm. **(C)** After the silver enhancement, a second antigen in the
same section can be labeled by an Ab (dark hatched) raised in the same species as was
the Ab (white) against first antigen. The gold labeled antispecies Ab is the same as used
in the first labeling step. EM picture: double-labeled poliovirus-infected cell. First label
was with anti-2C Ab, gold grains enlarged by the silver enhancement (arrows) as in (B).
Second label (small grains, arrowheads) was with MAb against the viral protein VP1
and the same gold marker GAM G10 as in (A). Bar: 500 nm.

tion. Thus, it leads to an autocatalytic increase in size of the gold label during
the developing process.

The EM-silver enhancement procedure may not only be used for IEM double
labeling, but also for double *in situ* hybridization (ISH), or a combination of
IEM and ISH *(6)*. In addition, the EM-silver enhancement *per se* is also useful
when IEM preparations are to be photographed at low magnifications. The
immunocytochemical labeling can be done with 5- or 10-nm gold grains, which
provide good labeling efficiency, and the size of the marker can afterward be
reproducibly adjusted at will. Ultrasmall (1-nm) gold grains, however, cannot
be reproducibly enlarged *(6)*.

2. Materials

1. IEM specimens: use sections of material, fixed and embedded (e.g., in Lowicryl K4M, LR White or LR Gold) in order to retain antigenicity (*see* Note 1) It is essential to use gold grids, since the chemicals involved in the procedures react with copper or nickel. The use of negatively stained, unfixed material (subcellular fractions, viruses, and so on) is not recommended, since the EM-silver enhancement affects the structure of such specimens.
2. Antibodies: the type of primary Ab is determined by the antigens to be detected. The secondary antispecies Ab should ideally be labeled with 5- or 10-nm gold, and good-quality Ab can be obtained commercially from several suppliers (*see* Note 2).
3. TBS-bovine serum albumin (BSA) buffer (washing buffer): 0.9% NaCl and 0.1% BSA in 20 mM Tris, adjusted with HCl to pH 8.2.
4. Blocking buffer: normal serum of the species in which the secondary Ab was raised, is used diluted to 5% in TBS-BSA to block nonspecific binding sites.
5. To dilute the primary Ab, blocking buffer is used that contains only 1% serum.
6. The developer for EM-silver enhancement ("Agfa-Gevaert-developer," ref. *2*) is freshly made up by dissolving 0.075 g of Metol (4[methylamino]-phenolsulfate, Fluka, Buchs, Switzerland), 0.05 g of sodium sulfite (anhydrous), and 0.02 g of potassium thiocyanate in 10 mL of distilled water. The final pH is 6.3.
7. Silver ions: Ilford L4 nuclear research emulsion, gel form.
8. Safelight illumination: Ilford filter S902.
9. Glutaraldehyde (2%) in phosphate-buffered saline is used to fix the sections. Sections are stained with a 4% aqueous solution of uranyl acetate.

3. Methods

3.1. Immunocytochemical Labeling of First Antigen

All steps are performed at room temperature.

1. Float the grids with the sectioned cells for 10 min on distilled water.
2. Then block nonspecific binding sites by floating for 20 min on blocking buffer.
3. Follow this by incubation on the primary Ab (e.g., hybridoma culture supernatant, diluted appropriately in blocking buffer containing 1% serum) for 1 h.
4. Wash the grids by floating them on TBS-BSA in a watch glass on a gyrotary shaker for 2 × 5 min.
5. Then incubate them for 1 h on the gold-labeled secondary Ab, diluted in TBS-BSA according to the manufacturer's instructions.
6. Rinse again twice on TBS-BSA as above, and "jet-wash" with distilled water.

3.2. EM-Silver Enhancement

Perform all steps in the darkroom with safelight illumination turned on:

1. To prepare the developing solution (physical developer), weigh 100 mg of L4 emulsion (silver donor) into a watch glass, and add 2.5 mL of the freshly pre-

pared "Agfa-Gevaert" developer. Alternatively, put an estimated amount of L4 emulsion into a light tight container in the darkroom, and weigh outside the darkroom before adding the amount of developer required to obtain the proportion of 40 mg of emulsion/mL of developer.

2. Stir the freshly prepared physical developer with a small magnetic stirring bar for 5 min. Only part of the emulsion will dissolve; for reproducible results, keep the stirring time constant, and record the temperature of the developer (preferably 20–21°C).
3. Place the gold-labeled sections, moistened with distilled water on the surface of the developer, and stir continuously for 4–6 min.
4. To stop the action of the developer, wash the grids by quickly dipping them several times in distilled water. The final size of the silver-coated gold grain depends on the amount of emulsion used, the stirring time during which some of the emulsion is dissolved, the temperature of the developer, and the developing time (*see* Note 3).

3.3. Immunocytochemical Labeling of the Second Antigen

The grid is now ready for repeating the immunocytochemical labeling using a primary Ab directed against another antigen. The procedure is performed exactly as described in Section 3.1.

3.4. Staining of Sections

1. To avoid loss of gold-labeled Ab during staining with the acidic uranium acetate, fix the sections with glutaraldehyde for 15 min.
2. Then rinse them with distilled water, and stain with uranium acetate for 30 min at 37°C for Lowicryl and 15 min at room temperature for LR White and LR Gold. They may then be stained further with a conventional lead stain (*see* Note 4).

4. Notes

1. The IEM double-labeling method described was performed with cells fixed in 2% paraformaldehyde and 0.04% glutaraldehyde, and embedded in Lowicryl K4M, LR White, or LR Gold. Other fixation and embedding procedures should work equally well, provided that the specimen resists the chemicals used in the silver enhancement.

    Some embedding media, such as Lowicryl, evaporate to a certain extent under the electron beam. Thus, when the section is monitored after the first labeling step, extensive irradiation should be avoided. Otherwise, evaporated methacrylate might become deposited in the vicinity of the irradiated area. In such regions of the section, the gold grains are no longer accessible to the photographic developer.

    If the sections have been dried during the procedure, e.g., for viewing in the EM, they must be rehydrated with water before proceeding to the next step to avoid increased background.

2. When labeling the first and second antigen, the same gold-coupled, secondary Ab can be employed. Owing to enlargement of the first label, first and second labels can easily be distinguished. It is, however, necessary that the colloidal

gold used to label the secondary Ab, be very uniform in diameter, so that after enhancement no overlapping in size between the two labels occurs. Although we did not test it, the method should also work for gold-labeled protein A instead of an antispecies secondary Ab.

3. To allow a clear-cut distinction between the two labeled antigens after silver enhancement, the final size of the developed silver grains should be rather homogeneous and accurately predictable. The following parameters influence size, variation in size, and shape of the final grain:

   a. Developer: Metol, a slow-working fine-grain developer produces silver grains of uniform size and of round or slightly oval form. Hydrochinone, a coarse grain developer, which is used widely in light microscopic immunocytochemistry, leads in the EM to silver grains of irregular size and outlines. The same holds true for the IntenSE M-procedure (Amersham, Little Chalfont, Amersham, UK).

   b. Source of silver ions: Different silver ions were tested, but it was found that only pieces of Ilford L4 emulsion as silver ion donor, in combination with the Metol developer as described in Section 3.2. above, lead to compact silver grains of predeterminable, uniform size (coefficient of variation <10%). We do not know why the L4 emulsion is superior to all other silver donors tested, since its exact composition is not known to us.

   c. The useful concentration of emulsion is in the range of 20–50 mg of emulsion/mL of developer. It should be noted, however, that the number of emulsion pieces influences the developing speed, because the silver halide in the emulsion is only slowly soluble in the sodium sulfite incorporated in the developer, and the larger surfaces of several small emulsion pieces accelerate the dissolution of the silver halide. Similarly, the time of stirring the developer, before the section is put on, influences the concentration of silver ions and, thus, the developing speed.

   d. If the gold grains need only to be enlarged to be more easily visible in low-magnification work, silver bromide (10–20 mg/mL) can be substituted for L4 emulsion, or the commercial IntenSE M-procedure can be performed. As mentioned above, both methods yield very heterogeneously sized grains, so that they cannot be used for double labeling experiments.

   e. Developing time and temperature: the grain size increases linearly with the developing time, doubling its diameter at 20–21°C in approx 4 min *(1)*. For double labeling, it is convenient to obtain a two- to threefold increase in size of the gold grain. Smaller grains may be hard to distinguish from the unenlarged grains of the second labeling step, and larger grains obscure underlying details. Changes in temperature influence the developing speed considerably. Note in this respect that magnetic stirrers may give off heat.

4. For sufficient contrast, most specimens will require lead staining after the uranium acetate stain. Although all conventional lead stains can be used, we found staining with Millonig's lead hydroxide for 2 min under N_2 best for Lowicryl and LR Gold embedded material.

References

1. Bienz, K., Egger, D., and Pasamontes, L. (1986) Electron microscopic immuno-cytochemistry: silver enhancement of colloidal gold marker allows double labeling with the same primary antibody. *J. Histochem. Cytochem.* **34,** 1337–1342.
2. Kopriwa, B. M. (1975) A comparison of various procedures for fine grain development in electron microscopic radioautography. *Histochemistry* **44,** 201–224.
3. Bienz, K. (1977) Techniques and applications of autoradiography in the light and electron microscope. *Microsc. Acta* **79,** 1–22.
4. Holgate, C. S., Jackson, P., Cowen, P. N., and Bird, C. C. (1983) Immunogold-silver staining: new method of immunostaining with enhanced sensitivity. *J. Histochem. Cytochem.* **31,** 938–944.
5. Moeremans, M., Daneels, G., van Dijck, A., Langanger, G., and De Mey, J. (1984) Sensitive visualization of antigen-antibody reactions in dot and blot immune overlay assays with immunogold and immunogold/silver staining. *J. Immunol. Methods* **74,** 353–360.
6. Egger, D., Troxler, M., and Bienz, K. (1995) Light- and electron microscopic *in situ* hybridization: nonradioactive labeling and detection, double hybridization, and combined hybridization—immunocytochemistry. *J. Histochem. Cytochem.* **42,** 815–822.

33

Flow Cytometric Analysis
of Cell Surface Antigen Density

R. Adrian Robins

1. Introduction

Analysis of cell surface antigen density and, thus, the distribution of cell surface molecules among individual members of complex cell populations can be achieved rapidly and accurately by flow cytometry. This approach has been revolutionized over the last 20 yr by the codevelopment of monoclonal antibodies (MAb) to an ever-wider selection of cell-associated molecules, novel fluorochromes, and flow cytometric technology backed by increasingly powerful computers. This combination of technologies allows the simultaneous measurement of independent fluorochrome markers as well as light scatter parameters of individual cells as they pass through an intense focused light source. The multiple analysis of individual cells enabled by flow cytometry has facilitated the definition of functional subpopulations of many cell types, and some aspects of this approach are discussed in Chapter 34. In this article, the potential of flow cytometric analysis for quantitative purposes is considered, exemplified by discussion of factors important for the measurement of antigen density by quantitation of antibody binding.

1.1. Theoretical Considerations

Antibodies interact noncovalently with their target epitope, and the "strength" of this interaction is characterized by the kinetics of association and dissociation of the antibody. Antibody–antigen interactions are in principle reversible, and appropriate conditions must therefore be selected for a given antibody to bind with reproducible stoichiometry to its target antigen. Linkage of the antibody to an appropriate fluorochrome will mean that the number of antibody molecules bound will be reflected by the fluorescence intensity/cell.

From: *Methods in Molecular Biology, Vol. 80: Immunochemical Protocols, 2nd ed.*
Edited by: J. D. Pound © Humana Press Inc., Totowa, NJ

Appropriate application of flow cytometric methods allows cellular fluorescence to be measured and calibrated accurately. In this way, flow cytometric analysis of target antigen density can be undertaken.

1.1.1. Antibody Association and Dissociation

The amount of antibody initially bound to antigen will be determined by the association rate and incubation time, and of course by the level of antigen expression. The association rate is influenced by the association rate constant, antibody concentration, and temperature. Other factors, such as salt concentration and pH, are also important, but these are usually controlled within physiological limits. Further processes before analysis (washing, fixation, storage) may result in loss of some of the antibody initially bound; the amount lost will depend on the dissociation rate and valency, and will also be influenced by temperature.

1.1.2. Stoichiometry of Antigen–Antibody Interactions

Determination of antigen density from the numbers of antibody molecules bound clearly requires knowledge of the stoichiometry of the antibody–antigen interaction. The first requirement is for the antibody to be in excess, so that antigen sites are saturated. However, at "saturation" the stoichiometry between antigen and antibody may be controlled by characteristics of the antibody (e.g., valency) and the antigen (e.g., valency, density, and mobility). For example, a low-density immobile antigen may only be available for monovalent binding, because epitopes are too widely separated to be bridged by a divalent antibody. This will result in a 1:1 stoichiometry between antigen and antibody. Similarly, procedures that change mobility of antigens, such as prefixing to stabilize antigen expression *(1)*, may affect valency of binding by preventing antigen movement in the cell membrane that might be necessary for divalent binding. Conversely, higher-density antigens may give rise to predominantly divalent binding, with a stoichiometry of 2:1 for antigen:divalent IgG antibody. The stoichiometric ratio may effectively be higher in cases with closely spaced antigen, where steric obstruction of antigen by antibody bound to adjacent sites can occur. Counting the number of antibodies bound as a measure of antigen would in these circumstances lead to a marked underestimation of antigen expression.

It should also be noted that the valency of binding at equilibrium may also be influenced by antibody concentration *(2)*. Thus, high divalent antibody concentrations drive binding to a predominantly monovalent state, whereas at lower concentrations, the binding may be predominantly divalent; this obviously varies the antigen–antibody stoichiometry from near 2:1 to approaching 1:1. The best compromise when this effect is in operation may be to use an antibody concentration on the initial plateau of a saturation curve. Increases in binding above this plateau probably reflect valency change, and the predominantly monovalent binding observed at high antibody concentrations is more difficult to measure because of the increased dissociation rate with this form of binding *(2)*. For critical determination of antigen density, however, the mode of binding may need to be determined.

Unless all these factors are taken into account, it is usually more appropriate to refer to the results of a flow cytometric analysis in terms of "antibodies bound per cell" rather than "antigens per cell." Stoichiometry will be even less certain with multivalent IgM antibodies; the usually low monovalent affinity and strong role of avidity in the binding of IgM antibodies make them of limited value for antigen quantitation. Theoretically, the most precise alternative would be the use of directly labeled monovalent antibody fragments, which would avoid problems of variable stoichiometry. However, in addition to the inconvenience of producing suitable labeled monovalent antibody fragments, the increased "off rate" of monovalently bound antibody may make analysis more difficult.

1.1.3. Fluorochrome Selection

Choice of fluorochrome for antigen quantitation is influenced by sensitivity of detection required, availability of reagents, accuracy of calibration desired, and strategy for cell identification envisaged.

1.1.3.1. SENSITIVITY

The quantum efficiency of a given fluorochrome ultimately determines the sensitivity attainable. Thus protein fluorochromes derived from marine algae, such as phycoerythrin, have very high quantum efficiency in comparison to small chemical fluorochromes, such as fluorescein. For analysis of low antigen densities, phycoerythrin is to be preferred.

1.1.3.2. AVAILABILITY

If the antibody you intend to use is not available as a directly labeled conjugate, then the choice is between indirect fluorescence or synthesis of conjugate. The small chemical fluorochromes are advantageous here, because coupling methods are simple and reproducible *(2)* (*see* Section 2.2.2.).

1.1.3.3. CALIBRATION

Small chemical fluorochromes, such as fluorescein, have an advantage in this case because of the stability and predictability of their conjugates. Although methods for calibration of phycoerythrin-labeled antibodies are now available, a wider range of options is available for fluorescein (*see* Section 3.3.5.).

1.1.3.4. Cell Identification

The analysis of a complex population of cells may call for the identification of the cells of interest with one MAb, and quantitation of antigen expression on these cells with a second antibody. The choice of fluorochrome for each purpose may be influenced by relative levels of expression of the markers involved, as well as the factors referred to above. There is a degree of spectral overlap between fluorochromes, and this may make sensitive quantitation of a low level antigen difficult in the presence of high level labeling of the first antibody used for cell identification. This can be mitigated to some extent by selection of the more sensitive fluorochrome (e.g., phycoerythrin) for the low level quantitation. In any event, quantitative analysis requires careful adjustment of spectral overlap; an adjustment procedure for multiple fluorochromes appears in Chapter 34, and quantitative adjustment of compensation is illustrated in Section 3.4.

1.1.4. Flow Cytometry

1.1.4.1. Amplification of Fluorescence

The signal derived from the fluorescence of each individual cell is amplified before being transformed to a numerical scale by analog to digital conversion. This conversion essentially divides the whole range of possible signals into a series of categories (channels), each of which corresponds to a (more or less) narrow range of signal intensities. In this way, the intensity of fluorescence of each cell can be reduced to a number, and since computers work with binary numbers, this number will be 8 digits (bits) long to give a decimal channel number between 0 and 255. Some instruments use a number 10 bits long to give a scale between 0 and 1023. This seemingly obscure information is important because it emphasizes that when the fluorescence signal is converted to a number, precision is lost. The amplification method used (logarithmic or linear) affects the way in which this loss of precision occurs. The properties and advantages of logarithmic and linear scales therefore need to be considered to make an appropriate choice for the application intended. Logarithmic scales accommodate a wide dynamic range, but the scale is compressed as signal intensity increases. Linear scales are not compressed in this way, and are therefore good for comparing high levels of antibody binding, but have a narrower range of measurement. This is illustrated in Fig. 1, in which the logarithmic and linear amplified analyzes are superimposed for a set of 5 fluorescent beads of differing intensity. The logarithmic amplified peaks (open) are marked with upper-case letters, and the corresponding linear amplified peaks (filled) are marked with the same letters in lower-case. The top two peaks (D and E) are separated by only 19 channels on a logarithmic scale, but the corresponding linear peaks (d and e) are separated by over half the scale.

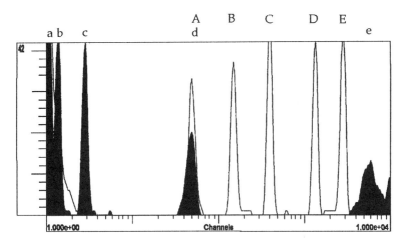

Fig. 1. Analysis of fluospheres (Dako Ltd.) using logarithmic (open peaks) and linear (filled peaks) amplification. Logarithmically amplified peaks are identified by upper-case letters, and the corresponding bead peak amplified on a linear scale by lower-case letters. The linear scale discriminates between bright signals (for example, d and e) better than the log scale (D and E), but the range of fluorescence covered by the log scale is much greater than the linear scale.

A second consideration with logarithmic amplifiers is that because of the complex way in which they operate *(3)*, quantitative data often require reconversion to a linear scale before further calculations can be done. This process requires information about the exact number of channels/decade, and any deviation from true logarithmic behavior *(4)*. Such deviations are sometimes found, particularly in the lowest decade.

1.1.4.2. STANDARDIZATION

Reproducible measurement over a period of time clearly requires that the flow cytometer is maintained to a high standard, and that the sensitivity of the instrument is checked on a daily basis. To ensure reproducibility, a stable standard for each scatter and fluorescence parameter must be established.

1.1.4.3. CALIBRATION

Refining the standardized measurement referred to above to provide a calibrated scale is a more difficult task, although calibration beads of various types now available facilitate the process. Beads with manufacturer's reported equivalent fluorescein content have been available for some time (Flow Cytometry Standards Corporation, San Juan, Puerto Rico), and these are useful for calibration of measurements using fluorescein-labeled antibodies, although knowledge of the fluorescein:protein ratio of the antibody conjugates used is required to calculate the number of antibody molecules bound. For commercial fluorescein conjugates, information concerning the fluorochrome:antibody ratio can usually be obtained from the supplier on request. Note that it is usually not possible to determine the ratio by optical density measurements (as in Section 2.2.2.), because carrier protein is often added to the labeled antibody for stability. External verification of calibrated standards may be required if batch variation occurs *(5),* but this is not a simple matter. In our own studies, an antibody double labeled with radioactive iodine and fluorescein has been used for this purpose *(2,6),* but this is a somewhat lengthy procedure.

A more versatile standard is a set of beads with calibrated numbers of anti-mouse immunoglobulin binding sites (e.g., Simply Cellular Beads, Flow Cytometry Standards Inc, available through Sigma, Poole, UK), referred to in Section 3.2. The mixture of beads provided can be taken through any standard staining protocol (direct or indirect) involving a mouse MAb "first layer." The mean fluorescence of each bead population in the mixture can then be used to construct a calibration curve, from which the mean number of "first layer" antibody molecules corresponding to any measured level of fluorescence can be extrapolated. As indicated above, this approach is particularly useful for calibration of indirect techniques, especially those involving phycoerythrin-labeled antibodies. For example, this methodology has been used to measure estrogen receptor expression on breast cancer cells *(7).*

The methods outlined below include protocols for direct and indirect immunofluorescence staining, that can be adapted easily for the cell type of interest as indicated in the relevant notes. The principal approaches to flow cytometric analysis, standardization and calibration are then given, followed by two more detailed protocols illustrating quantitation using direct immunofluorescence, and a competitive binding assay, which demonstrates the application of linear amplification of fluorescence.

2. Materials

2.1. Solutions

1. Dulbecco's phosphate-buffered saline (PBS), made by dissolving buffer tablets (Oxoid Ltd., Basingstoke, UK) in distilled water.
2. Nutrient culture medium, such as RPMI 1640.
3. Bovine serum albumin ([BSA], 10% stock solution in distilled water) may be added to wash media to give a final concentration of 0.1% (w/v).
4. Fetal bovine serum may be added to wash media to give a final concentration of 2% (w/v).
5. Stock solution of propidium iodide (PI) at 50 μg/mL: This is stable if stored refrigerated in the dark (*see* Note 1).

6. Sodium azide (10% stock solution in distilled water) may be added to media at a final concentration of 0.1% to reduce capping and internalization of surface-bound antibodies; it also inhibits microbial growth. Store at 4°C (*see* Note 1).
7. 2% Formaldehyde fixative solution, made by diluting 40% stock formaldehyde in PBS (*see* Note 1).
8. Carbonate buffer, pH 9.5, containing 150 mM sodium chloride, 30 mM sodium carbonate, and 50 mM sodium bicarbonate.

2.2. Antibodies
2.2.1. Commercial Antibodies

1. A very wide range of antibodies, unconjugated or conjugated to a variety of fluoro-chromes, is now available. These reagents are generally of high quality, and are usually supplied at a concentration suitable for labeling 10^6 cells with 10–20 µL of antibody.
2. Isotype-matched unconjugated or fluorochrome-labeled antibodies unreactive with mammalian cells are available as control reagents from many suppliers.
3. Fluorochrome-labeled anti-immunoglobulin antibody: labeled F(ab')$_2$ fragments should be selected for target cells that express Fc receptors.

2.2.2. Preparation of Labeled Antibodies

1. Dissolve fluorescein isothiocyanate (FITC) in acetone at 1 mg/mL, add 100 µL to a glass vial, and dry to leave a film of FITC.
2. Dialyze 1 mg of antibody at 1 mg/mL against carbonate buffer, pH 9.0.
3. Add antibody solution to a vial containing FITC, and roll gently for 1 h at room temperature in the dark.
4. Separate labeled antibody unconjugated FITC using a small column of Sephadex G25 equilibrated with PBS. Prepacked columns (PD10, Pharmacia, Milton Keynes, UK) may be used according to the manufacturer's instructions.
5. Determine the concentration and fluorescein:protein ratio of the labeled antibody by optical density measurements at 495 and 280 nm, respectively *(2)*.
6. Check the immunoreactivity of the labeled antibody by binding to target cells known to express the relevant antigen (*see* Note 2). An accurate assessment of the relative binding activity of the antibody before and after labeling can be made by competition experiments *(8)*, illustrated in Section 3.5.

2.3. Standards and Calibrators

1. Standard beads with broad-spectrum emission (e.g., FluoroSpheres, Dako Ltd., High Wycombe, UK).
2. Calibrator beads with known fluorescence intensity defined in terms of equivalent molecules of soluble fluorochrome (e.g., Quantum Beads, Flow Cytometry Standards Corporation).
3. Calibrator beads with known binding activity for mouse immunoglobulin (e.g., Simply Cellular Beads available through Sigma).

3. Methods

3.1. Direct Immunofluorescence

1. Dispense 100 μL of fluorochrome-labeled antibody solution (10 μg/mL) into tubes (*see* Note 3). Control fluorochrome-labeled antibody of the same isotype should be used in control tubes at the same concentration.
2. Add 100 μL of target cell suspension containing 10^6 cells/mL; mix carefully.
3. Incubate for 45 min at 4°C (*see* Note 4).
4. Add 1 mL of wash medium (*see* Note 5); centrifuge at 400*g* for 5 min; remove supernatant; resuspend cells by gently tapping tube.
5. Repeat wash procedure in step 4 twice more (*see* Note 6).
6. Resuspend cells in wash medium for immediate flow cytometric analysis or in formaldehyde fixative for storage before analysis (*see* Note 7). Keep tubes at 4°C and in the dark.

3.2. Indirect Immunofluorescence (see Note 8)

1. Dispense 100 μL of unlabeled primary antibody solution (10 μg/mL) into tubes (*see* Note 9). Unlabeled control antibody of the same isotype as the primary antibody should be used in control tubes at the same concentration.
2. Add 100 μL of target cell suspension containing 10^6 cells/mL; mix carefully.
3. Incubate for 45 min at 4°C (*see* Note 4).
4. Add 1 mL of wash medium (*see* Note 5); centrifuge at 400*g* for 5 min; remove supernatant; resuspend cells by gently tapping tube.
5. Repeat wash procedure in step 4 twice more (*see* Note 10).
6. Add 100 μL of fluorochrome-labeled anti-immunoglobulin reagent, diluted in wash medium (*see* Note 11).
7. Incubate for 45 min at 4°C
8. Wash cells as in steps 4 and 5.
9. Resuspend cells in wash medium for immediate flow cytometric analysis, or in form-aldehyde fixative for storage before analysis. Keep tubes at 4°C and in the dark.

3.3. Flow Cytometric Analysis

Having considered conditions for the binding of fluorochrome-labeled antibody to reflect antigen density, the most appropriate flow cytometric analysis method can then be selected. Some of these considerations will be specific to particular manufacturers' flow cytometers and cannot be addressed in detail here; there are, however, common approaches, that are generally applicable, and appreciation of the principles involved will at least allow some of the more obvious pitfalls to be avoided.

3.3.1. Scatter Gating

1. Pass a sample of cells through the flow cytometer, displaying on a "dot plot" measurement of light scattered from cells at a narrow angle (forward scatter

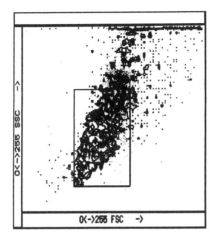

Fig. 2. Scatter gating of colorectal cancer cells from cell culture. The FSC and SSC gates are set to eliminate a small amount of debris on the left of the gate, and cell clumps above and to the right of the gate. Many of the clumps accumulate at the top of the SSC scale.

    [FSC]), strongly related to cell size) against light scattered at a wide angle (side scatter [SSC], which is influenced by cell structure and granularity).
2. Adjusting the gain on each of the scatter channels to ensure that single cells of interest are on scale.
3. Define a "gate" on the FSC vs SSC dot plot to identify single cells (Fig. 2), eliminating both cell clumps and debris from the analysis (*see* Note 12).

3.3.2. Viable Cell Gating

1. Add 5 μL of PI stock solution to each tube after immunofluorescence staining.
2. Pass a sample of cells through the flow cytometer, recording red fluorescence in addition to FSC and SSC.
3. Construct a gate to exclude cells with high red fluorescence from the analysis (*see* Note 13).

3.3.3. Amplification of Fluorescence Signal

3.3.3.1. LOGARITHMIC AMPLIFICATION

1. Analyze antigen-negative control cells using the scatter gates set above, displaying the logarithmic fluorescence measurement as a dot plot against FSC.
2. Adjust the photomultiplier tube (PMT) voltage to ensure that the cells of interest are in the lowest quarter of the scale.
3. Analyze a sample of the most strongly stained cells in the experiment.
4. Ensure that the signals from these cells is on scale; reduce the PMT voltage if necessary.
5. Analyze all the experimental tubes with these settings.

3.3.3.2. LINEAR AMPLIFICATION

1. Analyze antigen-negative control cells using appropriate scatter gates, displaying the linear fluorescence signal against FSC.
2. Adjust the linear "multiplier" gain to maximum (e.g., 9.99 on FacScan, Becton Dickinson, Cowley, UK).
3. Adjust PMT voltage to ensure that cells of interest are on scale. They should form a tight group at the bottom of the scale.
4. Analyze a sample of the most strongly stained cells in the experiment.
5. Reduce the "multiplier" gain to ensure that the cells are on scale. If the lowest gain available leaves more than 5% of the cells in the highest channel, reduce the PMT voltage accordingly.
6. Analyze all the experimental tubes without further adjustment of the PMT voltage setting. For each tube, adjust the "multiplier" gain to the highest setting that keeps at least 95% of the cells on scale.
7. By taking account of the "multiplier" gain used, normalize measurements to a constant gain, to provide an extended linear scale *(5)*; *see also* Section 3.5.

3.3.4. Standardization

1. Ensure flow cytometer is set up for intended analysis (appropriate scatter and fluorescence amplifier settings).
2. Run sample of broad-spectrum microbeads.
3. Set FSC and SSC gates to confine the analysis to single beads.
4. Adjust the photomultiplier high-voltage setting to ensure that the bead signal(s) appears in standardized channels. Figure 1 illustrates the distribution of FluoSpheres (Dako) in the green fluorescence channel (FL1, FacScan, Becton Dickinson).

3.3.5. Calibration

1. Subject an aliquot of "Simply Cellular" beads to the staining procedure to be standardized.
2. Run the stained bead preparation on the flow cytometer in parallel with the cell samples stained in the same experiment (*see* Note 14).
3. Set FSC and SSC gates for the bead sample to confine the analysis to single beads.
4. Plot a histogram of the fluorescence distribution of the gated beads.
5. Determine the mean peak position for each of the bead populations in the mixture, by setting a narrow window around each peak in turn.
6. Plot the peak positions against the manufacturer's specified antibody binding capacity for each bead in the mixture to create a standard curve. Figure 3 illustrates curves for Simply Cellular beads stained with a PE-labeled antibody in a direct assay (A), and in an indirect assay with a PE-labeled antimouse IgG (B). The increased sensitivity of the indirect assay is evident from the rightward shift of the curve.
7. Interpolate fluorescence intensity of experimental samples from the standard curve.

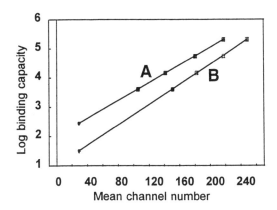

Fig. 3. Calibration of phycoerythrin (PE) staining using Simply Cellular Beads. Bead antibody binding capacity was plotted against the corresponding bead's channel position, after (A) direct staining with PE-antireceptor mouse MAb, and (B) after staining with mouse MAb and PE-antimouse IgG. The higher sensitivity of the indirect method is reflected in the rightward shift of the calibration curve.

3.4. Quantitation Using Direct Immunofluorescence

This method illustrates quantitation of a receptor using a PE-labeled antibody in a mixed cell population, using a FITC-labeled antibody to identify the cell population. As indicated in Section 1.1.3.4., one of the critical issues here is adjustment of compensation for fluorescence overlap between the FITC marker antibody and the PE measuring antibody.

3.4.1. Adjustment of Fluorescence Compensation

1. Prepare cell suspension from epithelial tissue by collagenase digestion; resuspend cells in RPMI + 2% fetal calf serum at 10^6 cells/mL. Use this medium throughout.
2. Prepare duplicate tubes with (a) control PE-labeled antibody + antiepithelial cell antibody (BerEP4-FITC, Dako Ltd.) and (b) control PE-labeled antibody alone.
3. Add 100 µL of cell suspension to each tube.
4. Incubate at 4°C for 30 min
5. Add 1 mL of ice-cold medium, mix, and centrifuge at 200*g* for 5 min; decant supernatant and resuspend cells.
6. Repeat wash step 5 twice.
7. Add 1 mL of formaldehyde fixative.
8. Run tubes through the flow cytometer, recording FSC, SSC, fluorescence 1 (FITC and fluorescence 2 [PE]). Fluorescence channels should be set to log amplification; in this experiment, the flow cytometer was set to conditions routinely used for analysis of lymphocytes.

Table 1
Effect of Changing Fluorescence Compensation

| Compensation | Mean channel number | | | |
| | Control FL1 antibody | | BerEP-4 FITC antibody | |
FL1 → FL2	FL1	FL2	FL1	FL2
25.2	124	124	176	103
22.5	125	125	177	118
21.5	124	125	174	122
20.0	125	126	176	126
17.5	124	126	177	133

9. Compare fluorescence 2 mean channel value in tubes a and b. If the value in a is >b, FITC fluorescence in a is not compensated fully, and the FL1 → FL2 compensation should be increased. Conversely, a lower value in b indicates overcompensation, and the compensation should be reduced. Table 1 illustrates the effect of different compensation settings; the standard lymphocyte setting (25.2) overcompensated when analyzing epithelial cells.
10. Repeat steps 8 and 9 until values for FL2 mean fluorescence are the same in a and b; a value of 20.0 was selected for this experiment (Table 1).

3.4.2. Estimation of Antibody Molecules Bound

1. Stain epithelial cell containing suspension as described in Section 3.4.1., including tubes containing PE-antireceptor antibody in combination with FITC-BerEP4. Also stain Simply Cellular Beads with PE-antireceptor antibody in parallel.
2. Run the tubes through the flow cytometer with optimized fluorescence compensation as described above.
3. Set gates to restrict the analysis to FITC positive (epithelial) cells.
4. Determine mean fluorescence channel number in PE channel.
5. Analyze the tube containing Simply Cellular Beads, setting FSC and SSC gates to restrict the analysis to single beads.
6. Determine mean fluorescence of each bead population, and plot a standard curve as described in Section 3.3.5.

The resulting determination of the numbers of antireceptor antibody molecules bound/epithelial cell are shown in Table 2. The value for the control antibody represents the autofluorescence of the target cells in terms of the equivalent number of fluorescent-labeled antibody molecules, rather than binding of the control antibody. Thus, a similar value was obtained for target cells with and without control antibody (not shown).

Table 2
Determination of Numbers
of Antireceptor Antibody Molecules Bound to Epithelial Cells

	Mean fluorescence 2	Mean antibodies/cell
Control PE antibody	48	538
Antireceptor PE antibody	111	4939

Table 3
Competition Between Fluorescein-Conjugated Antibody
and Unlabeled Antibody Analyzed by Flow Cytometry

Antibody added, µg/tube			Mean channel, duplicate tubes	Mean channel, adjusted for gain	% Maximum fluorescence
FITC-791T/36	Unlabeled 791T/36	Gain			
0	0	10	2, 2	2	0
1	0	2.5	112, 110	444	100
1	0.5	2.5	70, 70	280	63.3
1	1	5	110, 114	224	50.6
1	2	5	83, 81	164	37.1
1	4	10	114, 110	112	25.3

3.5. Competitive Binding Between a Fluorescein-Labeled Antibody and Unlabeled Antibody (see Section 2.2.2.)

This method illustrates well the precision with which antibody binding can be measured by flow cytometry, and the use of linear amplification of the fluorescence signal.

1. Harvest tumor cells (791T) from culture, and suspend at 10^6 cells/mL in RPMI+2% fetal calf serum, used as a diluent throughout.
2. Dilute fluorescein-labeled antibody (791T/36), which binds to 791T cells, to 10 µg/mL.
3. Dilute unlabeled 791T/36 antibody to 40, 20, 10, and 5 µg/mL
4. Prepare mixtures of 100 µL of labeled and unlabeled antibodies in duplicate, together with controls with labeled antibody + diluent and diluent alone.
5. Add 100 µL of target cell suspension to each tube, mix, and incubate for 1 h at 4°C.
6. Analyze cells using a flow cytometer, using forward and side scatter gating to restrict the analysis to single cells. In this example, the fluorescence 1 detector was used at 600 V with linear amplification on a 256-channel scale to measure fluorescein-labeled antibody binding. The resulting mean channel numbers and the gain setting used to extend the linear scale (*see* Section 3.3.3.2.) are shown in Table 3,

together with the values calculated from them. Note that under these experimental conditions, washing of the cells was not required.

The concentration of labeled antibody used is saturating, so that in mixtures of labeled and unlabeled antibody, there is competition for available antigenic sites. The reduction in fluorescence/cell observed (for example, about 50% maximum fluorescence with 1 µg of labeled and 1 µg of unlabeled antibody) is that expected if the labeled and unlabeled antibody molecules are binding equally well to antigen.

4. Notes

1. Propidium iodide and ethidium monoazide are suspected mutagens and should be handled accordingly. Sodium azide and fixatives are toxic, and should be handled with particular care.
2. Loss of binding activity after labeling can sometimes be avoided by modification of the coupling conditions, but the binding activity of some antibodies is very sensitive to standard labeling reagents, presumably because an easily substituted amino group is present in the binding site of the antibody. If this is the case, alternative labeling strategies might be considered, such as labeling carbohydrate moieties of the antibody *(9)*.
3. The association rate constant is characteristic of individual antibody–antigen interactions, but with typical association rate constants, antibody concentrations of 10–100 nM (about 1–10 µg/mL) are usually sufficient to drive binding to an adequate level of saturation in 30 min at 4°C. Unless high cell concentrations (>10^6 cells/mL) or high levels of antigen expression (>10^6 antigens/cell) are involved, antibody will be in excess under these conditions.
4. Incubation time together with antibody concentration should be chosen to achieve saturation binding, and incubation times may need to be long (possibly several hours) to allow equilibrium to be reached. If the nature of the system precludes extended incubation times (for example, antigen expression is not stable), antibody concentrations should be titrated carefully, and a sufficiently high concentration chosen to ensure that it is not the "on rate" of the antibody, rather than the level of antigen, which is limiting the amount of antibody bound.
5. When conditions are being established for analysis of a cell type not previously tested, it is useful to analyze the scatter characteristics (Section 3.3.1.) of freshly prepared cells, which have not been subjected to antibody labeling, washing, or fixation. This analysis can then be used as the benchmark to ensure that the cells are not being damaged (for example, undergoing apoptosis) during the staining procedure. Appropriate medium and supplements (Section 2.1.), and other experimental conditions, such as length and temperature of incubations, can then be selected to ensure that the cells are recovered in their original condition and high yield at the end of the labeling procedure.
6. Unbound fluorochrome-labeled antibody may need to be removed to allow the analysis of cell-bound labeled antibody. However, it should be noted that with

some systems, it is possible to analyze cells without washing, as described in the seminal paper of Sklar and Finney, which provides a basis for many aspects of quantitative analysis of ligand binding by flow cytometry *(10)*. The unbound antibody in the supernatant may be sufficiently separated from the bound antibody on the cells as the cells are drawn down into a fine stream for flow cytometric analysis. Parallel analysis of antigen-negative cells incubated with fluorochrome-labeled antibody will allow the signal derived from supernatant antibody to be estimated. If this is sufficiently low, the washing step can be dispensed with, avoiding the possibility of antibody dissociation.

If washing is essential, the extent of change in bound antibody between the binding stage and the analysis stage of the experiment depends on the dissociation kinetics, valency of binding and temperature, as well as the washing procedure used. To minimize dissociation, temperature should be kept as low as possible (holding cells on ice, using ice cooled wash medium, and refrigerated centrifuge), and cells analyzed as soon as practicable after washing. If dissociation of a fluorochrome-labeled antibody is a significant problem (for example, the antibody used is of low affinity or predominantly monovalently bound), one strategy is to stabilize binding immediately after washing by incubation with unlabeled antiimmunoglobulin antibody.

The dissociation rate constant of an antibody–antigen interaction is characteristic of individual antibodies, but as discussed above, the rate at which antibody "falls off" the cell also depends on the valency of binding. Monovalent dissociation rates are faster than divalent dissociation rates, and the reassociation of a divalent interaction (i.e., of an antibody already bound by one binding site) is favored in comparison with monovalent association from the fluid phase. This avidity effect means that divalently bound fluorochrome-labeled antibodies are shed more slowly when fluid-phase antibody is removed by washing.

7. Fixation of biological samples prior to analysis is good practice for safety reasons, and allows delayed flow cytometric analysis of samples, which is advantageous in a busy laboratory. Paraformaldehyde solutions used in the same way as formaldehyde are recommended for some cell types; the preparation of paraformaldehyde solutions from solid requires good fume hood facilities. Other fixatives are not used frequently in flow cytometry, other than for specialized purposes. For example, glutaraldehyde is the most effective fixative for neutrophils for analysis of shape change by flow cytometry *(11)*. However, use of glutaraldehyde precludes concurrent analysis with fluorochrome markers because of nonspecific broad-band fluorescence induced by this fixative.

8. Indirect fluorescence is usually taken to mean use of an unlabeled primary antibody quantitated by binding of a fluorochrome-labeled antiglobulin reagent, although related methods, for example using biotin-labeled primary antibody quantitated by binding of fluorochrome-labeled avidin, can also be used to estimate antigen expression. Both approaches require that reproducible binding and washing of the primary antibody is obtained, and that conditions to give constant stoichiometry between the primary antibody and fluorochrome-labeled reagent

are established. Use of multiple steps may mean that reproducibility may not be as good as with direct methods *(12)*. Because the stoichiometry between the primary antibody and fluorochrome-labeled reagent will depend on the precise reagents and conditions in use, estimates of absolute numbers of primary antibodies bound based on assumptions about primary antibody per secondary antibody stoichiometry will be approximate. However, this difficulty can be overcome by use of commercially available beads with known numbers of antimouse immunoglobulin binding sites per bead *(see* Section 3.3.5.). This allows the relationship to be determined between the number of primary antibodies bound and the resulting fluorescence signal. This methodology is applicable to both standard indirect immunofluorescence and to biotin-labeled primary antibodies; it is also suitable for any fluorochrome.

9. Factors important for directly labeled antibody binding apply equally well to the "first layer" antibody in an indirect technique; the antibody should be titrated to ensure a reproducible level of saturation under the incubation conditions selected.

10. The appropriate washing conditions should be selected to preserve the binding of the primary antibody as fully as possible. Some degree of washing is usually required to prevent unbound primary antibody blocking the fluorochrome-labeled antibody in solution, reducing the efficiency of binding to the cell-surface-associated primary antibody. If target cells are not stable in repeated washing (for example, platelets), compromise conditions in which the minimum amount of primary antibody is used can be employed, followed by an excess of the secondary antibody *(13)*.

11. Considerations of association kinetics and choice of saturating concentrations also apply to the fluorochrome-labeled second antibody. In this case, however, loss of bound antibody during washing is not usually a problem, because the high affinity of these reagents and increased avidity resulting from crosslinking make the cell binding of the second antibody virtually irreversible.

12. Changes in scatter signals can indicate damage to target cells, which may require modification of the conditions used to prepare the cells for analysis. For example, apoptosis of some cell types is accompanied by an increase in side scatter and a decrease in forward scatter. Any changes in light scatter characteristics of target cells should be viewed with suspicion, and their causes identified.

13. It is important to exclude nonviable cells from the analysis as dead cells may have changed antigenic characteristics, and may also take up fluorochrome-labeled antibodies nonspecifically. Light scatter may be used to identify damaged cells as discussed above, but with some cell types, nonviable cells are not easily distinguishable by their scatter characteristics, and use of a viability stain may be valuable. PI is frequently used for this purpose, since it is excluded from live cells, but penetrates dead cells where it intercalates with DNA and fluoresces red. PI fluorescence is usually detected above 600 nm, but significant spillover of fluorescence occurs in the 550–600 nm region used to detect phycoerythrin fluorescence, but since nonviable cells are usually excluded from the analysis, this does not necessarily preclude simultaneous use of a phycoerythrin marker. A

practical limitation is that PI-stained preparations are not stable to fixation and must be analyzed fresh. An alternative is a photoactivatable marker (ethidium monoazide), which has similar staining characteristics to PI, but the marker can be crosslinked to DNA in nonviable cells by light exposure, and the excess dye washed away before fixing and storage of the cells *(14)*.

14. A similar method is used for beads with defined fluorochrome content (e.g., Quantum beads, Flow Cytometry Standards Corporation), except that the beads are not subjected to the antibody-staining procedure. The number of fluorochrome molecules per cell is deduced from the standard curve, and is converted to bound antibody molecules from knowledge of the fluorochrome:protein ratio of the conjugate.

Acknowledgments

I would like to acknowledge the contribution of many collaborators in the Cancer Research Laboratories and Departments of Immunology, Clinical Oncology, Obstetrics and Gynecology, Surgery, and Therapeutics at Nottingham University. This work was supported by the Cancer Research Campaign (UK).

References

1. Macey, M. G. and McCarthy, D. A. (1993) Quantitation of adhesion molecules and other function associated antigens on peripheral blood leucocytes. *Cytometry* **14,** 898–908.
2. Roe, R., Robins, R. A., Laxton, R. R., and Baldwin, R. W. (1985) Kinetics of divalent monoclonal antibody binding to tumor cell surface antigens using flow cytometry—standardization and mathematical analysis. *Mol. Immunol.* **22,** 11–21.
3. Gandler, W. and Shapiro, H. (1990) Logarithmic amplifiers. *Cytometry* **11,** 447–450.
4. Schmid, I., Schmid, P., and Giorgi, J. V. (1988) Conversion of logarithmic channel numbers into relative linear fluorescence intensity. *Cytometry* **9,** 533–538.
5. Pallis, M. and Robins, R. A. (1995) What you need to know when you go with the flow: pitfalls in the use of flow cytometry. *Ann. Rheumat. Dis.* **54,** 785,786.
6. Pallis, M., Robins, R. A., and Powell, R. J. (1996) Peripheral blood adhesion molecule deployment in the immune response. *Scand. J. Immunol.* **43,** 304–313.
7. Brotherick, I., Lennard, T. W. J., Cook, S., Johnstone, R., Angus, B., Winthereik, M. P., and Shenton, B. K. (1995) Use of the biotinylated antibody Dako-Er 1d5 to measure estrogen-receptor on cytokeratin positive cells obtained from primary breast cancer cells. *Cytometry* **20,** 74–80.
8. Robins, R. A., Laxton, R. R., Garnett, M., Price, M. R., and Baldwin, R. W. (1986) Quantitation of antitumor antibody and antibody conjugate binding activity by competition with fluorochrome-labelled antibody. *J. Immunol. Methods* **90,** 165–172.
9. Duijndam, W. A. L., Wiegant, J., Vanduijn, P., and Haaijman, J. J. (1988) A simple method for labelling the carbohydrate moieties of antibodies with fluorochromes. *J. Immunol. Methods* **109,** 289,290.
10. Sklar, L. A. and Finney, D. A. (1982) Analysis of ligand–receptor interactions with the fluorescence activated cell sorter. *Cytometry* **3,** 161–165.

11. Cole, A. T., Garlick, N. M., Galvin, A. M., Hawkey, C. J., and Robins, R. A. (1995) A flow cytometric method to measure shape change of human neutrophils. *Clin. Sci.* **89,** 549–554.

12. Traill, K. N., Bock, G., Winter, U., Hilchenbach, M., Jurgens, G., and Wick, G. (1986) Simple method for comparing large numbers of flow-cytometry histograms exemplified by analysis of the CD4 (T4) antigen and LDL receptor on human peripheral-blood lymphocytes. *J. Histochem. Cytochem.* **34,** 1217–1221.

13. Johnston, G. I., Heptinstall, S., Robins, R. A., and Price, M. R. (1984) The expression of glycoproteins on single blood-platelets from healthy individuals and from patients with congenital bleeding disorders. *Biochem. Biophys. Res. Comm.* **123,** 1091–1098.

14. Reidy, M. C., Muirhead, K. A., Jensen, C. P., and Stewart, C. C. (1991) Use of a photolabelling technique to identify nonviable cells in fixed homologous or heterologous cell populations. *Cytometry* **12,** 133–139.

34

Multiple Immunofluorescence Analysis of Cells Using Flow Cytometry

R. Adrian Robins

1. Introduction

As indicated in Chapter 33, flow cytometry has developed rapidly to provide a powerful means of characterizing complex cell populations, both in terms of quantitative analysis of functional cell-associated molecules, and, as is considered here in more detail, the simultaneous analysis of combinations of markers that can be used to identify functional subpopulations of cells. Many of the considerations discussed in the previous chapter are relevant, but issues particularly pertinent to this type of analysis relate to the independence of the markers used, both at the level of the labeling process and at the level of cytometric analysis.

1.1. Fluorochrome Selection

The scope for multiparameter immunofluorescence analysis has been increased greatly in recent years by the development of fluorochromes that can be excited by a single wavelength of light, but which have sufficiently distinct fluorescence emission spectra to allow each to be measured in the presence or absence of the other(s). Fluorescein isothiocyanate (FITC) remains a standard fluorochrome, excited effectively by the 488 nm (the strongest wavelength emitted by argon-ion lasers), with a green fluorescence emission centered on 515 nm. The first of a new generation of fluorochromes was phycoerythrin (PE), a member of the phycobilins, a family of fluorescent proteins derived from marine algae. These fluorochromes have very high quantum efficiency (they emit almost as much light as they absorb), which means that they can be detected with high sensitivity. PE has almost ideal characteristics for single laser flow cytometry with effective excitation by the 488 nm line of the argon laser, and a narrow band

From: *Methods in Molecular Biology, Vol. 80: Immunochemical Protocols, 2nd ed.*
Edited by: J. D. Pound © Humana Press Inc., Totowa, NJ

of emission centered on 575 nm. The combination of FITC and PE has allowed two-color flow cytometric analysis to become routine in many laboratories.

The addition of a third color is desirable for many investigations, but this could previously only be achieved using a second wavelength for excitation. This entailed expensive flow cytometers equipped with a second laser, and complex setup and alignment procedures, restricting this approach to a few specialized laboratories. The first generation of new fluorochromes attempting to overcome this limitation were conjugates of PE and Texas red, in which the energy of the light absorbed by PE was transferred to Texas red instead of being emitted directly. Texas red emits fluorescence with a wavelength longer than 600 nm, allowing this fluorescence to be distinguished from that of PE. These conjugates have now been succeeded by newer materials, such as Peridinin-Chlorophyll Protein (PerCP, Becton Dickinson, Cowley, UK) or PE-Cy5 (Dako Ltd., High Wycombe, UK), which have superior stability and reduced overlap of fluorescence emission. The increasing availability of reagents labeled with these fluorochromes means that three-color analysis is now routinely achievable with a single laser flow cytometer.

The potential for multi-fluorochrome analysis has increased further with the availability of dyes excited by shorter wavelengths (such as Cascade blue) and longer wavelengths (such as Allophycocyanin and Texas red). With multiple laser flow cytometers, five cell-surface antigens *(1)* or more may be analyzed simultaneously. In principle, these methods are a natural extension of the methods outlined here, but require more sophisticated flow cytometers, and much more powerful computer facilities to explore the exponentially more complex data sets arising from such multiparameter analyses.

1.2. Staining Methods

1.2.1. Direct Labeling

Direct labeling methods are the simplest approach to multiple parameter fluorescence analysis. If suitable antibody conjugates are available for the combination of antigens of interest, a mixture of two or three antibodies can be incubated with the target cells. This approach is illustrated by a method for staining lymphocytes in whole blood (*see* Section 3.1). A suitable concentration of each antibody has to be determined to ensure that each is saturating its respective antigen. A comprehensive set of control combinations of antibodies should be investigated to ensure that unexpected interactions between the labeling of target antigens is not occurring. These should include substitution of each antibody in turn with an isotype/fluorochrome-matched control, and testing each antibody alone. The total percentage of cells stained by each antibody should be the same in each combination in which it is included.

1.2.2. Indirect Labeling

When one or more of the desired antibodies is not available as a direct conjugate and a conjugate cannot be synthesized, indirect methods have to be used. The simplest variation is to use a biotin-labeled antibody as a "first layer," and then after washing the cells, incubate with fluorochrome-labeled streptavidin, and additional directly labeled antibodies labeled with complementary fluorochromes. The additional streptavidin step does not usually cause difficulty.

Primary antibodies originating in different species may be coanalyzed using fluorochrome-labeled species-specific anti-immunoglobulin reagents. There is however considerable potential for crossreactivity in such systems, particularly if the anti-immunoglobulin reagents are themselves from different species. Controls to check for crossreactions should be carefully designed. For example, with rat and mouse primary monoclonal antibodies (MAbs) labeling human lymphocytes, antimouse Ig may crossreact with rat Ig, the antirat Ig antibody, or human Ig on the target lymphocytes; similar reactivities could occur with the antirat Ig reagent. Good-quality commercial reagents are now available, with some suppliers affinity-purifying and absorbing anti-immunoglobulin reagents to eliminate specified interspecies crossreactivities. Careful choice of reagents may therefore avoid the problem. If crossreactivity is observed, it may be possible to achieve specific staining by using normal serum of the appropriate species to block cross-species binding.

If an unlabeled mouse MAb is to be used in conjunction with a labeled mouse monoclonal, one possibility is to seek monoclonals of differing isotype with the desired specificity. In this way, an isotype-specific anti-immunoglobulin conjugate (for example, anti-IgG2a-PE) could be used to stain the unlabeled IgG2a MAb, and the mouse antibody of different isotype (e.g., IgG1-FITC) coincubated without crossreactivity. Careful controls should be performed to ensure the specificity of the anti-IgG2a-PE reagent for the appropriate mouse isotype and lack of reactivity with the species of origin of the target cells.

In some cases, the choice of antibodies is very limited, and only a combination of labeled and unlabeled antibodies of the same species and isotype is available. In this case, the indirect staining with unlabeled mouse antibody followed by fluorochrome-labeled antimouse IgG has to be completed, followed by free binding sites for mouse IgG on the labeled cells blocked by addition of unlabeled mouse immunoglobulin. Normal mouse serum will serve this purpose. The directly labeled mouse MAb can then be added, and the staining procedure completed. A protocol illustrating this approach is given in Section 3.2., in which a cell suspension containing lymphoid and nonlymphoid cells was stained with an antireceptor antibody and PE-conjugated antimouse IgG; lymphoid cells were then identified using FITC-labeled anti-CD45 antibody. Receptor expression on lymphoid and nonlymphoid cells could then be compared.

1.3. Multiparameter Flow Cytometry

Many of the considerations relating to measurement of expression of one fluorochrome (Chapter 33) also apply to multiparameter analysis. For example, forward angle scatter (FSC) and side scatter (SSC) are almost invariably used to restrict the analysis to a particular component of a mixture of cells. The emphasis in multiparameter analysis is usually on identifying discrete subpopulations of cells, each of which is characterized by a specific combination of surface markers. The level of expression of a marker may contribute to this phenotype, but absolute measurement of antigen expression is usually a secondary objective. These priorities dictate the almost exclusive use of logarithmic amplification of the fluorescence signals in multifluorescence analysis, because the wide dynamic range and compression of high levels of fluorescence into a single scale allow easy visualization of stained populations.

The complexity of the data generated by multiparameter flow cytometric analysis means that the scatter and fluorescence measurements from individual cells are stored on the computer in the form of a list (list mode data). This means that the relationships between measurements on individual cells is preserved, and these relationships can be explored by effectively rerunning the analysis on the computer.

1.4. Identification of Positive Cells

Distinguishing positive from negative cells is unequivocal with clearly stained populations. Where there is overlap between positive and negative cells, the situation is less clear *(2)*. The best option may be to apply a more sensitive staining method *(3)*, although the computer programs available for some flow cytometry systems are designed to model overlapping populations. If none of these options are possible, a cutoff point can be established with an appropriate control sample, which is then applied to determine the number of positive cells.

2. Materials
2.1. Solutions

1. Dulbecco's phosphate-buffered saline (PBS), made by dissolving buffer tablets (Oxoid Ltd., Basingstoke, UK) in distilled water.
2. Nutrient culture medium, such as RPMI 1640.
3. Bovine serum albumin ([BSA], 10% stock solution in distilled water) may be added to antibody diluent/wash medium to give a final concentration of 0.1% (w/v).
4. Fetal bovine serum may be added to diluent/wash medium to give a final concentration of 2% (v/v).
5. Sodium azide (10% stock solution in distilled water) may be added to media at a final concentration of 0.1% to reduce capping and internalization of surface-bound antibodies; it also inhibits microbial growth. Store at 4°C *(see* Note 1).

6. Red cell lysing solution (e.g., FACS Lysing Solution, Becton Dickinson) (*see* Note 1).
7. 2% Formaldehyde fixative solution, made by diluting 40% stock formaldehyde in PBS (*see* Note 1).
8. Normal mouse serum to block nonspecific binding.
9. Fluorochrome-labeled streptavidin.

2.2. Antibodies

1. A very wide range of antibodies is now available unconjugated, biotin-conjugated or conjugated to FITC, PE, or red-light-emitting fluorochromes, such as PerCP or PE-Cy5. These reagents are generally of high quality, and are usually supplied at a concentration suitable for labeling 10^6 cells with 10–20 μL of antibody.
2. Isotype-matched unconjugated, biotin-conjugated, or fluorochrome-labeled antibodies unreactive with mammalian cells are available as control reagents from many suppliers.
3. Fluorochrome-labeled anti-immunoglobulin antibody: labeled F(ab')$_2$ fragments should be selected when studying target cells that express Fc receptors.

3. Methods

3.1. Direct Immunofluorescence

1. Carefully dispense into 5 μL tubes of each labeled antibody to give the experimental combinations to be used. Include tubes with negative control conjugates and CD45-FITC/CD14-PE mixture as a gate control, and each of the antibodies to be used singly. To aid initial adjustment of the flow cytometer, cells stained singly with a highly expressed marker, such as CD8, are valuable.
2. Add 25 μL of whole blood to each tube, and mix carefully.
3. Incubate for 30 min at 4°C in the dark.
4. Add 1 mL of red cell lysing solution to each tube.
5. Incubate for 10 min at room temperature.
6. Centrifuge at 200*g* for 5 min; decant supernatant and resuspend cells
7. Add 1 mL of PBS containing 0.1% azide, and repeat step 6.
8. Repeat wash of step 7 once more.
9. Add 500 μL of fixative, and mix carefully. Store at 4°C in the dark until analyzed.

3.2. Multiple-Labeling Indirect Immunofluorescence

1. Prepare target cell suspension and dilute to 10^6 cells/mL in RPMI containing 2% fetal calf serum. Use this medium as diluent, and wash medium throughout.
2. Dispense 5 μL of unlabeled antireceptor antibody into tubes. A suitable dilution of antibody to achieve saturation was used. Control tubes contained 5 μL of control antibody at the same concentration.
3. Add 100 μL of cell suspension/tube, and mix carefully.
4. Incubate for 30 min at room temperature.
5. Add 1 mL of medium, and centrifuge at 200*g* for 5 min; decant supernatant and resuspend cells.
6. Repeat wash step 5 twice more.

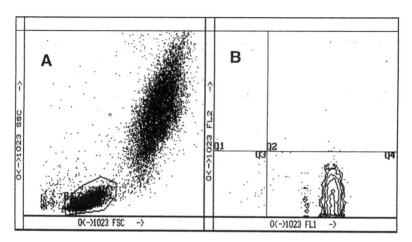

Fig. 1. Analysis of lysed whole blood stained with FITC-anti-CD45 and PE-anti-CD14. **(A)** Scatter analysis, showing the position of a gate to restrict the analysis to lymphocytes. **(B)** Gated fluorescence analysis, showing that over 98% of the gated cells are in quadrant 4 (Q4). Monocytes would appear in quadrant 2 (Q2) and nonleukocytes in quadrant 3 (Q3). With suboptimal cell preparations, the position of the lymphocyte scatter gate can be determined by "back-gating"; that is, examining the scatter distribution of cells gated by quadrant 4.

7. Add 50 μL of diluted antimouse IgG-PE conjugate (F[ab'])₂ PE reagent [Dako Ltd, High Wycombe, UK] can be diluted 1/40).
8. Incubate for 30 min at room temperature.
9. Wash cells according to step 5 three times.
10. Add 10 μL 1/10 diluted normal mouse serum.
11. Incubate for 10 min.
12. Without washing, add 5 μL of anti-CD45-FITC antibody.
13. Incubate for 20 min at room temperature.
14. Wash cells according to step 5 three times.
15. Resuspend cells in 500 μL of formaldehyde fixative. Store at 4°C in the dark before analysis.

3.3. Flow Cytometry

Analysis of samples of whole blood stained with directly labeled antibodies (Section 3.1.) will be used to illustrate cytometric analysis of multiple fluorochromes.

3.3.1. Scatter Gating

1. Analyze the FSC and SSC signals of a sample stained with CD45-FITC/CD14-PE.
2. Identify the lymphocyte population (Fig. 1A), and set a gate to identify these cells.

3. Analyze the FITC (FL1) and PE (FL2) signals using logarithmic amplification. Ensure that the majority of the gated cells are positive for FITC and negative for PE (Fig. 1B).

4. When subsequently recording data from cells, use the scatter gate as a "live gate" if your flow cytometer has this facility. This ensures that most of the list mode data recorded relates to lymphocytes.

5. During subsequent data analysis, gate the cells positive for CD45 and negative for CD14 onto the FSC vs SSC dot plot to refine the optimal position for the lymphocyte scatter gate. This method is known as "back-gating."

3.3.2. Analysis of Individual Fluorochromes

1. Analyze a control sample (FITC/PE/PE-Cy5 control antibody incubation) using the scatter gate to restrict the analysis to lymphocytes.

2. Plot FL1 against FSC, and adjust photomultiplier voltage to ensure cells are in the first quarter of the FL1 scale.

3. Analyze a sample stained singly with an FITC-labeled antibody, for example, anti-CD8.

4. Ensure that the positive cells are on scale on the FSC vs FL1 dot plot.

5. Repeat steps 1–4 for the FL2 channel, using PE-CD8 antibody.

6. Repeat steps 1–4 for the FL3 channel, using PE-Cy5-CD8 antibody.

3.3.3. Fluorescence Compensation (see Note 2)

1. Analyze an FITC single-stained tube, such as FITC-CD8, scatter gating to restrict analysis to lymphocytes.

2. On the FL1 vs FL2 dot plot, adjust the FL1 → FL2 compensation so that the FL1-positive cells, which initially spill into the FL2 scale (Fig. 2A), run horizontally (Fig. 2C); overcompensation results in the samples exhibiting lower FL2 signals as FL1 increases (Fig. 2B).

3. Analyze a PE single-stained tube, such as PE-CD8, using scatter gating to restrict the analysis to lymphocytes.

4. On the FL1 vs FL2 dot plot, adjust the FL2 → FL1 compensation to bring the cells that initially spill into FL1 (Fig. 2D) to run vertically (Fig. 2E).

5. On the FL3 vs FL2 dot plot, adjust the FL2 → FL3 compensation so that FL2 does not spill into FL3 (Fig. 2F).

6. Analyze a PE-Cy5 single-stained tube, again using scatter gating.

7. On the FL2 vs FL3 plot, adjust the FL3 → FL2 compensation to move the PE-Cy5-stained cells from spilling into the FL2 scale (Fig. 2G), to run parallel to the FL3 scale (Fig. 2H).

8. On the FL1 vs FL3 plot, note that there should be no spillover of FL3 into FL1 (Fig. 2I); similarly, there should be no spillover of FL1-stained cells into the FL3 scale (not shown).

Note that any change in the photomultiplier voltages of the fluorescence channels requires the compensation to be readjusted using the above procedure.

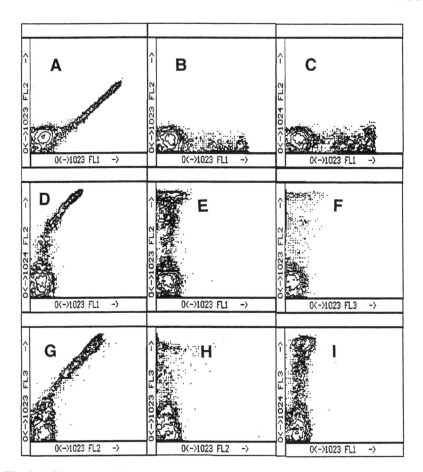

Fig. 2. Adjustment of fluorescence compensation. Lymphocytes stained with FITC-anti-CD8 **(A–C)**, PE-anti-CD8 **(D–F)** and PECy5-anti-CD8 **(G–I)** were analyzed, to compensate FL1, FL2 and FL3, respectively. The effects of under- (A) and over- (B) compensation are illustrated. The compensation network is adjusted systematically to adjust for FL1 fluorescence in FL2, FL2 spilling into FL1 and FL3, and FL3 spilling into FL2.

3.4. Three-Color Analysis

Analysis of the CD4-positive lymphocytes in whole blood for their expression of the CD45 isoforms RA and RO may be achieved as follows:

1. Stain whole blood according to Section 3.1., using negative control, CD45/CD14 gate control, and CD45RA-FITC/CD45RO-PE/CD4-PE-Cy5 antibodies.
2. Record list mode data, using the flow cytometer set up as in Section 3.3.
3. Analyze CD45/CD14 gate control data, setting the lymphocyte gate by "back-gating" the CD45-positive CD14-negative cells (Section 3.3.1.).

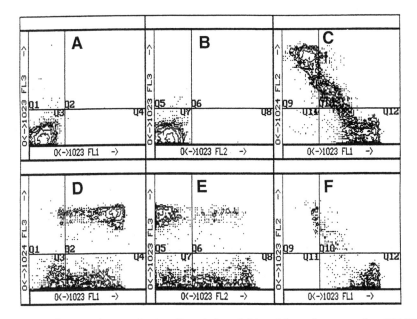

Fig. 3. Three-color analysis of peripheral blood lymphocytes for CD45RA, CD45RO, and CD4. Lymphocytes were stained with antibodies directly labeled with FITC, PE, and PECy5, respectively. The distribution of control labeled cells is shown in **A** and **B**, and labeled cells in **C–F**. The relationship between CD45RA and CD45RO in CD4-positive cells is shown in (F), which is gated for PECy5-positive cells.

4. Analyze data from control antibody tube; determine cutoff for quadrant analysis (Fig. 3A,B).
5. Analyze data from CD45RA/RO/CD4-stained cells. The relationship between CD4 and CD45RA (Fig. 3D) and CD4 and CD45RO (Fig. 3E) can be examined in the FL3 vs FL1 and FL3 vs FL2 plots, respectively. By adding a gate on CD4-positive cells, the relationship between CD45RA and CD45RO among CD4-positive cells can be visualized (Fig. 3F), and compared with ungated cells (Fig. 3C).

4. Notes
1. The notes to Chapter 33 apply to the similar techniques in this chapter.
2. Fluorescence compensation for FITC/PE analysis of lymphocytes may also be performed using Autocomp beads (Becton Dickinson). Refinement of this adjustment will be necessary if target cells other than lymphocytes are analyzed.

Acknowledgments
I would like to acknowledge the contribution of many collaborators in the Cancer Research Laboratories and Departments of Immunology, Clinical Oncology, Obstetrics and Gynecology, Surgery, and Therapeutics at Nottingham University. This work was supported by the Cancer Research Campaign (UK).

References

1. Beavis, A. J. and Pennline, K. J. (1994) Simultaneous measurement of 5-cell sur-face-antigens by 5-color immunofluorescence. *Cytometry* **15,** 371–376.
2. Pallis, M. and Robins, R. A. (1995) What you need to know when you go with the flow: pitfalls in the use of flow cytometry. *Ann. Rheum. Dis.* **54,** 785,786.
3. Zola, H. (1992) Studies of cytokine receptor expression by cells of the immune system—a waste of time? *Immunol. Today* **13,** 419,420.

35

Flow Cytometric Methods of Analyzing Apoptotic Cells

Anne E. Milner, J. Michaela Levens, and Christopher D. Gregory

1. Introduction

Apoptosis is a physiological, programmed mode of cell death, which is necessary for tissue modeling and organogenesis in embryonic development and in the control of homeostasis in a diversity of tissue types *(1)*. The distinct morphological features of apoptosis clearly distinguish it from the passive mode of cell death, necrosis, which is an unprogrammed response to toxic stimuli. The diagnosis of apoptosis relies on detection of these morphological changes, i.e., condensation and fragmentation of chromatin, cell shrinkage associated with cytoplasmic condensation, and retention of cell membrane integrity. These changes may be accompanied by the fragmentation of the cell into membrane-bound apoptotic bodies containing cytoplasmic organelles, nuclear components, or both *(2)*. Classical methods of diagnosing apoptosis include light and electron microscopy in which the above morphological changes can be visualized, and internucleosomal DNA fragmentation assays in which the fragmentation of DNA can be seen after gel electrophoresis as a ladder pattern representing the generation of multiple oligonucleosomal fragments. The widespread use of in vitro systems for studying cell death has led many researchers to turn to flow cytometry as an alternative to the classic methods of analyzing apoptosis, since it offers the advantages of rapid analysis of individual cells, low cell number requirement, and the opportunity for simultaneous measurement of several cellular parameters.

Four methods of quantitating apoptosis by flow cytometry are described in this chapter. The two-dimensional light scatter assay measures the reduction in cellular volume and increase in cell density that are observed during apoptosis and that are revealed by a decrease in forward light scatter and an increase in

From: *Methods in Molecular Biology, Vol. 80: Immunochemical Protocols, 2nd ed.*
Edited by: J. D. Pound © Humana Press Inc., Totowa, NJ

90° light scatter *(3–5)*. The subdiploid DNA peak assay and the multiparameter light scatter and DNA assay analyze the condensation and fragmentation of chromatin that occur during apoptosis by detecting changes in the fluorescence emitted by the DNA binding fluorochrome, propidium iodide. This is a widely used method that has been utilized to assess apoptosis in many different cell types *(6–9)*. The *in situ* end-labeling assay is based on the visualization of the DNA strand breaks that accompany apoptosis. A variety of cell types stained with fluorescein isothiocyanate (FITC)-conjugated 2'-deoxyuridine-5'-triphosphate (dUTP) display an increase in FITC-generated fluorescence after induction of apoptosis in a manner that correlates with the onset of apoptosis *(10,11)*.

On a final note of caution, however, it should be stressed that no flow cytometric technique is yet able to diagnose apoptotic cells, and in all cases, if necrotic cells are present, they will cause inaccuracies in the results. Therefore, prior to flow cytometric analysis of apoptosis, diagnosis should be confirmed by light microscopy.

2. Materials

1. Phosphate-buffered saline (PBS): pH 7.4, 100 mM NaCl, 20 mM NaH$_2$PO$_4$, 80 mM Na$_2$HPO$_4$.
2. 1% Formaldehyde solution in PBS. Store at 4°C.
3. 1% Paraformaldehyde, 0.1% Triton-X 100 solution in PBS. Store at 4°C.
4. Propidium iodide solution: Dissolve 10 mg of propidium iodide (Sigma, Aldrich, Dorset, UK) in 10 mL distilled water. Store at 4°C in the dark.
5. 70% Ethanol: Store at –20°C.
6. Tris-buffered saline (TBS): 50 mM Tris. Adjust pH to 7.6 with concentrated HCl, and then add 150 mM NaCl. Store at 4°C.
7. Standard saline citrate (SSC), 20X concentration: 263 mM trisodium citrate, 3.08M NaCl.
8. Terminal deoxynucleotidyl transferase (TdT) buffer, 5X concentration: 500 mM sodium cacodylate, 10 mM cobalt chloride, 1 mM dithiothreitol. Add water to the sodium cacodylate, cool to 0°C on ice, add dithiothreitol, and then cobalt chloride dropwise, stirring continuously. Store in aliquots at –20°C.
9. Reaction mixture: For each reaction make up 80 μL of water, 20 μL of 5X concentration TdT buffer, 0.2 μL of 1 mM digoxigenin-11-dUTP (Boehringer Mannheim, Lewes, UK), and 10 U of TdT. Make up enough for all reactions then aliquot. Use immediately.
10. Staining buffer (100 mL): 10% Triton-X 100 (1 mL), 20X concentration SCC (20 mL), water (79 mL). Store at 4°C.
11. Freeze-dried nonfat milk (e.g., "Marvel," Premier Beverages, Stafford, UK).
12. Labeling mixture: For each reaction, make up 250 μL staining buffer, 0.1 μg antidigitoxin-FITC conjugated antibody (Boehringer Mannheim). Use immediately.

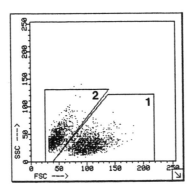

Fig. 1. Two-dimensional light scatter assay. Burkitt lymphoma cells induced into apoptosis by incubation with a MAb against IgM were assayed for forward light scatter (FSC) and 90° light scatter (SSC). Region 1, viable cells; Region 2, apoptotic cells.

3. Methods
3.1. Two-Dimensional Light Scatter Assay

1. Aliquot 5×10^5 cells in suspension into FACS tubes and centrifuge at 150g for 5 min. Discard the supernatant (*see* Note 1).
2. Resuspend the cells in 300 μL of 1% formaldehyde in PBS, and store at 4°C until analysis (*see* Notes 2–4).
3. Analyze with a flow cytometer set to any wavelength. Record the light scattered in a forward direction and at 90°.
4. Display a two-dimensional dot plot of forward vs 90° scattered light and draw gates around the live cells (high forward scatter, low 90° scatter) and apoptotic population (low forward scatter, high 90° scatter) as in Fig. 1 (*see* Notes 5 and 6).

3.2. Subdiploid DNA Peak Assay (see Notes 7 and 8)

1. Aliquot 5×10^5 cells in suspension into FACS tubes, and centrifuge at 150g for 5 min. Discard the supernatant (*see* Note 1).
2. Resuspend cells in 0.5 mL of 1% paraformaldehyde, 0.1% Triton-X 100 in PBS, and store at 4°C until analysis (*see* Note 9).
3. Add propidium iodide to a final concentration of 20 μg/mL. Mix well, and stand at 4°C for 30 min in order to allow the dye to equilibrate (*see* Note 10).
4. Analyze with a flow cytometer with an argon-ion laser tuned to 488 nm. Record the light emitted into the red fluorescence photomultiplier tube (PMT) using a 620-nm long pass filter in front of the PMT.
5. Display a histogram of red fluorescence and set a gate around the subdiploid peak (*see* Fig. 2).

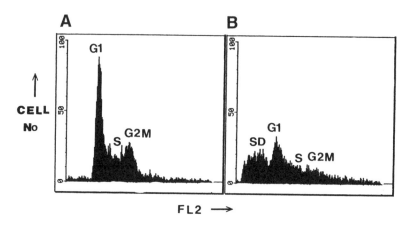

Fig. 2. Subdiploid DNA peak assay. Burkitt lymphoma cells were analyzed for cell cycle 24 h after irradiation with 4 Gy. Control cells **(A)** show a cycling population with the G1, S, and G2M phases clearly visible. Irradiated cells **(B)** have an additional peak with decreased fluorescence (the subdiploid peak [SD]) representing apoptotic cells.

3.3. Multiparameter Light Scatter and DNA Assay

1. Aliquot 5×10^5 cells in suspension into FACS tubes, and centrifuge at 150g for 5 min. Discard the supernatant (*see* Note 1).
2. Resuspend the cells in 0.5 mL of 1% paraformaldehyde, 0.1% Triton-X 100 in PBS, and store at 4°C until analysis (*see* Note 9).
3. Add propidium iodide to a final concentration of 20 µg/mL. Mix well, and stand at 4°C for 30 min in order to allow the dye to equilibrate (*see* Note 10).
4. Analyze with a flow cytometer with an argon-ion laser tuned to 488 nm. Record the light scattered in the forward direction and into the red fluorescence PMT (using a 620-nm long pass filter in front of the PMT).
5. Display a two-dimensional dot plot of forward light scatter vs red fluorescence and set a gate around the apoptotic population (decreased red fluorescence) as in Fig. 3.

3.4. In Situ *End-Labeling Assay* (see Note 11)

1. Aliquot 1×10^6 cells in suspension into FACS tubes and centrifuge at 130g for 5 min. Discard the supernatant, resuspend the cells in 100 µL ice-cold PBS, and mix in 1 mL of 1% formaldehyde in PBS (*see* Notes 1 and 12).
2. Incubate on ice for 15 min. Centrifuge at 170g for 5 min. Discard the supernatant, and resuspend in 1 mL ice-cold PBS. Centrifuge at 170g for 5 min. Discard the supernatant.
3. Resuspend the cells in 100 µL of ice-cold PBS, and mix in 1 mL 70% ethanol at −20°C. Either incubate on ice for 1 h or store at 4°C until needed.
4. Centrifuge at 170g for 10 min. Discard the supernatant, and resuspend in 100 µL of TBS (*see* Note 13). Centrifuge at 170g for 5 min. Discard the supernatant.

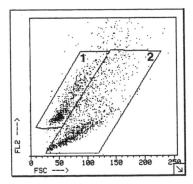

Fig. 3. Multiparameter light scatter and DNA assay. Burkitt lymphoma cells induced into apoptosis by irradiation with 4 Gy were analyzed for forward light scatter (FSC) and propidium iodide fluorescence (FL2). Region 1, viable cells; Region 2, apoptotic cells.

5. Resuspend the cells in 100 μL of reaction mixture. Incubate at 37°C for 35 min. Remove and place on ice for 3 min. Centrifuge at 170*g* for 5 min. Discard the supernatant.
6. Resuspend the cells in 500 μL staining buffer + 5% (w/v) Marvel. Centrifuge at 170g for 5 min. Discard the supernatant.
7. Resuspend the cells in 250 μL labeling mixture. Incubate for 35 min at 37°C. Centrifuge at 170*g* for 5 min. Discard the supernatant.
8. Resuspend the cells in 0.5 mL of 1% formaldehyde in PBS. Store at 4°C until use.
9. Analyze with a flow cytometer with an argon laser tuned to 488 nm. Record the light scattered in the forward direction and into the green fluorescence PMT (using a 520 nm band pass filter in front of the PMT).
10. Display a two-dimensional dot plot of forward light scatter vs green fluorescence, and set a gate around the viable population (negative fluorescence) and apoptotic population (positive fluorescence) as shown in Fig. 4.

4. Notes
4.1. All Methods
1. For all methods samples must be in a single cell suspension before analysis. Large clumps of cells or debris will block the nozzle of the flow cytometer and prevent analysis. Small clumps of cells will give inaccuracies in the results.

4.2. Two-Dimensional Light Scatter Assay
2. The two-dimensional light scatter assay can be equally well carried out on viable cells.
3. Fixation of cells in 1% formaldehyde in PBS will change their light scatter characteristics slightly. Therefore, when comparing samples over a time-course, it is important that all samples should be fixed for at least 24 h before analysis.

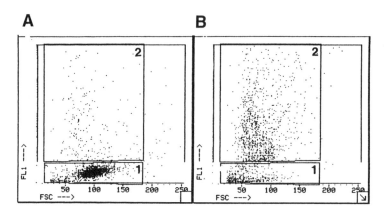

Fig. 4. *In situ* end-labeling. Forward light scatter (FSC) vs FITC fluorescence (FL1) of (**A**) viable and (**B**) apoptotic Burkitt lymphoma cells. Cells were induced into apoptosis by incubation with the calcium ionophore, ionomycin. Region 1, viable cells; Region 2, apoptotic cells.

4. Samples fixed in 1% formaldehyde in PBS can be kept for at least 2 wk at 4°C.
5. We have observed in our cell systems, when comparing the two-dimensional light scatter assay with light microscopy of acridine orange-stained cells, that at early time-points (<12 h), the flow cytometric method gives an underestimate of the percentage of apoptosis present. For time-points later than this, the light scatter assay is very accurate.
6. To ensure that the changes in light scatter that occur in apoptotic cells are not masked by the light scatter profiles from a second cell type, the two-dimensional light scatter method tends to be limited to populations that, in their viable state, show little size variation and consist predominantly of a single cell type.

4.3. Subdiploid DNA Peak Assay and Multiparameter Light Scatter and DNA Assay

7. The main limitation of the subdiploid DNA peak assay is that it cannot be used accurately on a cycling population, since the fluorescence from apoptotic S and G2M cells overlays the fluorescence from viable G1 cells. However, this limitation can be largely overcome by the use of the multiparameter light scatter and DNA assay.
8. Another important limitation to be aware of is that the induction of apoptosis in a population of cells will not always result in a clearly distinct subdiploid peak *(12)*. We have seen this particularly when apoptosis is induced in Burkitt lymphoma cells by serum deprivation. After approx 2 wk, all cells are apoptotic as can be clearly seen by the two-dimensional light scatter assay and confirmed by microscopic analysis of acridine orange-stained cells, but the cell-cycle profile gives the appearance of a mainly viable population (Fig. 5).

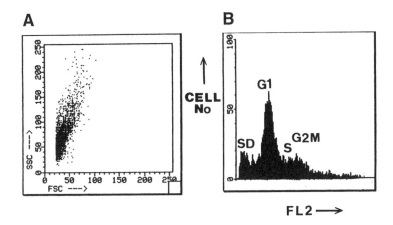

Fig. 5. Comparison of two-dimensional light scatter assay with subdiploid DNA peak assay. Burkitt lymphoma cells were serum-deprived for 14 d and then assayed for **(A)** forward light scatter (FSC) versus 90° light scatter (SSC) or **(B)** cell cycle. Note that although all the cells are clearly apoptotic as shown by the light scatter assay, there is only a small subdiploid peak (SD) present in the cell-cycle analysis, demonstrating that in this case, cell-cycle analysis alone would grossly underestimate the extent of apoptosis present in the cell population.

9. When making up the cell-cycle fixative, add 1% paraformaldehyde to the PBS first, and warm the solution to allow it to dissolve (this may take some time). Finally, add 0.1% Triton-X 100.
10. The subdiploid DNA peak assay can be used in conjunction with staining for surface/cytoplasmic antigens with an FITC-labeled antibody, but when doing this, it is advisable to decrease the propidium iodide concentration from 20 to 5 µg/mL to minimize quenching of FITC by propidium iodide.

4.4. In Situ *End-Labeling Assay*

11. The nick translation method can be used in conjunction with cell-cycle analysis to determine which phases of the cell-cycle the apoptotic cells are in. To do this, add 5 µg/mL propidium iodide to the samples 30 min prior to analysis.
12. Include one sample of viable cells to assay as a negative control.
13. TBS is used instead of PBS, since phosphate chelates the cobalt in the TdT buffer.

References

1. Wyllie, A. H. (1992) Apoptosis and the regulation of cell numbers in normal and neoplastic tissues: an overview. *Cancer Metastasis Rev.* **11,** 95–103.
2. Wyllie, A. H., Beattie, G. J., and Hargreaves, A. D. (1981) Chromatin changes in apoptosis. *Histochem. J.* **13,** 681–692.
3. Swat, W., Ignatowicz, L., and Kisielow, P. (1991) Detection of apoptosis of immature CD4+8+ thymocytes by flow cytometry. *J. Immunol. Methods* **137,** 79–87.

4. Dive, C., Gregory, C. D., Phipps, D. J., Evans, D. L., Milner, A. E., and Wyllie, A. H. (1992) Analysis and discrimination of necrosis and apoptosis by multiparameter flow cytometry. *Biochim. Biophys. Acta* **1133,** 275–285.

5. Illera, V. A., Perandones, C. E., Stunz, L. L., Mower, D. A., and Ashman, R. E. (1993) Apoptosis in splenic B lymphocytes. *J. Immunol.* **151,** 2965–2973.

6. Rodriguez-Tarduchy, G., Collins, M., and Lopez–Rivas, A. (1990) Regulation of apoptosis in interleukin-3-dependent haemopoietic cells by interleukin-3 and calcium ionophores. *EMBO. J.* **9,** 2997–3002.

7. Telford, W. G., King, L. E., and Fraker, P. J. (1991) Evaluation of glucocorticoid-induced DNA fragmentation in mouse thymocytes by flow cytometry. *Cell Proliferation* **24,** 447–459.

8. Ormerod, M. G., Collins, M. K. L., Rodriguez-Tarduchy, G., and Robertson, D. (1992) Apoptosis in interleukin 3-dependent haemopoietic cells. *J. Immunol. Methods* **153,** 57–65.

9. Garvy, B. A., Telford, W. G., King, L. E., and Fraker, P. J. (1993) Glucocorticoids and irradiation-induced apoptosis in normal murine bone marrow B-lineage lymphocytes as determined by flow cytometry. *Immunology* **76,** 270–277.

10. Gorczyca, W., Melamed, M. R., and Darzyńkiewicz, Z. (1993) Apoptosis of S-phase HL-60 cells induced by topoisomerase inhibitors: detection of DNA strand breaks by flow cytometry using the *in situ* nick translation assay. *Toxicol. Lett.* **67,** 249–258.

11. Gold, R., Schmied, M., Rothe, G., Zischler, H., Breitschopf, H., Wekerle, H., and Lassmann, H. (1993) Detection of DNA fragmentation in apoptosis: application of *in situ* nick translation to cell culture systems and tissue sections. *J. Histochem Cytochem.* **41,** 1023–1030.

12. Allday, M. J., Inman, G. J., Crawford, D. H., and Farrell, P. J. (1995) DNA damage in human B-cells can induce apoptosis, proceeding from G(1)/S when p53 is transactivation competent and G(2)/M when it is transactivation defective. *EMBO J.* **14,** 4994–5005.

36

Flow Cytometric Detection of Proliferation-Associated Antigens, PCNA and Ki-67

George D. Wilson

1. Introduction

The rapid evolution of monoclonal antibody (MAb) technology has resulted in an ever-growing repertoire of proteins becoming accessible for study using immunohistochemical techniques. Nuclear antigens represent a class of proteins of increasing significance and diversity; they are intimately associated with important cellular functions, such as cell-cycle regulation and DNA replication and repair. The control of growth of any tissue is a complex series of coordinated mechanisms. Deregulation of this control is a fundamental feature of most common neoplasms. Knowledge of proliferative activity in human tumors should give important information for evaluating both biological behavior and potential treatment strategies.

Many proliferation-associated antigens have been reported as clinically useful indicators of proliferative activity (1). Of these, the so-called proliferating cell nuclear antigen (PCNA) and Ki-67 have been identified as the most useful in both immunohistochemistry (see Chapter 27) and flow cytometry (FCM). PCNA is an auxiliary protein to DNA polymerase δ (2,3) and is intimately associated with DNA replication, but also DNA repair (4,5). Ki-67 is a large protein associated with nuclear nonhistone proteins (6,7), and is expressed in all actively proliferating cells (8,9). Expression of these two proteins, in a cell population should equate to the growth fraction, i.e., the proportion of cells involved in an active cell cycle. However, there are apparent inconsistencies when these two proteins have been compared with one another (10) and with other methods of assessing cell proliferation (11).

From: *Methods in Molecular Biology, Vol. 80: Immunochemical Protocols, 2nd ed.*
Edited by: J. D. Pound © Humana Press Inc., Totowa, NJ

Although FCM offers the attractive possibility of simultaneously studying the cell-cycle distribution and coexpression of proliferation-associated antigens, the nuclear localization of these proteins represents a significant challenge for the cytometric technique, because unlike the detection of surface antigens, for which antibody access and saturation of binding sites can be achieved relatively easily, the cellular and nuclear membrane barriers to both antibodies and fluorochromes must be overcome in order to detect nuclear antigens. This must be achieved with minimum disruption of the antigen of interest and maximal sensitivity. Furthermore, these potential problems may be compounded by the existence of regions of hydrophobicity within the nucleus, alteration of the protein conformation by permeabilization, and the occurrence of some nuclear antigens as multiprotein complexes.

Both Ki-67 and PCNA show variability in their localization throughout the cell cycle. In the G1 phase, Ki-67 is predominantly localized to the perinuclear region, whereas in later stages of the cell cycle, it is detected throughout the nuclear interior, but mainly in the nuclear matrix. During mitosis, Ki-67 is present on all chromosomes, but undergoes rapid degradation during anaphase and telophase, suggesting that it has a biological half-life of <1 h. Early studies of immunohistochemical detection of the protein were only successful on frozen sections, and it was suggested that the epitope for Ki-67 may be fragile or labile. However, this was not found to be a problem for flow cytometric detection, which employed acetone or alcohol fixation. Study of the reactivity of antibodies raised against recombinant Ki-67 *(12)* suggested that these earlier discrepancies were more associated with epitope access rather than fragility. In comparison to Ki-67, PCNA has a long biological half-life (approx 30 h), however, it is known to exist in at least two forms, one that is loosely bound in the nucleoplasm and one that is tightly bound at sites of DNA replication or repair. These latter characteristics are an important consideration in the choice of antigen-detection method and interpretation of the data obtained.

A fundamental prerequisite for detection of intranuclear antigens by FCM is fixation and/or permeabilization to facilitate access of antibodies to their epitopes. Since most studies will be carried out in conjunction with DNA staining, the preparation and staining procedures must meet the following criteria:

1. Minimal cellular clumping and loss of morphology (for intact cells).
2. High resolution of the DNA profile.
3. Accessibility and preservation of the nuclear epitope to produce well-defined immunofluorescent staining patterns with minimal autofluorescence.
4. Relatively quick and simple preparative procedures.

As with all biological systems, there is no universal method able to satisfy all these criteria for different proteins, antibodies, and source material. Fixa-

PRE-FIXATION   **PERMEABILISATION**   **POST-FIXATION**

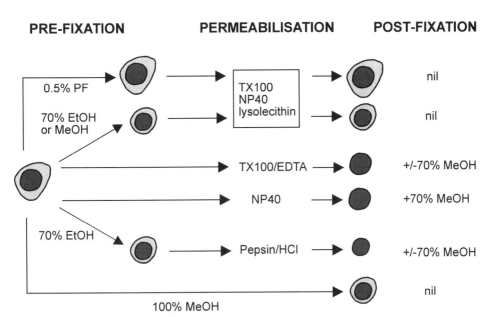

Fig. 1. Scheme showing the basic strategies available for the detection of nuclear antigens by flow cytometry. PF, paraformaldehyde; EtOH, ethanol; MeOH, methanol.

tion can affect antigens through epitope destruction, loss or leaching, masking, and redistribution. Destruction may occur when the epitope depends on secondary protein structure or as a result of the action of proteolytic enzymes or from formation of the Schiff base by interaction of aldehydes and peptidyl primary amine groups within the epitope. Loss can occur by extraction using alcoholic fixation or leaching by changing the chemical environment within the cell using permeabilizing agents. Epitope recognition can be affected by protein unfolding and loss of tertiary structure.

The starting point for most studies will be the intact cell, either from cell cultures or dissociated by mechanical or enzymatic methods from experimental or human tissues and tumors. Figure 1 summarizes some of the basic strategies that can be used to detect nuclear antigens. This chapter will describe three protocols for detection of PCNA and Ki-67: a simple method involving combined fixation and permeabilization by methanol, and two methods of detergent permeabilization that have been optimized for specific applications.

2. Materials

1. Methanol (high-purity): absolute and 70% (v/v).
2. Phosphate-buffered saline (PBS) pH 7.5: 0.14M NaCl, 2.7 mM KCl, 1.5 mM KH$_2$PO$_4$, 8.1 mM Na$_2$HPO$_4$.

3. Lysing solution 1: (0.25% [v/v] Nonidet P-40 (NP40), 0.33 mM CaCl$_2$ calcium chloride, 0.25M sucrose). Dissolve sucrose completely before adding calcium chloride, and add NP40 last.
4. Lysing solution 2: PBS containing 0.5% (v/v) Triton X-100, 0.5 μM disodium EDTA, and 1% (w/v) bovine serum albumin (BSA).
5. Antibody staining buffer: PBS containing 0.5% (v/v) Tween-20 and either 1% (w/v) BSA (for direct antibody conjugates), or 0.5% (v/v) normal goat serum when a second antibody is used.
6. Propidium iodide.
7. Ribonuclease A.
8. MAb to PCNA and Ki-67 with the appropriate isotypic antibody controls—secondary antibodies if a two step staining is required.

3. Methods
3.1. Fixation with Organic Solvents

Despite the harshness of these reagents (*see* Note 1), the organic solvents are the simplest and most rapid method to fix and permeabilize cells. Methanol is preferable to ethanol in many cases. The basic fixation procedure outlined below is suitable for the detection of total PCNA within the cell and for Ki-67 in most cells.

1. Resuspend a concentrated cell pellet (10^6 cells) in 200 μL of PBS.
2. Fixation is best achieved by adding 2 mL of 100% methanol, precooled to –20°C, dropwise while continually vortexing. Fixation is allowed to proceed for 10 min at –20°C.
3. For storage, prior to staining, the solution is diluted to 70% with distilled water, and stored at 4°C (*see* Note 2).

3.2. Permeabilization with NP40

Alcohol fixation does not permit detection of tightly bound PCNA. Permeabilization, which results in enucleation, using detergents (*see* Note 3) is required to achieve the best results. The method described below has been optimized for PCNA *(13)*.

1. Aliquot 1–2 × 10^6 cells into a 10-mL polystyrene conical bottom tube.
2. Centrifuge at 200g for 5 min at 4°C.
3. Wash in 5 mL of ice-cold PBS, and centrifuge again at 200g for 5 min at 4°C.
4. Resuspend pellet in 2 mL of ice-cold lysing solution 1, mix thoroughly, and leave for 10 min on ice.
5. Add 5 mL cold PBS, and centrifuge at 200g for 5 min at 4°C.
6. Resuspend pellet in 200 μL of cold PBS (*see* Note 4), add 3.5 mL of 100% methanol (cooled to –20°C), and fix for 10 min at –20°C.
7. Add 1.3 mL of distilled water to give a final methanol concentration of 70%, and store at 4°C (*see* Note 2) prior to staining.

3.3. Permeabilization with Triton X-100.

This procedure is suitable for both Ki-67 and tightly bound PCNA. This procedure can be used to stain PCNA, Ki-67, and DNA content simultaneously (*see* Note 5).

1. Aliquot 1–2 × 10^6 cells into a 10-mL polystyrene conical bottom tube.
2. Centrifuge at 200g for 5 min at 4°C.
3. Wash in 5 mL ice-cold PBS, and centrifuge at 200g for 5 min at 4°C.
4. Add 2 mL of lysing solution 2, thoroughly mix, and leave to stand on ice for 15 min.
5. Add 5 mL PBS, and centrifuge at 200g for 5 min.
6. Resuspend pellet in 200 µL of PBS, and fix as in steps 6 and 7 of previous protocol (*see* Note 6).

3.4. Immunochemical Staining

Directly conjugated MAbs can be used to detect PCNA and Ki-67, since these proteins are present in the nucleus at relatively high levels.

1. Centrifuge cells or nuclei out of fixative at 400g for 5 min.
2. Wash once with 5 mL of PBS, and centrifuge again at 400g for 5 min.
3. Resuspend pellet in 90 µL of antibody staining buffer containing BSA (Section 2.), and add 10 µL (*see* Note 7) of MAb. The recommended antibodies are PC10-FITC (DAKO F863) and Ki-67-FITC (DAKO F788). The appropriate directly conjugated isotypic control antisera are also available from DAKO. The suspensions are incubated for 1–2 h at room temperature and protected from light.
4. Add 5 mL of PBS, and centrifuge at 400g for 5 min.
5. Resuspend in 1 mL of PBS containing 10 µg/mL of propidium iodide and 1 mg/mL of Ribonuclease A. Analyze on the flow cytometer after 15 min.

3.5. Cytometric Analysis

The procedure described below is based on the use of a FACScan (Becton Dickinson) using LYSYS II software with doublet discrimination.

1. DNA fluorescence (propidium iodide) is collected into FL3, doublets, and so forth, excluded by gating on the area vs width dot plot. As a guideline, the FL3 voltage should be ~400.
2. The antibody signals are collected into FL1 using either linear or log amplification, depending on the intensity of the signal. No compensation should be required if the DNA signal is collected into FL3.
3. As with most FCM, 10,000 events should be recorded.
4. Examples of typical staining patterns are shown in Fig. 2. These profiles are analyzed for positivity by setting a lower limit of detection based on the isotypic control sample. In our laboratory, we would normally set a region on the control that includes <1% of positive events and transpose this region to the MAb-stained samples.

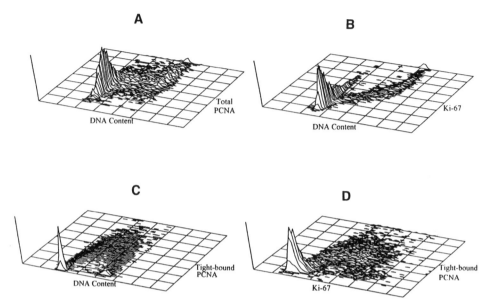

Fig. 2. Typical flow cytometry profiles obtained in HT29 cells for **(A)** total PCNA detection using methanol fixation, **(B)** Ki-67 expression using methanol fixation, **(C)** demonstration of tightly bound PCNA using NP-40 extraction, and **(D)** simultaneous staining of tightly bound PCNA and Ki-67 using Triton X-100 extraction. In D, PCNA was detected using PC10-FITC, whereas Ki-67 was labeled using a phycoerythrin-conjugated second antibody.

3.6. Cytometric Profiles

Figure 2 shows a series of profiles obtained in HT29 human colon carcinoma cells using the described staining protocols. In panels A and B, Ki-67 and total PCNA profiles are shown, respectively, after methanol fixation of intact cells. In panel A, Ki-67 expression shows a steady increase throughout S phase and is greatest in G2 + M. In G1, there would appear to be a population with slightly higher Ki-67, which may represent recently divided cells; the Ki-67 level then decreases as cells progress through G1 in preparation for S-phase. In this cell line, there are no cells in G0: studies using solid tumors and stimulated peripheral blood lymphocytes show universal lack of Ki-67 in noncycling cells. In panel B, there is a similar but different expression of total PCNA throughout the cell cycle. There appears to be a much more uniform increase in expression as cells progress from G1 to mitosis without the variation in G1 and G2 + M observed for Ki-67. Although PCNA is synthesized during late G1 and S-phase, it is present throughout the cell cycle owing to its long half-life. This characteristic might also result in apparent expression in cells that recently have left the cell cycle. There is also evidence of PCNA expression, in the absence of cell proliferation, in response to growth factors *(14)*. These properties and the involvement of PCNA in other cellular processes make it a less robust marker of growth fraction than Ki-67.

In panel C, the NP40 detergent extraction procedure has been used to demonstrate tightly bound PCNA. The profile resembles that obtained by pulse-labeling with a DNA precursor, such as bromodeoxyuridine, in which the S-phase cells have been highlighted by their expression of PCNA at replication sites. This staining technique should provide better functional information concerning the S-phase fraction than single-parameter DNA staining. This method has been used to detect nucleotide excision repair *(15)*.

The combination of PCNA and Ki-67 staining using a Triton X-100 detergent extraction is shown in panel D. This profile is similar to that which has been obtained using an autoantibody to PCNA and a monoclonal to Ki-67 as described in ref. *16*. This double-staining technique has many advantages: The combination of the two markers allows the investigator to exploit the ability of Ki-67 to discriminate G0 from G1, early G1 from late G1 and G2 and mitosis, whereas PCNA provides the discrimination of S-phase cells. This technique has been used *(17)* to show that newly recruited cells into the cycle do not express Ki-67 until the end of G1 and is a potentially useful method to study recruitment and repopulation of cells in response to DNA damaging agents.

4. Notes

1. Alcoholic fixatives, such as methanol, ethanol, and acetone, in the concentration range 50–100%, simultaneously fix and permeabilize cells by dehydration, lipid extraction, and protein precipitation. Cells tend to shrink, which can impair their light-scattering characteristics on the flow cytometer. Two potential problems can occur: first, detection of many surface antigens may be impaired, and second, cells are prone to clumping. The latter can usually be overcome using the protocol described by keeping the volume of resuspended cells small, adding fixative dropwise with constant vortexing, and keeping everything cold. Alcohols are usually inefficient below 50%.

2. After fixation, it is usually best to stain and run the samples as soon as possible, and certainly within a few days, since there is evidence to suggest that some proteins are susceptible to degradation in longer-term storage. With the enucleated samples, there is a tendency for further clumping to occur in storage.

3. The detergents NP-40 and Triton X-100 are nonionic, strong membrane solubilizers. Cell membranes become highly permeable to proteins, and this has the effect of reducing light scatter and refractive index. In order to prevent extreme solubilization of cellular membranes and the possibility of total cell lysis, the concentration of detergent is restricted to the range 0.01–0.5% (v/v) and usually incubated for short times at low temperature. In some case, the addition of

mild membrane agents, such as saponin, Tween-20, lysolecithin, or streptol-ysin O can aid the detection of nuclear proteins.
4. This step is particularly prone to clumping, and syringing may be required.
5. The protocol outlined in this section uses permeabilization followed by fixation. Several techniques have been developed for the staining of Ki-67 and PCNA. A particularly useful method if cell numbers are limiting is that described in ref. *18,* where a washless, unfixed staining can be achieved.
6. A precipitation sometimes forms at this stage owing to the presence of alcohol and BSA, but this does not affect subsequent staining.
7. When using directly conjugated antibodies, the dilution should be as recom-mended by the supplier. Overdilution will result in loss of signal and positivity. If nonconjugated MAbs are used, then the appropriate concentration should be optimized from a dilution curve. In our experience, a dilution of 1:50 is suitable for both antibodies.

References

1. Hall, P. A. and Woods, A. (1990) Immunohistochemical markers of cell prolifera-tion. Achievements, problems and prospects. *Cell Tissue Kinet.* **23,** 531–549.
2. Bravo, R. and Bravo, H. (1985) Changes in the nuclear distribution of cyclin (PCNA) but not its synthesis depend on DNA replication. *EMBO J.* **4,** 655–661.
3. Prelich, G., Kostura, M., Marshak, D. R., Matthews, M. B., and Stillman, B. (1987) The cell-cycle regulated proliferating cell nuclear antigen is required for SV40-DNA replication in vitro. *Nature* **326,** 471–475.
4. Celis, J. E. and Madsen, P. (1986) Increased cyclin/PCNA antigen staining of non S-phase transformed human amnion cells engaged in nucleotide excision DNA repair. *FEBS Lett.* **209,** 277–283.
5. Toschi, L. and Bravo, R. (1988) Changes in cyclin/proliferating cell nuclear anti-gen distribution during DNA repair synthesis. *J. Cell Biol.* **107,** 1623–1628.
6. Verheijen, R. H., Kuijpers, J. H., Schlingemann, R. O., Boehmer, A. L. M., van Driel, R., Brakenhoff, J. G., and Raemakers, F. C. S. (1989) Ki-67 detects a nuclear matrix-associated proliferation-related antigen. I. Intracellular localization dur-ing interphase. *J. Cell Sci.* **92,** 123–130.
7. Schluter, C., Duchrow, M., Wohlenberg, C., Becker, M. H. G., Key, G., Flad, H.-D., and Gerdes, J. (1993) The cell proliferation-associated antigen of anti-body Ki-67: a very large, ubiquitous nuclear protein with numerous repeated elements, representing a new kind of cell-cycle-maintaining proteins. *J. Cell Biol.* **123,** 513–522.
8. Gerdes, J., Schwab, U., Lemke, H., and Stein, H. (1983) Production of a mouse MAb reactive with a human nuclear antigen associated with cell proliferation. *Int. J. Cancer* **31,** 13–20.
9. Gerdes, J., Lemke, H., Baisch, H., Wacker, H.-H., Schwab, U., and Stein, H. (1984) Cell-cycle analysis of a proliferation-associated human nuclear antigen defined by the MAb Ki-67. *J. Immunol.* **133,** 1710–1715.

10. Steck, K. and El-Naggar, A. K. (1994) Comparative flow cytometric analysis of Ki-67 and proliferating cell nuclear antigen (PCNA) in solid neoplasms. *Cytometry* **17,** 258–265.

11. Scott, R. J., Hall, P. A., Haldane, J. S., van Noorden, S., Price, Y., Lane, D. P., and Wright, N. A. (1991) A comparison of immunohistochemical markers of cell proliferation with experimentally determined growth fraction. *J. Pathol.* **165,** 173–178.

12. Key, G., Becker, M. H. G., Baron, B., Duchrow, M., Schluter, C., Flad, H.-D., and Gerdes, J. (1993) New Ki-67 equivalent murine monoclonal antibodies (MIB 1-3) generated against bacterially expressed parts of the Ki-67 cDNA containing three 66bp repetitive elements encoding for the Ki-67 epitope. *Lab Invest.* **68,** 629–635.

13. Wilson, G. D., Camplejohn, R. S., Martindale, C. A., Brock, A., Lane, D. P., and Barnes, D. M. (1992) Flow cytometric characterization of proliferating cell nuclear antigen using the MAb PC10. *Eur. J. Cancer* **28A,** 2010–2017.

14. Hall, P. A., Levison, D. A., Woods, A. L., Yu, C. C.-W., Kellock, D. B., Watkins, J. A., Barnes, D. M., Gillett, C. E., Camplejohn, R. S., Dover, R., Waseem, N. H., and Lane, D. P. (1990) Proliferating cell nuclear antigen localization in paraffin sections: an index of cell proliferation with evidence of deregulated expression in some neoplasms. *J. Pathol.* **162,** 285–294.

15. Prosperi, E., Stivala, N. A., Sala, E., Scovassi, A. I., and Bianchi, L. (1993) Proliferating cell nuclear antigen complex formation induced by ultraviolet irradiation in human quiescent fibroblasts as detected by immunostaining and flow cytometry. *Exp. Cell Res.* **205,** 320–325.

16. Landberg, G., Tan, E. M., and Roos, G. (1990) Flow cytometric multiparameter analysis of proliferating nuclear antigen/cyclin and Ki-67: a new view of the cell cycle. *Exp. Cell Res.* **187,** 11–118.

17. Landberg, G. and Roos, G. (1991) Expression of proliferating cell nuclear antigen (PCNA) and Ki-67 antigen in human malignant hematopoietic cells. *Acta Oncol.* **30,** 917–921.

18. Larsen, J. K., Christensen, I. J., Christiansen, J., and Mortensen, B. J. (1991) Washless double-staining of unfixed nuclei for flow cytometric analysis of DNA and a nuclear antigen (Ki-67 or bromodeoxyuridine). *Cytometry* **12,** 429–437.

37

Sorting of Human Peripheral Blood T-Cell Subsets Using Immunomagnetic Beads

Eddie C. Y. Wang

1. Introduction

Immunomagnetic beads are uniform, polymer particles coated with a polystyrene shell that provides both a smooth, hydrophobic surface to facilitate absorption of molecules, such as antibodies, and surface hydroxyl groups that allow covalent chemical binding of other bioreactive molecules, such as streptavidin, lectins, and peptides. Iron (III) oxide (Fe_2O_3) deposited in the core gives the beads superparamagnetic properties that lead to consistent and reproducible reactions to a magnetic field without permanent magnetization of the particles. These are the two qualities on which immunomagnetic separation (IMS) depends.

IMS is a fast, simple method for separating a range of targets, and principally involves the removal of an indirectly magnetized target by a permanent magnet. "Magnetization" is achieved using beads coated with a target-specific, bioreactive molecule, and removal occurs by the application of a neodynium-iron boron or similar magnet. With respect to cell-sorting, "target-specific, bioreactive molecules" consist of monoclonal antibodies (MAbs) specific to certain cell subsets. Thus, OKT8 and OKT4 (used in this chapter) are mouse antihuman MAbs to the T-cell markers CD8 and CD4 that target the cytotoxic/suppressor and helper T-cell subsets, respectively.

Although this chapter will only discuss IMS in relation to cell-sorting, this approach has also been adapted for DNA sequencing (1), purification of DNA binding proteins (2), immobilization and isolation of nucleic acids (3), tissue-typing (4,5), quantification of lymphocyte subsets directly from blood (6), bone marrow T-cell depletion (7), depletion of malignant neuroblastoma cells from

From: *Methods in Molecular Biology, Vol. 80: Immunochemical Protocols, 2nd ed.*
Edited by: J. D. Pound © Humana Press Inc., Totowa, NJ

bone marrow *(8,9)*, and the selective enrichment of microorganisms *(10,11)* and other cell types, such as Langerhans cells *(12)*, antigen-specific B-cells *(13)*, endothelial cells *(14)*, villous trophoblast *(15)*, reticulocytes *(16)*, osteoclasts *(17)*, epithelial cells *(18)*, megakaryocytes *(19)*, or anterior pituitary cells *(20)*. IMS is, therefore, a highly versatile procedure.

The advantages of this technique over other separation methods can be summarized as follows:

1. The procedure is very rapid.
2. Beads are easy to work with under sterile conditions.
3. The procedure is cheaper than fluorescence-activated cell-sorting (FACS).
4. The magnetic particles, once coated, may be stored for at least several months at 4°C.
5. Both positive and negative selection of cells can be achieved.
6. Unlike FACS, cell viability can be measured during the separation procedure using ethidium bromide and acridine orange.
7. The method can be used in large-scale isolations.

There are two major disadvantages: first, isolation of subsets defined by more than one cell-surface marker is difficult to achieve with immunomagnetic beads and requires two positive selection steps. In these circumstances, although FACS is more expensive and is performed on a smaller scale, the ability to define markers with different fluorescent dyes allows a one-step procedure that gives rise to very high-purity isolations. Second, the full effects of having polymer beads in close association with cells is still unknown, and isolation still involves the use of MAb, which may trigger functional changes in target cells. IMS has enormous potential, but understanding of bead–cell interactions is currently limited. A related product that uses the same principles as IMS, but employs smaller beads and magnetic columns for separation, is the magnetic cell-sorting (MACS) system from Miltenyi Biotec Inc. (Auburn, CA), details of which are given in Note 1. That method is not discussed here, but its use for positive selection warrants serious consideration.

IMS consists of the following steps:

1. Preparation of beads.
2. Preparation of cells for use with either immunomagnetic beads preconjugated with MAbs or immunomagnetic beads coated with antimouse IgG antibodies.
3. Immunomagnetic separation.

Ideal conditions for cell separation using immunomagnetic beads differ for the cell types and antibodies employed, and can only be identified by experimentation. This chapter gives sample protocols for isolating subsets of human peripheral blood T-cells and discusses technical points that may be of wider relevance to cell separation by this approach.

2. Materials

1. Immunomagnetic beads: Dynabeads M-450 coated with sheep antimouse IgG, sheep or rat antimouse IgG subclass (Fc-specific), or preconjugated with MAbs specific for CD4 and CD8 (available from Dynal, Wirral, Merseyside, UK). A broad range of other preconjugated beads are now supplied by Dynal and are summarized in Note 2. They will remain stable for up to 1 yr when stored at 2–8°C. Thiomersal (0.01% [w/v]), or sodium azide (0.02% [w/v]) is used as preservative. **Hazard warning:** Both sodium azide and thiomersal are irritants to the skin and eyes, and are toxic if inhaled or ingested. Handle with care.
2. Phosphate-buffered saline (PBS), pH 7.4: 8.0 g of NaCl, 0.2 g of KH_2PO_4, 2.9 g of $Na_2HPO_4 \cdot 12H_2O$, 0.2 g of KCl, and 0.2 g of NaN_3. Make up to 1 L with sterile, distilled water. Alternatively, PBS tablets can be obtained from Sigma or Oxoid, Unipath Ltd., Basingstoke, UK. Each tablet is dissolved in a known volume (as recommended by suppliers) of sterile, distilled water. Store at room temperature.
3. PBS/BSA: PBS containing 0.1% bovine serum albumin (BSA). Store at 4°C.
4. Hank's Balanced Salt Solution (HBSS), pH 7.4 (Gibco, Paisley, Scotland). Store at 15–30°C.
5. Permanent magnet: Dynal Magnetic Particle Concentrator (MPC-1, MPC-2, MPC-6, or MPC-Q) (Dynal, UK), or equivalent magnet (e.g., from Biolab, Belgium).
6. 0.05M Tris-HCl buffer, pH 9.5. Store at 4°C.
7. Specific monoclonal or polyclonal antibody to cell subsets. OKT8 (Leu 2) recognizes the CD8 marker on cytotoxic/suppressor T-cells. OKT4 (Leu 3) recognizes the CD4 marker on helper T-cells. Store at 4°C.
8. Heparin: Make to 50 U/mL with PBS. Use 5 U/mL of blood. Store at 4°C.
9. Ficoll-Hypaque: Ficoll and sodium metrizoate/diatrizoate solution of density 1.077 g/mL, supplied as Ficoll Paque (Pharmacia), Histopaque (Sigma), or Lymphoprep (Nycomed AS, Pharma Diagnostic Division, Oslo, Norway), Store at 4°C protected from light.
10. Ethidium bromide/acridine orange: stock solutions consist of 50 mg of ethidium bromide and 15 mg of acridine orange, dissolved in 1 mL of 95% ethanol and made up to 50 mL with distilled water. Store at –20°C.

    For use in viability counts, stocks are diluted 1:100 with PBS. Stored at room temperature in the dark. The solution has a shelf-life of at least 2 mo. **Hazard warning:** both ethidium bromide and acridine orange have mutagenic properties, are combustible, toxic, and irritants to the skin, eyes, and respiratory system. Handle with care.

3. Methods
3.1. Preparation of Beads

The following protocol should be used to remove preservatives, such as thiomersal or sodium azide, which may affect cell viability.

1. Suspend the immunomagnetic beads using a pipet or shake lightly.
2. Take out an appropriate volume of beads. For depletion, recommended bead:target ratios range from 10:1–40:1. For positive selection, a bead:target cell ratio of 3:1 is sufficient.
3. Make up to 10 mL with PBS/BSA.
4. Collect beads using a strong permanent magnet (the magnets suggested in Section 2. are supplied with useful holding devices for test tubes/universal bottles). This process takes approx 2 min.
5. Discard the supernatant while the tube is still held against the magnet.
6. Repeat three times, and resuspend in the original volume in PBS/BSA.

3.2. Preparation of Cells

3.2.1. Preparation of Cells for Use with Immunomagnetic Beads Preconjugated with MAb

Prepare peripheral blood mononuclear cells (PBMC) from heparinized blood, by Ficoll-Hypaque density centrifugation *(21)* as follows:

1. Carefully layer anticoagulated blood onto Ficoll-Hypaque (in a 4:3 ratio of blood to Ficoll-Hypaque), such that there is no mixing of blood and density separation medium. After centrifugation at 800g for 15 min without braking, mononuclear cells form a distinct band at the interface between the sample layer and Ficoll-Hypaque, whereas erythrocytes aggregate and sediment. Harvest mononuclear cells using a Pasteur pipet.
2. Wash PBMC three times with 10 mL of PBS by spinning down first at 800g for 10 min, and then twice at 400g to remove excess Ficoll-Hypaque and platelets from the sample. Resuspend the cells at $\leq 10^7$/mL in PBS/BSA.
3. Make viability counts by diluting a 50-μL sample of cells with an equal volume of ethidium bromide/acridine orange. Under UV illumination, viable cells appear green, and nonviable cells, red *(22)*.

The cells are now ready for use with immunomagnetic beads preconjugated with MAb.

3.2.2. Preparation of Cells for Use with Immunomagnetic Beads Precoated with Sheep Antimouse IgG

In order to label antigen-positive cells, treat PBMC prepared as in Section 3.2.1. with OKT4 or OKT8 MAb of the appropriate specificity as follows:

1. Resuspend PBMC at 4×10^7 cells/mL in PBS in a universal bottle.
2. Add sufficient MAb to saturate the antigenic binding sites on the cells (*see* Note 3).
3. Incubate at 4°C for 25 min.
4. Wash with PBS by centrifuging at 400g for 5 min to pellet cells. Aspirate off supernatant, and resuspend the cells in 5 mL of PBS. Repeat this twice to remove excess antibody.
5. Resuspend the cells at $\leq 10^7$/mL in PBS/BSA.

3.3. Immunomagnetic Separation (see Note 4)

1. Add an appropriate number of prepared beads (*see* Section 3.1.) to the cells prepared as described in Sections 3.2.1. or 3.2.2. For depletion, a bead:target cell ratio of 10:1–40:1 is recommended (*see* Notes 5 and 6 for discussion on separation efficiency). For positive selection, a bead:cell ratio of 3:1 is sufficient.
2. Incubate at 4–20°C for 30–60 min, with slow tilting and rotation (*see* Notes 1 and 2).
3. Make up to 5 mL with HBSS.
4. Remove beads by applying the magnet for 2 min to the side of the tube and pouring off the supernatant. To obtain higher yields, wash the beads twice by adding another 5 mL of HBSS and repeat the separation.
5. Perform the separation procedure on the supernatant to remove as many carried over beads as possible.
6. A small sample should be passed through a flow cytometer to assess the efficiency of depletion.

3.4. Positive Selection Using Immunomagnetic Beads (see Notes 7 and 8)

Positively selected cells attached to the beads after incubation can be collected by overnight incubation at 37°C and then application of a magnet to remove the dissociated beads.

An alternative approach for some human cell-surface markers (CD4, CD8, CD19, and CD34) is the use of "Detachabead," which is an anti-Fab polyclonal antiserum that causes dissociation of bound MAbs preconjugated to Dynabeads (*see* Note 9). For protocols detailing use of Detachabead *see* refs. *23–33.*

4. Notes

1. MACS (Miltenyi Biotec) uses considerably smaller beads (50-nm diameter) made of iron oxide and polysaccharide *(34)*. Beads can be supplied preconjugated with MAbs specific for CD3, CD4, CD8, CD11b (monocytes, granulocytes, and NK cells), CD14, CD15, CD16, CD19, CD33 (myeloid cells), CD34, CD45RA, CD45RO, and CD71. MACS has been used to isolate a broad range of human cell types *(35–41)*. These smaller beads have the following advantages when compared to Dynabeads:
   a. Reduced carryover.
   b. Less physical disturbance to the cells during separation.
   c. According to the manufacturers, nontoxic and biodegradable.
   This alternative approach to IMS may therefore resolve some of the problems encountered using Dynabeads.
2. Dynal supplies Dynabeads conjugated with MAbs to the following human markers: CD2 (pan T-cell), CD3 (pan T-cell), CD19 (pan B-cell), CD4, CD8, CD14 (monocytes/macrophages), CD15 (myeloid cells), CD34 (hematopoietic progenitor cells), CD45 (pan leukocyte), CD71 (transferrin receptor), and antihuman MHC II. In addition, Dynal also supplies Dynabeads conjugated with polyclonal

Abs specific for mouse IgG, rat IgG, and rabbit IgG, and MAb specific for mouse IgG1, IgG2a, IgG2b, IgG3, and IgM. The majority of MAb to human cell markers are derived from mouse. Therefore, the range of Dynabeads conjugated with secondary antibodies allows cell-sorting of most human cell subsets. This has virtually eliminated the need to adsorb MAbs physically onto uncoated or "tosylactivated" Dynabeads (beads with a surface activated by tosyl chloride that triggers bonding via secondary-OH groups, thus allowing chemical binding to protein ligands). However, detailed methods describing the use of tosylactivated beads can be obtained directly from Dynal (42). The conjugation of MAbs to uncoated beads has been described (43), but it should be noted when considering this method that only IgM, and not IgG, results in efficient antibody–antigen complex formation, probably because of the effects of steric hindrance on IgG antibody–antigen interactions.

3. This will depend on the affinity of the MAb and the density of the antigen on the cells, but a final concentration of 5 μg/mL will be adequate for most commercially available MAbs. If necessary, the concentration can be determined empirically by using serial dilutions of MAb and analyzing uptake by flow cytometry (*see* Chapter 33).

4. Sequential depletions may be more efficient. This involves two or more separation procedures using decreased bead:cell ratios and shorter incubation periods, e.g., a 3:1 bead:cell ratio repeated three times with 20-min incubation periods at 4–20°C. This gives around 95% or greater depletion and use of lower bead:cell ratios may decrease carryover effects.

5. A major problem when using IMS to deplete cell subsets is the loss of cells owing to nonspecific binding and entrapment with the beads during separation. This loss can be as high as 70% if incubations are performed at room temperature. Nonspecific binding is reduced at lower temperatures, e.g., 4°C, though incubation periods have to be increased correspondingly to allow for the slower kinetics of interaction (*see* Figs. 1 and 2). However, high temperatures favor depletion of cells expressing very low levels of the specific antigen of interest (e.g., CD8); these remain in suspension when using incubations at 4°C, independently of the number of separations carried out. Incubations at 37°C lead to high levels of nonspecific binding. The optimal temperature for separation is dependent on the individual cell, antibody, and protocol used in addition to the goal of any particular experiment.

   Carriage of some cells with beads by entrapment is almost inevitable. This can be kept to a minimum by diluting mixtures before each separation procedure. Washing and application of the magnet on bead–cell mixtures several times after initial separation also help recapture as many carried cells as possible. Even with these precautions, between 30 and 50% of the original number of cells is usually lost.

6. A small minority of beads are not captured by the magnet and remain in the supernatant; such residual may pose a problem if a cell population depleted by IMS is to be cultured. Although the beads will be phagocytosed by any macroph-

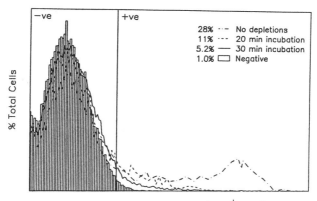

Fig. 1. Effect of incubation time on deletion of CD8+ cells. PBMC were prepared from anticoagulated peripheral blood and stained with OKT8 as in Section 3.2. Beads were added at a 20:1 bead:target cell ratio. The mixture was left for varying incubation times (10, 20, or 30 min) at room temperature, after which samples were made up to 10 mL in HBSS and a magnet applied for 2 min to gather bead:CD8+ cell rosettes. The supernatant was collected, cells spun down, resuspended in 150 µL of PBS, and stained with antimouse Ig fluorescein isothiocyanate (FITC)-conjugated secondary antibody. After 25 min of incubation at room temperature, samples were washed three times with PBS and passed through an EPICS-Profile flow cytometer (Coulter) to measure the CD8+ cells remaining. Negative controls included an unstained sample (negative) and a sample stained with the antimouse Ig FITC conjugate only (not shown). The positive control was a sample that had not been passed through a depletion cycle (no depletions). Results show the total depletion of cells expressing high levels of CD8 independent of the incubation period, but increased depletion of cells expressing low levels of CD8 with the 30-min incubation (solid line) compared to 20 min (dashed line). However, a small percentage of low expressing CD8+ cells still remain.

ages present, their numbers can be minimized by applying the separation procedure to the supernatant a number of times. The use of HBSS for these washes rather, than PBS has been reported to give significantly better yields, though the reason for this is unclear. The use of lower bead:cell ratios (Fig. 2) with a greater number of separation procedures should also be considered (Fig. 3). Although this would increase total loss of cells by nonspecific binding and carriage with the beads, there would be fewer beads carried over with the supernatant, resulting in "cleaner" cultures.

7. Overnight incubation at 4°C causes beads to dissociate from positively selected cells. However, up to 50% of the selected cells can be lost when magnetic separation is performed, resulting in low yields of bead-free cells. Furthermore, cell viability can be reduced following close contact with the beads. In the author's laboratory, it has been found that positively selected T-cells often do not survive

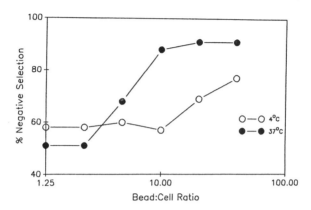

Fig. 2. Effect of temperature and bead:cell ratio on negative selection. PBMC were prepared from anticoagulated peripheral blood as described in Section 3.2. Cells were either unstained, incubated with excess OKT8, or excess antimouse Ig FITC-conjugated secondary antibody (control for nonspecific binding of this Ab). Beads were added at varying bead:cell ratios (from 40–1.25:1). Mixtures were left for 20 min with agitation every 5 min at 4°C (open circle) or 37°C (filled circle). Samples were then made up to 10 mL in HBSS and a magnet applied for 2 min to gather bead:CD8⁺ cell rosettes. The supernatant was collected, cells spun down, resuspended in 150 μL, and stained with antimouse Ig FITC-conjugated secondary antibody, using the same procedure as with OKT8. Samples were washed three times with PBS and passed through an EPICS-Profile to measure the CD8⁺ cells remaining. Percentage negative selection was calculated as follows: (%CD8⁺ cells in depleted samples –% + ve cells in antimouse Ig FITC control)/(%CD8⁺ cells in undepleted samples –% + ve cells in antimouse Ig FITC control) × 100. Results show a marked increase in depletion as the bead:cell ratio and the temperature increases.

longer than 48 h in culture after shedding beads, although use of apparently the same protocol has also yielded T-cells capable of good, though possibly reduced, proliferative responses to stimulants, such as OKT3 and phytohemagglutinin (PHA). The responses of positively selected cells have not been thoroughly investigated, but a number of groups have reported that cell function and viability are not adversely affected by positive selection using IMS (e.g., ref. *44*).

8. The use of enzymes, such as papain, to cleave bead:cell rosettes has also been investigated: chymopapain, used at 200 U/mL of cells (10⁷/mL in TC199 tissue-culture medium) for 10 min at 37°C, has been found to be most effective and least toxic to KG1a human leukemia cells, giving 100% recovery of viable cells *(45)*.

9. Detachabead is available from Dynal for positive selection of CD4⁺, CD8⁺, CD19⁺, and CD34⁺ cell subsets *(23–30)*. This reagent has also been used to select positively for CD45⁺ cells *(31)*, HLA-DR⁺ Langerhans cells *(32)*, and c-kit⁺ human lung mast cells *(33)*. However, its suitability for dissociation of beads coated with MAbs of other specificities should always be assessed by the user in a pilot study.

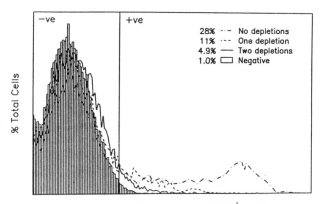

Log Green Fluorescence (CD8⁺cells)

Fig. 3. Effect of number of cycles of depletion on deletion of CD8⁺ cells. PBMC were prepared from anticoagulated peripheral blood as described in Section 3.2. Cells were either unstained, incubated with excess OKT8, or excess antimouse Ig FITC-conjugated secondary antibody (control for nonspecific binding of this Ab). Beads were added at a 20:1 bead:cell ratio. Samples were incubated for 20 min at 4°C with agitation every 5 min, and then made up to 10 mL in HBSS and a magnet applied for 2 min to gather bead:CD8⁺ cell rosettes. The supernatant was collected, cells spun down, resuspended in 150 µL, and beads added to the two depletion samples for a second 20-min incubation period and washes (as above). Antimouse Ig FITC-conjugated secondary antibody was then added, and incubated at room temperature for 25 min. Samples were washed three times with PBS and passed through an EPICS-Profile to measure the CD8⁺ cells remaining. Negative controls included an unstained sample (negative) and an antimouse Ig FITC-conjugated secondary antibody stain only (not shown). Positive control was an OKT8-stained undepleted sample (no depletion). Results show that two cycles of depletion (solid line) reduce the numbers of low-expressing CD8⁺ cells remaining compared with one cycle (dashed line).

References

1. Hultman, T., Stahl, S., Hornes, E., and Uhlen, M. (1989) Direct solid phase sequencing of genomic and plasmid DNA using magnetic beads as solid support. *Nucleic Acids Res.* **17,** 4937–4946.
2. Gabrielsen, O. S., Hornes, E., Kornes, L., Ruet, A., and Oyen, T. B. (1989) Magnetic DNA affinity purification of yeast transcription factor T—a new purification principle for the ultrarapid isolation of near homogenous factor. *Nucleic Acids Res.* **17,** 6253–6267.
3. Uhlen, M. (1989) Magnetic separation of DNA. *Nature* **340,** 733,734.
4. Hansen, T. and Hannestad, K. (1989) Direct HLA typing by rosetting with immunomagnetic beads coated with specific antibodies. *J. Immunogenet.* **16,** 137–139.

5. Laundy, G. J., Peberdy, M., Klouda, P. T., and Bradley, A. (1989) Applications of automated simultaneous double fluorescence (SDF). II. HLA class I phenotyping using immunomagnetically separated T-lymphocytes. *J. Immunogenet.* **16,** 141–148.
6. Brinchmann, J. E., Leivestad, T., and Vartdal, F. (1989) Quantification of lymphocyte subsets based on positive immunomagnetic selection of cells directly from blood. *J. Immunogenet.* **16,** 177–183.
7. Gee, A. P., Mansour, V., and Weiler, M. (1989) T-cell depletion of human bone marrow. *J. Immunogenet.* **16,** 103–115.
8. Combaret, V., Favrot, M. C., Chauvin, F., Bouffet, E., Philip, I., and Philip, T. (1989) Immunomagnetic depletion of malignant cells from autologous bone marrow graft: from experimental models to clinical trials. *J. Immunogenet.* **16,** 125–136.
9. Kemshead, J. T., Heath, F., Gibson, F. M., Katz, F., Richmond, F., Treleaven, J., and Ugelstad, J. (1986) Magnetic microspheres and monoclonal antibodies for the depletion of neuroblastoma cells from bone marrow: experiences, improvements and observations. *Br. J. Cancer* **54,** 771–778.
10. Lund, A., Helleman, A. L., and Vartdal, F. (1988) Rapid isolation of K88+ Escherichia coli by using immunomagnetic particles. *J. Clin. Microbiol.* **26,** 2572–2575.
11. Widjojoatmodjo, M. N., Fluit, A. C., Torensma, R., and Verhoef, J. (1993) Comparison of immunomagnetic beads coated with protein A, protein G, or goat antimouse immunoglobulins. *J. Immunol. Methods* **165,** 11–19.
12. Schmitt, D. A., Hanau, D., and Cazenaze, J-P. (1989) Isolation of epidermal Langerhans cells. *J. Immunogenet.* **16,** 157–168.
13. Ossendorp, F. A., Bruning, P. F., van den Brink, J. A. M., and de Boer, M. (1989) Efficient selection of high affinity B-cell hybidomas using antigen-coated magnetic beads. *J. Immunol. Methods* **120,** 191–200.
14. Jackson, C. J., Garbett, P. K., Nissen, B., and Schrieber, L. (1990) Binding of human endothelium to Ulex europaeus I-coated Dynabeads: application to the isolation of microvascular endothelium. *J. Cell Science* **96,** 257–262.
15. Loke, Y. W., Gardner, L., and Grabowska, A. (1989) Isolation of extravillous trophoblast cells by attachment to laminin-coated magnetic beads. *Placenta* **10,** 407–415.
16. Brun, A., Gaudernack, G., and Sandberg, S. (1990) A new method for isolation of reticulocytes: positive selection of human reticulocytes by immunomagnetic separation. *Blood* **76,** 2397–2403.
17. Collin-Osdoby, P., Gursler, M. J., Webber, D., and Osdoby, P. (1991) Osteoclast-specific monoclonal antibodies coupled to magnetic beads provide a rapid and efficient method of purifying avian osteoclasts. *J. Bone Miner. Res.* **6,** 1353–1365.
18. Joplin, R., Strain, A. J., and Neuberger, J. M. (1989) Immuno-isolation and culture of biliary epithelial cells from normal human liver. *In Vitro Cell Dev. Biol.* **25,** 1189–1192.
19. Tanaka, H., Ishida, Y., Kaneko, T., and Matsumoto, N. (1989) Isolation of human megakaryocytes by immunomagnetic beads. *Br. J. Hematol.* **73,** 18–22.
20. Wynick, D. and Bloom, S. R. (1990) Magnetic bead separation of anterior pituitary cells. *Neuroendocrinology* **52,** 560–565.

21. Timonen, T., Ortaldo, J. R., and Herberman, R. H. (1981) Characteristics of human large granular lymphocytes and relationships to natural killer and K cells. *J. Exp. Med.* **153,** 569–582.

22. Parks, D. R., Bryan, V. M., Oi, V. I., and Herzenberg, L. A. (1979) Antigen-specific identification and cloning of hybridomas with a fluorescent-activated cell sorter (FACS). *Proc. Natl. Acad. Sci. USA* **76,** 1962–1966.

23. Rasmussen, A. M., Smeland, E., Erikstein, B. K., Caignault, L., and Funderud, S. (1992) A new method for detachment of Dynabeads from positively selected B lymphocytes. *J. Immunol. Methods* **146,** 195–202.

24. Schandene, L., Namias, B., Crusiaux, A., Lybin, M., Devos, R., Velu, T., Capel, P., Bellens, R., and Goldman, M. (1993) IL-5 in post-traumatic eosinophilic pleural effusion. *Clin. Exp. Immunol.* **93,** 115–119.

25. Santiago-Schwartz, F., Belilos, E., Diamond, B., and Carsons, S. E. (1992) TNF in combination with GM-CSF enhances the differentiation of neonatal cord blood stem cells into dendritic cells and macrophages. *J. Leuk. Biol.* **52,** 274–281.

26. Jenkinson, E. J., Anderson, G., and Owen, J. J. T. (1992) Studies on T cell maturation on defined thymic stromal cell populations *in vitro*. *J. Exp. Med.* **176,** 845–853.

27. Wengler, G. S., Allen, R. C., Parolini, O., Smith, H., and Conley, M. E. (1993) Nonrandom X chromosome inactivation in natural killer cells from obligate carriers of X-linked severe combined immunodeficiency. *J. Immunol.* **150,** 700–704.

28. Ljungquist, C., Lundeberg, J., Rasmussen, A.-M., Hornes, E., and Uhlen, M. (1993) Immobilization and recovery of fusion proteins and B-lymphocyte cells using magnetic separation. *DNA Cell Biol.* **12,** 191–197.

29. Schwella, N., Zingsen, J., and Eckstein, R. (1992) Effective derosetting of mononuclear cells isolated by immunomagnetic beads. *Infusionstherapie* **19,** 149–150.

30. Geretti, A. M., van Els, C. A. C. M., Poelen, M. C. M., and Osterhaus, A. D. M. E. (1993) Preservation of phenotype and function of positively selected virus-specific CD8+ T lymphocytes following anti-Fab detachment from immunomagnetic beads. *J. Immunol. Methods* **161,** 129–133.

31. Anderson, G., Jenkinson, E. J., Moore, N. C., and Owen, J. J. T. (1993) MHC class II-positive epithelium and mesenchyme cells are both required for T-cell development in the thymus. *Nature* **362,** 70–73.

32. Barrett, A. W., Ross, D. A., and Goodacre, J. A. (1993) Purified human oral mucosal Langerhans cells function as accessory cells *in vitro*. *Clin. Exp. Immunol.* **92,** 158–163.

33. Okayama, Y., Hunt, T. C., Kassel, O., Ashman, L. K., and Church, M. K. (1994) Assessment of the anti-*c-kit* MAb YB5. B8 in affinity magnetic enrichment of human lung mast cells. *J. Immunol. Methods* **169,** 153–161.

34. Miltenyi, S., Muller, W., Weichel, W., and Radbruch, A. (1990) High gradient magnetic cell separation with MACS. *Cytometry* **14,** 231–238.

35. Abts, H., Emmerich, M., Miltenyi, S., Radbruch, A., and Tesch, H. (1989) CD20 positive human B lymphocytes separated with the magnetic cell sorter (MACS) can be induced to proliferate and antibody secretion *in vitro*. *J. Immunol. Methods* **125,** 19–28.

36. Kleine, H. D., Schienichen, Lux, E., Poliwoda, H., and Freund, M. (1993) A constant flux system using "magnetic cell separator" (MACS) for highly efficient T-cell depletion. *Anal. Cell. Pathol.* **5,** 125–128.

37. Koegler, G., Capdeville, A. B., Hauch, M., Bruester, H. T., Goebel, U., Wernet, P., and Burdach, S. (1990) High efficiency of a new immunological magnetic cell-sorting method for T cell depletion of human bone marrow. *Bone Marrow Transplant.* **6,** 163–168.

38. Manyonda, I. T., Soltys, A. J., and Hay, F. C. (1992) A critical evaluation of the magnetic cell sorter and its use in the positive and negative selection of CD45RO$^+$ cells. *J. Immunol. Methods* **149,** 1–10.

39. Pflueger, E., Mueller, E. A., and Anderer, F. A. (1990) Preservation of cytotoxic function during multicycle immunomagnetic cell separations of human NK cells using a new type of magnetic bead. *J. Immunol. Methods* **129,** 165–173.

40. Schmitz, J., Petrasch, S., van Lunzen, J., Racz, P., Kleine, H. D., Hufert, F., Kern, P., Schmitz, H., and Tenner-Racz, K. (1993) Optimizing follicular dendritic cell isolation by discontinuous gradient centrifugation and use of the magnetic cell sorter (MACS). *J. Immunol. Methods* **159,** 189–196.

41. Semple, J. W., Allen, D., Chang, W., Castaldi, P., and Freedman, J. (1993) Rapid separation of CD4$^+$ and CD19$^+$ lymphocyte populations from human peripheral blood by a magnetic activated cell sorter (MACS). *Cytometry* **14,** 955–960.

42. Dynal Ltd. (1996) Cell separation and protein purification, in *Technical Handbook,* 2nd ed.

43. Guadernack, G., Leivestad, T., Ugelstad, J., and Thorsby, E. (1986) Isolation of pure functionally active CD8$^+$ T cells: positive selection with monoclonal antibodies directly conjugated to monosized magnetic microspheres. *J. Immunol. Methods* **90,** 179–187.

44. Leivestad, T., Guadernack, G., Ugelstad, J., Vartdal, F., and Thornsby, E. (1987) Isolation of pure and functionally active T4 and T8 cells by positive selection with antibody-coated monosize magnetic microspheres. *Transplantation Proc.* **19,** 265–267.

45. Civin, C. I., Strauss, L. C., Fackler, M. J., Trischmann, T. M., Wiley, J. M., and Loken, M. R. (1990) Positive stem cell selection—basic science. *Prog. Clin. Biol. Res.* **333,** 387–402.

38

Preparation and Use
of Nonradioactive Hybridization Probes

Victor T.-W. Chan

1. Introduction

1.1. Preparation of Nonradioactive Hybridization Probes

Molecular hybridization is a useful technique for identifying specific target sequences even when they are present as a single copy in a complex population of highly heterogeneous gene sequences. It can be performed either on a solid matrix on which pure DNA (or RNA) is bound (blot hybridization) or on tissue section *(in situ* hybridization). Until recently, the probes used in hybridization were usually labeled with radioisotopes. However, the short half-life, disposal, and safety problems of radioactive probes stimulated the development of nonradioactive hybridization techniques. In these, the probes are labeled with nonradioactive reporter molecules, which can be haptens, proteins, digoxigenin, biotin, and so forth. These reporter molecules can then be detected by enzyme-labeled antibodies or streptavidin (in the case of biotinylated probes). Of these reporter molecules, biotin and digoxigenin have several advantages over the other because of their small size. Therefore, they minimally interfere with hybridization efficiency. In addition, the high affinity of the binding of biotin and streptavidin ($K_d = 10^{-15}M$) is almost equivalent to covalent bonds. In fact, the biotin system was the first nonradioactive hybridization technique sensitive enough for routine use on blot hybridization *(1)* and *in situ* hybridization *(2)*.

In the original system, biotin is attached to the deoxy analog of rUTP via a spacer arm. Biotinylated dUTP is incorporated into DNA strands by a conventional labeling reaction, nick translation, which was also widely used to pre-

From: *Methods in Molecular Biology, Vol. 80: Immunochemical Protocols, 2nd ed.*
Edited by: J. D. Pound © Humana Press Inc., Totowa, NJ

pare radioactive probes *(3)*. The presence of a spacer arm between biotin and dUTP separates these two molecules far apart, and thus, reduces the steric hindrance caused between them. Therefore, the efficiency of labeling, hybridization, and detection is greatly increased.

The principle of nick translation *(3)* is based on the ability of deoxyribonuclease I (DNase I) to attack each strand of the DNA molecule independently in a random fashion, resulting in single-stranded nicks at low enzyme concentration in the presence of Mg^{2+}. *Escherichia coli* DNA polymerase I (Pol I) synthesizes DNA complementary to the intact strand in a 5'–3' direction using the 3'-OH termini of the nicks as primers. At the same time, the 5'–3' exonuclease activity of Pol I removes nucleotides in the same direction. The result of these two enzyme reactions is the replacement of the original nucleotides with new nucleotides, and the movement of the nicks in a 5'–3' direction along the DNA strands whose nucleotide sequences remain unchanged. If one of the deoxyribonucleotide triphosphates included in the reaction is labeled, the original nucleotide will be replaced by labeled counterparts and the DNA is thus labeled. Since DNase I introduces nicks to both strands in a random fashion, theoretically, the probe is uniformly and almost completely labeled. Practically, nick translation is, however, less reproducible simply because it depends on the combination of the reactions of two enzymes that may be selectively inhibited by different contaminants in the DNA samples. Under optimal conditions, this method can be used to label all different forms of double-stranded DNA molecules with very high sensitivity.

Biotinylated dUTP can also be used to label DNA probes by a different method, namely random-primed labeling *(4)*. The principle of this method is based on the reannealing of hexadeoxyribonucleotide primers, which have random specificity, to the single-stranded (denatured) DNA molecules. The DNA to be labeled has to be linearized and denatured before the strands are used as templates in the labeling reaction. The complementary strands are synthesized from the 3'OH termini of the reannealed hexanucleotides by the Klenow fragment of *E. coli* DNA polymerase I. The primers reanneal at random sites of the template strands, so that the synthesis of the complementary strands is primed at random positions. If one of the deoxyribonucleoside triphosphates present in the reaction mixture is labeled, the newly synthesized strands will become labeled by the incorporation of the labeled nucleotides. The end product of this reaction is a mixture of unlabeled (template) and labeled (synthesized) DNA strands. However, this method is more reliable and reproducible than nick translation, because only the Klenow fragment of Pol I is used, which is rather resistant to the inhibition caused by various contaminants in the DNA samples. This method can only be used to label linear DNA molecules. Supercoiled DNA has to be linearized before being labeled. In general, the sensitivity of probes labeled by this method can also be very high.

Another development of the biotin system is the synthesis of biotinylated UTP that can be used to prepare single-stranded biotinylated RNA probes. The success of this technique is based on two important components: (1) the synthesis of a biotinylated derivative of rUTP, and (2) the fact that this derivative of rUTP is a good substrate for T3 and T7 RNA polymerase (but not SP6 RNA polymerase). The DNA to be transcribed is cloned into a vector containing phage transcription promoters (e.g., T3 and T7) that can initiate the in vitro transcription of the DNA insert in the presence of the respective phage RNA polymerase. In some cases, two different phage transcription promoters are placed on either side of the polylinker cloning region of the vector in opposite orientation, so they can initiate the transcription of the coding and noncoding strands of the DNA insert, respectively. In general, hybrids of target sequences and RNA probes have a higher melting temperature T_m) than that of DNA probes. Furthermore, after hybridization, the nonspecifically bound RNA probes can be selectively removed by RNase treatment. All these turn out to be the advantages of this method, which enhance its sensitivity and specificity.

Soon after the demonstration of the general utility of the biotin system in molecular hybridization, a photoactivatable biotin analog (photobiotin) was synthesized *(5)*. A cationic spacer arm is placed between a photoactivatable group and biotin to enhance the efficiency of labeling. The photoactivatable group of this molecule is extremely reactive on exposure to light and with a wide range of chemical groups. Therefore, it can be used to label various biomolecules (e.g., DNA, RNA, and protein).

In addition to biotin, a digoxigenylated derivative of dUTP was also synthesized. This derivative of dUTP can be incorporated into DNA by Pol I (or the Klenow fragment of Pol I). Therefore, digoxigenin-labeled DNA probes can be prepared by nick translation or random primed-labeling methods developed for the biotin system. It is almost certain that more nonradioactive alternatives to biotin and digoxigenin will be developed in the future. Chemiluminescent methods for nonradioactive probe detection are now widely being used.

Chemically modified DNAs can also be used as hybridization probes, provided that the modification does not interfere with the formation of hybrid DNA molecules. A psoralen biotin label has also been developed. Psoralen is a photoactivable agent that can intercalates into single- or double-stranded nucleic acids. On irradiation at 365 nm, it will covalently bind to the probes. This labeling reaction is simple and straightforward. However, the reagents for labeling and detection are only available in a kit format.

2. Materials

2.1. Nick Translation

1. Nucleotides/buffer mixes:
   a. Nucleotides/buffer mix I (for dUTP analog): 0.2 mM dATP, 0.2 mM dCTP, 0.2 mM dGTP in 500 mM Tris-HCl, pH 7.5, containing 50 mM MgCl$_2$, 10 mM β-mercaptoethanol; or
   b. Nucleotides/buffer mix II (for dATP analog): 0.2 mM dTTP, 0.2 mM dCTP, 0.2 mM dGTP in 500 mM Tris-HCl, pH 7.5, containing 50 mM MgCl$_2$, 10 mM β-mercaptoethanol.
2. Enzyme mix: 0.5 U of DNA polymerase I/μL, 50 pg of DNase I/μL in 100 mM KHPO$_4$, pH 6.5, containing 1 mM dithiothreitol (DTT), 500 μg of BSA/mL, and 50% glycerol.
3. Analogs:
   a. dUTP analog: 0.2 mM Biotin-dUTP, or 0.2 mM digoxigenin-dUTP in 50 mM Tris-HCl, pH 7.5; or
   b. ATP analog: 0.2 mM Biotin-7-dATP in 50 mM Tris-HCl, pH 7.5.
4. Template DNA.
5. TE Buffer: 10 mM Tris-HCl, 1 mM EDTA, pH 8.0.
6. Stop solution: 150 mM EDTA, pH 8.0.
7. 3M Sodium acetate (NaOAc), pH 5.2.
8. Carrier DNA: Sonicated salmon sperm DNA, 10 mg/mL in double-distilled water.
9. 100% Ethanol.

2.2. Random-Primed Labeling

1. Nucleotides/buffer mixes:
   a. Nucleotides/buffer mix I (for dUTP analog): 0.5 mM dATP, 0.5 mM dCTP, 0.5 mM dGTP, 50 U of pd(N)$_6$ (hexanucleotides)/mL in 2M HEPES, pH 6.6 containing 50 mM MgCl$_2$, 10 mM β-mercaptoethanol; or
   b. Nucleotides/buffer mix II (for dATP analog): 0.5 mM dTTP, 0.5 mM dCTP, 0.5 mM dGTP, 50 U of pd(N)$_6$ (hexanucleotides)/mL in 2M HEPES, pH 6.6 containing 50 mM MgCl$_2$, 10 mM β-mercaptoethanol.
2. Klenow fragment of Pol I: 0.5 U/μL in 100 mM KH$_2$PO$_4$, pH 6.5, containing 1 mM DTT, 500 μg of BSA/mL, and 50% glycerol.
3. Analogs:
   a. dUTP analog: 0.5 mM Biotin-dUTP, or 0.5 mM digoxigenin-11-dUTP in 50 mM Tris-HCl, pH 7.5; or
   b. dATP analog: 0.5 mM Biotin-7-dATP in 50 mM Tris-HCl, pH 7.5. Materials in Section 2.1., items 4–9 are also required for this protocol.

2.3. In Vitro Transcription

1. Nucleotides/buffer mix: 4 mM rATP, 4 mM rGTP, 4 mM rCTP in 400 mM Tris-HCl, pH 8.0, containing 80 mM MgCl$_2$, 20 mM spermidine, and 500 mM NaCl.
2. 0.75M DTT.

3. Human placental ribonuclease inhibitors.
4. T3 or T7 RNA polymerase: 10 U/µL in 20 mM KH$_2$PO$_4$, pH 7.7, containing 100 mM NaCl, 0.1 mM EDTA, 1 mM DTT, 0.01% Triton X-100, and 50% glycerol.
5. rUTP Analog: 4 mM Biotin-11-rUTP in 10 mM Tris-HCl, pH 7.5.
6. DNase I (RNase-free): 10 U/µL in 10 mM Tris-HCl, pH 7.6, containing 10 mM CaCl$_2$, 10 mM MgCl$_2$ and 50% glycerol.
7. Phenol/chloroform (1:1).
8. Chloroform.
9. DNA in a suitable vector. Materials in Section 2.1., items 5–9 are also required for this protocol.

2.4. Photobiotinylation

1. Photobiotin: 1 mg/mL in water (it should be kept in dark all the time).
2. 100 mM Tris-HCl, pH 9.0.
3. 2-Butanol.
4. Sunlamp: For example, General Electric Model no. RSM, 275W. Also required are materials in Section 2.1., items 4, 5, 7–9.

3. Methods
3.1. Nick Translation (see Notes 1–3)

1. Transfer 1 µg of DNA (500 µg/mL in TE) to an Eppendorf tube.
2. Add 5 µL of nucleotides/buffer mix I or II and 5 µL of the appropriate labeled nucleotide. Add sterile distilled water to give a final vol of 45 µL.
3. Mix the sample thoroughly, and keep it on ice.
4. Add 5 µL of enzyme mix, and mix the sample gently.
5. Incubate at 14°C for 1–2 h (*see* Note 3).
6. Add 5 µL of stop solution and 5 µL of 3M NaOAc, pH 5.2.
7. Add 2 µL of carrier DNA.
8. Add 140 µL of ethanol to precipitate the DNA.
9. Dissolve the DNA pellet in 20 µL of TE.

3.2. Random-Primed Labeling (see Notes 4–6)

1. Transfer 0.05–1.0 µg of linearized DNA (2 µL) to an Eppendorf tube.
2. Add water to 35 µL.
3. Heat-denature the DNA sample at 100°C for 10 min.
4. Incubate the sample on ice for 5 min, and then spin it briefly in a microcentrifuge.
5. Add 5 µL of nucleotides/buffer mix.
6. Add 5 µL of labeled nucleotide, and mix the sample thoroughly.
7. Add 5 µL of Klenow fragment of Pol I, and mix the sample gently.
8. Incubate at room temperature for 6–16 h, or at 37°C for 1–4 h (*see* Note 6).
9. Add 5 µL of stop solution and 5 µL of 3M NaOAc, pH 5.2.
10. Add 2 µL of carrier DNA.
11. Add 140 µL of ethanol to precipitate the DNA.
12. Dissolve the DNA pellet in 20 µL of TE.

3.3. In Vitro Transcription (see Notes 7–10)

1. Transfer 1 µg of RNase-free digested DNA (100 µg/mL in TE) to an Eppendorf tube (*see* Note 7).
2. Add 3 µL of nucleotide/buffer mix, and 3 µL of labeled nucleotide.
3. Add 1 µL of 0.75M DTT and 25 U of RNase inhibitor.
4. Add water to 29 µL, and mix the sample thoroughly.
5. Add 1 µL of RNA polymerase, and mix sample gently (*see* Note 8). Incubate at 37°C for 30 min.
6. Add 1 µL of RNase-free DNase I and incubate the sample for another 15 min at 37°C.
7. Extract the sample with phenol/chloroform (1:1) once, then with chloroform once.
8. Add 1.5 µL of carrier DNA and 3 µL of 3M NaOAc, pH 5.2.
9. Add 85 µL of ethanol to precipitate the labeled RNA.
10. Dissolve the RNA pellet in 20 µL of TE containing 25 U of RNase inhibitor (*see* Note 9).

3.4. Photobiotinylation (see Notes 11 and 12)

1. Transfer the DNA or RNA sample (1 mg/mL in water) to be labeled to an Eppendorf tube.
2. Add an equal volume of photobiotin stock solution.
3. Mix thoroughly, and keep the sample on ice.
4. Initiate the labeling reaction by irradiating the reaction mix 10 cm below the sunlamp for 15 min.
5. Add 150 µL of 100 mM Tris-HCl, pH 9.0, to the sample.
6. Extract the sample with equal volume of 2-butanol.
7. Discard the upper phase, and repeat the extraction twice.
8. Add 3 µL of carrier DNA and 1/10 vol of 3M NaOAc, pH 5.2.
9. Add 2.5× the volume of ethanol to precipitate labeled nucleic acids.
10. Dissolve the pellet in an appropriate amount of TE.

4. Notes

4.1. Nick Translation

1. Nick translation is probably the most sensitive method to prepare nonradioactive DNA probes. In general, it is simple, easy, and reasonably reliable. However, in order to achieve reproducible results, use of reagents and DNA samples of the highest quality is strongly recommended.
2. The reaction can be either scaled up or scaled down proportionally.
3. The incubation time in Section 3.1., step 5 should be optimized experimentally for different DNA samples to give highest sensitivity.

4.2. Random-Primed Labeling

4. The end product of the random-primed labeling reaction is a mixed population of unlabeled and labeled strands. Even if the reaction achieves completion, the labeled (synthesized) strands only account for 50% of the DNA strands. This is probably

the reason why probes labeled by this method are not as sensitive as optimally nick-translated probes. However, this method is more reliable and reproducible than nick translations.

5. This method can only be used to label linear DNA molecules. It is particularly useful for the DNA samples extracted from agarose gels, especially short DNA fragments, for which nick translation usually gives poor results.

6. The incubation time in Section 3.2., step 8 should be optimized experimentally for different amounts of DNA and different DNA samples to give highest sensitivity.

4.3. In Vitro Transcription

7. The vector should be linearized with a restriction enzyme before the transcription reaction in order to obtain transcripts of a defined length. Using intact plasmid DNA as template for transcription will result in heterogeneous transcripts of different sizes.

8. Excessive amounts of RNA polymerase should not be used with the vector containing both T3 and T7 promoters. Otherwise, transcription may not be promoter-specific (strand-specific). Nonspecific initiation of RNA transcripts may also occur at the ends of the DNA template. This is most prevalent with a 3'-protruding terminus. Nonspecific initiation may be reduced by increasing the final NaCl concentration in the transcription buffer to 100 mM. When possible, restriction enzymes that leave blunt or 5'-protruding ends should be used.

9. The addition of RNase inhibitor is to preserve the full-length single-stranded RNA transcripts.

10. Since SP6 polymerase cannot use bio-rUTP efficiently, it is not suitable for preparing biotinylated RNA probes.

4.4. Photobiotinylation

11. Photobiotinylation is a simple and inexpensive method to prepare large quantities of nonradioactive hybridization probes. The advantage of this method is that the same reagents can be used to label DNA as well as RNA molecules.

12. The sensitivity of probes labeled by this method is not as high as for those labeled by enzymatic methods. Furthermore, photobiotinylated probes usually give higher nonspecific background owing to the cationic spacer arm of photobiotin, which nonspecifically binds to anionic molecules (e.g., DNA and RNA).

Acknowledgment

Work done in this laboratory was supported in part by National Cancer Institute Grant CA60154.

References

1. Chan, W. T.-W., Fleming, K. A., and McGee, J. O'D. (1985) Detection of subpicogram quantities of specific DNA sequences on blot hybridization with biotinylated probes. *Nucleic Acids Res.* **13,** 8083–8091.

2. Burns, J., Chan, V. T.-W., Joasson, J. A., Fleming, K. A., Taylor, S., and McGee, J. O'D. (1985) A sensitive method for visualizing biotinylated probes hybridized *in situ:* rapid sex determination on intact cells. *J. Clin. Pathol.* **38,** 1085–1092.

3. Rigby, P. W. J., Dieckmann, M., Rhodes, C., and Berg, P. (1977) Labelling deoxyribonucleic acid to high specific activity in vitro by nick translation with DNA polymerase I. *J. Mol. Biol.* **113,** 237–251.

4. Feinberg, A. P. and Vogelstein, B. (1983) A technique for radio-labeling DNA restriction endonuclease fragments to high specific activity. *Anal. Biochem.* **132,** 6–13.

5. Forster, A. C., McInnes, J., Skingle, D. C., and Symons, R. H. (1985) Nonradioactive hybridization probes prepared by chemical labeling of DNA and RNA with a modified novel reagent, photobiotin. *Nucleic Acids. Res.* **13,** 745–761.

39

Cellular Human and Viral DNA Detection by Nonisotopic *In Situ* Hybridization

C. S. Herrington

1. Introduction

In situ hybridization may be defined as the detection of nucleic acids *in situ* in cells, tissues, chromosomes, and isolated cell organelles. The technique was described in 1969 by two separate groups who demonstrated repetitive ribosomal sequences in nuclei of *Xenopus* oocytes using radiolabeled probes *(1,2)*. Refinements in recombinant DNA technology and the development of nonisotopic probe labeling and detection *(3)* obviate the need for radiation protection and disposal facilities, and have converted nonisotopic *in situ* hybridization (NISH) from a purely research technique to one that can be used in routine laboratory testing.

Nonisotopic reporter molecules, such as biotin, digoxigenin, mercury, and acetylaminofluorene (AAF), can be detected using either affinity or immunocytochemical techniques. The reporters can be detected by fluorochromes and enzyme/chromogen combinations, although the former require expensive equipment and are less suitable for routine analysis. The immunoenzymatic procedures, however, can be combined with routine tissue and cytological staining, enabling simultaneous analysis of nucleic acid content within intact cells and tissues. By combining NISH and immunocytochemistry (ICC), individual cells can be genotyped and phenotyped *(4,5)*. Similarly, more than one nucleic acid can be detected in individual cells within tissue sections *(6)*. These techniques and their combination can be applied to a variety of experimental and clinical situations (for reviews, *see* refs. *7* and *8*). A more recent modification of conventional *in situ* hybridization techniques is their combination with target DNA amplification using the polymerase chain reaction (PCR) (for review, *see* ref. *9*). This involves either PCR amplification of target DNA

From: *Methods in Molecular Biology, Vol. 80: Immunochemical Protocols, 2nd ed.*
Edited by: J. D. Pound © Humana Press Inc., Totowa, NJ

followed by *in situ* hybridization (as described below), or the incorporation of labeled nucleotides into the PCR reaction followed by direct detection. The former approach has generally gained more favor, since it excludes problems owing to nonspecific polymerase elongation either of nicks present within cellular DNA or from inappropriately annealed primers. The technical details are complex and beyond the scope of this chapter: further details can be found in ref. *9* and references therein.

NISH has four elements:

1. Choice of probe/reporter and probe labeling: The reporter molecule is determined by considerations of sensitivity, specificity, safety, and practicability. Sensitivity is dependent not only on the reporter, but also on all other components of the NISH procedure, particularly nucleic acid unmasking and detection. Specificity can be enhanced by using reporters that are not normally present in cells. For example, biotin (vitamin H)-labeled probes produce unacceptable background noise in tissues containing high levels of endogenous biotin (e.g., liver). Biotin is the most widely used reporter in NISH and was originally chosen because of its high affinity for, and tetravalent binding to, avidin. Many alternatives have been formulated, including mercury, acetylaminofluorene, bromodeoxyuridine, sulfones (for review, *see* ref. *3*), and digoxigenin *(7,10)*. Many have intrinsic disadvantages. For example, mercuric cyanide is toxic and acetylaminofluorene carcinogenic. However, digoxigenin, a derivative of the therapeutic cardiac glycoside digoxin, is safe, produces low background, and can be incorporated into nucleic acids in the same way as biotin. These alternatives can be used in place of, or in addition to, biotin. The choice depends on the experimental situation.

    Multiple *in situ* nucleic acid detection can be achieved in two ways: by sequential hybridization with probes labeled with the same reporter and by simultaneous hybridization using probes labeled with different reporters. Any of the reporters listed above can be combined to allow dual nucleic acid detection, but we have found biotin and digoxigenin to be the most generally useful, since they are safe and sensitive. Probes labeled with these reporters can be combined in NISH and detected differentially according to the scheme presented in Fig. 1 *(6)*.

2. Pretreatment of cells/tissues: Having chosen the reporter and incorporated it into a probe, the cell/tissue to be analyzed is prepared for hybridization. The following requirements must be met to allow a successful hybridization reaction to take place:
    a. The cell/tissue and its nucleic acid content must be fixed in such a way that cell/tissue morphology is preserved and nucleic acids retained during the reaction.
    b. The cell/tissue sample must be sufficiently permeable to allow the labeled probe to reach its target nucleic acid.

    The latter is dependent on interplay between the degree of permeability of the cell/tissue and the size of the probe. In practice, probes with a median size of 200–400 bp are suitable for cells/tissues fixed in aldehyde and subjected to varying degrees of proteolysis (*see* Section 3.). I have found that fixation of cells in aldehyde followed by mild proteolysis produces the best results.

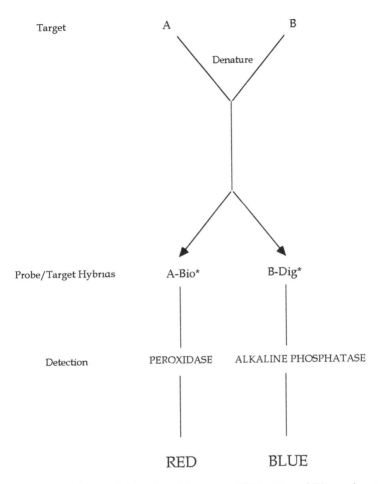

Fig. 1. Dual nucleic acid detection. The target DNAs (A and B) are denatured and hybridized with complementary DNA probes labeled with biotin (Bio*), or digoxigenin (Dig*). Biotin and digoxigenin residues are detected, respectively, with avidin peroxidase (red) and antibody to digoxigenin labeled with alkaline phosphatase (blue).

3. Denaturation/hybridization: Hybridization of probe to target requires that both probe and cellular target are denatured to form single stranded molecules. Denaturation can be achieved by treatment with alkali or heat. The former is inappropriate for probes labeled with many nonisotopic labels, since the ester linkage between reporter and nucleotide undergoes alkaline hydrolysis. Hybridization occurs when the reaction temperature falls below the melting temperature (T_m) of the duplex formed between probe and target. Stringency conditions, which determine the degree to which a probe crosshybridizes with closely related sequences, can be varied according to individual requirements (for full discussion, *see* refs. *11–13*).

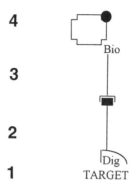

4

3

2

1   TARGET

Fig. 2. Diagrammatic representation of three-step digoxigenin detection. The target nucleic acid (1) is labeled with digoxigenin (Dig.). Monoclonal antidigoxigenin (2) is linked via biotinylated (Bio) rabbit antimouse (3) to avidin alkaline phosphatase (4).

4. Detection of signal: The principles employed in the detection of nonisotopic probe labels are similar to those used for ICC; the main differences between NISH and ICC are the degree of unmasking required to render nucleic acids available for hybridization and the hybridization reaction itself. Affinity and immunohistochemical techniques are used for probe detection employing avidin conjugates for the detection of biotin-labeled probes and antibody-based systems for the detection of digoxigenin. Combining affinity and immunohistochemical systems produces hybrid detection systems of high sensitivity. Thus, biotinylated linker antibodies are used as a bridge between monoclonal antibodies to the reporter molecule and an avidin conjugate (Fig. 2). Similarly, the alkaline phosphatase-antialkaline phosphatase (APAAP) system can be applied to the detection of both biotin- and digoxigenin-labeled probes. The latter has the advantage that it is biotin-independent.

   In this chapter, methods developed for the detection of human papillomaviruses and repetitive genomic DNA sequences (individually and in combination) in cultured cells and routinely processed surgical biopsies are described.

2. Materials

1. Aminopropyltriethoxysilane (2% [v/v]): mix 12 mL of aminopropyltriethoxysilane with 588 mL of acetone immediately prior to use.
2. CaSki cells can be obtained from the American Type Culture Collection (ATCC, Rockville, MD).
3. Complete medium: 50 mL of fetal calf serum, 5 mL of glutamine (29.2 g/L), 5 mL of penicillin (10,000 U/mL), 5 mL of streptomycin (10 mg/mL) and 435 mL of RPMI 1640 medium. Store at 4°C.
4. Phosphate-buffered saline (PBS), pH 7.4: 8.0 g of NaCl, 0.2 g of KH_2PO_4, 2.9 g of $Na_2HPO_4 \cdot 12H_2O$, 0.2 g of KCl.
5. PBS/glycine: dissolve 0.2 g of glycine in 100 mL of PBS.

6. Tris-buffered saline (TBS): 50 mM Tris-HCl, 100 mM NaCl, pH 7.2.

7. TBT: TBS containing 3% (w/v) bovine serum albumin (BSA) (Fraction V) and 0.05% (v/v) Triton X-100.

8. Alkaline phosphatase substrate buffer: 50 mM Tris-HCl, 100 mM NaCl, 1 mM MgCl$_2$, pH 9.5.

9. Tris-EDTA buffer (TE), pH 8.0: 10 mM Tris-HCl, 1 mM EDTA.

10. Paraformaldehyde (4% [w/v]): boil 100 mL of PBS containing 4 g of paraformaldehyde in a fume cupboard. Cool on ice prior to use. The final pH of this solution should be 7.2–7.4 without adjustment.

11. Methanol/acetic acid (3:1 [v/v]): add 25 mL of glacial acetic acid to 75 mL of methanol in a fume cupboard and mix by inversion. Store on ice for up to 4 h or at –20°C indefinitely.

12. Sodium azide/hydrogen peroxide solution: 0.1% (w/v) sodium azide in 0.3% (v/v) hydrogen peroxide. This solution must be prepared in a fume cupboard and handled with care.

13. Proteinase K/pepsin: The source used is important: the activity of these enzymes varies according to manufacturer and lot. I have found the proteinase K supplied by Boehringer Mannheim (Mannheim, Germany) the most consistent, and the details quoted in Section 3. refer to that source. I find that pepsin obtained from Sigma (Poole, Dorset, UK) is superior to that from Boehringer and can be used at 0.1% (w/v) compared with 0.4% (w/v) in PBS.

14. Pepsin solution: dissolve 0.1 g of pepsin in 96 mL of distilled water prewarmed to 37°C, and add 4 mL of 5M HCl slowly.

15. Standard saline citrate (1X SSC): 150 mM NaCl, 15 mM sodium citrate.

16. Hybridization mix (HM) is prepared by adding 1 mL of 50% (w/v) dextran sulfate in distilled H$_2$O and 1 mL of 20X SSC to 5 mL of deionized formamide. This mix is adjusted to pH 7.0 using 5M HCl, and stored at 4°C. Under these conditions, it lasts up to 1 yr.

17. Four-spot multiwell slides: In my laboratory, these are used for most *in situ* hybridizations. These allow the analysis of four samples (under identical conditions) on the same slide and require a smaller volume of reagent per section than conventional microscope slides. Since the spot diameter is 12-mm, 14-mm cover slips are used to cover the section without adjacent aliquots of reagent running together. These can be obtained from Chance Ltd. (Raymond Lamb, UK).

18. Microtiter or Terasaki plates (Gibco/Nunc, Paisley, UK): Proteolysis, denaturation, and hybridization are carried out in these plates. They can be floated in a 37°C water bath or incubated in a moist environment at 42 or 95°C. Two slides can be accommodated in each plate.

19. All antibody and conjugate dilutions are determined by experiment using reagents from Dako (High Wycombe, UK) unless otherwise stated: monoclonal antibiotin; biotinylated rabbit antimouse (F[ab']$_2$ fragment) (this is used to reduce background staining further); monoclonal antidigoxin, Sigma; rabbit antimouse immunoglobulin; APAAP complex; streptavidin–peroxidase; avidin (or streptavidin) alkaline phosphatase; antidigoxigenin alkaline phosphatase (Boehringer Mannheim).

20. Enzyme substrates: A variety of different substrates for both alkaline phosphatase and peroxidase are available. In this chapter, only the alkaline phosphatase substrate nitroblue tetrazolium/bromochloroindolylphosphatase (NBT/BCIP) and the peroxidase substrate 3-amino-9-ethyl carbazole (AEC) are described. Other substrates can be found in textbooks of histochemistry (*see also* Chapter 24).

   a. NBT/BCIP is made in advance, and stored at –20°C. After equilibration of 30 mL of alkaline phosphatase substrate buffer at 37°C, 10 mg of NBT are dissolved in 200 µL of dimethylformamide (DMF), and added to 1 mL of the prewarmed substrate buffer. The mixture is added dropwise to the remaining substrate buffer. BCIP (5 mg), dissolved in 200 µL of DMF, is then added slowly, and the whole preparation stored in 4-mL aliquots at –20°C.

   b. AEC is prepared fresh daily by dissolving 2 mg of AEC in 1.2 mL of dimethyl-sulfoxide in a glass tube. The mixture is added to 10 mL of 20 m*M* acetate buffer, pH 5.0–5.2. Immediately prior to use, 1 µL of 30% (v/v) hydrogen peroxide is added. The final mix may require filtration prior to use.

21. Glycerol jelly is used as an aqueous mountant (*see* Note 1). Ten grams of gelatin are dissolved in 60 mL of distilled water on a hot stirrer. Glycerol (70 mL) and phenol (0.25 g) are added, and the mountant is thoroughly mixed. Glycerol/gelatin can be stored at room temperature (solid), or at 42°C (liquid).

3. Methods

3.1. Preparation of Slides for Archival Material

1. Place multiwell slides in a slide rack, and immerse in 2% Decon 90 at 60°C for 30 min.
2. Rinse thoroughly in distilled water, and then acetone, and air-dry (*see* Note 2).
3. Immerse in 2% (v/v) aminopropyltriethoxysilane in acetone for 30 min.
4. Rinse in acetone, wash in distilled water, and air-dry at 37°C.
5. Slides prepared in this way can be stored indefinitely at room temperature.
6. Cut 5-µm sections from routine paraffin embedded blocks onto slides prepared as above.
7. Bake the sections either overnight at 60°C, or for 45 min at 75°C.
8. Store slides at room temperature.
9. Dewax the sections by heating to 75°C for 15 min (*see* Note 3).
10. Then plunge them into xylene and wash for 2 × 5 min.
11. Remove xylene by washing in 99% ethanol (industrial-grade) for 5 min at room temperature.
12. Wash in distilled water.

Unmasking of nucleic acids is achieved by using either proteinase K or pepsin HCl (*see* Note 4).

3.1.1. Proteinase K

1. Dilute lyophilized proteinase K to 500 µg/mL in PBS, and spot onto the slides (100 µL/spot), put in Terasaki plates, and float in water bath at 37°C for 15 min.
2. Wash in distilled water, and air-dry at 75°C.

3.1.2. Pepsin HCl

1. Incubate sections in pepsin solution in a coplin jar for 15 min at 37°C.
2. Wash in distilled water, and air-dry at 75°C.

3.2. Preparation of Slides Using CaSki (or Other Adherent Cultured) Cells

1. Grow CaSki cells to midlog phase in complete medium.
2. Subculture onto four-spot multiwell slides, and grow almost to confluence.
3. Fix in 4% paraformaldehyde (*see* Note 5) for 15 min at room temperature.
4. Rinse in 0.2% (w/v) in PBS/glycine (5 min), PBS (5 min), and air-dry.
5. Unmask nucleic acids using proteinase K. Dissolve 1 mg of proteinase K in 1 mL of PBS.
6. Add 100 μL to 100 mL PBS prewarmed to 37°C to give a final concentration of 1 μg/mL.
7. Incubate slides in this solution in coplin jar for 15 min at 37°C.

3.3. Preparation of Cervical Smears (14)

This method applies to both stained and unstained routinely collected smears. If previously stained (e.g., with Papanicolau stain) and mounted, the cover slip and most of the stain can be removed by soaking the slides in xylene (this may take up to 48–72 h). Following this, the xylene should be removed using 99% (industrial-grade) ethanol, and the slides then soaked in distilled water and air-dried.

1. Fix the slides in ice-cold methanol/acetic acid (3:1 [v/v]) for 10 min at room temperature.
2. Transfer the slides directly to 4% paraformaldehyde (*see* Note 5), and fix for 15 min at room temperature.
3. Rinse in 0.2% (w/v) in PBS/glycine (5 min), PBS (5 min), and air-dry.
4. Incubate slides in sodium azide/hydrogen peroxide solution for 20 min at room temperature (*see* Note 6).
5. Wash in PBS for 5 min.
6. Proceed from step 5 of Section 3.2.

3.4. Probe Preparation/Hybridization

This and the following methods sections apply to slides prepared by any of the three methods described above.

1. Add 1 μL (10–20 ng) of each of biotin and/or digoxigenin labeled probe to 7 μL of HM.
2. Excess carrier DNA may be added at this state (*see* Note 7).
3. Add TE to a total volume of 10 mL.
4. Spot 8 μL of the mixture onto each well (*see* Note 8).

5. Cover each spot with a 14-mm cover slip (*see* Note 9).
6. Place slides in Terasaki plates (2 slides/plate).
7. Denature in a convection hot air oven at 95°C for 15 min. A hot plate is also satisfactory.
8. Hybridize at 42°C in a hot air oven for 2 h.

3.5. Stringency Washing and Blocking Procedure

1. Wash slides in 4X SSC at room temperature for 2 × 5 min.
2. Wash in the appropriate solution for stringency, e.g., 50% formamide/0.1X SSC, if required for discriminating closely homologous sequences (*see* refs. *11–13*). Adjust all washing solutions to pH 7.0 with 5*M* HCl. The temperature of the solution should be monitored directly using a mercury thermometer. Washing should be carried out for 30 min.
3. Wash in 4X SSC at room temperature for 5 min.
4. Incubate for 10–15 min in blocking solution (TBT).

All incubations in antibody/avidin/enzyme conjugates described below are carried out at room temperature for 30 min unless otherwise stated. The substrate reactions are carried out at room temperature, and signal development monitored by light microscopy. The substrate incubation times are, therefore, determined empirically for each experiment. All slides are finally washed in distilled water, air-dried at 42°C, and mounted in glycerol jelly.

3.6. Detection of Biotinylated Probes

3.6.1. Conventional Signal Detection

1. Incubate the slides in avidin alkaline phosphatase (or streptavidin alkaline phosphatase) diluted 1:100 in TBT.
2. Remove unbound conjugate by washing twice in TBS for 5 min.
3. Incubate in NBT/BCIP for 15–20 min.
4. Terminate the reaction by washing in distilled water for 5 min (*see* Note 10).

3.6.2. Amplified Signal Detection

1. Incubate the slides in monoclonal antibiotin diluted 1:50 in TBT.
2. Wash twice in TBS for 5 min.
3. Incubate in biotinylated rabbit antimouse (F[ab']$_2$ fragment) diluted 1:200 in TBT.
4. Wash twice in TS for 5 min.
5. Incubate in avidin alkaline phosphatase diluted 1:50, or avidin peroxidase diluted 1:100 in TBT, containing 5% (w/v) nonfat milk (e.g., Marvel).
6. Wash in TBS, and develop the signal using either NBT/BCIP or AEC/H$_2$O$_2$.

3.6.3. APAAP Detection System

1. Incubate the slides in monoclonal antibiotin diluted 1:50 in TBT.
2. Wash twice in TBS for 5 min.

3. Incubate in rabbit antimouse immunoglobulin diluted 1:50 in TBT, and wash in TBS.
4. Incubate in APAAP complex diluted 1:50 in TBT.
5. Develop the signal using NBT/BCIP.

3.7. Detection of Digoxigenin-Labeled Probes

3.7.1. Conventional Detection

1. Incubate the slides in alkaline phosphatase-conjugated antidigoxigenin diluted 1:600 in TBT.
2. Wash in TBS, and develop the signal using NBT/BCIP as described for detection of biotinylated probes.

3.7.2. Amplified Signal Detection

1. Incubate the slides in monoclonal antidigoxin diluted 1:10,000 in TBT.
2. Wash in TBS.
3. Incubate in biotinylated rabbit antimouse (F[ab']2 fragment) diluted 1:200 in TBT.
4. Wash in TBS (5 min), and incubate in avidin alkaline phosphatase diluted 1:50 or avidin peroxidase diluted 1:100 in TBT containing 5% (w/v) nonfat milk.
5. Wash in TBS (5 min), and incubate in either alkaline phosphatase or peroxidase substrate.

3.7.3. APAAP Detection System

1. Incubate in monoclonal antidigoxin diluted 1:10,000 in TBT.
2. Proceed as for APAAP detection of biotinylated probes from step 2 in Section 3.6.3.

3.8. Double-Probe Detection

1. Incubate the slides in a mixture of avidin–peroxidase conjugate diluted 1:100 and alkaline phosphatase-conjugated antidigoxigenin diluted 1:600 in TBT; in practice, 1 μL of antibody and 6 μL of avidin are added to 600 μL of TBT.
2. Remove any unbound conjugate by washing twice in TBS for 5 min.
3. Incubate in AEC for 30 min at room temperature.
4. Terminate the reaction by thorough washing in TBS.
5. Wash in alkaline phosphatase substrate buffer for 5 min at room temperature.
6. Incubate in NBT/BCIP for 20–40 min.
7. Terminate the reaction by washing in distilled water for 5 min.

4. Notes

1. The NBT/BCIP and AEC reaction products are soluble, and/or crystallize out, in organic solvent-based mountants.
2. It is important that the slides dry completely, since aminopropyl-triethoxysilane is insoluble in water.

3. It is important to preheat the sections prior to dewaxing: this leads to more effective dewaxing of nucleic acids.

4. We have noted that the proteolysis step appears to be the most critical in the whole technique. Variability in signal intensity is virtually always caused by incomplete or excessive proteolysis; the only remedy is repetition of the experiment! Silane is an effective adhesive for most cells and sections, although occasionally, high concentrations of proteinase K can cause repeated section dehiscence. Under these circumstances, reduction of the proteinase K concentration or, alternatively, the use of pepsin HCl may prove more effective; these, however, reduce the sensitivity of the method.

5. The fixation of CaSki cells in aldehyde has been shown to enhance the sensitivity of the detection of human papillomavirus type 16 by *in situ* hybridization compared with fixation by acid/alcohol *(9)*.

6. Sodium azide/hydrogen peroxide solution blocks endogenous peroxidase enzyme activity. This is important in cervical smears where large numbers of neutrophil polymorphs and red blood cells are present. Although often not essential when analyzing cultured cells or biopsies, incubation in this solution is equally effective with these sample types.

7. Carrier DNA (e.g., salmon sperm) can be added to the reaction mix in excess to reduce nonspecific probe binding. I have not found this necessary for the detection of human papillomaviruses in archival surgical biopsies, but it is often necessary for cultured cells and cervical smears *(14)*.

8. The volume of probe mixture required to cover the section without adjacent aliquots running together varies inversely with the size of the section. Thus, large sections require as little as 6 μL of mixture and small ones up to 8.5 μL.

9. I have found that sealing the cover slips with rubber cement is not necessary.

10. The NBT/BCIP reaction can be terminated chemically by lowering the pH (e.g., by rinsing in TBS, pH 7.2), adding phosphate ions (e.g., PBS), or by chelating Mg ions using EDTA. However, I find that thorough rinsing in distilled water is as effective.

Acknowledgment

This work was supported by grants from the Cancer Research Campaign, UK.

Suggested Readings

Herrington, C. S. and McGee, J. O'D. (eds.) (1992) *Diagnostic Molecular Pathology: A Practical Approach,* vols. 1 and 2. Oxford University Press, Oxford, UK.

Levy, E. R. and Herrington, C. S. (eds.) (1995) *Nonisotopic Methods in Molecular Biology: A Practical Approach.* Oxford University Press, Oxford, UK.

References

1. Gall, J. G. and Pardue, M. L. (1969) Formation and detection of RNA–DNA hybrid molecules in cytological preparations. *Proc. Natl. Acad. Sci. USA* **63,** 378–383.

2. John, H. A., Birnstiel, M. L. and Jones, K. W. (1969) RNA–DNA hybrids at the cytological level. *Nature* **223,** 582–587.

3. Hopman, A. H. N., Speel, E. J. M., Voorter, C. E. M., and Ramaekers, F. C. S. Probe labeling methods, in *Nonisotopic Methods in Molecular Biology: A Practical Approach* (Levy, E. R. and Herrington, C. S., eds.), Oxford University Press, Oxford, UK, pp. 1–24.

4. Graham, A. K., Herrington, C. S., and McGee JO'D. (1991) Sensitivity and specificity of monoclonal antibodies to human papillomavirus Type 16 Capsid protein: comparison with simultaneous viral detection by nonisotopic *in situ* hybridization. *J. Clin. Pathol.* **44,** 96–101.

5. Mullink, H., Vos, W., Jiwa, N. M., Horstman, A., Rieger, E., and Meijer, C. J. L. M. (1995) Combination of nonradioactive *in situ* hybridization and immunocytochemistry, in *Nonisotopic Methods in Molecular Biology: A Practical Approach* (Levy, E. R. and Herrington, C. S., eds.), Oxford University Press, Oxford, UK, pp. 111–144.

6. Herrington, C. S., Burns, J., Graham, A. K., Bhatt, B., and McGee J, O'D. (1989) Interphase cytogenetics using biotin and digoxigenin labeled probes 11: simultaneous detection of two nucleic acid species in individual nuclei. *J. Clin. Pathol.* **42,** 601–606.

7. Herrington, C. S. and McGee, J. O'D. (1992) Principles and basic methodology of DNA/RNA detection by *in situ* hybridization., in *Diagnostic Molecular Pathology: A Practical Approach,* vol. 1 (Herrington, C. S. and McGee, J. O'D., eds.), Oxford University Press, Oxford, UK, pp. 69–102.

8. Klinger, K. (1995) Cytogenetic analysis, in *Nonisotopic Methods in Molecular Biology: A Practical Approach* (Levy, E. R. and Herrington, C. S., eds.), Oxford University Press, Oxford, UK, pp. 25–50.

9. O'Leary, J. J., Browne, G., Bashir, M. S., Landers, R. J., Crowley, M., Healy, I., Lewis, F., and Doyle, C. T. (1995) Nonisotopic detection of DNA in tissues, in *Nonisotopic Methods in Molecular Biology: A Practical Approach* (Levy, E. R. and Herrington, C. S., eds.), Oxford University Press, Oxford, UK, pp. 51–83.

10. Herrington, C. S., Burns, J., Graham, A. K., Evans, M. F., and McGee, JO'D (1989) Interphase cytogenetics using biotin and digoxigenin labeled probes 1: relative sensitivity of both reporters for detection of HPV 16 in CaSki cells. *J. Clin. Pathol.* **42,** 592–600.

11. Herrington, C. S., Burns, J., Graham, A. K., and McGee, JO'D (1990) Discrimination of closely homologous HPV types by nonisotopic *in situ* hybridization: definition and derivation of tissue Tms. *Histochem. J.* **22,** 545–554.

12. Herrington, C. S., Anderson, S. M., Graham, A. K., and McGee, J. O'D (1993) The discrimination of high risk HPV types by *in situ* hybridization and the polymerase chain reaction. *Histochem. J.* **25,** 191–198.

13. Herrington, C. S. and McGee, J.O'D. (1994) Discrimination of closely homologous genomic and viral sequences in cells and tissues: further characterization of Tm^t. *Histochem. J.* **26,** 545–552.

14. Herrington, C. S., de Angelis, M. L., Evans, M. F., Troncone, G., McGee, J. O'D. (1992) Detection of high risk human papillomavirus in routine cervical smears: strategy for screening. *J. Clin. Pathol.* **45,** 385–390.

40

Biotinylated Probes in Colony Hybridization

Michael J. Haas

1. Introduction

Colony hybridization is a procedure that allows the detection of cells containing nucleic acid sequences of interest *(1)*. In this method, microbial colonies grown on, or transferred to, a supporting membrane are lysed and their nucleic acids denatured to single strands and fixed in place on the membrane. The membrane is then exposed to a similarly denatured "probe" sequence, which is identical or homologous to all or part of the target sequence, under conditions favoring reannealing. Probe sequences hybridize to complementary sequences on the membrane. Positive hybridization events are then detected by determining the presence and location of probe sequences on the membrane.

The original colony hybridization method described the use of radiolabeled probes and the detection of positive hybridization events by autoradiography *(1)*. However, because of the high waste disposal costs, short half-lives, long autoradiographic exposures, and potential health hazards associated with radioisotopes, there is interest in alternative methods to detect positive hybridizations.

Nonradioactive technology involves the attachment to the nucleic acid probe of a ligand that can subsequently be detected by chemical or enzymatic methods. The vitamin biotin is one such ligand. Biotin can be covalently incorporated into nucleic acids in a manner that does not interfere with their ability to hybridize with homologous sequences. This is accomplished by replacing a nucleoside triphosphate with its biotinylated analog in an in vitro DNA replication or transcription reaction, generating a biotinylated probe sequence *(2,3)*. Hybridization of such a probe to a homologous sequence immobilized on a membrane results in the retention of biotin at that site. Positive hybridization events can then be detected by assaying for biotin.

From: *Methods in Molecular Biology, Vol. 80: Immunochemical Protocols, 2nd ed.*
Edited by: J. D. Pound © Humana Press Inc., Totowa, NJ

Enzymatic reaction schemes that generate insoluble colored products at sites where biotin is bound to the filters have been developed for the purpose of biotin detection in these applications. These detection reactions employ either avidin or streptavidin, two functionally identical proteins that bind to biotin with very high affinities and specificities. These proteins are retained at sites where biotinylated probes have hybridized to homologous sequences. Avidin and streptavidin have multiple biotin binding sites per molecule. They therefore retain biotin binding capability even after binding to probe sequences on the membranes. Incubation with a biotinylated form of an enzyme (e.g., alkaline phosphatase) for which there exists an assay that generates an insoluble, colored product results in the retention of signal enzyme at sites of positive hybridization. These sites are detected by applying the histochemical assay for the signal enzyme.

To facilitate our work on plasmids with no known phenotype, we have developed a method for the use and detection of biotinylated probes in colony hybridization. It is suitable both for the detection of rare positive hybridization events over a background of nonreactive colonies and for the detection of nonhybridizing colonies in a population containing sequences homologous to the probe. The latter capability could be useful in such applications as the detection of cured (i.e., plasmid-free) cells in a bacterial population containing plasmids.

2. Materials

1. Nitrocellulose filters (82-mm diameter, BA 85) are obtained from Schleicher & Schuell (Keene, NH). (Products from other suppliers may be acceptable.)
2. Formamide: deionized by stirring for 30 min with 10% (w/v) of a mixed-bed ion exchange resin (e.g., Bio-Rad AG 501-X8, 20-50 mesh, Bio-Rad, Hercules, CA), filtering twice through Whatman (Clifton, NJ) no. 1 paper and storing single-use aliquots at $-80°C$.
3. Bovine serum albumin ([BSA], Fraction V, Sigma, St. Louis, MO) is used as obtained. Fatty acid-free albumin gives poor results.
4. Denatured herring sperm DNA is prepared by dissolving in water (10 mg/mL) with stirring at room temperature, shearing by 10 passages through an 18-gage needle, and immersing in boiling water for 10 min. Aliquots are stored at $-20°C$. Just prior to use, these are incubated for 10 min in a boiling water bath and chilled in ice water.
5. 20X SSC buffer: $3M$ sodium chloride, $0.3M$ sodium citrate, pH adjusted to 7.0 with sodium hydroxide. Sterilize by autoclaving, store at room temperature.
6. Proteinase K is obtained from Beckman (Somerset, NJ). Other sources may be acceptable. In using alternate sources, the occurrence of blue backgrounds between colonies, and oversize, blurry signals at colony sites after the final color development step indicates insufficient proteolytic activity. Prepare a solution of 200 μg/mL in 1X SSC.

7. 50X Denhardt's solution: 1% (w/v) Ficoll, 1% (w/v) polyvinyl pyrrolidone, 1% (w/v) BSA. Filter-sterilize. Store aliquots at –20°C. Do not flame the pipets used to transfer this solution. Denaturation and precipitation of the protein result from the use of hot pipets at this stage.

8. Template DNA for the production of hybridization probes must be pure. Standard methods, such as dye-buoyant density ultracentrifugation, generate acceptable products. Ethidium bromide and cesium chloride are removed prior to use of the DNA *(4)*.

9. Biotin-11-deoxyuridine-5'-triphosphate (BiodUTP) and reagents for its incorporation into DNA by nick translation are obtained commercially. The products from Bethesda Research Laboratories (BRL, Gaithersburg, MD) are acceptable. BRL now provides a prepackaged kit (BioNick) containing necessary supplies and employing biotin-14-dATP as the source of biotin. The concentration of the resulting biotinylated DNA is determined by the histochemical method for biotin *(below)*. Adequate instructions are provided with these kits.

10. Prehybridization solution: 50% formamide, 5X SSC, 5X Denhardt's solution, 25 mM sodium phosphate, pH 6.5, 300 µg/mL freshly denatured sheared herring sperm DNA. Filter through Whatman no. 1 paper on a Buchner funnel, then through a sterile 0.45-µm filter. Store 10-mL aliquots in glass at –20°C. Use only once.

11. Hybridization solution: 45% Formamide, 5X SSC, 5X Denhardt's solution, 20 mM sodium phosphate, pH 6.5, 300 µg/mL freshly denatured, sheared, herring sperm DNA, 200 ng of biotinylated DNA/mL. Before its addition, the biotinylated probe DNA is denatured by incubating for 10 min in a boiling water bath and quick-chilling in an ice bath. Shearing to reduce size is unnecessary, since the products generated by nick translation are sufficiently small. Filter and store the hybridization solution as was done for the prehybridization solution. Hybridization solution can be recovered after use and stored at –20°C. The solution can be reused at least 10 times over a time-span of at least 5 mo, without noticeable reduction in performance. The solution is heat-denatured as described for the herring sperm DNA preparation immediately before each use.

12. Reagents for the detection of filter-bound biotin are obtained from BRL (BlueGene Nonradioactive Nucleic Acid Detection System). Comparable materials are available from Bio-Rad Laboratories.

13. Special equipment required for this protocol are a vacuum oven, a slab gel dryer, a device for the heat sealing of plastic bags (e.g., Seal-A-Meal, Sears Seal-and-Save), thin rubber sheet (such as dental sheet, A. H. Thomas, Philadelphia, PA), and a filtration device designed for the washing of nitrocellulose filters. The latter was originally described by Grunstein and Hogness *(1)* and is available from Schleicher and Schuell as the "Screen-It" colony filter hybridization device.

14. 90% (w/w) Ethanol.

15. Chloroform: Reagent grade.

16. Solutions for the posthybridization washing of filters:
    a. 0.1% (w/v) Sodium dodecylsulfate (SDS) in 2X SSC.
    b. 0.1% (w/v) SDS in 0.2X SSC.

    c. 0.1% (w/v) SDS in 0.16X SSC.
    d. 2X SSC.

3. Methods
3.1. Filter Preparation and Cell Growth

1. Use a soft lead pencil to label nitrocellulose filters with a hash mark and letter or number on one edge to allow subsequent identification and orientation (*see* Note 1).
2. Place the labeled filters between sheets of filter paper, wrap in aluminum foil, and autoclave for 10 min.
3. Seal the packets of sterile filters in an air-tight bag and store at 4°C.
4. To inoculate, place a filter on top of solidified media in a Petri dish and spread an appropriately diluted bacterial culture over the surface.
5. Incubate the plates until the cells are approx 1–3 mm in diameter (*see* Note 2). Cell densities of approx 800/82 mm diameter filter are compatible with single colony discrimination after hybridization and color assay. If one is attempting to locate positively hybridizing sequences in a generally nonreacting population, and single colony resolution is not required in the first detection step, as many as 10^5 cells can be applied to each filter.
6. Invert the filter and gently lay it onto fresh media just prior to lysis to create a replica of the colony pattern of the filter. (Mark the plate to indicate the orientation of the filter on it.) After an appropriate incubation, this becomes a master plate from which viable analogues of desirable colonies, as identified on the filter after hybridization and processing, can be recovered.

3.2. Cell Lysis

All operations are conducted at room temperature unless otherwise noted. After steps 1–3, gentle suction is applied to the filters (*see* Note 3). Steps 2–4 are conducted in glass Petri dishes, one filter per dish. It has not been determined if these steps can be done batchwise. It is difficult to process more than 12 filters at a time.

To achieve lysis, incubate the filters in the following fashion (*see* Note 4):

1. Incubate 7 min, colony-side up, on filter paper sheets stacked to a thickness of 4 mm and saturated with fresh $0.5M$ NaOH.
2. Incubate 5 min in $1.5M$ sodium chloride, $0.5M$ Tris-HCl, pH 7.4, 30 mL/filter.
3. Incubate 1 h in prewarmed proteinase K in 1X SSC, 30 mL/filter, 37°C.
4. Incubate 2 × 2 min in 90% (w/w) ethanol, 30 mL/filter (*see* Note 5).
5. Air-dry, 20 min.
6. Wash each filter with 100 mL of chloroform using the Screen-It colony hybridization device. A single sheet of filter paper is used as an underfilter.
7. Air-dry (approx 15 min).
8. Sandwich the filters individually between filter paper, wrap loosely in aluminum foil, and bake at 80°C *in vacuo* for 2 h.
9. Store the filters in a vacuum desiccator at room temperature.

3.3. Prehybridization, Hybridization, and Detection of Hybridization

1. For prehybridization, place pairs of filters containing lysed, fixed colonies back to back in sealable plastic bags. Add 20 mL of prehybridization solution, seal the bag, seal it within a second bag, and incubate at 42°C for 2 h. Maintain the proper temperature by submersion in a water bath.

2. After prehybridization, replace the liquid with 20 mL of hybridization solution, exclude air bubbles, reseal the bags, and immerse in the water bath. Brief incubations (1 h) are sufficient for the detection of relatively abundant sequences, such as unamplified plasmid pBR322 in *E. coli*. More extensive incubations (45 h) may be necessary to detect less abundant sequences.

3. Following hybridization, wash the filters sequentially:
   a. Twice in 250 mL of 0.1% (w/v) SDS in 2X SSC, 3 min per wash, room temperature;
   b. Twice in 250 mL of 0.1% (w/v) SDS, 0.2X SSC, 3 min per wash, room temperature;
   c. Twice in 250 mL of 0.1% (w/v) SDS, 0.16X SSC, 15 min per wash, 50°C; and
   d. Briefly in 2X SSC at room temperature.

4. Detection of the sites of hybridization-dependent binding of biotinylated probe to the filters is most readily conducted with commercially available kits. Favorable results have been obtained with the BluGene Nonradioactive Nucleic Acid Detection System from BRL. Follow the manufacturer's instructions when carrying out the following steps. After washing, sequentially expose the filters to streptavidin and biotinylated alkaline phosphatase (or to a conjugate of these two proteins). This causes the immobilization of alkaline phosphatase at sites of positive hybridization.

5. Incubate the filters with 5-bromo-4-chloro-3-indolylphosphate (BCIP) and nitroblue tetrazolium (NBT). Indoxyl generated from BCIP by the action of alkaline phosphatase condenses to form indigo (blue). Indigo then reacts with NBT to form insoluble diformazan (purple).

6. Terminate the reaction when reacting colonies are intensely purple (*see* Note 6) by replacing the dye solution with 20 m*M* Tris-HCl, 5 m*M* EDTA, pH 7.5. Nonreactive colonies should be light blue on a white background.

7. Store the moist filters in sealed bags. The elapsed time from the end of hybridization to the termination of color development is approx 3 h. Figure 1 illustrates typical results obtained with this method.

4. Notes

1. Cellulose filters give unacceptably diffuse colony patterns after lysis and should not be used. Nylon filters should be acceptable, although we have not examined their suitability.

2. The lysis of colonies larger than specified above is generally acceptable. However, with relatively mucoid strains, such as *Xanthomonas*, the lysis of oversize colonies results in smeared colony patterns. The researcher should investigate the performance of younger cells if such behavior is experienced.

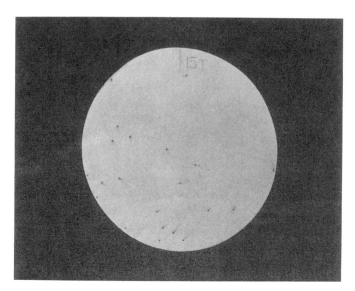

Fig. 1. Specific identification of *E. coli* containing plasmid pBR322. Approximately 225 colonies, consisting of a 10:1 mixture of plasmid-free and plasmid-containing cells, was grown on a nitrocellulose filter. The filter was subjected to the lysis protocol described here, followed by a hybridization with biotinylated pBR322. Sites of positive hybridization were detected by means of streptavidin and alkaline phosphatase. The dark sites correspond to colonies harboring pBR322. Plasmid-free cells give the faint signals present at numerous sites on the filter.

3. The application of gentle suction to the filters following steps 1–3 of the lysis protocol reduces the dispersion of cells from their sites, promoting tighter patterns and stronger signals, and reducing the interference of signals from adjacent colonies with one another. Suction is applied by means of a slab gel dryer and a gentle vacuum source. A single sheet of filter paper serves as an underfilter. On this sheet is placed a template made by cutting into a sheet of flexible rubber holes slightly smaller than the nitrocellulose filters. The filters are placed over these holes and vacuum is applied. A brief suction suffices to remove excess moisture from the filters and to pull lysed colonies down onto them. Six filters can be treated at a time with a standard commercially available gel dryer with an 18 × 34 cm suction surface.

4. In our initial studies, the filters were swirled in the lysis solutions in an attempt to ensure lysis. After hybridization and application of the color assay, it was found that positively reacting colonies had "tails" extending away from them in a circular pattern across the filters. These tails obscured the signals of adjacent colonies. Tailing was eliminated by omitting the swirling action during lysis. This omission did not noticeably reduce the efficiency or sensitivity of the detection reaction.

5. The ethanol concentration in step 4 of the lysis protocol is a w/w concentration. Ethanol solutions made up v/v, or otherwise in excess of 90% w/w, exceed the ethanol tolerance limits of some batches of nitrocellulose. Filters washed in such solutions may become brittle and be reduced nearly to powder by the end of the hybridization-color assay procedure. The appropriate solution can be made from 100% ethanol.

6. The final color development step must be conducted under dim light (i.e., incubated in a drawer) since the reagents are light sensitive. Examine the filters at frequent intervals (10 min) during this incubation. Stop the reaction when the color of positively reacting colonies is deep purple. Further incubation past this point allows the color of nonreacting colonies to darken to such a degree that they are mistaken for positives. Overdevelopment is the greatest single factor contributing to the appearance of false-positive signals.

7. The minimal probe concentration necessary for efficient detection of target sequences has not been determined. It has been noted, however, that probe concentrations of 10–20 ng/mL, when coupled with overnight hybridizations, are too low to give strong signals for nonreiterated target DNAs 3 MDa or larger in size. Maas *(5)* reported a simple modification of the Grunstein-Hogness protocol *(1)*, which is reported to increase the sensitivity of the colony hybridization method by 100-fold. This could increase the ability to detect single copy sequences.

8. Nucleic acids can also be biotinylated by nonenzymatic methods with photobiotin, a photoactivatable biotin analog *(6)*, which can be commercially obtained from BRL, Sigma, and other commercial sources. I have not compared the suitability of this method of biotin incorporation with that reported here, but expect that the method would be fully acceptable. FMC (Rockland, ME) markets an alternate nonradioactive sequence detection kit known as Chemiprobe. The basis of this system is a chemical modification of cytosine residues in the probe DNA. After hybridization, the probe is detected by means of a monoclonal antibody that specifically recognizes the sulfonated DNA. Detection of the bound monoclonal antibody is achieved by means of an alkaline phosphatase-conjugated second antibody.

References

1. Grunstein, M. and Hogness, D. S. (1975) Colony hybridization: a method for the isolation of cloned DNAs that contain a specific gene. *Proc. Natl. Acad. Sci. USA* **72,** 3961–3965.
2. Langer, P. R., Waldrop, A. A., and Ward, D. C. (1981) Enzymatic synthesis of biotin-labeled polynucleotides: novel nucleic acid affinity probes. *Proc. Natl. Acad. Sci. USA* **78,** 6633–6637.
3. Brigati, D. J., Myerson, D., Leary, J. J., Spalholz, B., Travis, S. Z., Fong, D. K. Y., Hsiung, G. D., and Ward, D. C. (1983) Detection of viral genomes in cultured cells and paraffin-embedded tissue sections using biotin-labeled hybridization. *Virology* **126,** 32–50.

4. Boffey, S. A. (1984) Plasmid DNA isolation by the cleared lysate method, in *Methods in Molecular Biology,* vol. 2: *Nucleic Acids* (Walker, J. M., ed.), Humana, Clifton, NJ, pp. 177–183.

5. Maas, R. (1983) An improved colony hybridization method with significantly increased sensitivity for detection of single genes. *Plasmid* **10,** 296–298.

6. Forster, A. C., McInnes, J. L., Skingle, D. C., and Symons, R. H. (1985) Nonradioactive hybridization probes prepared by the chemical labeling of DNA and RNA with a novel reagent, photobiotin. *Nucleic Acids Res.* **13,** 745–761.

41

Nonisotopic *In Situ* Hybridization

Gene Mapping and Cytogenetics

Bhupendra Bhatt, Tulin Sahinoglu, and Cliff Stevens

1. Introduction

With the advent of nonradioactive probes during the past decade, *in situ* hybridization has become an immensely valuable tool in the hands of:

1. Developmental biologists and cell biologists for the detection of mRNA in cells and tissue sections *(1–7)*;
2. Virologists for detection of viral DNA and RNA *(8)*; and
3. Molecular cytogeneticists in detecting chromosome aberrations in interphase cells (Interphase Cytogenetics, especially Cancer Genetics, *9–11*), sex determination *(12,13)*, and gene mapping by nonisotopic *in situ* hybridization (NISH, *14,15*).

In NISH, the probe labeled with a nonradioactive reporter, such as biotin, digoxigenin, or fluorescein, is hybridized to chromosome spreads, and the label is detected by indirect immunocytochemistry. Nonfluorescent reporters are either detected by an enzymatic conversion of a substrate into a colored precipitate or by fluorescence *(14,15)*. In fluorescent *in situ* hybridization (FISH), the probe may be directly labeled with either a fluorescent nucleotide (fluorescein 11-dUTP) or with nonfluorescent nucleotides, such as biotin-11-dUTP or digoxigenin-11-dUTP. When a nonfluorescent label is used, the signal is detected by reporter-specific antibodies or, in the case of biotin, by avidin/streptavidin conjugated to a fluorescent dye. FISH offers greater sensitivity over nonfluorescent immunocytochemical detection methods. Apart from conventional single-copy gene mapping and interphase cytogenetics, FISH has been used in high-resolution mapping of several genes simultaneously *(16)*. It has also been used in resolving the order of sequences within the human muscular dystrophy gene

From: *Methods in Molecular Biology, Vol. 80: Immunochemical Protocols, 2nd ed.*
Edited by: J. D. Pound © Humana Press Inc., Totowa, NJ

(17). The major disadvantage of FISH is that the fluorescent signal is only analyzable on photographs. However, when confocal laser microscopy and digital densitometric analysis of the signal are available, FISH affords a level of sensitivity where it is possible to resolve the order of sequences within a gene (e.g., the human muscular dystrophy gene; *17,18*), or to clone specific chromosomal regions by microdissection *(19)*. Another recent addition to the list of methods for gene mapping is popularly referred to as primed *in situ* labeling (PRINS). It involves hybridization of unlabeled synthetic oligonucleotide primers to chromosome spreads and subsequent amplification of the specific chromosomal regions with *Taq* DNA polymerase. The label is incorporated during amplification. This method is a combination of *in situ* hybridization and polymerase chain reaction (PCR), which is covered by US patents owned by Hoffman La Roche [Nutley, NJ], *20–22*). Both FISH and PRINS methods are described here. In addition, detection by fluorescence, as well as by the DAB/gold/silver method is described. Although the methods described in this chapter refer to biotin-11 dUTP for labeling the probe, with appropriate modifications, other labels, such as digoxigenin, and fluorescein, will work equally well.

There are several steps involved in mapping genes on chromosomes by either of the methods. The following are common to both methods:

1. Preparation of metaphase spreads from whole blood cultures.
2. Fixation of slides.
3. Immunocytochemical detection of signal.
4. Chromosome banding.

2. Materials

2.1. Tissue Culture and Slide Preparation

1. Complete medium (CM): 76 mL of RPMI 1640, 20 mL of fetal bovine serum, 2 mL of phytohemagglutinin (M form), 1 mL of antibiotic/antimycotic solution (100X = 10,000 U penicillin, 10,000 U streptomycin and 25 µg fungizone), and 1 mL of 100X L-glutamine (100X = 30 mg/mL) (Gibco, Paisely, UK).
2. 5'-Bromo-2-deoxyuridine (BUdR): Dissolve 10 mg/mL in distilled water. Sterilize by filtration with a 0.2-µm filter. Store in aliquots at –20°C.
3. Thymidine: Dissolve to a concentration of 250 µg/mL in distilled water. Filter-sterilize, and store in aliquots at –20°C.
4. Colcemid: Dissolve 5 µg/mL of distilled water. Filter-sterilize, and store in aliquots at –20°C.
5. Hypotonic solution: Dissolve 560 mg of potassium chloride (KCl) in 100 mL distilled water. Prepare fresh, and keep at 37°C.
6. Fixative: Mix three parts methanol with one part glacial acetic acid. Prepare fresh, and keep on ice.

2.2. Labeling of the Probe for FISH

1. DNase I: 1 μg/μL in DNase buffer (50% glycerol, 150 mM NaCl, 10 mM NaH$_2$PO$_4$, pH 7.2, 0.1% [w/v] bovine serum albumin [BSA], 1.0 mM dithiothreitol). Store in aliquots at –20°C.
2. DNA polymerase I: store at –20°C.
3. 10X Nick translation buffer: 500 mM Tris-HCl, pH 7.5, 50 mM MgCl$_2$, 10 mM β-mercaptoethanol. Store at 4°C.
4. Cot-1 DNA.
5. Glycogen: mussel glycogen at 20 mg/mL in sterile distilled water.
6. 1 mM Biotin-11-dUTP.
7. dNTP mixture: 10 mM of each of dATP, dCTP, and dGTP.
8. 10 mM dithiothreitol (dTT).
9. 0.2M EDTA: Dissolve 7.4 g ethylenediaminetetracetic acid (disodium salt) in 100 mL distilled water. Raise the pH to 8.0, and autoclave.
10. TE buffer: Dissolve 10 mM Tris-HCl and 1 mM EDTA (pH 8.0) in sterile distilled water. Do not autoclave.

2.3. Evaluation of Labeling by Gel Electrophoresis

1. NBT/BCIP:
    a. Dissolve 10 mg nitroblue tetrazolium (NBT) in 200 μL of dimethyl formamide (DMF), and add to 1 mL substrate buffer (0.1M NaCl, 0.1M Tris-HCl, pH 9.6, 0.01M MgCl$_2$). Add the mixture to 29 mL of substrate buffer.
    b. Dissolve 5 mg of bromochloro indolylphosphatase (BCIP) in 200 μL DMF, and add to (a).
2. TBE buffer: 10.8 g Tris, 5.5 g boric acid, and 0.93 g EDTA dissolved in 1 L of distilled water.
3. Agarose: Dissolve agarose 1.6% (w/v) in TBE buffer by boiling in microwave oven.
4. Ethidium bromide (EtBr): Dissolve 10 mg of EtBr in sterile distilled water. Dilute to 0.5 μg/mL of distilled water for staining the gel. EtBr is a suspected carcinogen. Handle with care in a fumehood.
5. 6X Loading buffer: Dissolve 4 g sucrose and 2.5 mg bromophenol blue in 6.0 mL of TE buffer. Store at 4°C.
6. 100-bp and 1.0-kb DNA ladders: these are used as size markers for the labeled probes. Aliquot and store at –20°C.

2.4. Hybridization for FISH

1. 10X SSC buffer: 3.0M sodium chloride, 0.3M sodium citrate. Adjust pH to 7.4, and autoclave.
2. Deionized formamide: Mix 5.0 g mixed-bed ion-exchange resin (Bio-Rad [Hercules, CA] AG501-x8, 20–50 mesh) with 50 mL formamide. Stir for 45 min, and filter with Whatman's filter paper. Store in aliquots at –20°C.
3. 100X Denhardt's solution: 0.2 g BSA, 0.2 g ficoll, 2 g glycine, 0.2 g polyvinyl pyrrolidone, sterile distilled water to 10 mL. Store in aliquots at –20°C.

4. Dextran sulfate: 50% (w/v) in sterile distilled water.
5. Hybridization buffer (HB): 600 μL deionized formamide, 100 μL 100X Denhardt's solution, 200 μL 50% dextran sulfate, 100 μL 20X SSC. Store at 4°C.
6. Human placental DNA: 10 mg/mL in sterile distilled water. Stir for 1–2 h, shear by passing through 18-gage needle, or sonicate. Place in boiling water bath for 10 min. Store in aliquot at –20°C.
7. Gene Framer™ (Advanced Biotechnologies, Surrey, UK): This is an adhesive frame that forms a seal around the section or chromosomal spread, and prevents loss of solutions as well as forming a boundary around the area of interest.

2.5. Immunocytochemical Detection and Chromosome Staining

1. Wash buffer: 4X SSC containing 0.5% (v/v) Tween-20.
2. Blocking buffer: 5% skimmed milk powder (e.g., Marvel) in wash buffer.
3. Avidin-FITC.
4. Peroxidase-conjugated mouse monoclonal antifluorescein antibody.
5. Streptavidin-gold conjugate: streptavidin conjugated to 1.0-nm gold particles. Store in aliquots at –20°C.
6. Peroxidase substrate (DAB): 2.5 mg of 3,3'-diaminobenzidine tetrahydrochloride dissolved in 5 mL phosphate-buffered saline (PBS). Add 2 μL of 30% hydrogen peroxide (H_2O_2). DAB powder should be handled only in a fume cupboard.
7. Sodium chloroaurate (gold-sodium-chloride, BDH Chemicals Ltd. [Poole, UK]): make a 10% solution in distilled water, and store at 4°C. For the working solution, dilute 1:100.
8. Sodium sulfide (Na_2S): dissolve 100 mg in 10 mL distilled water. Add 560 μL $1M$ HCl. Handle in fume cupboard.
9. Silver solution: follow manufacturer's instructions.
10. Tris-buffered saline (TBS), pH 7.2: $0.1M$ Tris-HCl, $0.1M$ NaCl.
11. TBST: TBS containing 0.05% Tween-20 (or Triton X-100).
12. Hoechst 33258: prepare 100X stock solution by dissolving 5 mg in 10 mL of methanol and store in dark at 4°C. Working solution: dilute the stock 1:100 in 2X SSC.
13. Giemsa stain: make a 5% (v/v) solution in PBS at pH 6.8.

2.6. Primed In Situ Labeling (PRINS)

1. *Taq* polymerase: supplied at 5 U/μL. Store aliquots at –20°C. Dilute to 1–2.5 U/μL in sterile distilled water for working concentration. In the author's laboratory, Red Hot Polymerase™ (Advanced Biotechnologies) works best at 0.2 U/μL.
2. 10X *Taq* Polymerase buffer: 500 mM KCl, 100 mM Tris-HCl, pH 9.0, 1.0% Triton X-100. Store at –20°C.
3. 25 mM MgCl.
4. dNTP Mixture (*see* Section 2.2.) *(7)*.
5. dTTP Mixture (*see* Section 2.2.) *(8)*.
6. 1 mM Fluorescein-11-dUTP. Store at –20°C.

3. Methods

3.1. Preparation of Metaphase Chromosomes

1. Add 0.8 mL of heparinized human venous blood to each culture bottle containing 10 mL of CM. Incubate at 37°C for 72 h.
2. Add 100 μL BUdR to each culture and incubate for another 16–17 h at 37°C.
3. Centrifuge the cultures at 700g for 10 min. Discard supernatant, and resuspend the pellet in 10 mL RPMI 1640 or PBS.
4. Repeat step 3.
5. Resuspend pellet in CM containing 2.5 μg thymidine. Incubate at 37°C for another 6 h.
6. Add 100 μL colcemid solution to each culture, and incubate at 37°C for another 20 min.
7. Centrifuge the cultures at 600g, and resuspend the pellet in hypotonic solution. Incubate at 37°C for 7 min.
8. Centrifuge, and discard supernatant. Resuspend the pellet in 1 mL fresh, chilled fixative. Bring the volume to 10 mL with fixative. Keep on ice for at least 20 min.
9. Wash the pellet several times in fresh fixative by repeated centrifugation and resuspension of pellet in fresh chilled fixative.
10. Cells may be left in the fixative indefinitely at –20°C.
11. Centrifuge, resuspend the pellet in 0.5–1.0 mL of fresh chilled fixative, and keep on ice.
12. Soak precleaned microscope slides in distilled water.
13. Place the wet slides on a hotplate maintained at 60°C, and immediately drop 10–20 μL of the cell suspension on the slide from a distance of 15–20 cm. Allow to dry.
14. Slides may be examined under phase contrast to select areas of well-spread metaphase or prometaphase chromosomes.

3.2. Labeling the Probe for FISH

Label 1.0 μg of probe with biotin-11-dUTP by the nick translation reaction according to the following protocol.

1. Make serial dilutions of DNase I in sterile distilled water to 10 ng, 1 ng, 100 pg, and 10 pg DNase/μL.
2. Aliquot 1.0 μL of probe DNA in each of four Eppendorf tubes.
3. Add 1 μL 10X nick translation buffer.
4. Add 1 μL of DNase I (10 ng in the first tube, 1 ng in the second, and so on).
5. Add sterile distilled water to 10 μL.
6. Incubate at 37°C for 16 h or overnight.
7. Add the following reagent volumes to each of the tubes:

Nick translation buffer	4.0 μL
dNTPs	5.0 μL
Biotin-II-dUTP	2.5 μL
dTTP	4.5 μL
DNA polymerase	11.0 μL
H$_2$O	23.0 μL

8. Incubate at 14°C for 3 h.
9. Add 5 µL of 0.2M EDTA, and incubate at 70°C for 5 min to inactivate the enzymes.

3.3. Size Fractionation and Evaluation of the Probe

3.3.1. Gel Electrophoresis

1. Add the following reagents to Eppendorf tubes:
   Labeled probe   3.0 µL
   TE buffer   1.0 µL
   0.4M NaOH   6.0 µL
   6X loading buffer, dye   2.0 µL
2. Add the following reagents to a separate tube:
   100-bp DNA ladder   2.0 µL
   TE buffer   1.0 µL
   6X loading buffer   2.0 µL
   H_2O 7.0 µL
3. Incubate at 65°C for 5 min, and chill on ice. (Do not incubate the DNA ladder at 65°C.)
4. Run the samples on an agarose gel electrophoresis unit.
5. Stain the gel with EtBr solution (0.5 µg/mL of distilled water) and observe over a UV box.
6. Transfer the DNA probes to nitrocellulose filter by Southern transfer (23). Small fragments normally transfer within 4–6 h.
7. Bake the filter in a vacuum oven at 80°C for 1 h.
8. Store at room temperature.

3.3.2. Detection of Label

1. Wet the nitrocellulose filter in distilled water.
2. Incubate in TBS for 5 min.
3. Incubate in TBT solution for 5 min.
4. Incubate in avidin alkaline phosphatase for 10 min.
5. Wash the filter in TBT for 5 min.
6. Wash in developing buffer for 5 min
7. Incubate in 10 mL of NBT/BCIP in a dark box.
8. Color development (bluish purple) occurs within 10 min.
9. The intensity of the color as judged by the eye is normally a good indicator of labeling efficiency. Alternatively, the labeling efficiency may be checked by scanning with a densitometer.

3.4. In Situ Hybridization

1. Add 20–100 µg (1–5 µL) of labeled probe to 5.0 µL of human placental DNA.
2. Add HB to a final volume of 40 µL.
3. Apply 30 µL of this mixture to chromosomal preparation under a cover slip, and seal with Gene Frame™.

4. Place the slides in Terasaki plates, and incubate at 75°C for 7 min.
5. Incubate at 37–42°C for 16 h or overnight.
6. Remove cover slips, and incubate the slides in 50% formamide in 2X SSC at 42–45°C for 20 min.
7. Rinse in 2X SSC for 20 min at 42°C.
8. Rinse in 0.1X SSC at room temperature for 20 min.

3.5 Visualization of Label on Chromosomes

3.5.1. Fluorescent Detection of Label

1. Incubate the slides in TBS for 10 min at room temperature.
2. Incubate in TBST for 10 min at room temperature.
3. Add 100 μL of TBST containing 1 ng/mL avidin-FITC, and incubate for 30 min at room temperature.
4. Rinse slides in wash buffer 3× for 5 min.
5. Add 100 μL of TBST containing 1 ng/mL of biotinylated antiavidin to the slides, and incubate for 30 min.
6. Rinse in wash buffer 3× for 5 min.
7. Add 100 μL of TBST containing 1 ng/mL avidin-FITC, and incubate for 30 min.
8. Wash 3× for 5 min in wash buffer.
9. Stain slides with Hoechst 33258 for 10 min, and mount in antifade solution.
10. Observe under fluorescence microscope.

3.5.2. Detection by the Gold/Silver Method

1. Incubate slides in TBS for 10 min at room temperature.
2. Incubate in TBST for 10 min at room temperature.
3. Add 100 μL of TBST containing 1 ng/mL of streptavidin-gold, and incubate at room temperature for 30 min.
4. Rinse in TBS 3× for 5 min.
5. Place a few drops of the silver solution on each slide, and monitor under light microscope. Silver grains take 5–10 min to develop.

3.5.3. Detection by DAB/Gold/Silver Method

1. Incubate in TBS for 10 min at room temperature.
2. Incubate in TBST for 10 min at room temperature.
3. Add 100 μL of TBST containing 1 ng/mL avidin-FITC, and incubate for 30 min at room temperature.
4. Rinse in TBST for 5 min.
5. Add 100 μL of TBST containing anti-FITC-peroxidase, and incubate for 30 min at room temperature.
6. Rinse in TBS 3× for 5 min.
7. Prepare fresh DAB solution and immediately place a few drops on each slide. Incubate for 5 min at room temperature.
8. Rinse in distilled water 3× for 5 min.

9. Add 100 µL of gold solution to each preparation, and incubate for 5 min at room temperature.
10. Rinse in distilled water 3× for 5 min.
11. Place a few drops of Na_2S solution on each side, and incubate for 5 min at room temperature.
12. Rinse in distilled water 3× for 5 min.
13. Place a few drops of silver solution on each preparation and follow manufacturer's instruction.
14. Rinse in distilled water.

3.6. Replication Banding

1. Stain sides with 5.0 µg/mL of Hoechst 33258 in 2X SSC for 20 min.
2. Rinse in distilled water, mount in 2X SSC, and expose the slides to UV light for 1–16 h.
3. Rinse the sides in distilled water, and stain with Giemsa solution for 10 min.
4. Dry, and mount in DPX.

3.7. Primed In Situ Labeling (PRINS)

PRINS can be performed with synthetic oligonucleotides ranging in size from 18–30 bp *(24)*. Alternatively, the primer may be a double-stranded fragment of DNA (dsDNA) generated by PCR™ or from a plasmid. A method for detection of alphoid repeats at the centromeres of chromosome 17 *(23,25)* is described, although single-copy genes have also been mapped using this approach.

1. Prepare the reaction mixture as follows:

Taq polymerase buffer (10X)	5.0 µL
25 mM MgCl$_2$	3.0 µL
Forward primer (100 ng/µL)	2.0 µL
Reverse primer (100 ng/µL)	2.0 µL
dNTP mixture	1.0 µL
dTTP (1 mM)	1.0 µL
Fluorescein-II-dUTP (1 mM)	1.0 µL
Sterile distilled water to	49.0 µL
Taq polymerase enzyme (1.0 U/µL)	1.0 µL

2. Denver the mixture to the chromosome spreads under a cover slip, and seal with Gene Frame™.
3. Incubate the sides in a thermal cycler.
4. Incubate the sides at 95°C for 1.0 min, 58°C for 1.0 min, and 72°C for 4.0 min.
5. Remove cover slips, and wash in 2X SSC containing 0.01% Triton X-100 for 5 min.
6. For detection of label, *see* Sections 3.4. and 3.5.
7. Stain with propidium iodide (2.0 µg/mL), mount, and observe under fluorescent microscope. Typical examples are illustrated in Figs. 1 and 2.

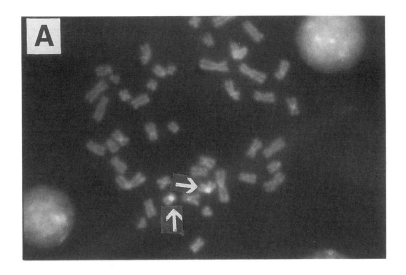

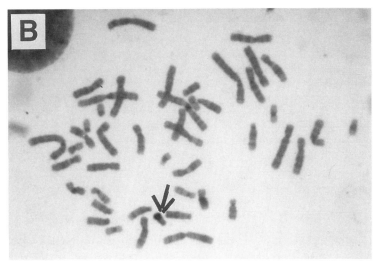

Fig. 1. Detection of chromosome aberrations and sex determination by PRINS: **(A)** A metaphase spread from peripheral blood of a patient with chronic myelogenous leukemia (CML) in lymphoid blast crisis. A set of 21-mer oligonucleotides specific for a satellite DNA at the centromere of chromosome 17 were used. White arrow shows isochromosome 17. The yellow arrow shows the normal chromosome 17. **(B)** Metaphase spread from peripheral blood of a male showing the Y chromosome. PRINS was performed with a set of 21-mer oligonucleotides specific for the Y chromosome. The signal was detected with streptavidin conjugated with 1-nm gold particles and enhanced with silver.

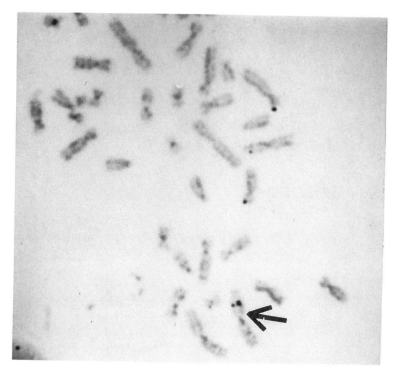

Fig. 2. Gene mapping by PRINS: Three sets of oligonucleotides were used to map the COL9A2 gene on chromosome 1p32. The signal was initially detected with avidin fluorescein and enhanced with antifluorescein peroxidase followed by DAB/gold/silver as described in the text.

4. Notes
4.1. Tissue Culture and Preparation of Chromosome Spreads

1. There is no reason why chromosome spreads for gene mapping should not be prepared from any type of dividing cells, including fibroblasts, epithelial cells, or lymphoblastoid cell lines. However, unless the karyotype of a given cell type is well characterized, or there is a specific reason for using a particular cell type, such as mapping chromosomal aberrations, it is best to use primary cell cultures e.g., skin fibroblasts.
2. PHA-induced lymphocytes provide an ample source of material for gene mapping primarily because of the ease of handbag short-term cultures, but also because the lymphocytes retain their normal diploid karyotype for a long time in culture.
3. Incorporation of BUdR for replication banding permits direct detection of bands and signal when stained with the Hoechst dye.
4. BUdR is sensitive to light. After addition of BUdR, the cultures should be handled in subdued light until the cells are fixed, in order to avoid extensive chromosomal

damage. Preparations used for PRINS must be handled with extreme care, because nicks in chromosomal DNA can act as primers for the amplification reaction. Fixing slides in 3% paraformaldehyde preserves the chromosomal architecture.

4.2. Probes for FISH

5. For repetitive DNA sequences, such as alphoid repeats, especially for identification of centromeric regions on chromosomes, as well as in interphase nuclei, I routinely prepare labeled probes by PCR™ using a centromeric DNA-specific set of primers. For single-copy gene mapping by FISH, it is essential to use DNA cloned into either cosmids or in yeast artificial chromosome vectors (YAC) in order to obtain the level of sensitivity that will enable visualization of signal with a fluorescence microscope.

6. Biotin- and/or digoxigenin-labeled probes are stable for more than a year when stored at 4°C. It is therefore possible to nick translate up to 5 µg of the probes and store a good batch. When compared with tritium (5 ng), the amount of probe used is much larger (typically 20–100 ng).

4.3. Denaturation/Hybridization and Stringency Washes for FISH

7. Inclusion of formamide is essential for lowering the melting temperature of DNA. It is necessary to perform denaturation and hybridization of probe and chromosomal DNA at a lower temperature to ensure preservation of chromosomal architecture. Similarly, inclusion of formamide in the stringency washes increases the stringency without having to increase the temperature.

8. Reducing the salt concentration (from 2X SSC to 0.1X SSC) during washing also increases the stringency.

4.4. Detection

9. A fluorescent microscope equipped with filter blocks for fluorescein, rhodamine, and Hoechst 33258 (or DAPI) is ideal. Confocal laser scanning microscope will enable visualization and analysis of high-resolution mapping, but is not strictly essential for routine *in situ* hybridization. Assignment of signal on chromosome is best done on photographs. It is possible to hybridize more than one probe to a slide as long as the probes are labeled with different reporters, e.g., fluorescein and rhodamine, biotin and fluorescein, or biotin and digoxigenin. It is possible to visualize the signal with the FISH method and then process the preparations for DAB/gold/silver. However, the silver method does increase the signal-to-noise ratio.

4.5. PRINS

10. The method described here is ideally suited for detection of both alphoid repeats at the centromeric regions of all chromosomes, and moderately repetitive DNA sequences within the arms and telomeric regions.

11. For mapping single-copy genes, the incubation times in the thermal cycler should be longer. The anneal log temperature should be between 54–60°C. The incubation time may be extended to 10 min. The primer extension step at 72°C should be extended to 30 min.

12. A mixture of more than one set of forward and reverse primers specific for the gene of interest will enhance the signal.

13. The primers should be tested in preliminary PCR™ reaction to establish the annealing temperature, as well as the authenticity of the PCR™ product *(26)*. It may be necessary to use laser scanning confocal microscopy and a digitized image enhancer if the signal is too weak to be detected by conventional fluorescent microscope. Alternatively, the DAB/gold/silver detection method will enhance the signal, although it will also increase background noise (Fig. 2).

References

1. Heniford, B. W., Shum-Siu, A., Leonberger, M., and Hendler, F. J. (1993) Variation in cellular EGF receptor mRNA expression demonstrated by *in situ* reverse transcriptase polymerase chain reaction. *Nucleic Acids Res.* **21,** 3159–3166.

2. Schmidt, J. E., Suzuki, A., Ueno, N., and Kimehnan D. (1995) Localized BMP-4 mediates dorsal/ventral patterning in the early *Xenopus* embryo. *Dev. Biol.* **169,** 37–50.

3. Harvey, M. B., Leco, K. J., Arcellana-Panlilio, M. Y., Zhang, X., Edwards, D. R., and Schultz, G. A. (1995) Proteinase expression in early mouse embryos is regulated by leukaemia inhibitory factor and epidermal growth factor. *Development* **121,** 1005–1014.

4. Affolter, M., Nellen, D., Nussbaumer, U., and Basler, K. (1994) Multiple requirements for the receptor serine/threonine kinase thick veins reveal novel functions of TGF beta homologues during *Drosophila* embryogenesis. *Development* **120,** 3105–3117.

5. Suzuki, A., Thies, R. S., Yamaji, N., Song, J. J., Wozuey, J. M., Murakami, K., and Ueno, N. (1994) A truncated bone morphogenetic protein receptor affects dorsal-ventral patterning in the early *Xenopus* embryo. *Proc. Natl. Acad. Sci. USA* **91,** 10,255–10,259.

6. Sassoon, D. and Rosenthal, N. (1993) Detection of messenger RNA by *in situ* hybridization. *Methods Enzymol.* **225,** 384–404

7. Pratt, G. D. and Kokaia, M. (1994) *In situ* hybridization and its application to receptor subunit mRNA regulation. (Review) *Trends Pharmacol. Sci.* **15,** 131–135.

8. Bettinger, D., Mougin, C., and Lab, M. (1994) Rapid detection of cytomegalovirus-infection by *in situ* polymerase chain reaction on MRC5 cells inoculated with blood specimens. *J. Virol. Methods* **49,** 59–66.

9. Nuovo, G. J., MacConnell, P. B., Simsir, A., Valea, F., and French, D. L. (1995) Correlation of the *in situ* detection of polymerase chain reaction-amplified metalloproteinase complementary DNAs and their inhibitors with prognosis in cervical carcinoma. *Cancer Res.* **55,** 267–275.

10. Anastasi, J., Thangavelu, M., Vardiman, J. W., Hooberman, A. L., Bian, M. L., Larson, R. A., and Le Beau, M. M. (1991) Interphase cytogenetic analysis detects minimal residual disease in a case of acute lymphoblastic leukemia and resolves the question of origin of relapse after allogeneic transplantation. *Blood* **77,** 1087–1091.

11. Cremer, T., Lichter, P., Borden, J., Ward, D. C., and Manuelidis, I. (1988) Detection of chromosome aberrations in metaphase and interphase tumour cells by *in situ* hybridization using chromosome specific library probes. *Hum. Genet.* **80,** 235–246.

12. Delhanty, J. D. A., Griffin, D. K., Handyside, A. H., Harper, J., Atkinson, G. H. G., Pieters, M. H. E. C., and Winston, R. M. L. (1993) Detection of aneuploidy and chromosomal mosaicism in human embryos during preimplantation sex determination by fluorescent *in situ* hybridization (FISH). *Hum. Mol. Genet.* **2,** 1183–1185.

13. Delhanty, J. D. A. (1994) Preimplantation diagnosis. *Prenat. Diag.* **14,** 1217–1227.

14. Bhatt, B., Burns, J., Flannery, D., and McGee, J. O'D. (1988) Direct visualization of single-copy genes on banded metaphase chromosomes by nonisotopic *in situ* hybridization. *Nucleic Acids Res.* **16,** 3951–3961.

15. Garson, J. A., van den Berghe, J. A., and Kemshead, J. T. (1987) Novel nonisotopic *in situ* hybridization technique detects small (1 kb) unique sequences in routinely G-banded human chromosomes: fine mapping of N-MYC and b-NGF genes. *Nucleic Acids Res.* **15,** 4761–4770.

16. Lichter, P., Chieh-Ju, C. T., Calls, K, Hermanson, G., Evans, G. A., Housman, D., and Ward, D. C. (1990) High-resolution mapping of human chromosome by *in situ* hybridization with cosmic clones. *Science* **247,** 64–69.

17. Lawrence, A. B., Singer, R. H., and McNeil, J. A. (1990) Interphase and metaphase resolution of different distances within the human dystrophin gene. *Science* **249,** 928–932.

18. Parra, I. and Windle, B. (1993) High-resolution visual mapping of stretched DNA by fluorescent hybridization. *Nature Genet.* **5,** 17–21.

19. Bailey, D. M., Carter, N. P., de Vos, D., Leversha, M. A., Perryman, M. T., and Ferguson-Smith, M. A. (1993) Coincidence painting: a rapid method for cloning region specific DNA sequences. *Nucleic Acids Res.* **21,** 5117–5123.

20. Cinti, C., Santa, S., and Maraldi, N. M. (1993) Localization of single-copy gene by PRINS technique. *Nucleic Acids Res.* **21,** 5799,5800.

21. Gosden, J. and Lawson, D. (1995) Instant PRINS: a rapid method for chromosome identification by detecting repeated sequences *in situ*. *Cytogenet. Cell Genet.* **68,** 57–60.

22. Therkelsen, A. J., Nielsen, A., Koch, J., Hindjaer, J., and Kølvraa, S. (1995) Staining of human telomeres with primed *in situ* labeling (PRINS). *Cytogenet. Cell Genet.* **68,** 115–118.

23. Sambrook, J., Fritsch, E. F., and Maniatis T. (1989) *Molecular Cloning: A Laboratory Manual.* Cold Spring Harbor Laboratory Press, Cold Spring Harbor, NY.

24. Hindkjaer, J., Koch, J., Mogensen, J., Kølvraa, S., and Bolund, L. (1994) Primed *in situ* (PRINS) labeling of DNA. *Methods Mol. Biol.* **33,** 95–107.

25. Waye, J. S. and Willard, H. F. (1986) Structure, organisation, and sequence of alpha satellite DNA from human chromosome 17: evidence for evolution by unequal crossing-over and an ancestral pentamer repeat shared with the human X chromosome. *Mol. Cell. Biol.* **6,** 3156–3165.

26. Erlich, H. A. (ed.) (1989) *PCR Technology. Principles and Applications for DNA Amplification.* Stockton Press, New York.

42

Expression of Recombinant Antibody Fusion Proteins in *E. coli*

Stephen M. Hobbs

1. Introduction

Conjugates of antibodies or antibody fragments with foreign proteins have attracted interest because of their therapeutic potential as antitumor agents in vivo. Localization of the complex to the target site is dependent on the specificity of the antibody moiety, and local cytotoxic action is determined by the foreign protein. Examples of this approach include immunotoxins, in which the effector protein is a plant or bacterial toxin *(1)*, and antibody-directed enzyme prodrug therapy (ADEPT), in which the foreign protein is a prodrug-activating enzyme that converts a systemically administered nontoxic prodrug into a cytotoxic species at the target site *(2)*.

The classical method of conjugating an antibody to a foreign protein is chemical crosslinking (Chapter 13), but this can have certain drawbacks: It may be difficult to control the degree and site of substitution; interference with the activity of either partner may occur; and it may be difficult to separate the final products. An alternative is to use recombinant DNA techniques to construct a fusion protein in which the antibody and effector proteins form part of the same peptide chain. With this approach, the site and nature of the linkage between the two proteins can be defined precisely, and complex manipulation of the product is not required. Extra peptide sequences can also be included to facilitate detection and/or purification of the product by affinity chromatography, either on a column of antibody directed against the tag sequence or on metal chelate columns if the tag is a polyhistidine sequence *(3)*. This technique is of course dependent on the availability of DNA coding sequences for the VH and VL regions of the antibody as well as the toxin or enzyme. Development of

From: *Methods in Molecular Biology, Vol. 80: Immunochemical Protocols, 2nd ed.*
Edited by: J. D. Pound © Humana Press Inc., Totowa, NJ

the reverse transcriptase polymerase chain reaction (RT-PCR) has simplified the isolation of antibody coding sequences from hybridoma cell lines and enabled easy incorporation of terminal restriction sites to facilitate subsequent cloning *(4)*.

The resultant chimaera is then cloned into a suitable expression vector for protein production in a variety of hosts, including bacterial *(5,6)*, yeast *(7,8)*, plant *(9)* and mammalian cells *(4,10,11)*. Expression of proteins in bacteria has the advantage that the system can be assembled rapidly and scaled up for large-scale induction in fermenters at high cell densities. However, since bacteria do not express whole-antibody molecules efficiently, smaller fragments, such as Fv, single-chain Fv (scFv), and Fab are generally used. This also simplifies the construction of the fusion gene and assembly of the final vector. Proteins expressed intracellularly tend to form insoluble inclusion bodies, which have to be redissolved and the protein renatured, reducing the recovery and biological activity of the product. These problems can be avoided by inclusion of an N-terminal hydrophobic leader sequence to direct secretion of the protein through the cell membrane into the periplasm. This mimics the cotranslational transport and folding of antibody chains in plasma cells *(12)*. Signal processing and disulfide bond formation also occur in the oxidizing environment of the periplasm *(13)*, and secretion of the product through the outer cell wall may occur on prolonged incubation. Soluble active product can then be isolated from the culture medium or from periplasmic extracts.

This chapter describes the construction of an Fab sequence bearing a foreign gene on the truncated antibody heavy chain, and gives a typical protocol for expression of the fused protein in *Escherichia coli*.

1.1. Vector Construction

There are several types of antibody expression vector available, an example of which is shown in Fig. 1. It is based on the vector pSW1–VHD1.3-VkD1.3 from the laboratory of G. Winter *(14)* and contains antibody heavy and light chain cDNA sequences cloned in frame with the pectate lyase B leader sequence from *Erwinia carotovora* for periplasmic secretion *(15)*. In this case, the foreign gene of interest is cloned in frame in place of the first cysteine codon in the upper hinge region of the antibody heavy chain. The resultant chimeric protein is shown in Fig. 2. The rest of the vector is based on pUC19 *(16)*, and includes an ampicillin resistance gene and origin of replication for growth and selection in bacteria, and a *lac* promoter for isopropylthio-β-D-galactoside (IPTG)-inducible gene expression. This type of vector is expressed in the strain BMH 71-18 *(14)*, which carries the *lacIq* gene *(17)*.

It is not possible to specify precisely the steps necessary to assemble such a vector, since they will depend on the structure of the particular antibody and

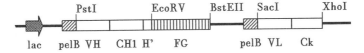

Fig. 1. Structure of the expression cassette of a typical bacterial expression plasmid designed to produce an antibody Fab linked to a foreign gene (FG), pelB leader sequences direct periplasmic secretion of the nascent chains. The remainder of the plasmid contains the ampicillin resistance gene and a plasmid origin of replication.

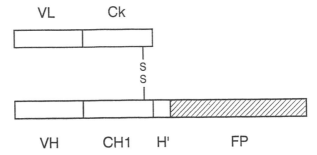

Fig. 2. Structure of the antibody Fab fusion protein expressed from the vector in Fig. 1. The antigen-binding region is formed by the VH and VL domains, the foreign protein (FP) fused to the truncated hinge region (H') may be a toxin or prodrug activating enzyme.

foreign gene of interest. PCR amplification of coding regions from cDNA, cloning, and sequencing are all carried out by standard procedures, and the reader is referred to several treatises on the subject *(18,19)*. However, a few general points are worth noting:

1. An open reading frame must be maintained at the end of the antibody heavy chain, and the foreign gene must be inserted so as to be translated in the correct frame as determined by the upstream start codon in the leader sequence. Any stop codons may be removed by reamplification of the gene by PCR with a suitably modified primer. If a C-terminal affinity tag is to be included for subsequent detection and/or purification of the product, the stop codon of the foreign gene must also be removed in a similar way and the correct reading frame maintained into the tag sequence.

2. The restriction sites used for cloning should ideally be unique, both in the vector and in all the sections to be conjugated. If such sites are not available, then several approaches are possible:
   a. A partial digest may be performed with limiting amounts of enzyme. A product of the correct size may then be isolated after agarose gel electrophoresis

of the digest. However, this becomes progressively more difficult as the number of sites increases.

b. Site-directed mutagenesis using specific oligonucleotides may be carried out either by PCR or by direct cloning using any of several proprietary kits. The gene of interest may first have to be subcloned into a suitable vector for this technique.

c. It may be possible to ligate in the gene as a blunt-ended fragment, using Klenow or T4 DNA polymerase to fill in the non compatible overhangs. This is again sequence-dependent, since correct framing of the final product must be maintained. Partial fill-ins may also be used, where a subset of dinucleotide triphosphates (dNTPs) is used to create compatible ends from pairs of otherwise noncohesive sites: examples include *Bam*HI/*Bgl*II-*Sal*I/*Xho*I and *Xba*I-*Hin*dIII. Certain pairs of enzymes also produce compatible ends, e.g., *Bgl*II-*Bam*HI, *Xho*I-*Sal*I, although the final ligated joint will not represent an endonuclease recognition site, so detection of cloned insert by restriction digest may be more difficult.

3. When using PCR to amplify existing clones to incorporate different terminal sequences, it is important to minimize the possibility of polymerase-induced copying errors. An error-correcting polymerase, such as Pfu (Stratagene, Cambridge, UK), may be used, and the number of amplification cycles kept to a minimum.

4. Depending on the complexity of the sequences, it may be necessary to assemble the final vector in stages. The various PCR products can be cloned into standard cloning vectors, such as pBluescript (Stratagene), and then combined into the expression vector separately.

In all cases, the junction between the two protein genes should be sequenced before expression is attempted to ensure that ligation has occurred correctly and that the proper reading frame has been maintained.

2. Materials

1. LB broth: 10 g/L Bacto-tryptone, 5 g/L Bacto-yeast extract, 10 g/L NaCl; adjusted to pH 7.0 with NaOH and sterilized by autoclaving.

2. LB agar: add 1.5g Bacto-agar/100 mL LB broth. Sterilize by autoclaving.

3. Ampicillin: Dissolve at 50 mg/mL in distilled water, sterilize by filtration through a sterile 0.22-μm disposable filter, and freeze in aliquots at −20°C.

4. Glucose: Make up at 20% in distilled water, and filter-sterilize.

5. $1M$ IPTG in distilled water: sterilize by filtration, and freeze in aliquots at −20°C.

6. Competent *E. coli* of the appropriate strain.

7. Sterile 250-mL conical flasks and 2-L baffled conical flasks.

8. An orbital incubator capable of operating at 30°C if lower temperature expressions are to be performed. This generally requires a refrigeration system to be fitted.

9. Columns for affinity chromatography, depending on the system in use.

3. Method

1. Transfect the final expression vector into competent *E. coli* strain BMH 71-18.
2. Plate the transformation mixture onto LB agar plates containing 100 µg/mL ampicillin and 1% glucose, and incubate overnight at 37°C.
3. Transfer a colony into 25 mL LB broth containing 100 µg/mL ampicillin and 1% glucose in a sterile 250-mL Erlenmeyer flask. Grow up overnight at 37°C in an orbital incubator.
4. Harvest the cells by centrifugation at 4000*g* for 20 min, and wash once in LB broth without glucose. Resuspend the pellet in 20 mL LB broth.
5. Inoculate 2-L baffle flasks containing 500 mL LB broth and 100 µg/mL ampicillin with 1 mL of the washed overnight culture, and grow at 30°C in an orbital incubator until the absorbance at 600 nm is approx 0.6.
6. Induce protein expression by adding IPTG to a final concentration of 1 m*M*. Continue incubation at 30°C for 6–16 h.
7. Cool the flasks on ice for 1 h, and then separate the cells and supernatant by centrifugation at 4000*g* for 20 min at 4°C. The supernatant should be sterilized by pressure filtration through a 0.45-µm membrane.
8. Concentrate the supernatant on a stirred pressure cell (e.g., Amicon, Stonehouse, Gloucs, UK) or a tangential membrane concentrator (e.g., Minitan from Millipore, Watford, UK) fitted with 10,000 M_r cutoff membranes. A preservative, such as sodium azide may be added to prevent unwanted bacterial contamination.
9. Fusion protein may be purified from the supernatant by affinity chromatography. The choice of immobilized ligand will depend on the specific circumstances, but may be the antigen to which the antibody was raised, an antibody to the antibody fragment or to the foreign gene (*see* Chapter 14), or if an affinity tag has been included at the C-terminus of the foreign gene, then this can also be used for purification on antibody or metal chelate columns as appropriate.

4. Notes

1. Expression and secretion of exogenous proteins can be damaging to bacterial cells. It is therefore necessary to use a promoter that can be tightly regulated, so that the cells can be grown to a suitable density without plasmid loss before expression is induced. For this reason, the IPTG/*lacIq* system is often used. A related system is the IPTG-inducible cascade T7 promoter as used in the pET series vectors *(20)*, the *lacIq* gene being carried in the vector. These vectors are expressed in the strains BL21(DE3) or BL21(DE3)pLysS.
2. Growth at lower temperatures (e.g., 30°C) may improve yield and activity of the secreted protein, possibly by allowing more time for membrane translocation and folding to occur *(21)*. Variation of IPTG concentration and duration of induction may also affect the final yield. It is beneficial therefore to carry out smaller scale expressions under various conditions to optimize these aspects.
3. The degree to which fusion protein may be processed and secreted from the periplasm into the medium may depend on the exact structure of the protein. The

factors that govern this are not fully understood. The distribution of the product among the cytoplasm, periplasm, and medium should be determined empirically by ELISA, RIA, or Western blotting before large-scale purification

4. Bacteria do not carry out posttranslational modifications such as glycosylation, so the resulting proteins may not be in their fully native state. It is important to test both parts of the purified fusion protein to make sure that biological activity is retained and that the foreign protein still functions when fused to an antibody chain.

References

1. Ghetie, M. A. and Vitetta, E. S. (1994) Recent developments in immunotoxin therapy. *Curr. Opinion Immunol.* **6,** 707–714.
2. Bagshawe, K. D. (1994) Antibody-directed enzyme prodrug therapy. *Clin. Pharmacokinet.* **27,** 368–376.
3. Porath, J. (1992) Immobilized metal ion affinity chromatography. *Protein Exp. Purification* **3,** 263–281.
4. Orlandi, R., Gussow, D. H., Jones, P. T., and Winter, G. (1989) Cloning immunoglobulin variable domains for expression by the polymerase chain reaction. *Proc. Natl. Acad. Sci. USA* **86,** 3833–3837.
5. Skerra, A. and Pluckthun, A. (1988) Assembly of a functional immunoglobulin Fv fragment in *Escherichia coli. Science* **240,** 1038–1041.
6. Better, M., Chang, C. P., Robinson, R. R., and Horwitz, A. H. (1988) *Escherichia coli* secretion of an active chimeric antibody fragment. *Science* **240,** 1041–1043.
7. Horwitz, A. H., Chang, C. P., Better, M., Hellstrom, K. E., and Robinson, R. R. (1988) Secretion of functional antibody and Fab fragment from yeast cells. *Proc. Natl. Acad. Sci. USA* **85,** 8678–8682.
8. Bowdish, K., Tang, Y., Hicks, J. B., and Hilvert, D. (1991) Yeast expression of a catalytic antibody with chorismate mutase activity. *J. Biol. Chem.* **266,** 11,901–11,908.
9. Ma, J. K., Lehner, T., Stabila, P., Fux, C. I., and Hiatt, A. (1994) Assembly of monoclonal antibodies with IgG1 and IgA heavy chain domains in transgenic tobacco plants. *Eur. J. Immunol.* **24,** 131–138.
10. Riechmann, L., Foote, J., and Winter, G. (1988) Expression of an antibody Fv fragment in myeloma cells. *J. Mol. Biol.* **203,** 825–828.
11. Gillies, S. D. (1992) Design of expression vectors and mammalian cell systems suitable for engineered antibodies, in *Antibody Engineering. A Practical Guide* (Borrebaeck, C. A. K., ed.), Freeman, New York.
12. Wulfing, C. and Pluckthun, A. (1994) Protein folding in the periplasm of *Escherichia coli. Mol. Microbiol.* **12,** 685–692.
13. Bardwell, J. C. (1994) Building bridges: disulfide bond formation in the cell. *Mol. Microbiol.* **14,** 199–205.
14. Ward, E. S., Gussow, D., Griffiths, A. D., Jones, P. T., and Winter, G. (1989) Binding activities of a repertoire of single immunoglobulin variable domains secreted from *Escherichia coli. Nature* **341,** 544–546.

15. Lei, S.-P., Lin, H.-C., Wang S.-S., Callaway, J., and Wilcox, G. (1987) Characterization of the *Erwinia carotovora* pelB gene and its product pectate lyase. *J. Bacteriol.* **169,** 4379–4383.

16. Yanisch-Perron, C., Vieira, J., and Messing, J. (1985) Improved M13 phage cloning vectors and host strains: nucleotide sequences of the M13mp18 and pUC19 vectors. *Gene* **33,** 103–119.

17. Gronenborn, B. (1976) Overproduction of the phage lambda repressor under control of the lac promoter of *Escherichia coli. Mol. Gen. Genet.* **148,** 243–250.

18. Sambrook, J., Fritsch, E. F., and Maniatis, T. (1989) *Molecular Cloning: A Laboratory Manual, 2nd ed.* (Ferguson, M., Ford, N., and Nolan, C., eds.). Cold Spring Harbor Laboratory Press, Cold Spring Harbor, NY.

19. Erlich, H. A. (ed.) (1989) *PCR Technology: Principles and Applications for DNA Amplification.* Stockton Press, New York.

20. Studier, F. W., Rosenberg, A. H., Dunn, J. J., and Dubendorff, J. W. (1990) Use of T7 RNA polymerase to direct expression of cloned genes. *Methods Enzymol.* **185,** 60–89.

21. Cabilly, S. (1989) Growth at sub-optimal temperatures allows the production of functional, antigen-binding Fab fragments in *Escherichia coli. Gene* **85,** 553–557.

43

Expression of Antibody Fusion Proteins in Mammalian Cells

Anita A. Hamilton, John R. Adair, and Simon J. Forster

1. Introduction

Recombinant DNA technology provides a means to mimic nature and build multidomain proteins that display several functions. This ability is being applied by the pharmaceutical industry to develop novel products. Fusion proteins of antibodies and enzymes formed one of the earliest examples of protein engineering *(1)*. By genetic engineering "magic bullets," comprising a targeting agent linked to an active agent can be produced in one step, without recourse to laborious conjugation chemistry. A wide range of recombinant molecules have now been constructed where the binding specificity of an antibody or T-cell receptor variable domain, cytokine, growth factor, or other protein ligand (e.g., CD4) is fused to another protein domain, for example, a toxin, enzyme, cytokine, or antibody constant region. Progress in this area is summarized in recent reviews *(2,3)*.

The ability to generate gene fusions of choice can also be applied to assist the purification of recombinant proteins. In this case, one or more of the domains in the protein acts as an affinity "handle," allowing rapid and efficient recovery of the product. This is beneficial where rapid initial analysis of protein variants is required, or where the final protein product is difficult to purify by standard methods and no direct affinity-purification process is available. For example, if the protein of interest is fused to the binding site of an antihapten antibody, the fusion can then rapidly be recovered by affinity chromatography on solid-phase hapten. The availability of a method for rapid affinity-purification means that a series of fusion points can be assessed to obtain the correct specific activity of the C-terminal fusion partner (for example, if a cytokine or enzyme is to be attached a spacer of varying length may have to be incorporated to allow the

From: *Methods in Molecular Biology, Vol. 80: Immunochemical Protocols, 2nd ed.*
Edited by: J. D. Pound © Humana Press Inc., Totowa, NJ

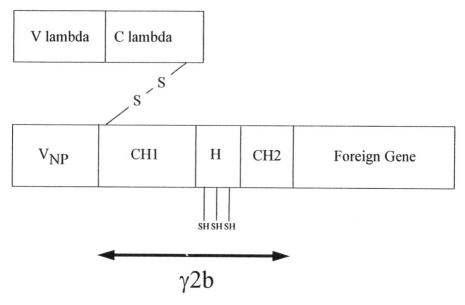

Fig. 1. Structure of the antibody fusion protein. The Fab-like form is formed from a λ light chain derived from the J558L cell line, and the chimeric heavy chain produced from the vector. The heavy chain consists of a variable region with NIP binding activity, C_H1, hinge and part of the C_H2 domain of murine γ2b heavy chain, and the foreign gene. The fusion protein may be secreted in this form or as an F(ab')$_2$-like form consisting of 2 Fab-like molecules linked at the hinge region by three disulfide bonds.

correct functioning of the cytokine or enzyme). Once the correct overall configuration has been established, the hapten recognition site can easily be replaced by a therapeutically useful binding site. An example is the anti-NP system described by Neuberger et al. *(1)*, which has been used in affinity-purification and analysis of antibody-ricin A fusions *(4)*.

Here we describe the basic system of gene assembly, expression and purification of such fusions. The gene to be expressed is inserted behind the hinge region of an antibody heavy chain gene in place of the C_H2 and C_H3 domains *(1,5)*. This hybrid heavy chain construct is transfected into a myeloma cell line that produces a compatible light chain, or cotransfected with a suitable antibody light chain gene. The recombinant antibody-like molecule (*see* Fig. 1) is secreted and can be purified using the corresponding antigen.

The fusion vector pSV-$V_{NP}γ2b$△(C_H2, C_H3) *(1,5)* is shown in Fig. 2. This plasmid is derived from pSV2*gpt* *(6)*. It contains the variable region, V_{NP}, the C_H1, hinge, and the N-terminal part of the C_H2 domain of the $γ_{2b}$ heavy chain of a mouse antibody that binds to the haptens NP (4-hydroxy-3-nitrophenecetyl) and NIP (5-iodo-4-hydroxy-3-nitrophenacetyl).

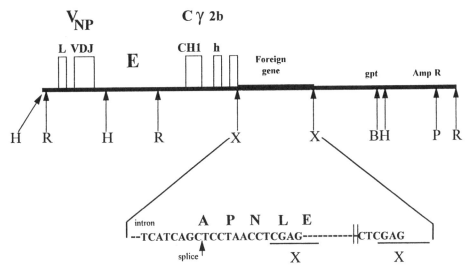

Fig. 2. Structure of the fusion vector pSV-$V_{NP}\gamma_{2b\triangle}(C_H2, C_H3)$. The V_{NP} and γ2b genes are inserted in pSV*gpt* between the *Eco*RI and *Bam*HI sites. The *Bam*HI site is converted to *Xho*I by the addition of linkers. B, *Bgl*II; H, *Hin*dIII; P, *Pvu*I; R, *Eco*RI; X, *Xho*I; E, immunoglobulin enhancer.

In the original description of the process *(1)*, the point of fusion was at an *Xho*I site within the N-terminal sequence of the C_H2 domain of the antibody heavy chain. The gene of interest was presented as a restriction fragment with an *Xho*I-compatible cloning sites. These could be added by linker adaptation or site-directed mutagenesis. However, using the polymerase chain reaction (PCR) *(7)*, gene fusions can now be constructed at any convenient point, no longer dictated by the availability of restriction enzyme sites in the DNA sequence (*see* Note 1). This provides far more scope for protein design. The sole requirement is that the final fused gene sequence has external 5'- and 3'-cloning sites for insertion into the expression vector. Use of PCR means that any signal sequence can be accurately removed, and if necessary, linking peptides can be included between the antibody portion and the downstream protein. This can be important if the N-terminus is involved in the function of the protein (*see* Note 2).

For the current purpose, an in-frame fusion at the *Xho*I site will be described. The termination codon is supplied by the inserted gene sequence. Polyadenylation signals are provided on the vector. The fusion gene is expressed from the immunoglobulin heavy chain promoter, and the immunoglobulin enhancer is included for high-level expression in myeloma cells. The vector contains the *Escherichia coli gpt* gene coding for the enzyme XGPRT for selection in mammalian cells with medium containing mycophenolic acid and xanthine.

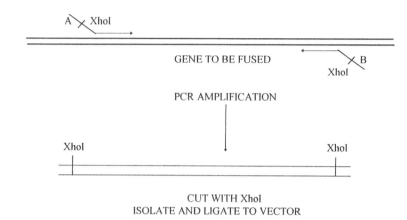

Fig. 3. Preparation of foreign gene for insertion into the fusion vector. The required DNA fragment is amplified by PCR with primers including *Xho*I sites.

Association of the pSV-V_{NP} heavy chain with light chains of the λ1 subgroup gives rise to hybrid antibody molecules that bind to the haptens NP and NIP (Fig. 1). A convenient source of light chain is the mouse plasmacytoma J558L, derived from J558 *(8)*. This line expresses a resident λ1 light chain, but no heavy chain. The fusion vector is transferred to the J558L host cell line by electroporation.

Once transfectomas have been generated, they must be screened for the production of the desired fusion. The binding site provided by the expression of the V_{NP} heavy chain in J558L cells and association of the heavy chain with the resident light chain means that the protein fusion can be "captured" on a solid phase by NP or NIP, and detected using commercially available antibody to mouse λ chain and an appropriate enzyme conjugate, in a simple ELISA screening procedure. Similarly, purification can be achieved by affinity adsorption of the fusion onto an NP matrix. An immunoblot method is described here for characterization of selected transfectomas, which allows the mol-wt of the fusion product to be estimated.

2. Materials

2.1. Preparation of Gene for Fusion

1. Two amplification/mutagenic oligonucleotides, A and B, 25 pmol/μL (Fig. 3).
2. Deoxyribonucleoside triphosphates (dNTPs). The stock contains 6.25 m*M* of each dNTP: The stock contains 6.25 m*M* of each dNTP.
3. Thermostable DNA polymerase (with a proofreading function).
4. 10X PCR reaction buffer as recommended by supplier.
5. Thermal cycler.

6. 1.5- and 0.5-mL Microcentrifuge tubes.
7. PCR-grade mineral oil.
8. Elutip D columns (Schleicher and Schuell, Dassel, Germany).
9. *Xho*I restriction enzyme and reaction buffer as provided by supplier.
10. Autoclaved, deionized distilled water.
11. Phenol/chloroform: 1:1 mixture of phenol (liquefied, washed with Tris buffer) and chloroform/isoamyl alcohol 24:1 (v/v). Note: phenol causes severe burns and should be handled with care. Store at 4°C.
12. 7.5*M* Ammonium acetate.
13. Ethanol (analytical-grade).

2.2. Insertion of Gene Into Fusion Vector

1. Plasmid pSV-V$_{NP}\gamma_{2b}\triangle$(C$_H$2, C$_H$3) *(1)*. Kindly supplied by M. Neuberger, Medical Research Council Laboratory of Molecular Biology, Cambridge, UK.
2. Enzymes: *Xho*I restriction enzyme, calf intestinal alkaline phosphatase, and T4 DNA ligase are available from commercial suppliers complete with reaction buffers. Follow the instructions for use, storage, and shelf-life.
3. DNA size standards (e.g., λ DNA *Hin*dIII digest).
4. 7.5*M* Ammonium acetate.
5. Ethanol (analytical-grade).
6. Geneclean™ kit: (BIO 101 Inc., La Jolla, CA).
7. TE buffer: 10 m*M* Tris-HCl, pH 8.0, 1 m*M* EDTA; autoclave and store at 4°C.
8. Transformation competent *E. coli* HB101 cells. These can be prepared as described in ref. *9,* or can be obtained from commercial suppliers.
9. Phenol/chloroform: prepared as in Section 2.1.
10. Chloroform/isoamyl alcohol 24:1 (v/v).
11. Kit for DNA sequencing: Available with protocol from commercial suppliers.
12. Kit for large-scale preparation of plasmid DNA: Available with protocol from commercial suppliers

2.3. Transfection into Mammalian Cells by Electroporation

1. J558L Mouse plasmacytoma cell line: Obtained from G. Koch, MRC Laboratory of Molecular Biology, Cambridge, UK.
2. Dulbecco's Modified Eagles Medium (DMEM) containing antibiotics (100 U/mL penicillin, 100 U/mL streptomycin, 0.25 µg/mL amphotericin B, 50 µg/mL gentamycin) and 10% (v/v) fetal bovine serum (FBS).
3. Selective DMEM: To 500 mL DMEM, add 5 mL 2.5 mg/mL xanthine in 0.5*M* NaOH and 160 µL 2.5 mg/mL mycophenolic acid in ethanol.
4. Electroporator and cuvets (e.g., Bio-Rad, Hercules, CA).
5. 24- and 96-Well tissue-culture plates.
6. *Pvu*I restriction enzyme and reaction buffer as provided by the manufacturer.

2.4. Screening, Analysis, and Purification

1. NIP caproate O succinimide (NIP-Cap-OSu) (Cambridge Research Biochemicals, Northwich, Cheshire, UK) *(see* Note 3): Dissolve 31 mg in 300 µL of

N,N'-dimethylformamide (DMF). Solid NIP-Cap-OSu should be stored desiccated at –20°C. DMF is toxic by inhalation and skin absorption, and should be handled with gloves in a fume hood. Prepare just prior to use.

2. 5 mg/mL Bovine serum albumin (BSA) in 1% (w/v) sodium bicarbonate: Prepare just prior to use.

3. NIP-Cap-BSA: Add 75 μL of NIP-Cap-OSu in DMF to 5 mL of BSA-bicarbonate solution, and leave stirring overnight at 4°C. Dialyze for 48 h against three changes of 2 L of PBS. Determine the protein concentration and coupling ratio by reading A_{280} and A_{430}. Protein concentration is:

$$[A_{280} - (0.59 \times A_{430})]/1.4 \text{ mg/mL} \tag{1}$$

and the coupling ratio (hapten:BSA) is:

$$(68 \times A_{430}) \, [4.85 \times (\text{BSA concentration in mg/mL})] \tag{2}$$

4. Phosphate-buffered saline (PBS), pH 7.2: 0.14M NaCl, 2.7 mM KCl, 1.5 mM KH_2PO_4, and 8.1 mM Na_2HPO_4.

5. PBS containing 0.1% (w/v) sodium azide: Sodium azide is toxic by ingestion and inhalation, and should be handled with gloves in a fume hood.

6. PBS containing 1 mM NIP-Cap-OH (Cambridge Research Biochemicals): Prepare just prior to use. Solid NIP-Cap-OH should be stored desiccated at –20°C.

7. Tris/saline: 10 mM Tris-HCl, 150 mM NaCl, pH 7.4.

8. Tris/saline/BSA: Tris/saline containing 3% (w/v) BSA.

9. Alkaline phosphatase substrate buffer: 0.1M Tris-HCl, 0.1M NaCl, 5 mM $MgCl_2$, pH 9.5.

10. 1M Iodoacetamide: Make only 1 mL and store at –20°C. Discard when a brownish tinge appears.

11. Blot buffer: 192 mM glycine, 12.5 mM Tris-HCl, pH 8.3, containing 10% (v/v) methanol. Store at –20°C.

12. Blot blocking solution: Tris/saline containing 3% (w/v) nonfat dried milk (e.g., Marvel). Store at –20°C.

13. Nitro blue tetrazolium (NBT) stock: 75 mg/mL in 70% (v/v) DMF. Store at –20°C.

14. 5-Bromo-4-chloro-3-indolyl phosphate (BCIP), *p*-toluidine salt, stock: 50 mg/mL in DMF.

15. 3% (w/v) Sodium bicarbonate: Prepare just prior to use.

16. ω-Aminohexyl Sepharose (Sigma, St. Louis, MO).

17. 1,4-Dioxan: 1,4-dioxan is toxic by ingestion and inhalation, and should be handled with gloves in a fume hood.

18. Small disposable plastic syringe or column (for example, Bio-Rad).

3. Methods

3.1. Preparation of Gene for Fusion

1. Synthesize two oligonucleotides, A and B, each encompassing the termini of the gene to be fused. These oligonucleotides include 15–20 nucleotides of homology

with the gene to be fused, and in A at the 5'-end the *Xho*I site, and in B, at the 5'-end
the complement of a stop codon and the 3'-cloning site (*see* Fig. 3).

2. Add together in a 0.5-mL microfuge tube:

Template DNA (100ng)	X μL
Primers	
(A) 25 pmol	1 μL
(B) 25 pmol	1 μL
10X PCR reaction buffer	5 μL
dNTP stock	2 μL
H₂O	49.5–X μL
Thermostable DNA polymerase	2.5 U

3. Overlay the mix with 50 μL of mineral oil.
4. Perform 20 cycles of 94°C for 1 min; 55°C for 1 min; 72°C for 1 min; followed
   by 72°C for 15 min using a thermal cycler.
5. Remove the reaction mixture from beneath the mineral oil, phenol/chloroform extract,
   chloroform extract, and precipitate the DNA by adding 25 μL 7.5*M* ammonium
   acetate and 150 μL ethanol. Precipitate at room temperature for 10 min.
6. Centrifuge for 10 min at 12,000 rpm in a microcentrifuge, wash the DNA pellet
   with 100 μL 70% ethanol, dry, and resuspend in 20 μL TE buffer.
7. Digest the DNA fragment with *Xho*I according to the supplier's instructions.

3.2. Insertion of Gene into Fusion Vector

1. To prepare the vector, digest 10 μg of pSV-V$_{NP}$γ$_{2b\Delta}$(C$_H$2, C$_H$3) vector DNA
   in 40 μL final volume in the buffer supplied by the manufacturer with an
   excess (20–50 U) of *Xho*I to ensure complete digestion. Check that the DNA
   is fully digested by electrophoresis of a 1-μL sample on a 0.8% (w/v) agarose
   minigel.
2. Precipitate one-half of the digested vector DNA with ethanol. Add 0.5 vol of
   7.5*M* ammonium acetate and 2 vol of 100% ethanol. Incubate at –20°C for 30
   min, then spin at full speed in a microcentrifuge for 10 min, wash the pellet with
   70% ethanol, dry, and resuspend in 10 μL of TE buffer.
3. Dephosphorylate the vector DNA by adding 5 μL of 10X phosphatase buffer,
   35 μL of water, and 0.02 U of calf intestinal alkaline phosphatase. Incubate at
   37°C for 30 min, then add another 0.02 U, and continue the incubation for a
   further 30 min. Extract with phenol/chloroform, followed by chloroform//isoamyl
   alcohol, and precipitate the DNA with ethanol as in step 2.
4. Load the *Xho*I-digested insert DNA (Section 3.1.) and the *Xho*I-digested,
   phosphatase-treated vector into separate wells on preparative agarose gels,
   and electrophorese until the fragments are well separated. Excise the vector
   and insert bands.
5. Purify these DNAs from the gels using Geneclean™ according to the manufacturers' instructions. Recover the DNA in a small volume of water. Inspect a small
   sample (10%) of each by electrophoresis on a 0.8% (w/v) agarose minigel along-
   side DNA size standards and estimate the concentrations.

6. Resuspend the DNA fragments in TE buffer at approx 200 μg/mL Set up a 20-μL ligation reaction in the ligase buffer provided by the manufacturer. The reaction should contain equimolar amounts of phosphatase-treated vector and DNA to be inserted, at a total DNA concentration of 40 μg/mL. Add 3 U of T4 DNA ligase, and incubate at 16°C overnight. Prepare parallel control reactions using only the *Xho*I-digested vector DNA and *Xho*I-digested, phosphatase-treated vector DNA as ligation/transformation controls.

7. Transform 10 μL each of the ligated DNAs into transformation-competent *E. coli* HB101 cells.

8. To identify colonies with inserts in the correct orientation, either perform colony PCR (*see* Note 4) or prepare plasmid DNA, and perform analytical restriction mapping to determine the orientation of the inserts (*see* ref. *10*).

9. Determine the DNA sequence to confirm that no spurious mutations have occurred during PCR (*see* Note 5).

10. Prepare plasmid DNA for transfection (*see* ref. *10*). Commercially available kits for large-scale preparation of plasmid DNA are convenient for this purpose.

3.3. Transfection into Mammalian Cells by Electroporation

1. Linearize 20 μg of the plasmid by digestion with *Pvu*I (*see* Note 6 if the inserted gene includes a *Pvu*I site). Precipitate the digested DNA with ethanol and dissolve in 50 μL sterile deionized H_2O.

2. Resuspend the cells from a semiconfluent culture, count the cells, and collect by centrifugation at 500*g* for 5 min at 4°C. Discard the supernatant.

3. Resuspend $1–3 \times 10^7$ cells in 0.5 mL DMEM, and transfer them to a Gene Pulser cuvet. Mix the DNA with the cells by gentle pipeting, and leave the cuvet on ice for 5 min.

4. Insert the cuvet between the electrodes of the Electroporator and apply a single pulse of 300 V, 960 μF.

5. Return the cuvet to ice for 20 min.

6. Transfer the cell suspension to a 75-cm^2 flask containing 20 mL of DMEM, and allow the cells to recover for 24 h at 37°C with 5% CO_2.

7. Harvest the cells by centrifugation at 500*g* for 5 min at 4°C and resuspend in 120 mL of selective DMEM. Dispense 1.5 mL to each well of two 24-well plates, and 200 μL to each well of two 96-well plates.

8. Approximately 10–15 d from the start of selection, colonies should be visible to the naked eye, and the culture supernatants from the wells should be assayed for antibody by ELISA (*see below*). Select cell lines for expansion on the basis of the level of recombinant antibody production, and the number and size of the colonies in the well. Wells with single colonies should be chosen.

9. Resuspend the cells from the designated wells by rubbing the end of a 1-mL pipet or pipeter tip across the surface of the well, and pipet up and down gently to dislodge the cells. Transfer all of the medium to a 25 cm^2 flask containing 4 mL fresh selective DMEM or to a 175-cm^2 flask containing 50 mL selective DMEM if colonies are being pooled.

10. As soon as practicable, stocks of cell lines should be preserved in liquid N_2.

3.4. Screening, Analysis, and Purification

3.4.1. Screening by ELISA for Cell Lines
Expressing and Secreting the Fusion Product

If antiserum to the foreign gene product is available, this can be used in the ELISA with an appropriate conjugate as the "revealing" reagent instead of anti-mouse λ chain antibody as described below.

1. Dilute NIP-Cap-BSA to 5 µg/mL in coating buffer. Dispense 200 µL/well to a microtiter plate, and incubate for at least 2 h at 37°C or overnight at 4°C.
2. Empty wells. Do not wash. Block wells by filling with 250 µL of Tris/saline/ BSA, and incubate for at least 2 h at 37°C or overnight at 4°C.
3. Empty wells, and wash three times with PBST.
4. Dispense 200-µL samples of conditioned medium to wells and incubate at 37°C for 1 h.
5. Wash three times with PBST.
6. Dilute goat antimouse λ chain antibody 1:1000 in PBST and dispense 200 µL/well. Incubate at 37°C for 1 h.
7. Empty wells and wash three times with PBST.
8. Dilute alkaline phosphatase conjugated rabbit antigoat IgG 1:1000 in PBST and dispense 200 µL/well. Incubate at 37°C for 1 h.
9. Empty wells and wash three times with PBST.
10. Develop color. Fill wells with 200 µL of substrate buffer containing 2.2 mg/mL of *p*-nitrophenyl phosphate. Incubate in the dark for 10–30 min. Read the plates at 405 nm. Positive wells should give a yellow color. The reaction can be stopped by adding 50 µL of $3M$ NaOH to each well.

3.4.2. Immunoblot Analysis of Fusion Products

If antisera or monoclonal antibodies are available to the fused gene product, these can be used in an immunoblot *(11)* to detect expression. As an alternative, $0.1M$ iodoacetate can be used instead of 2-mercaptoethanol in reducing SDS-PAGE. Under these conditions, the light-heavy chain disulfide bridge is not reduced, and the fusion protein is detected with an anti-λ chain antiserum. A gradient of 6–12.5% polyacrylamide has been found suitable to cover the range of molecular weights from free λ chains to large fusion products.

1. Electrophorese the samples on reducing SDS-PAGE according to standard methods *(12)*. If anti-λ antiserum is to be used as the detection method, the 2-mercaptoethanol should be replaced by iodoacetamide at final concentration of $0.1M$.
2. Transfer the separated proteins to nitro-cellulose paper following the instructions of the manufacturer of the blotting apparatus.
3. Block the surface of the blot with blocking solution for 1 h at room temperature, or overnight at 4°C.

4. Add the detection antiserum (for example, goat anti-λ chain antibody) at an appropriate dilution (normally 1:1000), and continue incubation for at least 1 h at room temperature or overnight at 4°C.

5. Wash the blot with multiple changes of Tris/saline, over 30 min.

6. Add the reveal antiserum (for example, rabbit antigoat IgG alkaline phosphatase conjugate) at an appropriate dilution (1:1000 in Tris/saline), and incubate for 1 h at room temperature.

7. Wash over 30 min as before, first with Tris/saline, and then with alkaline phosphatase substrate buffer.

8. Make up the substrate solution: for each 10 mL of substrate buffer, add 40 μL of NBT stock and 40 μL of BCIP stock, in that order, mixing between additions. Add the substrate solution to the blot, and allow color development to proceed. Stop the reaction by washing several times with water. Dry the blot between sheets of Whatman 3MM paper under a weight.

3.4.3. Affinity-Purification on NIP Columns (see Note 7)

1. Swell 10 g of ω-aminohexyl Sepharose by stirring for about 5 h at room temperature in 100 mL of 3% sodium bicarbonate.

2. Cool to 4°C and add 50 mg of NIP-Cap-OSu dissolved in 400 μL of 1,4-dioxan.

3. Stir overnight at 4°C.

4. Wash exhaustively with water and then PBS containing 0.1% azide.

5. Store at 4°C in PBS/azide.

6. Add an appropriate amount of NIP-Cap-Sepharose slurry into a small (2 mL) disposable column and allow to settle.

7. Block nonspecific binding sites by filling the column with Tris/saline/BSA and leaving for 30 min at room temperature.

8. Wash with PBS.

9. Pass the sample through the column.

10. Wash the column extensively with PBS.

11. Elute with 1 mM NIP-Cap-OH in PBS.

12. Analyze the eluted material by SDS-PAGE or by Immunoblot.

13. Dialyze against a large volume of PBS (no azide), overnight at 4°C.

14. Read the absorbance of the dialyzed material at 280 nm, and calculate the approximate protein concentration using A_{280} of 1.4 = 1 mg/mL.

4. Notes

1. If the sequence is known, fusions can be constructed between any two DNAs by two rounds of PCR. The procedure, termed "Gene Splicing by Overlap Extension" is described in ref. *13*. In the first PCR, gene I is amplified with primers A and B to give the product AB. Gene II is amplified with primers C and D to give the product CD. Primers B and C contain mismatches to the original sequences such that the ends of the PCR products are modified to include the same sequence. When these PCR products are mixed, denatured, and reannealed, the top strand of AB and the bottom strand of BC overlap and act as primers on one another.

The overlap is extended by polymerase and amplified in the second PCR with outside primers A and D.

2. Proteins with N-terminal signal peptides or C-terminal membrane anchor regions and proteins where the N terminus contributes to the biological properties of the protein require special attention to achieve a satisfactory fusion. A number of variants may need to be made and assayed. A protease-sensitive site may be designed into the amino acid sequence at the fusion point for eventual separation of the desired gene product from the fusion.

3. NIP-Cap-OSu comprises the NIP moiety with a five-carbon (caproic acid) spacer arm and an *N*-hydroxysuccinimidyl group that is reactive with amino groups, thus allowing attachment to BSA and ω-aminohexyl Sepharose. NIP-Cap-OH is the free acid form.

4. Colony PCR is a convenient method for identification of clones that contain inserted DNA in the correct orientation *(14)*. Use one oligonucleotide primer that anneals within the vector and one oligonucleotide primer that anneals within the inserted gene. The primers are oriented relative to each other, so that a defined-length PCR product will be generated if the insert has been cloned in the required orientation. For confirmation, use a PCR primer that anneals within the inserted gene, but on the opposite strand, in association with the first primer. No PCR product should be obtained with this primer pair unless the gene has been cloned in the wrong orientation.

5. For PCR, it is important to use a licensed thermostable enzyme with a proofreading facility and to reduce the cycle number to the minimum number that provides acceptable yield after the post-PCR manipulations. The precautions are necessary, because the error rate for some thermostable polymerases is quite high and the number of errors that accumulate increases with cycle number.

6. The transfection efficiency of linear DNA is higher than that of circular. It is generally convenient to linearize the fusion vector with *Pvu*I, since there is a single site in the ampicillin gene. If the inserted gene includes a *Pvu*I site, another site should be chosen that cuts in the pBR322-derived portion of the vector that is not required for expression in mammalian cells. Failing this, circular DNA can be used.

7. Although this expression system is designed to allow the fusion protein to be secreted as an antibody-like molecule, it is possible that a particular insert will give expression, but not secretion. This may be owing to incorrect folding, or the presence of a hydrophobic domain in the foreign protein. Provided that the fusion protein is not too rapidly degraded intracellularly, it may still be possible to characterize and purify it using the techniques described here, with slight modifications. The cells are harvested by centrifugation (150*g* for 10 min) and washed several times in PBS. The cells are lysed in a small volume of 50 m*M* Tris-HCl, 150 m*M* NaCl, 5 m*M* EDTA, pH 8.0, 1% (v/v) Nonidet-P40, 2 m*M* PMSF, and 5 m*M* NEM. The lysates should be clarified by centrifugation if necessary and can then be used in the methods given above, with the following modifications: for the ELISA screen, dilute lysates 1 in 5 with PBST before use; for purification on an NIP column, after blocking the column with Tris/saline/BSA, wash the col-

umn extensively with 50 m*M* Tris-HCl, 150 m*M* NaCl, 5 m*M* EDTA, pH 8.0, 1% (v/v) Nonidet-P40, load the sample, then wash again with this buffer, and elute with 1 m*M* NIP-Cap-OH in this buffer. No modification to the Western blot procedure is required.

References

1. Neuberger, M. S., Williams, G. T., and Fox, R. O. (1984) Recombinant antibodies possessing novel effector functions. *Nature* **312,** 604–608.
2. Adair, J. R. and King, D. J. (1995) Reconstruction of monoclonal antibodies by genetic engineering, in *Monoclonal Antibodies: The Second Generation* (Zola H., ed.), BIOS Scientific, Oxford, UK, pp. 67–92.
3. Pietersz, G. A. and McKenzie, I. F. C. (1995) The genetic engineering of antibody constructs for diagnosis and therapy, in *Monoclonal Antibodies: The Second Generation* (Zola H:, ed.), BIOS Scientific, Oxford, UK, pp. 93–117.
4. Spooner, R. A. and Lord, J. M. (1991) Expression of antibody-ricin A chain fusions in mammalian cells, in *Monoclonal Antibodies: Applications in Clinical Oncology* (Epenetos, A. A., ed.), Chapman and Hall Medical, New York, pp. 65–77
5. Williams, G. T. and Neuberger, M. S. (1986) Production of antibody-tagged enzymes by myeloma cells: application to DNA polymerase I Klenow fragment. *Gene* **43,** 319–324.
6. Mulligan, R. C. and Berg, P. (1981) Selection for animal cells that express the *Escherichia coli* gene coding for xanthine-guanine phosphoribosyl transferase. *Proc. Natl. Acad. Sci. USA* **78,** 2072–2076.
7. Saiki, R. K., Scharf, S., Faloona, F., Mullis, K. B., Horn, G. T., Erlich, H. A., and Arnheim, N. (1985) Enzymatic amplification of β-Globin genomic sequences and restriction site analysis for diagnosis of sickle cell anemia. *Science* **230,** 1350–1354.
8. Lundblad, A., Steller, R., Kabat, E. A., Hirst, J. W., Weigert, M. G., and Cohn, M. (1972) Immunochemical studies on mouse myeloma proteins with specificity for dextran or for levan. *Immunochemistry* **9,** 535–544.
9. Chuang, S.-E., Chen, A.-L., and Chao, C.-C. (1995) Growth of *E. coli* at low temperature dramatically increases the transformation frequency by electroporation. *Nucleic Acids Res.* **23,** 1641.
10. Sambrook, J., Fritsch, E. F., and Maniatis, T. (1989) *Molecular Cloning. A Laboratory Manual,* 2nd ed. Cold Spring Harbor Laboratory Press, Cold Spring Harbor, NY.
11. Harlow, E. and Lane, D. (1989) *Antibodies: A Laboratory Manual.* Cold Spring Harbor Laboratory Press, Cold Spring Harbor, NY.
12. Hames, B. D. (1981) An introduction to polyacrylamide gel electrophoresis, in *Gel Electrophoresis of Proteins: A Practical Approach* (Hames, B. D. and Rickwood, D. J., eds.), IRL, Oxford, UK, pp. 11–91.
13. Horton, R. M., Cai, Z., Ho, S. N., and Pease, L. R. (1990) Gene splicing by overlap extension: tailor made genes using the polymerase chain reaction. *Biotechniques* **8,** 528–535.
14. Gussow, D. and Clackson, T. (1989) Direct clone characterization from plaques and colonies by the polymerase chain reaction. *Nucleic Acids Res.* **17,** 4000.

44

Antibody Screening
of Bacteriophage λ gt-11 DNA Expression Libraries

Peter Jones

1. Introduction

Much of our current understanding of the molecular details of the activity and interactions of proteins has stemmed from the ability to isolate cDNA encoding these proteins. Computer-based analysis of deduced amino acid sequence allows predictions to be made about their structure and function that can then be tested experimentally. The starting point for all of this is the ability to isolate the specific cDNA encoding the protein of interest from libraries that contain on the order of 10^5–10^7 recombinants. There are many approaches that can be used to isolate cDNA clones, and the exact strategy applied really depends on the molecular tools available. If a cDNA encoding the particular protein of interest has already been cloned from one species, it can be used to probe cDNA libraries from other species using DNA hybridization techniques. Alternatively, degenerate oligonucleotides can be designed from amino acid sequences from regions of proteins that are conserved across species. The oligonucleotides can be used to screen cDNA libraries by hybridization or used as primers to amplify and clone the cDNA by using the polymerase chain reaction.

Often, when trying to isolate cDNAs encoding novel proteins, the only thing that can be used to any advantage has to be derived from the purified protein itself. The protein can be used for the generation of antibodies and to obtain amino acid sequence. Screening cDNA expression libraries, constructed in vectors like bacteriophage λ gt-11, with an antibody raised against the protein, represents one of the quickest approaches to isolate its cDNA. The cDNA is prepared from the appropriate source and ligated into the λ vector. It is ligated into a restriction site within the coding region of the β-galactosidase gene that

From: *Methods in Molecular Biology, Vol. 80: Immunochemical Protocols, 2nd ed.*
Edited by: J. D. Pound © Humana Press Inc., Totowa, NJ

has been engineered into the vector. Large amounts of β-galactosidase are expressed as transcription is driven by a strong promoter. Any coding region of a cDNA that is ligated into the β-galactosidase gene, in the correct orientation and reading frame, will be expressed as a fusion protein with β-galactosidase. Statistically, this will take place at a frequency of one in six ligation events, however, the probability of detecting a specific cDNA is largely determined by its abundance in the mRNA population.

The basic λ gt-11 expression system described by Young and Davis *(1,2)* now appears in many commercially available guises, which have been engineered to increase the number of cDNAs that are expressed or facilitate the recovery of cloned cDNAs by phage rescue. Although there have been improvements in the design of λ vectors, the basic protocols in screening the libraries with antibodies are very similar. Briefly, screening involves plating the λ library at a suitable dilution on a lawn of *Escherichia coli*. Expression of the β-galactosidase fusion proteins is then induced by overlaying the growing plaques with nitrocellulose filters that have been impregnated with isopropyl β-D-thiogalactopyranoside (IPTG), an inducer of β-galactosidase gene expression. The proteins expressed by λ gt-11 clones are transferred onto the nitrocellulose filters, and the filters processed for the detection of antigen in essentially the same way as they are after Western blotting.

The basic methodologies in constructing cDNA libraries are discussed in detail elsewhere *(3,4)*, but unless there is a need to make cDNA libraries from "exotic" sources or to generate a number of cDNAs libraries, it is more usual to purchase a cDNA library from a commercial supplier. The library is kept as a suspension of phage particles in a dilution buffer at a known titer in units of PFU/mL. The λ gt-11 can then be propagated in a host strain of *E. coli*, generally Y1090. This particular strain is used, since it is deficient in one of the major protease systems of *E. coli*, *lon*, thus minimizing the possibility of degradation of exogenous proteins.

2. Materials

1. *E. coli* strain Y1090 for library screening.
2. *E. coli* strain C600 for producing large amounts of the fusion protein.
3. Nutrient broth (100 mL): 1 g of Trypticase (BBL), 0.5 g of NaCl in water.
4. Top agar (100 mL): 1 g of Trypticase, 0.5 g of NaCl, 0.65 g of agar.
5. Bottom agar (100 mL): 1 g of Trypticase, 0.5 g NaCl, 1.5 g agar.
6. Ponceau S (Sigma, St. Louis, MO).
7. Chloroform.
8. IPTG.
9. Whatman paper 3MM.
10. Rabbit antiserum or affinity-purified antibody.

11. Swine immunoglobulins raised against rabbit immunoglobulins (Dako, Carpinteria, CA).
12. PAP (soluble complex of horseradish peroxidase and rabbit antihorseradish peroxidase, Dako).
13. PBS: $0.14M$ NaCl, 2.7 mM KCl, 1.5 mM KH_2PO_4, 8.1 mM Na_2HPO_4.
14. Tris/saline: 10 mM Tris-HCl, pH 7.5, 0.9% w/v NaCl.
15. Tris/saline/BSA: 10 mM Tris-HCl, pH 7.5, 0.9% w/v NaCl, 0.1% w/v bovine serum albumin (BSA).
16. Tris/saline/Marvel: 10 mM Tris-HCl, pH 7.5, 0.9% w/v NaCl, 3% w/v freeze-dried nonfat milk (e.g., "Marvel," Premier Beverages, Stafford, UK).
17. Tris/saline/Tween-20: 10 mM Tris-HCl, pH 7.5, 0.9% NaCl, 0.1% Tween-20.
18. DAB (3, 4, 3'-4'-tetra-amino biphenyl hydrochloride, BDH); add 20 mg of DAB to 1 mL of water, and mix until dissolved. Add to 99 mL of Tris/saline (*see* Note 3).
19. Nitrocellulose filters (Amersham International).
20. SM buffer (1 L): 5.8 g of NaCl, 2.0 g of $MgSO_4 \cdot 7H_2O$, 50 mL of $1M$ Tris-HCl, pH 7.5, 10 mg of gelatine. Autoclave to sterilize.
21. SM phage storage buffer: 10% v/v SM buffer in chloroform.

3. Methods

3.1. Primary Screen of a λ gt-11 Library

3.1.1. Plating of Library for Screening with Antibodies

1. Inoculate 10 mL of nutrient broth with Y1090. Add 0.1 mL of 20% maltose and 500 mg ampicillin. Grow overnight at 37°C with shaking (*see* Note 1).
2. Pellet cells by centrifugation at 4000g for 10 min at room temperature, and resuspend in 4 mL of sterile 10 mM $MgSO_4$.
3. A suitable number of plaques to screen/85-mm Petri dish is between 20 and 30,000. Dilute a portion of the library in SM buffer to 3×10^5 PFU mL, and add 200 µL of Y1090 to 100 µL of the diluted phage in a plastic universal bottle. Incubate at 37°C for 15 min to allow the phage to adsorb to the cell surface. The plaque size is affected by the amount of Y1090 cells used. If you require larger plaque sizes on subsequent rounds of screening, use 100 µL of Y1090 cells.
4. Add 4 mL of top agar (cooled to 50°C) to the cells, and pour onto the bottom agar plates. The addition of the agar is sufficient to mix the cell suspension, but be careful to avoid formation of air bubbles, which will make the top agar uneven. Prewarming the bottom agar plates at 42°C helps to avoid problems with the top agar setting before it is evenly spread. Allow the top agar to harden (~10 min). Number the bottom of the plates and incubate them at 42°C for 3 h to allow the plaques to form.
5. While the plates are incubating at 42°C, soak the nitrocellulose filters in 10 mM IPTG for 15 min. This may be carried out in one container, but ensure that all of the filters are properly wetted. Allow the filters to dry at room temperature for 1 h on Whatman 3MM paper. When the filters are dry, number the edges of the filters with a ballpoint pen.

6. The plaques will be very small at this stage and may not be visible to the naked eye. Place the IPTG-treated nitrocellulose filters onto the top agar, taking care not to trap any air bubbles between the top agar and the filter. This is best done by bowing out the center of the filter a little and touching it to the center of the plate first. Then allow the rest of the filter to be gently pulled down onto the plate.

7. Incubate the plates with the filters at 37°C for a further 2–3 h to allow sufficient expression of the cDNA insert.

8. Cool the plates to room temperature, and key the filters to the plate by pushing a syringe needle through the filter and agar of the plate. Mark the positions where the needle has passed through the agar with a marker pen on the underside of the plate. It is easier to align the position of the filters with these ink marks rather than the damaged agar. Remove the filters and perform the immunological screen.

9. Plates can be stored at 4°C for 2–3 wk.

3.1.2. Detection of Clones with Antibodies

1. Peel the filters off the plates, and place them plaque side up in a Petri dish (1/dish). Cover with Tris/saline/Marvel (about 5 mL), and incubate at room temperature for at least 45 min (or 4°C overnight) (*see* Note 2).

2. Remove the Tris/saline/Marvel, and wash the filters three times for 10 min in Tris/saline/Tween-20 (3 × 5 mL) on a rocking platform or similar device. Filters can be washed together in a large container if required.

3. After the final wash, add 5 mL of Tris/saline/Tween-20 containing 0.1% w/v BSA to each of the filters. If the primary antibody is in short supply, a number of filters can be screened in the same dish if care is taken not to trap air between the filters. Add the primary antibody to the appropriate dilution (*see* Note 3 to determine the optimum dilutions of antibody to use in screening the library), and incubate at room temperature for 2 h on a rocking platform or overnight at 4°C.

4. Remove the antibody solution. This can be kept at 4°C for use in further screens. The signal-to-noise ratio often increases with reuse of the antibody. Wash the filters as in step 2.

5. To each filter, add 5 mL of Tris/saline/BSA and the appropriate dilution of swine antirabbit antibody (usually about 1:300) to each filter, and incubate for 30 min at room temperature on a rocking platform.

6. Wash the filters as in step 2.

7. Add 5 mL of Tris/saline and the appropriate dilution of PAP, and incubate for 30 min at room temperature on a rocking platform.

8. Wash as in step 2.

9. Develop color on the filters by the addition of 5 mL of DAB solution to each filter and 2.5 μL of H_2O_2. Color develops in 0.5–5 min (*see* Note 4). It may be necessary to adjust the amount of H_2O_2 added to slow down the development times to allow the positive clones to become clearly visible before any background staining appears.

10. Stop color development by washing the filters in water.
11. Once the filters are dry, it is possible to align the filters with the original plates using the key marks that were made previously. Any putative positive plaques are then picked.
12. An agar plug from the region of the plate containing the recombinant phage is picked in the first instance with a 1-mL tip of a micropipet. The end of the pipet tip is cut to a diameter of approx 5 mm before picking the plug. The plug is removed by the suction that can be applied with the pipet. The agar plug containing the recombinant is then ejected into 1 mL of SM buffer containing 100 µL of chloroform (*see* Note 5) and the phage allowed to diffuse out of the plug for at least 4 h.
13. It is now necessary to carry out a further round of screening and purification at lower plaque densities until it is possible to pick a single, well-isolated plaque with the end of a Pasteur pipet. This usually requires a further two to three rounds of screening depending on the plaque densities used.

3.1.3. Plaque Purification and Titration

The approximate titer of the phage can be determined by a "spot titer" method:

1. Prepare a lawn of *E. coli* cells by adding 4 mL of molten top agar to 100 µL of cells resuspended in 10 mM MgSO$_4$ as described above. Pour the mixture over the bottom agar base, and allow it to set.
2. Make serial dilutions of 10^0, 10^{-3}, 10^{-6}, and 10^{-9} of the phage in SM buffer, and spot 5-µL aliquots of each dilution onto the solidified top agar. Tilt and rotate the plate to allow each spot to spread to a diameter of approx 10 mm, and allow the phage suspension to dry into the top agar. Incubate the plate overnight at 37°C. The approximate titer of the library is then be estimated from the number of plaques at each dilution.
3. Replate the eluted recombinant phage at a density of approx 500–1000 PFU/mL and rescreen with the antibody probe. Repeat the procedure of picking a positive plaque, eluting titrating, and replating at lower plaque densities until it is possible to pick a single well-isolated plaque.
4. Determine the titer of the purified phage, and store in 1 mL of phage storage buffer, in the dark, at 4°C. This can be kept for many years with little loss of phage viability.

3.1.4. Preparation of a High-Titer Stocks of Recombinant Phage

It is necessary to make high-titer stocks of the recombinant phage for the generation of stocks of phage to work with on a day-to-day basis, and also for the preparation of DNA for sequencing or for the preparation of protein lysates from recombinant phage. A relatively quick and easy method for the preparation of high-titer lysates is described below.

1. Infect Y1090 with the purified recombinant phage as described in the screening protocol, and plate at a density of about 50–100 PFU. Pick a single, well-isolated plaque with a Pasteur pipet, and remove the agar plug.
2. Add the agar plug to 50 μL of Y1090 cells resuspended in 10 mM MgSO$_4$ and incubate at room temperature for 5 min. Set up a control at the same time using 50 μL of uninfected Y1090 cells only.
3. Add 2 mL of nutrient broth containing 10 mM MgSO$_4$ to the tubes, and shake them vigorously at 37°C in an orbital shaker for 4–6 h or until lysis occurs. Lysis is complete when the solution becomes clear and contains string-like cell debris. Comparing the appearance of the infected culture with the control makes it easy to determine when this point is reached.
4. After lysis, add 50 μL of chloroform to the tube put on ice for 10 min. It is important to do this in chloroform-resistant containers.
5. Centrifuge the lysate at 4500g for 10 min to pellet the cell debris. Transfer the supernatant to a sterile container, and store in the dark at 4°C. Titers should be 10^{10} mL or better.

3.1.5. λ gt-11 Infection of E. coli Strain C600 for Western Blot Analysis of β-Galactosidase–cDNA Gene Fusion Products

Once a recombinant phage has been purified, it is expedient to analyze the β-galactosidase–cDNA gene fusion product by Western blotting to confirm the specific crossreaction of the antibody with the fusion protein. Preparative amounts of the fusion protein can be made by creating recombinant λ gt-11 lysogens, however a quicker and easier method is to take advantage of the amber mutation (S100) in the S gene of λ gt-11. This mutation renders λ gt-11 defective in lysing strains of *E. coli* which cannot suppress this mutation (*see* Note 7). A method is described below:

1. Add 0.1 mL of an overnight culture of *E. coli* strain C600, grown in nutrient broth containing 0.2% maltose, to 10 mL of fresh broth. Incubate the cells at 37°C, with shaking until they reach an absorbance of between 1.4–1.8 at 450 nm (A_{450} 0.64 = 2 × 10^8 cells/mL). This takes approx 2–3 h.
2. Pellet the cells from 1-mL aliquots of the culture by centrifugation at 12,000g for 2 min in a microfuge, and resuspend the bacterial pellets in 360 μL of nutrient broth containing 10 mM MgSO$_4$.
3. Dilute the recombinant λ gt 11 in 40 μL of SM buffer, and add the phage to each of the cell suspensions at a multiplicity of infection (M.O.I.) of 10, i.e., ratio of phage particles to bacterial cells is 10:1.
4. Incubate the mixture at 37°C for 3 h with occasional shaking.
5. Pellet the cells by centrifugation at 12,000g for 2 min in a microfuge, and resuspend the pellet in 100 μL of a loading buffer suitable for polyacrylamide gel electrophoresis. Boil the samples for 3 min, and remove any debris by a brief centrifugation. Load aliquots onto gels for analysis by Western blotting (generally, 50 μL contains approx 150 μg of protein).

3.1.6. Purification of Antibody Bound to Fusion Protein

Once a recombinant clone expressing a fusion protein has been purified and the fusion protein clearly shown to crossreact with the antibody by Western blotting, one can be reasonably confident that the cDNA isolated is the one required. Final proof of identity is ultimately dependent on sequencing the cDNA insert. The sequence of the cDNA is either compared with sequences in computer data bases (it is still possible to get a nasty surprise at this stage), or if the protein is novel, it is essential to find overlap be deduced amino acid sequences in the cDNA and peptide sequence from the purified protein. The latter approach is time-consuming and labor-intensive, and since many of the cDNAs initially isolated tend to be relatively small, it can take the sequences of many peptides to find overlaps. To gain further confidence that the time and effort in obtaining peptide data will be well invested, it is a worthwhile demonstrating that the fusion protein can be used to affinity-purify an antibody that will crossreact with the original antigen on a Western blot.

3.1.7. Affinity Purification of Antibody on Nitrocellulose Filters

1. Transfer the fusion protein from cell lysates to nitrocellulose by Western blotting. Load each track of the polyacrylamide gel with as much antigen as can be clearly resolved. The amount used has to be determined for the particular gel system used.
2. After blotting is complete, stain the nitrocellulose filter with Ponceau S for 5 min, and destain in water to detect the position of the fusion protein. Cut out the strip of nitrocellulose filter containing the fusion protein, and wash the filter for 10 min in PBS, 10% BSA, and 0.1% Triton X100. Repeat this washing step another two times.
3. Incubate the antibody (use 5X more concentrated than normal) with the nitrocellulose strip for 2–3 h at room temperature or 4°C overnight.
4. Wash the nitrocellulose filter as described in step 2, and then insert it into a precooled tube by curling it around the sides of the tube.
5. Elute the bound antibody by adding 1 mL of precooled $0.2M$ glycine-HCl, pH 2.2, and incubating the filter at 4°C for 5 min. Roll the tube to maximize the coverage of the filter.
6. Neutralize the solution by adding 30 μL of $2M$ Tris base, and then dialyze against PBS.
7. Dilute the antibody 1:10 for re-probing Western blots. The antibody can be reused several times if stored at 4°C in PBS, containing 5% w/v BSA.

4. Notes

1. Maltose is added to increase the amount of receptor for λ gt-11 on the cell surface of *E. coli*, but it is not essential.
2. The exact logistics of the number of filters screened and containers used for incubation with antibodies, and for washes can be decided individually. Generally,

we do not screen more than 10 filters (300,000 plaques) at a time and find it convenient to keep the filters in separate Petri dishes throughout the procedure.

3. Of the factors that determine the likelihood of success with this approach, assuming that the cDNA library contains a good representation of the mRNA population, by far the most important is the quality of the primary antibody used. In carrying out an antibody screen of a cDNA library, it is preferable to use a polyclonal antibody, since most of the cDNAs will probably be incomplete and may not contain the epitope recognized by a monoclonal antibody. Many of the problems associated with screening expression libraries stem from the crossreactivity of the other antibodies in the serum with *E. coli* proteins. This is quite a common occurrence, and it is useful to test the preimmune serum from a number of rabbits for crossreactivity with *E. coli* and phage proteins on a phage lift before starting an immunization regime. It is then possible to select rabbits to minimize any problems with high backgrounds or false positives. It is also worthwhile checking the secondary antibodies for crossreactivity. The optimum dilution of the primary antibody to be used in screening the library is one that allows the maximum sensitivity in detecting the antigen of interest without giving rise to high background staining. This optimum dilution can be determined by using segments (usually quarters) of a nitrocellulose filter taken from a plaque lift onto which serial dilutions of the antigen have previously been dried. The individual segments can then be incubated with different dilutions of the primary antibody to determine the optimum dilution. If antisera do produce high backgrounds in screening, it is possible to clean them up to some extent by subtracting antibodies that crossreact with *E. coli* proteins. This is most easily done by preincubating dilutions of antibody with nitrocellulose filters taken from plaque lifts before using them in screening.

4. DAB is a carcinogen, and should be handled and disposed of as dictated by the hazard data. There are a number of less hazardous substrates that can be used instead of the one described here. However, in our hands, DAB has worked best.

5. The chloroform is added to sterilize the phage suspension. Bacteriophage λ is resistant to the effects of chloroform as long as the chloroform is kept stored in the dark to prevent radical formation.

6. It is possible to grid the plate into 12 sections, allowing the titer of three plaque eluates to be determined on one plate. This is convenient, since it avoids the small mountain of plates, which can be generated if titering a number of putative positive plaques if separate plates are used for each dilution.

7. Preparative amounts of the fusion protein can be made from recombinant λ gt-11 lysogens in the *E. coli* strain Y1089. However, the isolation and purification of a lysogen are time-consuming and often impossible owing to mutations occurring in the λ repressor protein. By infecting an *E. coli* host strain, such as C600, which lacks the *supF* mutation, the phage will replicate many times without causing lysis. This results in high levels of the fusion protein being produced inside the cell, which is easily visible among the proteins of a cell lysate when analyzed by polyacrylamide gel electrophoresis. The very high numbers of λ gt-11 attained in

C600 result in the β-galactosidase fusion protein being expressed constitutively. If constitutive expression of fusion protein, or the fact that C600 is not *lon⁻*, affects the recovery of the protein or the viability of the C600, it is necessary to resort to forming a lysogen in Y1089.

References

1. Young, R. A. and Davis, R. W. (1983) Efficient isolation of genes by using anti-body probes. *Proc. Natl. Acad. Sci. USA* **80,** 1194.
2. Young, R. A. and Davis, R. W. (1983) Yeast RNA polymerase II genes: isolation with antibody probes. *Science* **222,** 778.
3. Huynh, T. V., Young, R. A., and Davis, R. W. (1985) Constructing and screening cDNA libraries in λ gt-10 and λ gt-11, in *DNA Cloning,* vol. 1 (Glover, D. M., ed.), IRL, Oxford, pp. 49–87.
4. Sambrook, J., Fritsch, E. F., and Maniatis, T. (1989) *Molecular Cloning, A Laboratory Manual.* Cold Spring Harbor Laboratory, Cold Spring Harbor, NY.

45

Display of Antibody Chains
on Filamentous Bacteriophage

Peter Jones

1. Phage Display

The construction of very large combinatorial libraries whereby antigen-binding functional domains of antibodies (Abs) are cloned and displayed on the surface of bacteriophage is proving to be a powerful technology in providing reagents for immunotherapy. Combinations of randomly assembled pairs of immunoglobulin heavy (H) and light (L) chain genes are cloned and expressed as fusions of bacteriophage coat proteins, allowing the bacteriophage expressing them to be selected by methods analogous to affinity chromatography. Purified phage can then be used for the production of large amounts of the pure antibody in a soluble form. Although phage-derived antibodies lack the effector functions of the parent antibodies since they have no Fc regions, these can subsequently be engineered into place or substituted with others, such as a toxin, with relative ease if required. Various antigen-recognition regions of the Ab can be cloned and selected, including:

1. Fv fragments that are noncovalently associated heterodimers of the heavy variable (VH) and light variable (VL) domains.
2. Single-chain Fv fragments (scFv) consisting of VH and VL regions linked by a flexible peptide.
3. Fabs that are noncovalently associated VH-CH and VL-CL pairings of Ab chains.

The selection of phage-expressing single heavy chains variable domains (dAbs), which make the major contribution to antigen binding, has also been reported (1). Although dAbs may have advantages in tissue penetration in therapeutic use, these domains have extensive hydrophobic surfaces, which present problems with specificity and limit their general use. The potential

From: *Methods in Molecular Biology, Vol. 80: Immunochemical Protocols, 2nd ed.*
Edited by: J. D. Pound © Humana Press Inc., Totowa, NJ

applications and some limitations of the phage display system can be better appreciated with some knowledge of the biology of filamentous bacteriophage. It is therefore the intention of this chapter to provide an introduction to bacteriophage biology and discuss, in general terms, the development of vectors and applications of the Ab phage display system, such as those described in Chapter 47. Potential "trouble spots" will also be highlighted, based on personal experience.

2. Biology of Filamentous Phage

Filamentous bacteriophage is a family of bacterial viruses that infect the host bacterium *Escherichia coli* which then continues to synthesize and export bacteriophage for as many generations as can be measured. The bacteriophage consist of a circular single-stranded DNA genome consisting of 10 genes *(Genes I–X)* encoding 10 proteins *(gp1–10)*. Five of the proteins are structural and form the phage coat, two are involved with the assembly of the phage particle, whereas the remaining three proteins participate in replication of the bacteriophage DNA. In addition to the coding regions of the bacteriophage genome, there is one main intergenic region (IR) that contains all of the sequences required for the initiation and termination of viral DNA synthesis, and for the morphogenesis of the bacteriophage particles. The protein coat consists of approx 2700 copies of *gp8* surrounding the main body of the particle, whereas small numbers of the minor coat proteins, *gp3*, *gp4*, *gp7*, and *gp9* are specifically located at each end.

The bacteriophage float freely in the extracellular milieu until making contact with a structure known as a sex pilus on the surface of *E. coli*. The pilus is effectively a protein tube that connects two *E. coli* together when they exchange DNA during conjugation. The proteins required for the assembly, structure, and transfer of DNA during conjugation are encoded by a large plasmid, called the F' plasmid. The presence of the F' plasmid in the host strain is absolutely essential for infection of *E. coli* by a filamentous phage, and its presence in host strains is indicated by the symbol "F'" in the description of the genotype. Adhesion to the pilus is mediated via *gp3*, of which there are five copies located at one of the ends of the bacteriophage particle. As the phage enters the pilus, the outer major coat protein is stripped off, and the phage DNA is transferred into the body of the bacterium. Thereafter, the single-stranded phage DNA (the "+" strand) is converted to a double-stranded form, known as the replicative form (RF), entirely by host enzymes.

After the formation of the RF, the bacteriophage-encoded *gp2* cleaves the positive strand within the intergenic region, which rolls off from the negative strand. During this process, both strands are again replicated to produce double-stranded RFs. This type of replication, known as the rolling circle

Table 1
Summary of Biology of Filamentous Bacteriophage

Filamentous bacteriophage can only be propagated in *E. coli* host strains that produce
   F'-plasmid encoded sex pili
Adhesion of the bacteriophage to the sex pili is through the minor coat protein *gp3*
   located at one of the ends of the phage particle
Infection of *E. coli* with filamentous phage is a chronic one in that the phage does not
   lyse the *E. coli*. It is therefore possible to maintain filamentous phage either as a
   phage-secreting *E. coli* strain or as a suspension of bacteriophage particles.

method, continues until there are some 200 copies of the RF form inside the
cell. During this time *gp5,* a single-strand DNA binding protein, accumulates
and sequesters the positive strand as it peels off the negative strand, thus preventing it from being converted to double-stranded DNA. The +DNA strand–
gp5 complex is then ready for assembly into virions.

Assembly of the progeny virus takes place at the membrane where *gp5* is
replaced by the virion structural proteins as the phage particles are extruded
through the phage envelope. Remarkably, this does not causes any damage to
the host. Although *gp3* is essential for the adsorption of the phage onto the tip
of the pilus during infection, DNA can be introduced into the host by other
routes in vitro, such as transfection using electroporation. Here the need for the
F factor is bypassed. A summary of the important points of the biology of
filamentous bacteriophage is given in Table 1.

3. Development of Filamentous Phage Vectors for Antibody Display

Filamentous phage display technology stems from the finding that filamentous phage could be used to display antigens on the virion surface *(2).* The two
coat proteins *gp3* and *gp8* will tolerate peptide inserts in their surface-exposed
N-terminal domains. Ab chains are therefore displayed as fusions of either *gp8*
or *gp3*. The *gp8* fusion system displays multiple copies of Ab chains leading to
phage selection on the basis of avidity rather than selection of antibodies with
high-affinity. As most applications of phage-derived antibodies require them
ideally to have the high affinities, the vector systems that have found the greatest application are those that create fusions with *gp3*.

Depending on the particular vector system used, *gp3* fusions can be displayed either multivalently for selection by avidity or monovalently to select
for binders with the highest affinity. By fusing VH or VL antigen binding
domains (Fv) or VH-CH and VL-CL (Fabs) to a bacterial leader sequence, the
Ab chains are directed through the cytoplasmic membrane into the gap between

this inner membrane and the outer membrane of *E. coli* known as the periplasmic space. The conditions in the periplasmic space provide an oxidizing environment that allows the antigen binding domains to fold correctly. In the case of scFv production, the VH and VL domains, held together with a linker peptide, are fused to *gp3*. In contrast, during Fab production, only one member of the pair is fused to *gp3*, whereas the other is secreted into the periplasmic space and is free to associate with the anchored chain. On extrusion of the phage DNA through the cytoplasmic membrane, the *gp3* fusions are incorporated onto the surface of the virion, and are displayed as either scFv or Fab fragments. The *gp3* protein consists of 406 amino acids and can be divided, roughly in half, into two functional domains. The N-terminal domain is necessary for infection of the phage and also confers immunity to superinfection by other filamentous phage. The C-terminal domain anchors the protein in the membrane, caps the trailing end of the extruded filament, and is required for normal morphogenesis (nonpolyphage).

Once phage display had been established, the phage-genome vectors were rapidly superseded with phagemid vectors because of their relative ease of handling and higher transformation efficiencies as a result of their smaller size. Phagemids are effectively plasmid vectors with plasmid origins of replication and genes that confer a selectable resistance to antibiotics. Phagemids differ from plasmids in that they also contain the major intergenic region of filamentous phage. This region was engineered into them to allow a single-strand copy of the phagemid to be rescued from *E. coli* if the host is subsequently transfected with another filamentous phage (helper phage), such as *VCSM13*. The helper phage supplies proteins that act at the intergenic region of the phagemid, in preference to their own, resulting in the phagemid DNA being replicated and packaged in coat proteins as if it were the RF form of a wild-type phage genome. Extruded phagemid viral particles are capable of infecting other *E. coli* with F pili, but cannot be released from the new host until that is coinfected with a helper phage. The propagation of phagemid DNA in this manner is very efficient, and by using the appropriate antibiotic selection for the phagemid vector, it is possible to select positively for transfected cells.

A number of phagemid display systems that fuse Ab chains to either full-length or N-terminally deleted *gp3* fusions have been described, along with the polymerase chain reaction (PCR) primer sets, restriction enzymes, and host strains required for the display of scFvs and Fabs *(3–7)*. Some systems are commercially available. There is an important difference in whether the Ab–*gp3* fusions are with the whole of the protein or with just the C-terminal domain. Fusions to the whole of *gp3* require that the expression of the fusion is suppressed until after it is infected with the helper phage because of the resistance to superinfection conferred by the N-terminal domain. Since expression of *gp3* is generally from a β-galactosidase promoter, it can be effectively repressed by growth in nutrient media containing glucose. Vectors that fuse the Ab chain directly to the C-terminus of *gp3* remove the strict necessity for suppression. The vector systems also have some mechanism of making the purified Fabs or scFvs soluble by removal of the C-terminal membrane-anchor sequence of *gp3*, resulting in secretion of the Ab chains into the periplasmic space.

Secretion of Fabs or scFvs is generally achieved by directly removing the *gp3* gene from the fusion with restriction enzymes followed by religation and transfection into *E. coli* or by transfer of the recombinant vector into a different host strain unable to suppress the effect of a translation stop codon at the junction between the Ab chains and the *gp3* protein (nonsuppressor strain). Potential problems can arise with either approach: the use of restriction enzymes to remove the *gp3* gene from the fusion increases the chances of cutting within the Ab chain, whereas the use of nonsuppressor strains can cause problems with premature termination of translation at stop codons that occur by chance in any degenerate or random primers used in scFv and Fab cloning or modification.

4. Construction of Antibody Libraries

Construction of combinatorial libraries consists of three steps:

1. Messenger RNA is isolated from the tissue source selected to contain the Ab-secreting cells. Spleen, bone marrow, tonsil, and lymph node have all been successfully used as a source. Copy DNA (cDNA) is then generated by reverse transcription and Fv or Fab regions amplified by PCR.
2. The amplification products are ligated into the phage or phagemid vectors after cutting with the appropriate restriction enzymes.
3. The recombinant vectors are introduced into *E. coli* by electroporation.

On a cautionary note, each of these stages appear deceptively simple when described by groups where the technology is established. Each requires time-consuming optimization, however, in order to ensure the successful generation of comprehensive libraries.

The isolation of RNA and production of cDNA from cells are now a routine procedure and do not generally present difficulty, particularly with an abundance of commercially available kits. The subsequent PCR reactions are carried out with primer sets specifically designed for producing scFvs or Fabs. Generally, the construction of scFvs requires the use of larger sets of PCR primers, since it is not possible to take advantage of conserved sequences in the constant regions of Ab chains for primer design. The generation of scFvs also requires a greater number of PCR reactions to be performed, since the VL and VH chains and linker peptide are joined together using the PCR-based technique of splicing by overlap extension *(8)*. The larger primer sets mean greater expense for their synthesis. Primers are designed using data bases for the alignment of IgG H and L chain sequences and identifying sequences that are relatively conserved at the 5'- and 3'-ends of the variable regions. The primers are then be divided into subsets for synthesis by applying a particular set of rules, e.g., the grouping together of those primer sequences that differ by only a small number of bases, but are identical at their 3'-ends. Fortunately, comprehensive primer sets for the production of murine and human antibodies are now well documented in the literature and are provided in commercial kits.

A number of protocols use a limited number of VH and VL variable region primers for the construction of libraries. The disadvantage of limited sets is that they may not amplify whole subsets of immunoglobulin gene sequences and consequently, will bias and decrease the diversity of any combinatorial library constructed with them. Deficiencies in primer sets only become apparent when trying to amplify L and H chains from cDNA isolated from a specific hybridoma when aberrant amplification or no amplification products are produced. Optimized sets of primers for mouse scFv repertoire and Fab display have been described *(9,10)*, including a full discussion on the factors taken into consideration in the design and use of their primer sets *(9)*. Usually, the amplification reactions present little difficulty, but a major hurdle often occurs at the stage of cloning the amplification products into the vector. This is largely owing to factors that affect the activity of restriction enzymes used in introducing sticky ends on the PCR fragments or vector. These factors include:

1. The range of efficiencies with which different restriction enzymes cleave at their restriction sites when they are close to the ends of linear DNA fragments. This can leave either the PCR fragments or the vector, which becomes a linear molecule once cut with the first restriction enzyme, with uncut ends unsuitable for ligation.
2. The presence of PCR primers in restriction digests, which inhibit the restriction enzyme.
3. The association of *Taq* polymerase with the ends of the PCR product sterically hindering the restriction enzyme.

The efficiency of these factors is reflected in the final size of the library generated after transfection of *E. coli* by electroporation. If commercial, quality-assured, electrocompetent cells are used in initial library constructions, then low numbers of transformants are likely to indicate problems at the earlier cutting and ligation steps. Libraries with large enough diversity to isolate antibodies against a particular antigen generally contain in the order of 10^7–10^8 transformants.

5. Library Sizes

In the immune system, antibodies with moderate affinities are selected from primary repertoires, and their affinities improved stepwise by rounds of somatic mutation and selection. The isolation of Fabs from combinatorial libraries essentially mimics this process, since Fabs isolated from libraries of 10^8 immunoglobulin genes have only a moderate affinity for their antigen, but this can often be improved by mutation followed by further rounds of selection. The size of the phage Ab repertoires ($\sim 10^8$) is limited by the efficiency of transformation of *E. coli*. This number represents only a small proportion of the natural Ab repertoire, and therefore, there is less chance of selecting an Ab against a specific antigen with a moderate to high affinity.

Fabs isolated from libraries containing 10^7–10^8 clones have dissociation constants in the range 10^{-6}–$10^{-7} M$ at best. This limitation in library size can be overcome through an approach known as combinatorial infection *(11)*. In this approach, *E. coli* are transfected with a repertoire of L chain genes harbored in a plasmid vector, and are then infected with phagemid particles harboring H chain sequences. Infection is extremely efficient, and most *E. coli* cells in exponential culture can be infected giving rise to a large combinatorial diversity. However, since the H and L chain genes are on separate vectors, they cannot be packaged together within the same phage particle and therefore cannot be coselected. This problem has been cleverly solved by taking advantage of the precise recombination events at specific DNA sequences catalyzed by recombinase enzymes of a number of bacteriophage.

By introducing a specific recombination site in the phage and phagemid vectors, site-specific recombination at that site precisely joins the L and H chain genes together on a single vector. Two such systems have been described to date. The *lox-Cre* system of bacteriophage P1 *(11)* where the two chains are combined on the same phage replicon within the bacterium by the *Cre* recombinase at *loxP* sites. The *Cre* enzyme is supplied in vivo by infecting the strain carrying the two vectors with bacteriophage P1. Using this approach, high-affinity human antibodies have been isolated directly from a library that consisted of close to 6.5×10^{10} Fab fragments displayed on filamentous phage *(12)*.

An analogous system using the (phage *att* recombination site on phage and plasmid vectors has been described by Geoffroy et al. *(13)*. In this system, the recombination event is catalyzed by the heat-inducible expression of λ phage integrase protein from the phage gene contained in the chromosome of a special host strain of *E. coli*. The latter system may prove to have some advantages in that the recombination event at the *att* site is irreversible, since enzymes other than integrase are required for the excision of DNA. In contrast, the *Cre* recombinase is present at all times in *P1* phage-infected cells, and can catalyze the excision of Ab genes as well as the integration.

6. Affinity Selection of Filamentous Phage (Panning)

The power of the phage display system comes from the fact that phage bearing Fabs or scFvs against a particular antigen are isolated by selection or panning in a process analogous to affinity chromatography rather than by screening. The first combinatorial libraries were constructed in bacteriophage λ vectors and required screening on nitrocellulose filters with labeled antigen to identify clones expressing Fabs capable of recognizing the antigen *(14)*. The library was of a moderate size (~10^6 members) and could be screened on a reasonable number of filters. Recent libraries of 10^{11} members would require an inordinate number of filters and amount of time to screen. In contrast, selection is fast, and in its simplest form, 10^{12} phage can be panned against an immobilized antigen in the well of a microtiter plate. After washing and elution of bound phage, the selected phage is then used to infect *E. coli*, where it is amplified and reselected by further rounds of panning and amplification.

A number of methods for the selection of bacteriophage displaying V gene products by affinity purification have been described including:

1. Binding to antigen-coated dishes or tubes.
2. Binding to antigen on a column matrix.
3. Binding to biotinylated antigen in solution followed by capture on streptavidin-coated beads.

Before choosing a particular approach to selection, it is worth considering what will be required from any Fab or scFv isolated from the library in terms of its binding kinetics and the nature of the antigen it will be required to detect. The binding of phage to an antigen is largely determined by three main factors:

1. The affinity of the VH–VL combination.
2. The avidity of binding of the phage, which is determined by whether a multivalent or monovalent display system is used
3. The on and off rates of binding.

How these factors may be exploited to distinguish between phage with closely related affinities is discussed by Hawkins et al. *(15)*. Without a rationally planned selection procedure, it is possible to lose any high-affinity binders present in a library among the greater numbers of bacteriophage that bind with a low-affinity, thus making it impossible to select phage from even the best combinatorial libraries.

7. Phage Evolution of Antibodies

Most of the affinities of Fabs or scFvs isolated from combinatorial libraries have affinities similar to those of antibodies found in the primary immune response in vivo (K_d 10^{-6}–$10^{-7}M$), but in vivo, these affinities are improved during affinity maturation. To realize the full therapeutic potential of Fabs or scFvs made in vitro, there is a need to mimic the affinity maturation process in some way. A number of approaches have been used successfully to achieve this.

Random mutations in the V regions in vitro can be made by error-prone PCR. By including manganese ions in the reaction buffers, *Taq* polymerase misincorporates nucleotides in the DNA strand being synthesized, creating random mutations (16). Phage display of antibodies with higher binding affinities are then selected under more stringent conditions than were used in initial pannings. This approach was successfully used to improve the binding of low-affinity Fabs derived from a nonimmune adult mouse and expressed multivalently. A multivalent display system was chosen to select low-affinity antibodies that were anticipated to predominate in an unprimed repertoire. Antibodies with initial binding affinities of $10^4 M^{-1}$ were improved (up to 30-fold) by subcloning the V regions into a *gp3*–fusion vector followed by error-prone PCR amplification on a mixture of templates (17). In another example, the affinity of an Fab for a small hapten was increased fourfold by mutating the H chain by error-prone PCR followed by phage selection (15).

An alternative method to increase the diversity of a restricted set of paired V chains and improve the affinities of primary phage antibodies from primary antibodies utilizes chain shuffling in which H and L chains are sequentially replaced with mutated chains. Phage-displaying Fabs with higher affinity are then selected (18,19). Generally, the L chains are shuffled first, followed by regions of the H chain containing the first two complementarity-determining regions (CDRs). H chain CDR3 is usually left intact, since this is the most hypervariable region in an Ab molecule and makes the largest contribution to the total accessible surface area of an Ab's antigen binding site. Retaining the integrity of VH CDR3 therefore maintains the key features of the antigen binding properties. Focusing mutational events on CDRs improved the affinity of an Ab isolated from a primary phage library for a small hapten from 10^6–$10^9 M^{-1}$ (18).

Where library size is a limiting factor in generating combinatorial diversity, Barbas et al. (20) described a chemical solution to increase diversity by using a semisynthetic approach controlled by oligonucleotide synthesis. Using a large primer spanning VH CDR3 and containing 18 bases complementary to the flanking framework regions of the CDR and a randomized 48-base sequence in the central region, there is the potential to generate vast numbers of CDRs (in the order of 10^{20}) for Ab H chains. Using this approach, a tetanus toxoid binding Ab was converted to a number of fluorescein binding antibodies, the best of which had K_d values of $10^{-7} M$ (20). In a modification of this method, termed "CDR walking," diversity is introduced in CDR regions of a defined Ab by making all the possible amino acid substitutions at a limited number of positions. CDR walking has been used to increase the affinity, but retain the broadly neutralizing property of a neutralizing human Ab to human immunodeficiency virus type 1, which are in general, two opposing characteristics *(21)*. This Ab may as a consequence find application in the passive immunization of subjects who have made accidental contact with HIV-1 infected blood. A wider range of applications in this continually expanding field have been covered in recent reviews *(22–24)*.

References

1. Ward, E. S., Gussow, D., Griffiths, A. D., Jones, P. T., and Winter, G. (1989) Binding activities of a repertoire of single immunoglobulin variable domains secreted from *Escherichia coli. Nature* **341,** 544–546.
2. Smith, G. P. (1985) Filamentous fusion phage. Novel expression vectors that display cloned antigens on the virion surface. *Science* **228,** 1315–1317.
3. Barbas, C. F., III, Kang, A. S., Lerner, R. A., and Benkovic, S. J. (1991) Assembly of combinatorial antibody libraries on phage surfaces: the gene III site. *Proc. Natl. Acad. Sci. USA* **88,** 7978–7982.
4. Garrard, L. J., Yang, M., O'Connell, M. P., Kelley, R. F., and Henner, D. J. (1991) Fab assembly and enrichment in a monovalent phage display system. *Biotechnology* **9,** 1373–1377.
5. Söderlind, E., Simonsson, A. C., and Borrebaeck, C. A. K. (1992) Phage display technology in antibody engineering. *Immunol. Rev.* **130,** 109–124.
6. Hoogenboom, H. R., Griffiths, A. D., Johnson, K. S., Chiswell, D. J., Hudson, P., and Winter, G. (1991) Multi-subunit proteins on the surface of filamentous phage: methodologies for displaying antibody (Fab) heavy and light chains. *Nucleic Acids Res.* **19,** 4133–4137.
7. Dübel, S., Breitling, F., Fuchs, P., Braunagel, M., Klewinghaus, I., and Little, M. (1993) A family of vectors for surface display and production of antibodies. *Gene* **128,** 97–101.
8. Horton, R. M., Hunt, H. D., Ho, S. N., Pullen, J. K., and Pease, L. R. (1989) Engineering hybrid genes without the use of restriction enzymes: gene splicing by overlap extension. *Gene* **77,** 61–68.
9. Ørum, H., Andersen, P. S., Øster, A., Johansen, L. K., Riise, E., Bjørnvad, M., Svendsen, I., and Engberg, J. (1993) Efficient method for constructing comprehensive murine Fab antibody libraries displayed on phage. *Nucleic Acids Res.* **21,** 4491–4498.
10. Zhou, H., Fisher, R. J., and Papas, T. S. (1994) Optimization of primer sequences for mouse scFv repertoire display library construction. *Nucleic Acids Res.* **22,** 888,889.
11. Waterhouse, P., Griffiths, A. D., Johnson, K. S., and Winter, G. (1993) Combinatorial infection and in vivo recombination: a strategy for making large phage antibody repertoires. *Nucleic Acids Res.* **21,** 2265,2266.
12. Griffiths, A. D., Williams, S. C., Hartly, O., Tomlinson, I. M., Waterhouse, P., Crosby, W. L., Kontermann, R. E., Jones, P. T., Low, N. M., Allison, T. J.,

Prospero, T. D., Hoogenboom, H. R., Nissim, A., Cox, J. P. L., Harrison, J. L., Zaccolo, M., Gherardi, E., and Winter, G. (1994) Isolation of high-affinity human antibodies directly from large synthetic repertoires. *EMBO J.* **13,** 3245–3260.

13. Geoffroy, F., Sodoyer, R., Aujame, L. (1994) A new phage display system to construct multicombinatorial libraries of very large antibody repertoires. *Gene* **151,** 109–113.

14. Huse, W. D., Sastry, L., Iverson, S. A., Kang, A. S., Alting-Mees, M., Burton, D. R., Benkovic, S. J., and Lerner, R. A (1989) Generation of a large combinatorial library of the immunoglobulin repertoire in phage lambda. *Science* **246,** 1275–1281.

15. Hawkins, R. E., Russell, S. J., and Winter, G. (1992) Selection of phage antibodies by binding affinity: mimicking affinity maturation. *J. Mol. Biol.* **226,** 889–896.

16. Leung, D. W., Chen, E., and Goeddel, D. V. (1989) A method for random mutagenesis of a defined DNA segment using a modified PCR chain reaction. *Technique* **1,** 11–15.

17. Gram, H., Marconi, LA., Barbas, C. F., III, Collet, T. A., Lerner, R. A., and Kang, A. S (1992) In vitro selection and affinity maturation of antibodies from a naive combinatorial immunoglobulin library. *Proc. Natl. Acad. Sci. USA* **89,** 3576–3580.

18. Marks, J. D., Griffiths, A. D., Malmqvist, M., Clackson, T., Bye, J. M., and Winter, G. (1992) Bypassing immunization-building high-affinity human antibodies by chain shuffling. *Biotechnology* **10,** 779–783.

19. Kang, A. S., Jones, T. M., and Burton, D. R. (1991) Antibody redesign by chain shuffling from random combinatorial immunoglobulin libraries. *Proc. Natl. Acad. Sci. USA* **88,** 11,120–11,123.

20. Barbas, C. F., III, Bain, J. D., Hoekstra, D. M. and Lerner, R. (1992) Semisynthetic combinatorial antibody libraries: A chemical solution to the diversity problem. *Proc. Natl. Acad. Sci. USA* **89,** 4457–4461.

21. Barbas, C. F., III, Hu, D., Dunlop, N., Sawyer, L., Cababa, D., Hendry, R. M., Nara, P. L., and Burton, D. R (1994) In vitro evolution of a neutralizing human antibody to human immunodeficiency virus type 1 to enhance affinity and broaden strain cross-reactivity. *Proc. Natl. Acad. Sci. USA* **91,** 3809–3813.

22. Burton, D. R. and Barbas, C. F., III (1994). Human antibodies from combinatorial libraries. *Adv. Immunol.* **57,** 191–280.

23. Barbas, S. M. and Barbas, C. F., III (1994) *Fibrinolysis* **8,** 245–252.

24. Winter, G., Griffiths, A. D., Hawkins, R. E., and Hoogenboom, H. R. (1994) Making antibodies by phage display technology. *Annu. Rev. Immunol.* **12,** 433–455.

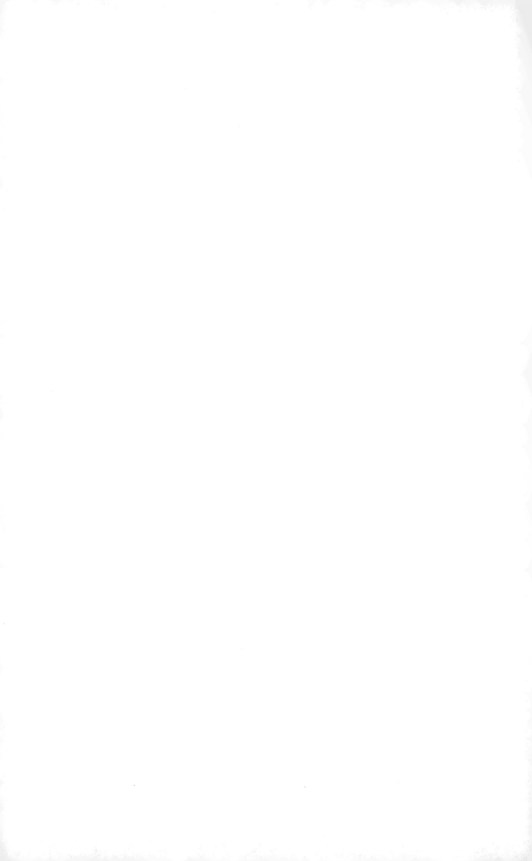

46

Production of Human Fab Antibody Fragments from Phage Display Libraries

J. Mark Hexham

1. Introduction
1.1. Principles of Phage Display

Phage display involves expression of a large library of diverse molecules as fusion proteins on the surface of filamentous bacteriophage. In this form, they may be subjected to biological or molecular selection to isolate molecules with the desired binding properties *(1) (see* review in ref. *2)*. Initially, the system was used for mapping antibody epitopes by expression of large libraries (10^7–10^8) of random peptides *(3–5)*. However, the approach has proved readily applicable to many types of molecular interaction, including the production or manipulation of antibodies *(6–10)*, enzymes, and their substrates *(11–13)*, general protein–protein interactions *(14–15)* and DNA binding proteins *(16–17)*.

All the above systems use filamentous phage of the M13, fd or fl phage, which have been modified to express the protein motif of interest on their surface as a fusion product with one of the viral coat proteins. The most widely exploited protein for this purpose is coat protein III, which gives monovalent display. This mode of expression ensures the linkage of the genes encoding a particular fusion protein on the surface of the phage that encodes it. For a fuller discussion of bacteriophage biology, the reader is directed to Chapter 45 in this volume.

1.2. Phage Library Vectors

Several systems exist for the expression and cloning of antibodies, as either Fab fragments (Fabs) or single-chain Fv fragments (scFvs) on the surface of

From: *Methods in Molecular Biology, Vol. 80: Immunochemical Protocols, 2nd ed.*
Edited by: J. D. Pound © Humana Press Inc., Totowa, NJ

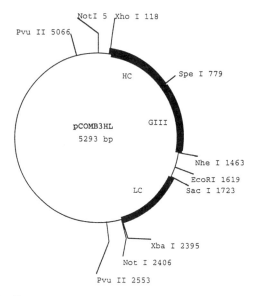

Fig. 1. Schematic diagram of *pComb3* vector containing HC and LC inserts. The heavy chain is expressed as a fusion protein with the C-terminal domain of the bacteriophage coat protein III gene (GIII).

phage (refs. *6–10* and Chapter 45). This chapter will focus on the production of human Fab-expressing libraries using the phage display vector *pComb3* (*7, see* Fig. 1). Clearly the system is also suited to the production of murine Fabs, given the use of appropriate primers. Other systems and approaches are discussed elsewhere in this volume (*see* Chapter 47).

To outline the procedure briefly, library construction begins with the isolation of lymphocyte RNA, obtained from the lymphocytes of a donor expressing the antibody specificity of interest. Reverse transcriptase polymerase chain reaction (RT-PCR) is then used to produce Fab-encoding fragments of DNA from the immunoglobulin (Ig) heavy chain (HC) and light chain (LC) genes. These fragments are then cloned sequentially into the vector (Fig. 1) to produce a Fab-expressing phage library. Screening to isolate phage-expressing antibodies of the desired specificity is carried out by repeated rounds of selection of the library on antigen-coated ELISA plates. Following this selection, individual Fab clones are isolated and expressed in bacterial culture to determine their binding characteristics. At this stage, clones may also be subjected to DNA sequence analysis.

The screening or panning procedure can also be carried out using cell lines expressing the antigen of interest either in a tissue-culture plate-based approach

(18) or using flow cytometry to separate phage bound to cell populations of interest *(19)*.

2. Materials

1. *Escherichia coli* strain *XL1-Blue* (Stratagene, La Jolla, CA).
2. VCSM13 (Stratagene) interference-resistant helper phage.
3. Carbenicillin.
4. Kanamycin.
5. SB medium (SB): 30 g/L Bacto-tryptone (Difco, Detroit, MI), 20 g/L yeast extract (Difco), 10 g/L MOPS (3-[*N*-morpholino]propanesulfonic acid), pH 7.0, containing 10 μg/mL tetracycline (Boehringer Mannheim, Indianapolis, IN).
6. SB containing 1.5% glucose.
7. Glycerol 10% (v/v) in water.
8. Transformation cuvets (2-mm gap, Bio-Rad [St. Louis, MO]).
9. SOC: 20 g/L Bacto-tryptone, 5 g/L yeast extract, 10 mM sodium chloride, 2.5 mM potassium chloride, 10 mM magnesium chloride, 10 mM magnesium sulfate, and 20 mM glucose, pH 7.0.
10. L-broth (LB).
11. Water treated with diethyl pyrocarbonate (DEPC) 0.05% (w/v) overnight at room temperature, and then autoclaved to remove DEPC.
12. RNA isolation kits (e.g., Stratagene).
13. Reverse transcriptase (Superscript II, BRL, Gaithersburg, MD).
14. rRNase inhibitor (Promega, Madison, WI).
15. Deoxynucleoside 5'-triphosphates (dNTPs) (Pharmacia, Uppsala, Sweden).
16. *Taq* polymerase (Promega).
17. 2 mM Magnesium chloride.
18. Mineral oil (Sigma, St. Louis, MO).
19. Restriction enzymes: *Spe*I, *Xho*I, *Sac*I, *Xba*I, and manufacturer's buffers (Boehringer Mannheim).
20. Ethanol.
21. Qiagen (tip 100) plasmid DNA extraction kit (Qiagen, Santa Clarita, CA).
22. PEG-8000.
23. Sodium chloride.
24. 1 mM Isopropyl β-D-thiogalactopyranoside (IPTG).
25. PBS: 0.14M NaCl, 2.7 mM KCl, 1.5 mM KH_2PO_4, 8.1 mM Na_2HPO_4.
26. PBS containing 1 and 3% bovine serum albumin (BSA).
27. PBS containing 0.05% (v/v) Tween-20.
28. 1M Sodium hydrogen carbonate.
29. 0.1M Glycine, pH 2.2.
30. 2M Tris base.
31. *Para*-nitrophenyl phosphate (PNP) substrate solution for ELISA: PNP (1 mg/mL) in 10% diethanolamine, pH 9.8, containing 0.5% w/v magnesium chloride, and 0.01% w/v sodium azide.
32. ELISA plates (Nunc Immunosorp strip modules are most useful).

3. Methods

3.1. General Methods

3.1.1. Preparation of Cells
for High-Efficiency Transformation by Electroporation

High-efficiency electrotransformation of bacteria is the key to generating a large library, although good-quality competent cells are commercially available from Stratagene and others, they are expensive. Sometimes it may be necessary to prepare them in the lab. Using this protocol, it is possible to generate cells with transformation efficiencies in the 10^8–10^9 colonies/µg range, which are ideal for library applications and approach that of the commercial preparations.

1. Grow *XL1-Blue*, from a single colony, overnight at 37°C with shaking in 10 mL SB.
2. On the next morning, inoculate 0.5 mL of this culture into 1 L of SB containing 1.5% glucose, and incubate with shaking at 37°C until an OD_{600} of between 0.5 and 0.8 is reached (4–6 h).
3. Chill the flask on ice for 15 min, and then harvest the cells by centrifugation at 4000g for 15 min at 4°C.
4. Wash the cells three times in 500, 250, and 100 mL of ice-cold 10% glycerol with centrifugation as before.
5. Resuspend in a final volume of 10 mL of 10% glycerol, aliquot (200–600 µL) into tubes on dry ice and store at −70°C.

3.1.2. Transformation by Electroporation

1. Thaw the cells slowly on ice, and then incubate 300 µL cells with the target DNA (0.5–2 µg in 10 µL water) in chilled transformation cuvets (2-mm gap) on ice for 5 min.
2. Electroporate at 2.5 kV with 25 µF capacitance and 400 Ω resistance (time constant should be 5-10 ms).
3. Resuspend the cells in 3 mL warm SOC (*see* Section 2.), and incubate at room temperature for 15 min.
4. Remove 1- and 10-µL aliquots of the cells, and grow up on carbenicillin (50 µg/mL) LB plates in order to calculate the transformation efficiency/library size.

3.1.3. Preparation of Helper Phage

Preparation of large amounts of high-titer helper phage stock is essential for phagemid rescue to generate viable libraries of Fab-expressing phage particles. The VCSM13 (Stratagene) interference-resistant helper phage is recommended.

1. Grow *XL1-Blue*, from a single colony, overnight at 37°C with shaking in 10 mL SB, containing 10 µg/mL tetracycline.
2. On the next morning, inoculate 300 µL of this culture into 100 mL SB (10 µg/mL tetracycline) and grown for 2 h.

3. Add 50 µL VCSM13 stock, and continue the incubation for a further hour.
4. Add kanamycin to 50 µg/mL, and continue the incubation for a further 4 h.
5. Harvest the cells by centrifugation at 4000g for 15 min at 4°C.
6. Incubate the supernatant, containing the free phage, at 70°C for 20 min, centrifuge as above, and store at 4°C.
7. Titer the phage stock by infecting fresh *XL1-Blue*, and grow overnight in top agar on LB agar plates. Typical titers are 10^{11-12} *pfu*/mL.

3.2. Construction of Antibody Libraries

3.2.1. Patient/Donor Selection and Lymphocyte Isolation

The source and quality of the lymphocytes and the antibody titer of the desired antibodies within an individual will influence the difficulty of producing antibodies from a library derived from that individual. The sources of lymphocytes that have been used successfully to produce human antibodies of the same specificity as the subject's serum antibodies have been peripheral blood lymphocytes from leukophoresis *(20)*, thyroid lymphocytes *(18,21)*, and lymphocytes from lymph nodes draining the site of the immune response *(22)*. The serum reactivity of the donor should be analyzed in as much detail as possible in order to clone Ig isotypes and subclasses responsible for the response of interest. Subclass-specific antisera can be used in antigen-specific ELISA to achieve this.

3.2.2. RNA Preparation

DEPC-treated water should be used for all RNA preparation solutions, gloves should be worn at all times, and "RNase-free" tips and tubes used. It is not necessary to purify mRNA, since total RNA prepared from freshly isolated or even frozen (liquid nitrogen or −80°C) lymphocytes is pure enough to carry out the RT-PCR reactions. A number of commercial kits are now available for RNA isolation (e.g., Stratagene), and use of one of these is recommended. Alternatively the single-step guanidinium thiocyanate/phenol extraction method of Chomczynski and Sacchi *(23)*, on which most kit protocols are based, should be employed. If the lymphocyte numbers are low (<5 × 10⁶), carrier RNA (100 µg of 16S ribosomal RNA) can be added at the start of this procedure to aid recovery. The preparation ends with a precipitation step using isopropanol, and the RNA may stored at −20°C in this form until required.

3.2.3. cDNA Synthesis

At least two separate reverse transcription reactions should be carried out, one to generate LC cDNA and another to generate HC (Fd) cDNA. At this point, the choice of the 3'-primers used will determine the range of Ig isotypes expressed in the library (for primers, *see* Table 1). For example, to generate a

Table 1
Primers for RT-PCR Amplification
of Human Ig HC (a, b) and LC (c, d, e, f) Genes

(a) HC variable domain 5'-primers
    VH1a 5'-CAGGTGCAG<u>CTCGAG</u>CAGTCTGGG-3' (24 mer)
    VH1f 5'-CAGGTGCAGCTG<u>CTCGAG</u>TCTGGG-3' (24 mer)
    VH2f 5'-CAGGTGCAGCTA<u>CTCGAG</u>TCGGG-3' (23 mer)
    VH3a 5'-GAGGTGCAG<u>CTCGAG</u>GAGTCTGGG-3' (24 mer)
    VH3f 5'-GAGGTGCAGCTG<u>CTCGAG</u>TCTGGG-3' (24 mer)
    VH4f 5'-CAGGTGCAGCTG<u>CTCGAG</u>TCGGG-3' (23 mer)
    VH4g 5'-CAGGTGCAGCTA<u>CTCGAG</u>TGGGG-3' (23 mer)
    VH6a 5'-CAGGTACAG<u>CTCGAG</u>CAGTCAGG-3' (23 mer)

(b) IgG HC isotype-specific 3'-primers
    CG1z 5'-GCATGT<u>ACTAGT</u>TTTGTCACAAGATTTGGG-3' (30 mer)   IgG1
    CG2a 5'-CTCGAC<u>ACTAGT</u>TTTGCGCTCAACTGTCTT-3' (30 mer)   IgG2
    CG3a 5'-TGTGTG<u>ACTAGT</u>GTCACCAAGTGGGGTTTT-3' (30 mer)   IgG3
    CG4a 5'-GCATGA<u>ACTAGT</u>TGGGGGACCATATTTGGA-3' (30 mer)   IgG4
    CM1   5'-GCTCAC<u>ACTAGT</u>AGGCAGCTCAGCAATCAC-3' (30 mer)   IgM
    CD1   5'-TGCCTT<u>ACTAGT</u>CTCTGGCCAGCGGAAGAT-3' (30 mer)   IgD
    CE1   5'-GCTGAA<u>ACTAGT</u>GTTGTCGACCCAGTCTGTGGA-3' (33 mer)   IgE
    CA1   5'-AGTTGA<u>ACTAGT</u>TGGGCAGGGCACAGTCAC-3' (30 mer)   IgA(1+2)

(c) κ LC variable region 5'-primers
    VK1a 5'-GACATC<u>GAGCTC</u>ACCCAGTCTCCA-3' (24 mer)
    VK1s 5'-GACATC<u>GAGCTC</u>ACCCAGTCTCC-3' (23 mer)
    VK2a 5'-GATATT<u>GAGCTC</u>ACTCAGTCTCCA-3' (24 mer)
    VK3a 5'-GAAATT<u>GAGCTC</u>ACGCAGTCTCCA-3' (24 mer)
    VK3b 5'-GAAATT<u>GAGCTC</u>AC(G/A)CAGTCTCCA-3' (24 mer)

(d) κ LC constant region 3'-primer
    CK1d 5'-GCGCCG<u>TCTAGA</u>ATTAACACTCTCCCCTGTTGAAGCTCTTTG-
          TGACGGGCGAACTCAG-3' (57 mer)

(e) λ LC variable region 5'-primers
    VL1   5'-AATTTT<u>GAGCTC</u>ACTCAGCCCCAC-3' (24 mer)
    VL2   5'-TCTGCC<u>GAGCTC</u>CAGCCTGCCTCCGTG-3' (27 mer)
    VL3   5'-TCTGTG<u>GAGCTC</u>CAGCCGCCCTCAGTG-3' (27 mer)
    VL4   5'-TCTGAA<u>GAGCTC</u>CAGGACCCTGTTGTGTCTGTG-3' (33 mer)
    VL5   5'-CAGTCT<u>GAGCTC</u>ACGCAGCCGCCC-3' (24 mer)
    VL6   5'-CAGACT<u>GAGCTC</u>ACTCAGGAGCCC-3' (24 mer)
    VL7   5'-CAGGTT<u>GAGCTC</u>ACTCAACCGCCC-3' (24 mer)
    VL8   5'-CAGGCT<u>GAGCTC</u>ACTCAGCCGTCTTCC-3' (27 mer)

(f) λ LC constant region 3'-primer
    CL2   5'-CGCCG<u>TCTAGA</u>ACTATGAACATTCTGTAGG-3' (30 mer)

---

[a]The restriction enzyme sites introduced to enable cloning of the amplified Ig genes are underlined and correspond to: *Xho*I (CTCGAG) for the HC 5' variable region primers (a), *Spe*I (ACTAGT)
for the HC 3' constant region primers (b), *Sac*I (GAGCTC) for the LC 5' variable region primers (c and
e), and *Xba*I (TCTAGA) for the LC 3' constant region primers (d and f).

complete IgG repertoire four different IgG primers (corresponding to sub-classes 1–4) should be used as well as the two LC primers for κ and λ LCs. Analysis of the donor serum reactivity using subclass-specific antisera can assist in choice of primers by determining which isotypes and subclasses are involved in a particular antigenic response.

1. RNA should be quantified spectrophotometrically and 5–50 µg used for each reaction.
2. Mix the primer (20 µ*M*) and RNA in a total volume of 25 µL, and anneal by heating to 75°C for 10 min and then incubating on ice for 5 min.
3. Add RT (Superscript II, 3 µL), rRNase inhibitor (Promega, 80 U), and 25 m*M* dNTPs in 50-µL total volume in the manufacturer's buffer.
4. Incubate for 1 h at 37°C. If the amount of RNA is low, then a longer incubation up to overnight can be employed.

3.2.4. PCR Amplification of Ig HC and LC Genes

PCR is used to amplify HC Fd regions and the entire light chain, enabling Fab library construction from the lymphocyte cDNA. The primers are designed to maintain the LC–HC disulfide bond in the Fabs. A wide range of 5'-primers is used to produce libraries that are representative of all the different human HC variable region (VH) and LC variable region (VL) gene families together with 3' primers specific for the different HC subclasses or LC isotypes (Table 1). The primers also contain restriction enzyme sites to facilitate cloning of the PCR products into the vectors.

1. Make up 100 µL PCR reactions containing 5 U *Taq* polymerase (Promega), 2 m*M* magnesium chloride, 2 µL cDNA (HC or LC), 200 µ*M* dNTPs, and 20 µ*M* of each of the 3'- and 5'-primers in the manufacturer's buffer. *See* Note 1.
2. Cover with two to three drops mineral oil.
3. Subject to 35 rounds of amplification beginning with denaturation at 95°C for 30 s, followed by annealing at 52°C for 2 min, and polymerization at 72°C for 2 min. Conclude with 10 min of polymerization at 72°C, and then cool to 4°C (*see* Note 2).

The HC Fd gives a PCR product of around 680 bp, whereas the LC gives a slightly smaller product of around 660 bp.

3.2.5. Digestion of PCR Products

The HC and LC PCR products are pooled separately, phenol/chloroform-extracted, and ethanol-precipitated. Following resuspension and, where appropriate, gel purification of PCR products, the DNA is quantitated, before restriction enzyme digestion and cloning into the *pComb3* vector. Gel purification (*see below* for methods) may be necessary when there are a high number of background bands in the PCR reaction. This tends to be more of a problem in HC amplifications. The equivalent amounts of enzyme required to digest the PCR product, calculated from the manufacturer's unit definitions (Boehringer-Mannheim), are as follows: *Spe*I, 17 U/μg; *Xho*I, 70 U/μg; *Sac*I, 35 U/μg; *Xba*I, 70 U/μg. The HC PCR products are digested with *Spe*I and *Xho*I in Boehringer-Mannheim Buffer H, and the LC products are digested in Boehringer-Mannheim Buffer A for at least 4 h at 37°C using at least a threefold excess of enzyme calculated from the above figures. Following digestion, the DNA is purified by 2% agarose gel electrophoresis, the appropriate bands are cut out, and the DNA purified. The best method of gel purification is a matter of debate and personal preference, but those that have been used successfully in this area are electroelution, Gene-clean (BIO-101), β-agarase (NEB) digestion of Nu-Sieve (Flowgen) agarose, electroelution, and phenol-phenol/chloroform extraction of Nu-Sieve (Flowgen) agarose.

3.2.6. Cloning of Ig Genes into the pComb3 Vector

1. Digest 10–20 μg of *pComb3* vector with the LC enzymes, *Sac*I (10 U/μg) and *Xba*I (20 U/μg) at 37°C for 2 h in Buffer A, using a twofold excess of enzyme (as defined by Boehringer-Mannheim) to prepare it to receive the LC insert.
2. Following digestion, purify the DNA by preparative electrophoresis on a 1% agarose gel. The cut vector band of 4.7 kb is excised, purified from the gel, precipitated, and quantitated.
3. Test the ligation efficiency of LC insert and vector by performing a small-scale ligation using around 200 ng of cut vector and 50 ng of insert in a 10-μL overnight ligation at 15°C.
4. Transform this ligation into competent bacterial cells, and compare to a control ligation of vector minus insert.
5. If the ligation is successful (i.e., vector + insert produces at least 5× more colonies than vector alone), then ligate 1 μg of cut vector with 200 ng of LC insert, overnight at 15°C, in a scaled-up volume (100–150 μL).
6. Ethanol-precipitate the ligation mixture, and wash the pellet in 70% ethanol.
7. Resuspend in 10 μL of water, and transform into 300 μL *XL1-Blue* by electroporation (*see* Section 3.1.2.).
8. Immediately following electroporation, add 3 mL of prewarmed SOC, and grow the cells for 1 h at 37°C.
9. Add 10 mL warm SB (containing 20 μg/mL carbenicillin), remove 1- and 10-μL aliquots from this culture, and grow overnight on LB agar plates containing 50 μg/mL carbenicillin to titer the library size. Continue growth of the main culture for 1 h at 37°C.
10. Increase the carbenicillin concentration to 50 μg/mL, and continue growth for 1 h.
11. Add the culture to 100 mL SB containing 50 μg/mL carbenicillin, and grow overnight.
12. Prepare plasmid DNA from this culture using the Qiagen (tip 100) method.
13. Test for the presence of LC insert by analytical digestion with *Sac*I and *Xba*I (this generates a 660-bp insert).

14. Perform DNA minipreps on several (e.g., 12) clones from the plates. These are then checked for the presence of insert by digestion with *Sac*I and *Xba*I as above and also with *Not*I (generates 2.5- and 2.9-kb fragments) to ensure the LC cloning has worked correctly. Once the LC library has been characterized, it can be digested with the HC enzymes prior to the cloning of the HC gene to create the Fab-expressing library.

15. Digest 10 μg LC library DNA with *Spe*I (6 U/μg) and *Xho*I (20 U/μg) at 37°C for 2 h in Boehringer Mannheim Buffer H to prepare it to receive HC insert. This corresponds to a twofold excess of enzyme. The HC insert is digested, ligated into the cut LC library-containing vector, and transformed as described above. However, following electroporation, the bacterial culture is grown to produce a library of phage-expressing Fabs on their surface, as opposed to plasmid DNA.

16. Immediately following electroporation, add 3 mL of prewarmed SOC, and grow the cells for 1 h at 37°C.

17. Add 10 mL of prewarmed SB containing 20 μg/mL carbenicillin, and again titer the library size by plating out 1- and 10-μL samples on LB agar (50 μg/mL carbenicillin) plates overnight. Continue growth of the culture for 1 h

18. Increase the carbenicillin concentration to 50 μg/mL, and continue growth for 1 h.

19. Add to 100 mL SB containing 50 μg/mL carbenicillin, and grow for a further 1 h.

20. Add 10^{12} *pfu* VCSM13 helper phage, and incubate for 2 h.

21. Add kanamycin to 70 μg/mL, and grow the phage overnight at 37°C with shaking.

22. Remove the cells by centrifugation at 4000*g* for 15 min at 4°C.

23. Transfer the supernatant to a clean flask, and add PEG 8000 (4% w/v) and sodium chloride (3% w/v) with stirring on ice to precipitate the phage. Continue to stir on ice for 30 min.

24. Sediment phage at 9000*g* for 20 min at 4°C, remove the supernatant carefully, and discard.

25. Resuspend the phage pellet in 2 mL PBS, and clarify by a short pulse of centrifugation in a microfuge.

26. The phage library stock may now be stored at 4°C. However, the selection procedure must be carried out with freshly prepared phage, since the antibody fusion protein may not be stable. To do this, the library can be reamplified by growth on *XL1-Blue* (Section 3.2.7., steps 7–17).

3.2.7. Screening of pComb3 Libraries

The screening procedure is an affinity selection process, is generally referred to as "panning" or "bio-panning," and is performed using four wells of an ELISA plate. The consecutive rounds of panning should ideally be performed on consecutive days so as to use fresh phage each time. Alternatively, the phage should be reamplified on the day before panning (steps 7–17 below).

1. Coat each of four ELISA wells with 100 μL antigen (1–10 μg/mL in 0.1*M* sodium hydrogen carbonate) overnight at 4°C.

2. Block the wells with 200 μL of PBS containing 3% BSA for 1 h at 37°C.

3. Remove the blocking solution, add 100 μL of freshly prepared phage library stock/well, and incubate at 37°C for 2 h.

4. Remove the unbound phage from the wells, and wash extensively (10 times) over 30 min.

5. Elute bound phage with 100 μL of 0.1*M* glycine, pH 2.2 for 10 min.

6. Neutralize immediately by adding 6 μL of 2*M* Tris base.

7. Pool the 4 × 100 μL aliquots of eluted phage, and use them to infect 2 mL of a fresh overnight culture of *XL1-Blue* grown in SB medium for 15 min at room temperature.

8. Add 10 mL of prewarmed SB containing 20 μg/mL carbenicillin, remove 1- and 10-μL samples for titration, and grow the culture for 1 h at 37°C.

9. Adjust the carbenicillin concentration to 50 μg/mL, and continue the incubation for 1 h.

10. Add the culture to 100 mL prewarmed SB containing 50 μg/mL carbenicillin and 10 μg /mL tetracycline, and incubate for a further h.

11. Add 10^{12} *pfu* of VCSM13 helper phage (typically 1–5 mL, *see* Section 3.1.3.) and continue the incubation for 2 h.

12. Add kanamycin (70 μg/mL) and grow the phage preparation overnight.

13. Centrifuge the bacterial cells down at 4000g for 15 min at 4°C.

14. Remove the supernatant, and add 4% w/v PEG–8000 and 3% w/v NaCl with stirring on ice. Continue stirring gently on ice for 30 min to precipitate the phage.

15. Harvest the phage by centrifugation at 9000g for 20 min at 4°C.

16. Remove the supernatant carefully and resuspend the pellet in 2 mL PBS. The phage pellet may be visible as a thin translucent coating on the wall of the tube, which may be removed by rinsing with PBS.

17. Clear the phagemid suspension with a short pulse of centrifugation in a microfuge, and store at 4°C. This stock is now ready for panning, and the panning process is repeated several (four to six) times until an appreciable enrichment (a recovery of 10^6–10^7 *pfu* from the four wells) is obtained. Typically, the recovery will be high on the first round because of background, lower on the second round and then on the third or fourth round, it should increase dramatically. Following the final round of panning, the culture can be used to make either phage particles or to make phagemid DNA for soluble Fab expression and DNA sequence analysis.

18. Titer the suspension on fresh *XL1-Blue* grown overnight in SB. The titration should be performed simultaneously with the panning.

3.2.8. Conversion of pComb3 Clones for Fab Expression

Phagemid DNA, prepared from the phage harvested from the final round of panning, may be converted from a surface-expressing mode to soluble Fab-expressing mode by a two-step digestion-religation process. In order to express free Fab, the coat protein III gene (GIII; *see* Fig. 1) is removed using the enzymes *Nhe*I and *Spe*I, which have compatible ends and can be religated to produce a soluble Fab-expressing vector.

1. Digest approx 5 µg of DNA with 1–2 equivalents of *Nhe*I and *Spe*I in buffer M (Boehringer Mannheim) for 3 h at 37°C.
2. Purify the DNA corresponding to the *pComb3* vector containing HC and LC (i.e., the 4.7-kb band), lacking GIII, from a 1% agarose gel.
3. Self-ligate the DNA and transform into *XL1-Blue* by any standard method, since high efficiency is not crucial, and plate out on LB agar plates containing 50 µg/mL carbenicillin. The resultant clones can then be tested for Fab expression under IPTG induction.

3.2.9. Fab Expression

1. Grow several colonies (e.g., 12) on a small scale in 2 mL SB containing 20 m*M* magnesium chloride and 50 µg/mL carbenicillin for 6–8 h at 37°C with shaking.
2. Remove 0.5 mL of each culture, and store as a glycerol stock.
3. Induce Fab protein expression by the addition of 1 m*M* IPTG and continue the incubation overnight.
4. Centrifuge the cells for 10 min at 10,000*g* at 4°C and remove the supernatant, and retain.
5. Resuspend the cells in 1 mL PBS, and lyse by three cycles of freeze/thawing. A cycle consists of 5 min in a dry ice/ethanol bath followed by 5 min at 37°C in a water bath.
6. Pellet the debris by centrifugation at 10,000*g* for 10 min at 4°C, and test the lysates by ELISA for Fab activity along with the culture supernatants.

3.2.10. ELISA Analysis of Fabs

1. Coat ELISA plates as for the panning procedure, and block with 200 µL PBS containing 1% BSA for 1 h.
2. Incubate with 100 µL potential Fab-containing cell lysates and supernatants for 1 h at room temperature.
3. Wash the plates five times in PBS containing 0.05% Tween-20.
4. Incubate with 100 µL of an antihuman Fab (IgG-specific) alkaline phosphatase antibody conjugate (Sigma) diluted to 1:1000 in PBS containing 1% BSA for 1 h.
5. Wash the plates again as above, and visualize the bound Fab using PNP substrate solution. Color development is carried out at 37°C for 15–60 min and measured at 405 nm using a suitable plate reader.

Once positive clones have been identified by ELISA they can be grown up on a larger scale for antibody production. Competition ELISA to determine specificity and affinity should be performed, and BIAcore (Pharmacia) analysis will enable the derivation of accurate kinetic constants for antigen–antibody interactions. The clones should also be grown up to produce plasmid DNA from which sequence can be derived to identify the antibody genes encoding the Fabs. Sequencing of diverse clones provides the definitive way of distinguishing them in the absence of clear differences in the binding data.

4. Notes

4.1. PCR Amplification of Ig HC and LC Genes

1. More cDNA, e.g., up to 10 μL, can be also added to optimize difficult amplifications.
2. The cycle conditions described provide an initial starting point for amplification. However, some reactions, particularly HC amplifications, can be more difficult and in these cases, the annealing temperature can be lowered slightly to optimize the reaction.

4.2. pComb3 *Vector*

3. In the initial version of this vector the HC and LC inserts were cloned into a *pComb3* plasmid containing short stuffer sequences between the HC and LC restriction sites. However, later, to increase the efficiency of enzyme digestion, a *pComb3* clone containing a well-characterized human anti-tetanus toxoid (TT) Fab *(20)* was used to prepare the vector to receive insert (*see* Fig. 1). The advantage of this method is that single-cut material is separable from double-cut and uncut vector on a preparative gel. In addition, the excised insert is clearly visible on the gel, indicating successful digestion. This is not apparent if the parent vector with no insert is used.
4. The current version of the vector is available from C. F. Barbas III at the Research Institute of Scripps Clinic, 10666 North Torrey Pines Road, La Jolla, CA 92037. This vector contains a number of modifications in the promoter regions designed to minimize recombination. In addition, the vector contains two different stuffer fragments (1200 and 300 bp) in the insertion sites, which is an improvement over using the TT antibody clone as the parent vector.

References

1. Smith, G. P. (1985) Filamentous fusion phage: novel expression vectors that display cloned antigens on the phage surface. *Science* **225,** 1315–1317.
2. Smith, G. P. (1993) Surface display and peptide libraries. *Gene* **128,** 1–2.
3. Parmley, S. and Smith, G. (1988) Antibody-selectable filamentous fd phage vectors: affinity-purification of target genes. *Gene* **73,** 305–318.
4. Cwirla, S., Peters, E., Barrett, R., and Dower, W. (1990) Peptides on phage: a vast library of peptides for identifying ligands. *Proc. Natl. Acad. Sci. USA* **87,** 6378–6382.
5. Scott, J. and Smith, G. (1990) Searching for peptide ligands with an epitope library. *Science* **249,** 386–390
6. McCafferty, J., Griffiths, A. D., Winter, G., and Chiswell, D. J. (1990) Phage antibodies: filamentous phage displaying antibody variable domains. *Nature* **348,** 552–554.
7. Barbas, C. F., Kang, A. S., Lerner, R. A., and Benkovic, S. J. (1991) Assembly of combinatorial antibody libraries on phage surfaces (Phabs): the gene III site. *Proc. Natl. Acad. Sci. USA* **88,** 7978–7982.

8. Hogrefe, H., Mullinax, R., Lovejoy, A., Hay, B., and Sorge, J. (1993) A bacteriophage lambda vector for the cloning and expression of immunoglobulin Fab fragments on the surface of filamentous phage. *Gene* **128,** 119–126.

9. Dubel, S., Breitling, F., Fuchs, P., Braunagel, M., Klewinghaus, I., and Little, M. (1993) A family of vectors for surface display and production of antibodies. *Gene* **128,** 97–101.

10. Griffiths, A., Williams, S., Hartley, O., Tomlinsom, I., Waterhouse, P., Crosby, W., Kontermann, R., Jones, P., Low, N., Allison, T., Prospero, T., Hoogenboom, H., Nissim, A., Cox, J., Harrison, J., Zaccolo, M., Gheradi, E., and Winter, G. (1994) Isolation of high affinity human antibodies directly from large synthetic repertoires. *EMBO J.* **13,** 3245–3260.

11. Corey, D., Shiau, A., Yang, Q., Janowski, B., and Craik, C. (1993) Trypsin display on the surface of bacteriophage. *Gene* **128,** 129–134.

12. Roberts, B., Markland, W., Ley, A., Kent, R., White, D., Guterman, S., and Ladner, R. (1992) Directed evolution of a protein: selection of potent neutrophil elastase inhibitors displayed on M13 fusion phage. *Proc. Natl. Acad. Sci. USA* **89,** 2429–2433.

13. Dennis, M. S. and Lazarus, R. A. (1994) Kunitz domain inhibitors of tissue factor-factor VIIa. II. Potent and specific inhibitors by competitive phage selection. *J. Biol. Chem.* **269,** 22,137–22,144.

14. Oldenburg, K., Longanathan, D., Goldstein, I., Scholtz, P., and Gallop, M. (1992) Peptide ligands for a sugar binding protein isolated from a random peptide library. *Proc. Natl. Acad. Sci. USA* **89,** 5393–5397.

15. Rickles, R.J, Botfield, M. C., Weng, Z., Taylor, J. A. Green, O. M., Brugge, J. S., and Zoller, M. J. (1994) Identification of Src, Fyn, PI3K, and Abl SH3 domain ligands using phage display libraries. *EMBO J.* **13,** 5598–5604.

16. Rebar, E. J. and Pabo, C. O. (1994) Zinc finger phage: affinity selection of fingers with new DNA-binding specificities. *Science* **263,** 671–673.

17. Choo, Y. and Klug, A. (1994) Toward a code for the interactions of zinc fingers with DNA: selection of randomized fingers displayed on phage. *Proc. Natl. Acad. Sci. USA* **91,** 11,163–11,167.

18. Portolano, S., McLachlan, S. M., and Rapoport, B. (1993) High affinity, thyroid-specific human autoantibodies displayed on the surface of phage use V genes similar to other autoantibodies. *J. Immunol.* **135,** 2839–2851.

19. DeKruif, J., Terstappen, L., Boel, E., and Logtenberg, T. (1995) Rapid selection of cell subpopulation-specific human monoclonal antibodies from a synthetic phage display library. *Proc. Natl. Acad. Sci. USA* **92,** 3938–3942.

20. Persson, M. A. A., Caothien, R. H., and Burton, D. R. (1991) Generation of diverse high-affinity human monoclonal antibodies by repertoire cloning. *Proc. Natl. Acad. Sci. USA* **88,** 2432–2436.

21. Hexham, J. M., Partridge, L. J., Furmaniak, J., Petersen, V. B., Colls, J. C., Pegg, C., Rees Smith, B., and Burton, D. R. (1994) Cloning and characterization of TPO autoantibodies using combinatorial phage display libraries. *Autoimmunity* **17,** 167–179.

22. Cha, S., Leung, P. S. C., Gershwin, M. E., Fletcher, M. P., Ansari, A. A., and Coppel, R. S. (1993) Combinatorial antibodies to dihydrolipoamide acetyltransferase, the major autoantigen of primary biliary cirrhosis. *Proc. Natl. Acad. Sci. USA* **90,** 2527–2531.

23. Chomczynski, P. and Sacchi, N (1987) Single-step method of RNA isolation by acid guanidinium thiocyanate phenol chloroform extraction. *Anal. Biochem.* **162,** 156–159.

47

Antibodies from Phage Display Libraries as Immunochemical Reagents

Dario Neri, Alessandro Pini, and Ahuva Nissim

1. Introduction

The display of a repertoire of recombinant antibodies on the surface of fila-mentous phage by fusion to a minor coat protein has provided a powerful meth-odology for isolating the desired binding specificities (*see* Chapter 45 and ref. *1*). Antibodies have typically been displayed on phage as single-chain Fv frag-ments (scFv *[2]*), in which the heavy chain variable region (VH) and the light chain variable region (VL) domains are linked together by a flexible polypep-tide *(3,4),* or as Fab fragments *(5).* In general, antibodies have been displayed either at the N-terminus of the minor coat protein pIII of filamentous phage *(2),* or at the C-terminal domain of pIII *(6).* For Fab fragments, one chain is fused to pIII, and the other assembles with the pIII-fused chain after leader peptide-mediated secretion in the bacterial supernatant.

Repertoires of recombinant antibodies have been derived from both immu-nized and unimmunized hosts. For the former source, the polymerase chain reaction (PCR) has been used to amplify V-genes *(7)* of populations of lym-phocytes from the spleen of immunized mice *(8–10),* the peripheral blood of immunized humans *(11),* and the bone marrow of virally infected patients *(12).* The exposure of the donor to the antigen(s) results in the repertoire enrichment for V-genes specific for the antigen, and typically results in the isolation of high-affinity antibodies *(10,12,13),* often with neutralizing activity *(14).* How-ever, libraries derived from an immunized source allow the isolation of anti-bodies against only a limited number of antigens.

Highly diverse antibody repertoires can also be derived from the rearranged V-genes of "unimmunized" humans (*naive repertoires*; *15,16*), or from semi-synthetic V-genes, created by PCR extension of V-germline genes using prim-

From: *Methods in Molecular Biology, Vol. 80: Immunochemical Protocols, 2nd ed.*
Edited by: J. D. Pound © Humana Press Inc., Totowa, NJ

ers, containing degenerate sequences in corresponding to the CDR3 (*synthetic repertoires; 17–20*). Naive and synthetic repertoires have allowed the isolation of hundreds of antibodies with different specificities, including those for conventionally "difficult" antigens, such as self-antigens, and highly conserved proteins (e.g., BiP and calmodulin; *18,19*). The affinity of antibodies isolated from these repertoires is to a large extent dependent on the size of the repertoire. Antibody libraries of size 5×10^8 have so far succeeded in producing the desired binding specificities against all purified challenging antigens (*18*), yet the antibody affinities are typically in the range $10^6–10^8 M^{-1}$. Higher affinities can be obtained by creating secondary repertoires, for example, by the use of error-prone PCR (*21*), by "chain-shuffling" (*22*), or by using very large (>10^{10} members) primary repertoires (*19*).

In this chapter, we focus on the methods for using (i.e., selecting, screening, and using for biochemical applications) antibodies from libraries produced at the MRC Centre, Cambridge (*18,19*) and distributed to hundreds of laboratories around the world. The methods for generation of such libraries are described in the original publications and will not be presented here.

The Nissim library (*18*) is cloned in the phagemid pHEN1 (*5*). This vector, derived from pUC119 (*23*), comprises the pIII fusion, plasmid, and phage origins of replication. Production of phage particles requires the presence of a helper phage, which provides the other genes and functions for single-stranded replication and packaging. Helper phages (such as VCS M13 and M13 K07, which are described in this chapter) are poorly packaged in comparison to phagemids owing to a defective origin (*24*). However, they do produce pIII not fused to antibody fragments and this competes with the phagemid pIII antibody fusion for incorporation into the phage coat. The majority of phage particles, therefore, display only one antibody molecule or none (*25,26*). Proteolytic cleavage of antibody–pIII fusion may also reduce the number of antibodies displayed. This fact must be considered when the antibody library on phage has to be stored for long periods. The *2-lox* library (*19*) is cloned in a phage vector, which encodes the pIII fusion, the antibiotic resistance, and contains all the genetic information for replication, packaging, and infection of bacteria.

The *lacZ* promoter, which is inhibited by glucose and induced by isopropyl β-D-thiogalactopyranoside (IPTG; *27*), controls the expression of the antibody–pIII fusion in the phagemid pHEN1. Since expression of pIII prevents infection of *Escherichia coli* with the helper phage, bacteria are typically grown in the presence of glucose until infection. After infection, bacteria are grown in the absence of glucose to promote pIII fusion expression and in the presence of ampicillin/kanamycin to ensure that the phagemid-containing bacteria have been infected by the helper phage conferring the kanamycin resistance. pHEN1 contains an amber codon at the junction between the antibody fragment gene and pIII. The use of *E. coli* nonsuppressor strains (such as HB2151; *28*) promotes the antibody secretion in the bacterial periplasmic space, in which the antibody disulfide bridges are formed and the antibody folds. After long expression times (typically >12 h), most of the antibody produced leaks from the bacterial periplasmic space into the culture supernatant, from which it can conveniently be purified. *E. coli* suppressor strains (such as TG1; *29*) favor the production of antibody–pIII fusion, but since suppression is never complete, soluble antibody fragments are typically found in large amounts even in TG1 supernatants.

It is easier to clone antibody repertoires in pUC-based phagemids rather than in phage vectors. With good electrocompetent cells, the efficiency of transformation for pUC vectors is typically 10^9 transformants/µg plasmid, and in the region between 10^7 and 10^8 transformants/µg plasmid cut and religated with an antibody gene insertion. Indeed, libraries >10^9 in size can be produced by repeated transfections with pUC-based phagemids. These libraries yield binders with affinity in the nanomolar range *(30)*.

Large libraries can be produced in phage vectors using recombination techniques. Griffiths et al. *(19)* have infected *E. coli* cells, containing a repertoire of antibody light chains, with phage particles, containing a repertoire of heavy chains cloned into a phage vector. The heavy and light chains have then been linked together in the same phage vector using asymmetric *loxP* sites and *Cre* recombinase *(31)*. This has allowed a combinatorial increase in library dimension, and the production of an antibody repertoire of approx 6.5×10^{10} distinct clones in the first attempt *(19)* and more recently repertoires larger than 10^{11} clones by using a 20-L fermenter (A. Griffiths, personal communication). It is worthwhile recalling, however, that in order to make full use of a library diversity, a number of bacteria (or phage) larger than library size has to be used. The relevant procedures are described in the protocols below; they are somewhat less user-friendly than the procedures needed for smaller libraries (<10^{10} members).

The *dimension* of an antibody library, typically defined as the number of clones bearing a suitable selectable marker (antibiotic resistance) and, containing the full-size antibody gene (detectable by PCR screening; *32*), does not necessarily correspond to the *functional dimension* of a library, which requires that the clones express properly folded antibodies. An approximation for the determination of the functional dimension of a library consists of determining what percentage of clones expresses antibodies, for example, using immunoblot techniques.

Selections are typically performed using purified antigen preparations, although direct panning on cells has been described *(20,33)*. Antigens are coated onto tubes ("Immunotubes") under similar conditions to those employed in ELISA.

Antibody phage libraries are then allowed to bind to the tube. Low-density antigen coating and extensive washings of the tube enrich for high-affinity binders *(22)*; high-surface density immunotube coating and less stringent washing procedures may otherwise be used to select also low-affinity antibodies *(34)*. To some extent, the avidity of antigen binding associated with the multivalent display of antibody fragments on phage makes it difficult to distinguish between medium- and high-affinity clones in the selection procedure. Selection schemes making use of biotinylated antigens and streptavidin-coated magnetic beads cancel avidity effects to a large extent and allow the imposition of conditions on the selection of antibodies with suitable K_d and kinetic constants *(21)*. In this case, however, a proportion of the antibodies isolated will be directed against streptavidin, rather than against the biotinylated antigen. The problem is typically negligible for large antigens, but may be serious for small biotinylated antigens, such as haptens.

Unlike Fab fragments, scFv fragments commonly form multimers by interchain (rather than intrachain) VH–VL pairing *(18,33,35)*. Purification of scFv fragments on protein A columns *(18)*, as well as freezing and thawing (D. Neri, unpublished observations) promotes multimerization. Alternatively, antibody oligomerization can be achieved by tagging recombinant antibodies with oligomerization domains, such as amphipatic helices *(36,37)*, CH3 immunoglobulin domains *(37a)*, or streptavidin *(38)*, at their C-terminus. Multimeric scFv fragments, as well as antibodies on phage, exhibit good performance as immunochemical reagents by virtue of their avidity *(18)*.

The selection procedure can conveniently be monitored by measuring the phage titer before and after selection. In the first couple of rounds, 10^5–10^6 phages are typically eluted after selection. The eluted phage titer may increase up to 10^9 as the phage population becomes enriched for binders, typically at the third or fourth round of panning. After a few rounds of panning, antibodies are typically screened for antigen binding by ELISA. Individual colonies can be picked and grown, in order to perform monoclonal ELISA with bacterial supernatants, containing either antibodies on phage or soluble antibody fragments. In the first case, antibodies against the major coat protein pVIII are used. The progress of a selection can also be monitored by polyclonal ELISA, using a population of phage or of antibody fragments. Immunodetection of soluble antibody fragments is performed using antibodies directed against a peptidic tag engineered at the C-terminus of scFv or Fab fragments.

Peptidic tags can also be used for antibody purification. For example, tags have been used for purification and detection of antibody fragments by binding to streptavidin *(39)*. Protein tags have also been employed, for example, calmodulin, a highly acidic protein that binds to peptide and organic ligands with high affinity ($K_d < 1$ nM) in a calcium-dependent manner. These properties

have been exploited for purification of calmodulin-tagged antibodies (with yields of 5–15 mg/L) from periplasmic lysates or supernatant in a single step by binding to anion-exchange resin, or to an organic ligand of calmodulin *(40)*. Both peptide and protein tags can be used for further characterization of antigen binding, for example, by competition ELISA, surface plasmon resonance *(41)*, or band shift *(40)*. Here, we present protocols for the use of two peptide tags for purification and detection of antibody fragment: the *c-myc* tag recognized by the MAb 9E10 *(42)* allowing both detection by ELISA and purification on affinity columns, and a hexahistidine tag that binds to immobilized metal chelates *(43)* allowing facile purification *(19,44)*. Antibodies of the VH3 family have also been purified on protein A columns *(17)*.

Since high-affinity recombinant antibodies are becoming easier to produce, it is important to be able to measure affinities with rigorous and reliable, yet user-friendly methods. Competition immunoassays *(45,46)* meet these criteria, but radioactive antibody labeling or use of fluorogenic or chemiluminescent substrates is needed for affinities $>10^9 \, M^{-1}$ owing to the limits of sensitivity in antibody detection using chromogenic substrates. A method exploiting similar principles, which has the advantage of visualizing the species involved in the binding equilibrium, is band-shift *(47–50)* using fluorescence- *(40)*, or ^{32}P- *(51)* labeled antibody. Surface plasmon resonance *(41)* is extremely useful for measuring antibody affinity, k_{off} and k_{on}. Care has to be taken that rebinding and multivalent binding are minimized in the experimental setup in order to obtain kinetically meaningful results *(18)*.

In pHEN1 phagemid vectors, the soluble antibody fragments are expressed and secreted directly using nonsuppressor strains of bacteria *(see above)*. However, for fd phage vectors, the antibody genes need to be subcloned into a pUC expression vector, either after PCR amplification *(19)*, or restriction digest of the fd replicative form. Details are not provided here, but can be obtained from the literature (e.g., refs. *6,10,19*). In our laboratory, antibody fragments have been produced from bacteria in shaker flasks with yields ranging from 0.2–70 mg/L, which can be harvested from the bacterial periplasm or from the culture supernatant. Both phage and soluble antibody fragments (scFv and Fab) can be used as monoclonal or polyclonal immunochemical reagents for Western blotting, immunoprecipitation, epitope mapping, and cell staining *(18)*. The reagents can be used directly, or after PEG precipitation (for phage), or affinity purification (for soluble fragments).

2. Materials
2.1. Buffers and Solutions

1. Phosphate-buffered saline (PBS), pH 7.2: 7.3 g NaCl, 2.3 g Na_2HPO_4 anhydrous, 1.3 g $NaH_2PO_4 \cdot 2H_2O$ made up to 1 L.

2. PBS, containing 0.1 and 0.05% (v/v) Tween-20.
3. PBS, containing 50 mM dithiothreitol.
4. PBS, containing 0.5M NaCl.
5. PBS, containing 2% fetal calf serum.
6. X% MPBS: PBS, containing X% (w/v) dried skimmed milk, for example, Marvel (Premier Beverages, Stafford, UK)
7. TBS, pH 7.4: 50 mM Tris-HCl, 100 mM NaCl.
8. TBSC, pH 7.4: 50 mM Tris-HCl, 100 mM NaCl, 1 mM CaCl$_2$.
9. TBS/EDTA, pH 7.4: 50 mM Tris-HCl, 100 mM NaCl, 1 mM EDTA.
10. TBS/Tween-20: TBS, pH 7.4, containing 0.05% Tween-20.
11. TBS/Tween-20/BSA: TBS/Tween-20, containing 3% (w/v) BSA.
12. HBS, pH 7.0: 50 mM HEPES, 100 mM NaCl.
13. 1M Tris-HCl, pH 7.4.
14. Tris/sucrose/EDTA: 30 mM Tris, pH 7.0, containing 20% (w/v) sucrose and 1 mM EDTA.
15. TE buffer, pH 7.4: 10 mM Tris-HCl, 1 mM EDTA.
16. Loading buffer for metal affinity columns: 50 mM phosphate-buffer, pH 7.5, 500 mM NaCl, 20 mM imidazole.
17. Elution buffer for metal affinity columns: 50 mM phosphate-buffer, pH 7.5, 500 mM NaCl, 100 mM imidazole.
18. Regeneration buffer for metal affinity columns: 50 mM phosphate-buffer, pH 7.5, 500 mM NaCl, 250 mM imidazole.
19. 0.2M glycine, pH 3.0.
20. PEG/NaCl: 20% polyethylene glycol (PEG) 6000 in 2.5M NaCl.
21. 100 mM Triethylamine: 700 µL triethylamine (7.18 M) in 50 mL water. Make up on day of use.
22. 5 mM MgSO$_4$.
23. 20 mM EGTA, pH 8.0.
24. Cobalt chloride, 1% (w/v).
25. Hydrogen peroxide 30% (v/v).

2.2. Growth Media

1. 5X M9 salts: 64 g of Na$_2$HPO$_4$ · 7H$_2$O, 15 g of KH$_2$PO$_4$, 2.5 g of NaCl, and 5 g of NH$_4$Cl made up to 1 L and autoclaved.
2. Minimal medium: 200 mL of 5X M9 salts, 20 mL of sterile glucose (20% w/v), 1 mL of 1M MgSO$_4$, 1 mL of vitamin B1 (2 mg/mL), and 750 mL of sterile water.
3. H-top agar: 7 g/L of agar dissolved in Bacto-tryptone (10 g/L), containing NaCl (8 g/L).
4. TYE medium: 10 g Bacto-tryptone, 5 g yeast extract, 8 g NaCl made up to 1 L. Adjust pH to 7.4 with 1M NaOH.
5. TYE agar: 15 g of agar dissolved in 1 L of TYE.
6. TYE-AMP-GLU: TYE, containing 100 µg/mL ampicillin and 1% (w/v) glucose.
7. 2X TY medium: 16 g Bacto-tryptone, 10 g yeast extract, 5 g NaCl made up to 1 L. Adjust pH to 7.4 with 1M NaOH.

8. 2X TY-AMP: 2X TY, containing 100 μg/mL ampicillin.
9. 2X TY-KAN: 25 μg/mL kanamycin.
10. 2X TY-AMP-KAN: 2X TY, containing 100 μg/mL ampicillin and 25 μg/mL kanamycin.
11. 2X TY-TET: 2X TY, containing 12.5 μg/mL tetracycline.
12. 2X TY-GLU: 2X TY, containing 1% (w/v) glucose.
13. 2X TY-X%-GLU: 2X TY, containing X% (w/v) glucose
14. 2X TY, containing 15% glycerol.
15. 2X TY-AMP, containing 9 m*M* IPTG.

2.3. Other Reagents

1. Streptavidin-coupled M-280 Dynabeads (Dynal, Oslo, Norway).
2. NHS-SS-Biotin (Picrce, Rockford, IL).
3. Horseradish peroxidase (HRP) conjugated anti-M13 MAb (Pharmacia, Uppsala, Sweden).
4. HRP substrate solution, e.g., BM blue POD substrate (Boehringer).
5. 9E10 MAb to detect *myc*-tagged antibody fragments (9E10 cell line is available from European Collections of Animal Cell Cultures)
6. HRP-conjugated monoclonal antimouse IgG Fc secondary antibody (e.g., cat. no. A-2554, Sigma, St. Louis, MO).
7. FITC conjugated monoclonal antimouse IgG Fc antibody.
8. Polyclonal rabbit IgG to human κ and λ light chains (Dako, Carpenteria, CA).
9. HRP-conjugated goat antirabbit IgG (Sigma).
10. 5/5 Mono-Q anion-exchange FPLC chromatography column.
11. Ni-NTA resin (Diagen) for metal affinity chromatography.
12. *N*-(6-aminohexyl)-5-chloro-1-naphtalensulfonamide-agarose (Sigma).
13. 3'3' diaminobenzidine (DAB) tablets (Sigma).
14. Normal swine serum.
15. Fast red (Sigma).
16. Acetone.

2.4. Bacteria and Phage (see Note 1)

1. Two bacterial strains are used:
   a. *E. coli* suppressor strain TG1 (K12, *[lac-pro], sup*E, *thi*, *hsd*△5/F'*tra*△36, *pro*A$^+$B$^+$, *lac*I^q, *lacZ*△M15) for propagation of phage particles, and
   b. HB21521 nonsuppressor strain (K12, *ara*, △*[lac-pro]*, *thi*/F'*pro*A$^+$B$^+$, *lac*I^{q}Z△M15) for expression of antibody fragments.
   Phage/phagemid infect $^{F+}$-*E. coli* via the sex pili. For sex pili production and efficient infection *E. coli* must be cultured at 37°C and be in the log phase of growth (OD [1 cm, 600 nm] = 0.4–0.5).
2. A variety of helper phages are available for the rescue of phagemid libraries. VCS M13 (Stratagene) and M13 K07 (Pharmacia) can be purchased in small aliquots: Large quantities for rescue of phagemid libraries can be prepared as described in Section 3.2.2.

For long-term storage at −70°C, bacteria, containing plasmids or phage replicative form are resuspended in 2X TY medium, containing 15% glycerol in 2-mL plastic vials (Biofreeze vials, Costar).

2.5. Equipment

1. Agar plates: round 9-cm diameter, or large square (243 × 243 mm) Nunc Bio-Assay dishes (Gibco-BRL, Gaithersburg, MD).
2. 0.45-μm Filters (Minisart NML; Sartorius).
3. 16-μm Filters (e.g., Filtron Technology Corporation ®Minisette© system).
4. Nunc 5-mL Immunotubes (Maxisorp, Gibco-BRL).
5. Magnetic particle concentrator: MPC-1 (Dynal).
6. MicroTest III flexible assay plates for ELISA (Falcon).
7. Ultrafree-MC filters (Millipore, Bedford, MA).
8. FPLC/HPLC chromatography system.
9. Polylysine-coated glass slides.
10. Cryostat.
11. Fluorescence-activated cell sorter (FACS), e.g., Becton Dickinson FACScan (*see* Chapters 33 and 34).

3. Methods
3.1. General

Unless otherwise stated:

1. Culture bacteria and phage in liquid media at 37°C in an orbital shaker at 250–300 rpm.
2. Culture agar plates at 30°C if time allows. Otherwise use 37°C.
3. Perform phage infections for 30 min in a 37°C water bath without shaking using exponentially growing bacteria.
4. Perform centrifugations at 4°C.
5. Perform OD measurements on bacterial suspensions at 600 nm in a 1-cm cuvet.

3.2. Bacteria and Helper Phage
3.2.1. Exponential Bacterial Cultures

1. Transfer a bacterial colony from a minimal media plate into 5 mL of 2X TY medium, and culture overnight.
2. On the next day, subculture by diluting 1:100 into fresh 2X TY medium. Culture until OD = 0.4–0.5, and then infect with phage. If necessary, the bacterial culture can be kept on ice for a short period before infection (<30 min; *see* Note 2).

3.2.2. Preparation of Helper Phage

1. Infect 200 μL *E. coli* TG1 at OD = 0.2 with 10-μL serial dilutions of helper phage in order to obtain well-separated plaques. Add to 3 mL H-top agar (42°C), and pour onto warm TYE plates. Allow to set, and then incubate overnight.

2. Pick a small plaque into 3–4 mL of an exponentially growing culture of *E. coli* TG1 (*see* Section 3.2.1.). Culture for about 2 h.
3. Inoculate into 500 mL 2X TY in a 2-L flask, culture for 1 h, and then add kanamycin (25 mg/mL in water) to a final concentration of 50–70 µg/mL. Culture for a further 8–16 h.
4. Centrifuge down bacteria at 10,800g for 15 min. To the phage supernatant add ¼ vol PEG/NaCl, and incubate for a minimum of 30 min on ice. Centrifuge 10,800g for 15 min.
5. Resuspend pellet in 2 mL TE buffer, and filter-sterilize the stock through a 0.45-µm filter.
6. Determine the titer of the stock, and then dilute to about 1×10^{12} PFU/mL. Store aliquots at –20°C.

3.3. Growth of Libraries

The libraries are generally stored at –70°C as bacteria harboring phagemid or phage DNA (at least 10^8 bacteria/10 µL in 2X TY-15% glycerol; *see* refs. *18* and *19*). In order to make phage for selection, the primary library is grown and the phage harvested. Generally, for a library comprised of 5×10^8 clones, at least 5×10^8 bacteria (50 µL stock, and preferably more) are inoculated; for a library of 10^{11} bacteria, at least 10^{11} clones (10 mL stock) are used. In the following examples, protocols for working with phagemid repertoires of 5×10^8 clones and phage repertoires of 10^{11} clones are described. For libraries of different sizes, it will be necessary to adapt the protocols accordingly.

3.3.1. Nissim Library (Phagemid Vector)

1. Inoculate 50 µL of bacterial library stock (5×10^8 clones) into 50 mL 2X TY-AMP-GLU (to give a 1/1000 dilution).
2. Culture to OD = 0.5. at 30°C (about 1–1.5 h). An aliquot of 40 mL can be taken at this stage to make a secondary stock (*see* Section 3.3.3.).
3. Infect the remaining 10 mL of culture with helper phage in a ratio of ~20:1 (phage:bacteria) (*see* Note 3).
4. Centrifuge the infected bacteria at 3300g for 10 min. Gently resuspend the pellet in 30 mL of 2X TY-AMP-KAN.
5. Add to 270 mL of 2X TY-AMP-KAN, and incubate at 30°C overnight.
6. Centrifuge down the culture at 10,800g for 10 min, and immediately precipitate the phage from the supernatant using PEG (*see* Section 3.4.). The phage, representing the library, should be used within 1 wk, or can be stored in aliquots at –20°C. These aliquots will be all of the same quality and will ensure the reproducibility of the selection procedure.

3.3.2. 2-lox Library (Phage fd Vector)

1. Inoculate 10 mL of bacterial library stock (10^{11} diversity) into 10 L 2X TY-TET.
2. Incubate at 30°C for 16 h.

3. Centrifuge down the bacteria at 7300g for 20 min, and keep the bacterial pellet for making a secondary stock (*see* Section 3.3.3.). Immediately precipitate the phage supernatant with PEG (*see* Section 3.4.). The phage, representing the library, should be used within 1 wk, or can be stored in aliquots at –20°C.

3.3.3. Secondary Stocks

An excellent secondary stock is the frozen phage library obtained from the primary stock. Antibodies on phage may undergo proteolysis or be denatured, but phage particles are resistant and maintain a good infectivity. A titer of phage larger than the library size can therefore be used to infect exponentially growing *E. coli* TG1 and produce a second generation of phage library. Secondary bacterial stocks can also be prepared from the primary library growths above. However, before using a secondary stock, it is recommended that the frequency of inserts be checked by PCR (*see* Section 1.).

3.3.3.1. PHAGEMID VECTORS

1. Take 40 mL of the 50-mL culture (primary phagemid library stock grown as described in Section 3.3.1.), and centrifuge down the bacteria at 3300g for 10 min.
2. Resuspend the bacteria in about 1 mL 2X TY.
3. Spread on a large Bio-Assay dish of TYE-AMP-GLU, and culture overnight.
4. Add 1–2 mL 2X TY-15% glycerol to the Bio-Assay dish, and loosen the bacteria with a glass spreader.
5. Store this stock (of about 1 × 10^8 bacteria/50 μL) at –70°C.

3.3.3.2. PHAGE FD VECTORS

1. Add 250 mL 2X TY-15% glycerol to the bacterial pellet of the primary phage fd library grown as described in Section 3.3.2.
2. Store this stock at –70°C.

3.4. Purification of Phage

The phage can be concentrated (and any soluble antibodies removed) by precipitation with PEG 6000. The protocol described here is appropriate for 300 mL phage-containing supernatant.

1. Add 75 mL PEG/NaCl to the phage supernatant. Mix well, and leave for a minimum of 1 h at 4°C.
2. Centrifuge at 10,800g for 30 min.
3. Resuspend the pellet in ~40 mL water (1 L for the supernatant of the fd library grown as described in Section 3.3.2.), and add ¼ vol PEG/NaCl. Mix, and leave for a minimum of 20 min at 4°C.
4. Centrifuge at 10,800g for 30 min, and aspirate off the supernatant.
5. Recentrifuge briefly, and aspirate off any remaining PEG/NaCl.
6. Resuspend the pellet. For the phagemid vectors, use 2 mL PBS (for the preparation of the fd library, use 15 mL PBS). Phage yields are normally 1–5 × 10^{13} t.u./mL phage.

7. Centrifuge at 3300g for 10 min or 11,600g for 2 min to remove any residual bacterial cell debris.
8. Store the phage supernatant either at 4°C for short-term storage or in PBS, containing 15% glycerol for longer-term storage at −70°C.

3.5. Selection of Phage

The phage libraries can be selected using "Immunotubes" (Nunc), biotinylated antigen in solution, or affinity chromatography. Here we present details for the first two methods, which are the most commonly used. The stringency of selection conditions can be adjusted; particularly during later rounds of selection, the stringency can be increased, for example, by reducing the density of coating of antigen to solid phase (*see* Section 1.). Skimmed powdered milk is added to prevent nonspecific binding of phage to surfaces.

3.5.1. Selection on Immunotubes

3.5.1.1. COATING IMMUNOTUBE WITH ANTIGEN

1. Coat a 5-mL Nunc Immunotube overnight using 4 mL of antigen. The efficiency of coating depends on the antigen concentration, the buffer, and the temperature employed. An antigen concentration in the range 10–100 μg/mL in PBS, pH 7.2, or 50 mM sodium hydrogen carbonate, pH 9.6, at room temperature is usually satisfactory.
2. Rinse the tube three times with PBS, and then block with 4 mL 2% MPBS at room temperature for 2 h.
3. Rinse the tube three times with PBS.

3.5.1.2. FIRST ROUND OF SELECTION

1. Add 10^{12}–10^{13} t.u. phage library in 2 mL PBS to Immunotube, containing 2 mL of 4% MPBS.
2. Seal the tube with Parafilm, and mix by repeated inversion at room temperature for 30 min.
3. Allow Immunotube to stand upright at room temperature for 1.5 h, and then discard the unbound phage in the supernatant.
4. Rinse the tube 10 times with PBS, containing 0.1% Tween-20, and then 10 times with PBS alone. Each washing step is performed by pouring in buffer, and then immediately pouring out.
5. Shake out excess PBS from the tube, and elute the bound phage by adding 1 mL 100 mM triethylamine.
6. Mix by repeated inversion at room temperature for 10 min (no longer).
7. Pour into a microfuge tube, containing 0.5 mL of 1M Tris HCl, pH 7.4, to neutralize the triethylamine, and vortex. Keep on ice until the TG1 bacteria reach OD = 0.4–0.5.
8. Infect 10 mL TG1 culture with 1 mL of collected phage (at further rounds of selection, 10 μL collected phage can be used to infect 1 mL exponential HB2151 for soluble ELISA screening; *see* Section 3.6.) (*see* Note 4).

9. Make a series of four to five 100-fold serial dilutions in 2X TY using new pipet tips each time. Plate 100 µL of each dilution on the appropriate selective TYE plates.
10. Centrifuge down the remaining infected TG1 at 3300*g* for 10 min.
11. Resuspend the pelleted bacteria in 0.5–1 mL 2X TY, and spread on a large Bio-Assay dish of the appropriate selective TYE agar.
12. Incubate at 30°C overnight or until colonies are visible.

3.5.1.3. FURTHER ROUNDS OF SELECTION (PHAGEMID VECTORS)

1. On the next day, monitor the titer of the selection by counting colonies on the plates from the dilution series. Add 1–2 mL 2X TY, containing 15% glycerol to the Bio-Assay dish, and loosen the bacteria with a glass spreader.
2. Store the bacteria at –70°C in 2X TY, containing 15% glycerol after inoculating 100 µL into 100 mL 2X TY-AMP-GLU for further selection.
3. Rescue as described in Section 3.3.1.
4. Precipitate with PEG as described in Section 3.4., and resuspend the second phage pellet in 2 mL of PBS.
5. Store a 1-mL aliquot of the phage at 4°C, and use the other 1-mL aliquot for the next round of selection. Repeat the selection for another three to four rounds.

3.5.1.4. FURTHER ROUNDS OF SELECTION (PHAGE FD VECTORS)

1. Add 2–5 mL 2X TY to a large Bio-Assay dish, and loosen bacteria with a glass spreader.
2. Inoculate into 200 mL 2X TY-TET, and culture at 30°C overnight.
3. Centrifuge the bacteria at 10,800*g* for 20 min. Add 2–5 mL 2X TY, containing 15% glycerol to the cell pellet, and store at–70°C.
4. Remove the supernatant and precipitate the phage with PEG (as described in Section 3.4.). Resuspend the second phage pellet in 2 mL of PBS.
5. Store a 1-mL aliquot of the phage at 4°C, and use another 1-mL aliquot for the next round of selection. Repeat the selection for another three to four rounds.

3.5.2. Selection Using Biotinylated Antigens

In this approach, the phage antibodies react with biotinylated antigen in solution, and the complex is then captured using Streptavidin coupled to Dynabeads.

3.5.2.1. BINDING PHAGE TO SOLUBLE BIOTINYLATED ANTIGEN

The antigen is first biotinylated with NHS-SS-Biotin according to the manufacturer's instructions (e.g., for FITC-BSA and NIP-BSA, *see* ref. *19*), and the phage is then bound to the biotinylated antigen (*see* Note 5).

1. Mix together: 2.5 mL of phage in PBS (10^{12}–10^{13} t.u.), 2.5 mL of 4% MPBS, 50 µL of Tween-20 and S-S-biotinylated antigen to give a final concentration of no more than 50 n*M* (for excess of streptavidin-Dynabeads over antigen)
2. Gently rotate on an inclined end-over-end mixer for 1 h at room temperature (*see* Note 6).

3.5.2.2. BLOCKING

1. Block 1.5 mL (per selection) streptavidin M-280 Dynabeads by adding 5 mL 4% MPBS, and rotate in a 15-mL tube on an end-over-end mixer for 5 min at room temperature.
2. Separate the beads from the MPBS with a magnetic particle concentrator for 4–5 min.
3. Pour off the supernatant, and add another 5 mL 4% MPBS. Rotate for 1 h at room temperature, and separate again with a magnetic particle concentrator.
4. Resuspend in 1.5 mL (per selection) of 2% MPBS.

3.5.2.3. SELECTION

1. Add 1.5 mL of blocked streptavidin Dynabeads to the phage bound to S-S biotinylated antigen.
2. Gently rotate for 15 min at room temperature.
3. Separate with the magnetic particle concentrator, and pour off the supernatant.
4. Resuspend in 1 mL 2% MPBS, and transfer to a 1.5 mL microfuge tube.
5. Wash twice with 1 mL PBS, and then once with 1 mL 2% MPBS; repeat this sequence of washes 15 times. For each wash, resuspend the beads, and separate using the magnetic particle concentrator.
6. Elute the phage from the beads by resuspending in 300 μL PBS, containing 50 mM dithiothreitol (*see* Note 7).
7. Stand for 5 min at room temperature, and separate the beads again with the magnetic particle concentrator.
8. Use 150 μL of the phage supernatant to infect 10 mL TG1, and store the remaining phage at 4°C.
9. Remove a small aliquot of the infected TG1, make a series of four to five 100-fold serial dilutions in 2X TY, and plate 100 μL each on the appropriate selective TYE plates.
10. Pellet the remaining bacteria by centrifuging for 10 min at 3300g.
11. Resuspend in 1 mL 2X TY, and spread on a large Bio-Assay dish with appropriate selective TYE agar.
12. Incubate at 30°C overnight or until colonies are visible, and then repropagate phage as described in Section 3.5.1.
13. Repeat the selection procedure another three to four times (use a 1-mL aliquot for selection, and store the remaining phage at 4°C). For the second and subsequent rounds of selection, mix 1 mL phage from the previous round of selection with 0.5 mL of 6% MPBS, 10 μL Tween-20, and biotinylated antigen to give a final concentration of 50 nM. Use only 300 μL of blocked streptavidin-coated Dynabeads.

3.6. Screening Phage by ELISA

It is recommended that after the third round of panning, the progress of the selection be monitored by ELISA, either with soluble antibodies or antibodies on phage. A polyclonal phage ELISA protocol, using phage produced at the end of each round of panning, is often chosen because the amount of antigen needed is minimal, since few wells must be coated. Alternatively, individual colonies of TG1 bacteria infected with phage from the desired round of panning can be used to produce phage particles in bacterial supernatants, which are then tested in ELISA.

The diversity of the selected phage MAb may be assessed by gel electrophoresis of PCR products (15,18), probing (52), or by sequencing of the vector DNA (whether as phage, phagemid, or plasmid).

3.6.1. Polyclonal Phage

1. Coat MicroTest III flexible assay plates with protein antigen (100 μL/well). Overnight incubation at room temperature with 10–100 μg/mL of antigen in either PBS, pH 7.2, or 50 mM sodium hydrogen carbonate, pH 9.6, is generally satisfactory.
2. Wash wells three times with PBS, and block with 200 μL/well of 2% MPBS for 2 h at room temperature.
3. Rinse wells three times with PBS. Add 10 μL PEG precipitated phage from the stored aliquot of phage at the end of each round of selection (about 10^{10} t.u.). Make up to 100 μL with 2% MPBS. Alternatively, 20 μL 10% MPBS and 80 μL phage-containing supernatants can be used. Incubate for 60 min at room temperature, and then discard well contents by inverting and shaking the plate over a sink. Wash three times with PBS, containing 0.05% Tween-20, and then three times with PBS.
4. Add appropriate dilution of HRP-anti-M13 (see Note 8). Incubate for 60 min at room temperature and wash as in step 3.
5. Develop with HRP substrate solution; if BM blue POD HRP substrate is used, add 100 μL to each well, and leave at room temperature for 10 min. The conversion product is colored blue.
6. Stop the reaction by adding 50 μL of 1M sulfuric acid. The color should change to yellow.
7. Read the OD at 650 and 450 nm to correct for light scatter. Subtract OD 650 nm values from those obtained at 450 nm.

3.6.2. Monoclonal Phage

For better aeration during phage growth or induction in 96-well plates, the plate lid may be removed.

3.6.2.1 PHAGEMID VECTORS

1. Inoculate individual colonies from the plates of phage-infected TG1 spread after the desired round of selection into 150 μL 2X TY-AMP-GLU into 96-well plates. Use a toothpick or a small pipet tip as inoculating device. After inoculation, use the same device to touch a replica 2X TY-AMP-GLU plate with a numbered grid

attached at the bottom. The colonies from the replica plate corresponding to positive clones in ELISA can be used to prepare a glycerol culture or to PCR-amplify the antibody gene.

2. Culture for 3 h.
3. To each well add 25 μL 2X TY-AMP-GLU, containing 10^9 PFU of helper phage.
4. Stand for 30 min at 37°C. Centrifuge at 1800g for 10 min, and then aspirate off the supernatant.
5. Resuspend bacterial pellet in 200 μL 2X TY-AMP-KAN. Culture overnight at 30°C.
6. Centrifuge at 1800g for 10 min, and use 50–100 μL of the supernatant in phage ELISA, as described in Section 3.6.1.

3.6.2.2. PHAGE FD VECTORS

1. Inoculate colonies from the plates of phage-infected TG1 spread after each round of selection into 200 μL 2X TY-TET in 96-well plates.
2. Culture at 30°C overnight.
3. Centrifuge at 1800g for 10 min.
4. Take 50–100 μL of phage supernatant for phage ELISA, as described in Section 3.6.1.
5. Make glycerol stocks of the remaining culture in the 96-well plates.

3.7. Screening Antibody Fragments by ELISA

ELISA for the antibody fragments either detects a peptide tag (for scFv and Fab fragments), or the heavy chain (for Fab only).

1. For detection of *myc*-tagged antibody fragments, use 9E10 MAb and HRP-conjugated monoclonal antimouse IgG Fc secondary antibody.
2. For detection of Fab antibody fragments, use a polyclonal rabbit IgG to human κ and λ light chains and HRP-conjugated goat antirabbit IgG (*see* Note 9).

3.7.1. Antibody Fragments from Phagemid Vectors

1. Infect 1-mL culture of HB2151 with 10 μL (about 10^5 t.u.) of the phage eluted and neutralized at the last round of selection. Plate 0.1, 1, 10, and 100 μL on TYE-AMP-GLU. Incubate overnight.
2. Inoculate individual colonies from the plates of phage-infected TG1 spread after the round of selection of interest into 150 μL 2X TY-AMP-0.1%GLU in 96-well plates using a toothpick or a small pipet tip as described in Section 3.6.2.1., step 1. Touch a replica 2X TY-AMP-GLU plate with a numbered grid attached at the bottom. The colonies from the replica plate corresponding to positive clones in ELISA can be used to prepare a glycerol culture or to PCR-amplify the antibody gene.
3. Culture for 3 h.
4. Add 30 μL 2X TY-AMP, containing 10 m*M* IPTG (to give a final concentration >1 m*M* IPTG). Continue shaking at 30°C for a further 16–24 h.
5. Centrifuge at 1800g for 10 min, and use 100 μL of the supernatant in ELISA.

3.7.2. ELISA of Supernatants

Washing and coating is as described in Section 3.6.1. This is a one-step procedure that works very well.

1. Coat MicroTest III flexible assay plates with 100 µL/well of protein antigen.
2. Rinse wells three times with PBS, and block with 200 µL/well of 2% MPBS for 1–2 h at room temperature. Rinse wells three times with PBS.
3. Add 20 µL 10% MPBS and 80 µL supernatant to each well. Then immediately, using a multichannel pipet, add 12 µL freshly prepared developing reagent (e.g., for *myc*-tag, containing antibodies: 9E10 [50 µg/mL] and antimouse HRP [1:100] in 2% MPBS).
4. Incubate for 20–60 min, and wash.
5. Develop with HRP substrate solution, e.g., with BM blue POD substrate.
6. Add 100 µL to each well, and leave at room temperature for 10 min.
7. Stop the reaction by adding 50 µL 1M sulfuric acid.
8. Read the OD at 650 and 450 nm. Subtract OD 650 nm values from those obtained at 450 nm.

3.8. Preparation of Antibody Fragments

After identifying polyclonal antibody or MAb fragments with binding activities, it is usually necessary to grow a larger culture in order to make enough antibody for use as a reagent. The fragments can be purified or used directly.

3.8.1. Cultures

For polyclonal antibody fragments from phagemid vectors, use an aliquot of pooled, scraped HB2151 bacteria infected with the selected pHEN1 phagemid; for MAb fragments, use individual colonies; for polyclonal antibody fragments from phage fd vectors, use an aliquot of pooled, scraped TG1 bacteria transformed with the cloned pUC expression vector, and for MAb fragments use individual colonies.

1. Inoculate either 10 µL of pooled, scraped bacteria (HB2151 or TG1 depending on the library), or single colonies into 2X TY-AMP-0.1% GLU (1 mL to 1 L medium, depending on the size of preparation needed).
2. Culture to OD = 0.9 and induce with 1 mM IPTG.
3. To harvest antibody fragments secreted into culture supernatant, incubate overnight at 30°C.

To harvest antibody fragments from *E. coli* periplasm, incubate for 3–16 h at 22°C.

3.8.2. Harvesting Fragments from Culture Supernatant

1. Centrifuge the induced bacterial culture at 10,800g for 15 min, and collect the antibody-containing supernatant.

2. For small-scale preparations (original culture volumes of <100 mL), the supernatant can either be taken directly for further purification (*see* Section 3.8.4.), or concentrated about 10-fold by dialysis against dry granular PEG-6000 and used without further purification.
3. For large-scale preparations, the antibody-containing supernatant can be purified further (*see* Section 3.8.4.). However, beforehand, it is recommended that:
    a. Supernatants from an original culture volume of up to 1 L are filtered through disposable 0.45-μm filters. Two to ten filters may be needed for 1 L, depending on the viscosity of the preparation (*see* Note 10). Initial centrifugation is an advantage.
    b. Supernatants from an original culture volume of over 1 L are ultrafiltered through a 16-μm filter, and then concentrated 5- to 10-fold using the same system equipped with a 10-kDa cutoff filter.

3.8.3. Harvesting Fragments from the Periplasm

1. Centrifuge the induced bacterial culture at 10,800g for 15 min.
2. Resuspend in $\frac{1}{20}$ the original volume of Tris/sucrose/EDTA, and leave for 20 min on ice.
3. Centrifuge at 10,800g for 15 min, and collect supernatant (periplasmic fraction) into a new tube.
4. Resuspend pellet in 50 mL of 5 mM MgSO$_4$, and incubate for 20 min on ice.
5. Take the supernatant, and centrifuge at 10,800g for 15 min. Take the supernatant (osmotic shock fraction), and add it to the periplasmic fraction.
6. Concentrate the pooled periplasmic preparation or filter depending on the initial culture volume (as with fragments from the culture supernatant).

3.8.4. Purification of Antibody Fragments

Antibody fragments from the *E. coli* periplasm or supernatant can be purified using a range of affinity matrices, the choice of which depends on the type of antibody fragment and the tag. We have so far mainly employed methods for antibody fragments that are coupled to either *myc* or *his-myc* tags. However, fragments can be subcloned into other expression vectors that use other tags, e.g., calmodulin. In this section, we provide three examples of approaches to purification of fragments.

Throughout these purifications, storage of the protein at 4°C or on ice is recommended, and if possible, fractionations should be performed in a cold room.

3.8.4.1. PURIFICATION USING A METAL AFFINITY COLUMN

Metal affinity columns can be used for the purification of antibodies with a hexa-Histidine tag. Immobilized metal affinity chromatography is incompatible, in our own experience, with direct loading of antibodies in supernatants onto the column: The supernatant must be exchanged into loading buffer, for example, by ammonium sulfate precipitation, or using an ultrafiltration device.

1. Preparations and supernatants:
    a. For periplasmic preparations: Dialyze the antibody preparation (10-kDa cut-off) against loading buffer overnight at 4°C.
    b. For bacterial supernatants: Exchange the supernatant into loading buffer at 4°C by ammonium sulfate precipitation followed by dialysis or using ultrafil-tration techniques.
2. Fill a column with 5 mL Ni-NTA resin.
3. Equilibrate the column with 50 mL loading buffer.
4. Load the antibody preparation onto the column.
5. Wash the column with 50 mL loading buffer.
6. Elute the protein with 20 mL elution buffer, and collect 1-mL fractions. Expect the antibody fragments to elute between 4 and 10 mL.
7. Dialyze the antibody fractions (detected by ELISA) against PBS or HBS to remove imidazole and NaCl (typical yields are 0.2–20 mg/L of culture). Some antibodies tend to precipitate during dialysis. The precipitation is associated with the presence of the *his*-tag. Addition of 20 mM EDTA to the antibody sample before dialysis often solves this problem.
8. Wash the column with 50 mL of regeneration buffer and equilibrate with 50 mL of loading buffer.
9. For small-scale rapid purification, Ni-NTA resin centrifuge columns (Qiagen, Hilden, Germany) can be used.

3.8.4.2. PURIFICATION USING PROTEIN A

Protein A-Sepharose can be used to purify antibody fragments encoded by VH segments from the VH3 family *(17)*. MAb 9E10 *(see* Section 3.7.) can be coupled to CNBr-activated Sepharose according to the manufacturer's instructions and used to purify *myc*-tagged fragments *(see* Note 11).

1. Pre-swell the protein A-Sepharose (or protein A-9E10–Sepharose) in PBS.
2. Fill a 10-mL plastic column with about 1 mL protein A-Sepharose, and equili-brate column with 50 mL PBS.
3. Load antibody preparation onto column.
4. Wash with five column volumes of first PBS and then PBS, containing 0.5M NaCl.
5. Elute the protein with about three column volumes of either 0.2M glycine, pH 3.0, or 100 mM triethylamine, collecting 1-mL fractions into 0.2 mL 1M Tris-HCl, pH 7.4, and mixing immediately.
6. Measure the OD at 280 nm *(see* Note 12), and dialyze sample overnight against PBS (10-kDa cutoff).
7. For small-scale purification, mix 5–10 mL of antibody fragments with 100–200 μL of pre-swollen protein A-Sepharose. Purify using ultrafree-MC filters following the above protocol, but wash with 1 mL of buffer, and elute with 100 μL of eluant.

3.8.4.3. PURIFICATION OF CALMODULIN FUSION ANTIBODIES

Since calmodulin is highly acidic, it allows the calmodulin-tagged antibody fragments to be purified on anion-exchange columns. Also, calmodulin-tagged antibodies can be purified by affinity chromatography, since calmodulin binds to several proteins, peptides and organic ligands with high affinity in a process inhibited by calcium chelators, such as EGTA *(40)*.

3.8.4.3.1. Anion Exchange. This purification is in the absence of calcium using a 5/5 Mono-Q anion-exchange FPLC chromatography column.

1. Equilibrate column extensively with TBS/EDTA, pH 7.4.
2. Load antibody preparation onto the column.
3. Elute the protein with TBS/EDTA, pH 7.4 and an NaCl gradient (100 mM to 1M). The fusion protein elutes in 0.5M NaCl.

3.8.4.3.2. Organic Ligands for Affinity Chromatography

1. Pre-swell N-(6-aminohexyl)-5-chloro-1-naphtalensulfonamide-agarose in TBSC, pH 7.4.
2. Fill a plastic 10-mL column with around 3 mL of slurry.
3. Equilibrate with TBSC, pH 7.4.
4. Load the antibody preparation onto the column.
5. Wash the column extensively with TBSC, pH 7.4, containing 0.5M NaCl.
6. Elute the protein with about 3 column volumes of 20 mM EGTA, pH 8.0.
7. Dialyze against TBS.

3.9. Antibody Fragments or Phage as Reagents

Antibody fragment preparations or PEG-precipitated phage can be used as immunochemical reagents.

3.9.1. Western Blotting

Polyclonal or monoclonal phage antibodies can be used as reagents to detect antigens on Western blots (*see* Chapter 20). Here we describe the detection of purified antigen, but the same protocol can be used for antigen present in complex protein mixtures.

1. Run 2 μg of each purified antigen on a 10 or 15% polyacrylamide gel, and then electrophoretically transfer proteins onto a nitrocellulose filter.
2. Block the filter for 1 h at room temperature in 2% MPBS, containing 0.05% Tween-20 (for antibody fragments), or 5–10% MPBS, containing 0.05% Tween-20 (for phage). The antibodies are generally dissolved in 2% MPBS, containing 0.05% Tween-20. However, according to the signal and background, the percentage Marvel and Tween-20 can be changed.
3. Add the antibody fragments (10 mg/mL of purified sample or 1:2 dilution of 10X concentrated supernatant), or phage (10^{11} t.u./mL) to the filter.

3.9.1.1. SOLUBLE ANTIBODIES

1. Add the antibodies needed for detection to the primary antibody solution for a one-step procedure. Choose the secondary antibodies from the following reagents:
   a. HRP-protein A (Sigma) in a 1:1000 dilution, for antibody fragments of the human VH3 family.
   b. MAb 9E10 (4 µg/mL) and HRP-conjugated goat antimouse IgG Fc antibody (*see* Note 8) to detect antibody fragments with a *myc*-tag.
   c. HRP-conjugated polyclonal sheep antihuman κ and λ light chain antiserum to detect the λ and κ light chains of Fab fragments.
2. Incubate with gentle agitation for 1–2 h at room temperature.

3.9.1.2. PHAGE

1. Wash filter twice in PBS, containing 0.05% Tween for 5 min and twice in PBS.
2. Detect binding by incubating the filter with HRP-conjugated anti-M13 at a 1:1000 dilution in 2% MPBS at room temperature.
3. Wash filter as in step 1.
4. Detect peroxidase activity using DAB by mixing 10 mg DAB (one tablet), 400 µL of 1% cobalt chloride, 20 mL PBS, and 20 µL 30% hydrogen peroxide. Pour onto the blot, allow to react, and then wash with water to block the staining reaction (*see* Note 13).

3.9.2. Immunocytochemistry

Phage and antibody fragments can both be used for cell staining, but phage particles penetrate membranes less effectively *(18)*. Here we present two protocols that employ soluble antibody fragments. The first is a method for staining tissue sections (for example, tumor sections) using antibodies in bacterial supernatants or purified preparations. The second is a one-step procedure for labeling cells with fluorescence, so that they can be analyzed by confocal laser microscopy or by fluorescence-activated cell sorter (FACS).

3.9.2.1. STAINING OF TUMOR SECTIONS

1. Cut 5–6 µm thick sections of frozen tumors with a Cryostat using standard procedures, and mount onto polylysine-coated glass slides.
2. Air-dry overnight.
3. Fix by immersion in cold acetone for 10 min (*see* Note 14).
4. Draw a circle with a glass pen around the sections, so that the area to be treated with the antibody solutions can readily be recognized.
5. Rehydrate the sections by immersion in TBS/Tween-20 for 5 min.
6. Block with normal swine serum diluted 1/5 in TBS/Tween-20 for 30 min at room temperature.
7. Drain out the liquid by touching the edge of the glass slide with paper.
8. Add antibody in bacterial supernatant (try three dilutions: undiluted, 1/10, and 1/100 in TBS/Tween-20/BSA. Incubate for 1 h at room temperature.

9. Wash gently three times with TBS/Tween-20 using a Pasteur pipet, and then immerse in TBS/Tween-20 for 10 min, changing the buffer three times.

10. Add secondary antibodies (as for ELISA and Western blotting, but use an alkaline-phosphatase conjugate instead of a HRP) in TBS/Tween-20/BSA. Incubate 30 min at room temperature.

11. Wash gently three times with TBS/Tween-20 using a Pasteur pipet, and then immerse in TBS/Tween-20 for 10 min, changing buffer three times.

12. Develop with Fast red for 20 min (*also see* manufacturer's instructions).

13. Wash by immersion in water to stop the reaction.

3.9.2.2. FLUORESCENT LABELING OF EUKARYOTIC CELLS FOR MICROSCOPY OR FACS ANALYSIS

1. Culture cells as appropriate in culture medium.

2. Detach cells from flask as appropriate (mechanically, by scraping, or using trypsin).

3. Centrifuge at 130g for 10 min, and resuspend the cells in antibody solution (try three dilutions: undiluted supernatant, 1/10, and 1/100 in PBS, containing 2% fetal calf serum.

4. Add secondary mouse MAb (for scFv with *myc*-tag, use 9E10 at 5–10 µg/mL) and FITC-conjugated antimouse IgG Fc tertiary antibody (*see* Note 15).

5. Wash cells 3 × 5 min in PBS.

6. Analyze by FACS or by pipeting the cells onto a microscope slide for confocal laser microscopy.

4. Notes

1. Phage contaminations in flasks, bottles, and so forth, may accumulate as one performs selections from phage display libraries. Precautions need to be taken throughout the protocol to avoid any carryover of phage. Autoclaving alone is not sufficient enough to remove all phage contamination. Wherever possible use dedicated pipets and disposable plasticware. Ensure that all nondisposable plasticware (e.g., centrifuge bottles) is completely phage-free by soaking the plasticware for 1 h in 2% (v/v) sodium hypochlorite, followed by extensive washing, and then autoclaving. If glassware is used, it should be baked at 200°C for at least 4 h. The use of polypropylene tubes is recommended, since phage may adsorb nonspecifically to other types of plastic.

2. If left for longer than 30 min, the F-pili may be lost.

3. An OD value of 1.0 is equivalent to ~8 × 10⁸ bacteria/mL.

4. Addition to the Immunotube of 200 µL of 1M Tris-HCl, pH 7.4, followed by 4 mL TG1 culture and then incubation for 30 min at 37°C for infection allows recovery of some phage that may have not been eluted by triethylamine. In general, however, this precaution is not required.

5. Sometimes, biotinylating reagents may lose their reactivity, typically by hydrolysis of the NHS-ester moiety, it is recommended that the quality of the reagent is checked by biotinylating 1 mg hen egg lysozyme at (3:1) biotin–protein ratio.

The biotinylated lysozyme can be analyzed on a native polyacrylamide gel (a conventional Laem mLi gel, but with the following differences:

a. No stacking gel.

b. No SDS in buffers

c. Using 80 mM γ-amino butyric acid (GABA), 20 mM acetic acid, pH 4.8, as gel and running buffer.

Run with reverse polarity (lysozyme is positively charged at pH 4.8). The unmodified lysozyme and lysozyme with 1, 2, 3, and so on, biotin molecules will migrate as distinct bands.

6. Shorter incubation times will favor the selection of antibodies with fast k_{on} values.

7. If NHS-LC-biotin is used as biotinylating reagent, the elution can be performed using 100 mM triethylamine.

8. We suggest that a dilution of 1/1000 be tried first.

9. Alternatively, use directly HRP-conjugated sheep antihuman κ and λ light chain antibodies (The Binding Site).

10. Millipore supplies a purpose-built 500-mL housing device for using disposable 0.45-μm filters.

11. In addition, 9E10 immobilized on protein A-Sepharose using dimethyl pimelimidate can be used for purification of these antibody fragments *(15)*.

12. An OD 280 nm value of 1.0 is equivalent to a fragment concentration of 0.8 mg/mL.

13. An ECL kit (Amersham) can also be used to detect peroxidase on Western blots (*see* Chapter 20).

14. These sections can be stored at –20°C for weeks to months, depending on the nature of the antigen.

15. We suggest a dilution of 1/200 be tried first.

References

1. Winter, G., Griffiths, A. D., Hawkins, R. E., and Hoogenboom, H. R. (1994) Making antibodies by phage display technology. *Annu. Rev. Immunol.* **12,** 433–455.

2. McCafferty, J., Griffiths, A. D., Winter, G., and Chiswell, D. J. (1990) Phage antibodies-filamentous phage displaying antibody variable domains. *Nature* **348,** 552–554.

3. Bird, R. E., Hardman, K. D., Jacobson, J. W., Johnson, S., Kaufman, B. M., Lee, S. M., Lee, T., Pope, S. H., Riordan, G. S., and Whitlow, M. (1988) Single-chain antigen-binding proteins. *Science* **242,** 423–426.

4. Huston, J. S., Levinson, D., Mudgetthunter, M., Tai, M. S., Novotny, J., Margolies, M. N., Ridge, R. J., Bruccoleri, R. E., Haber, E., Crea, R., and Oppermann, H. (1988) Protein engineering of antibody-binding sites—recovery of specific activity in an antidigoxin single-chain fv analog produced in *Escherichia coli. Proc. Natl. Acad. Sci. USA* **85,** 5879–5883.

5. Hoogenboom, H. R., Griffiths, A. D., Johnson, K. S., Chiswell, D. J., Hudson, P., and Winter, G. (1991) Multisubunit proteins on the surface of filamentous phage–methodologies for displaying antibody (Fab) heavy and light-chains. *Nucleic Acids Res.* **19,** 4133–4137.

6. Barbas, C. F., Kang, A. S., Lerner, R. A., and Benkovic, S. J. (1991) Assembly of combinatorial antibody libraries on phage surfaces—the gene-III site. *Proc. Natl. Acad. Sci. USA* **88,** 7978–7982.

7. Orlandi, R., Gussow, D. H., Jones, P. T., and Winter, G. (1989) Cloning immunoglobulin variable domains for expression by the polymerase chain-reaction. *Proc. Natl. Acad. Sci. USA* **86,** 3833–3837.

8. Ward, E. S., Gussow, D., Griffiths, A. D., Jones, P. T., and Winter, G. (1989) Binding activities of a repertoire of single immunoglobulin variable domains secreted from *Escherichia coli. Nature* **341,** 544–546.

9. Huse, W. D., Sastry, L., Iverson, S. A., Kang, A. S., Altingmees, M., Burton, D. R., Benkovic, S. J., and Lerner, R. A. (1989) Generation of a large combinatorial library of the immunoglobulin repertoire in phage-lambda. *Science* **246,** 1275–1281.

10. Clackson, T., Hoogenboom, H. R., Griffiths, A. D., and Winter, G. (1991) Making antibody fragments using phage display libraries. *Nature* **352,** 624–628.

11. Mullinax, R. L., Gross, E. A., Amberg, J. R., Hay, B. N., Hogrefe, H. H., Kubitz, M. M., Greener, A., Altingmees, M., Ardourel, D., Short, J. M., Sorge, J. A., and Shopes, B. (1990) Identification of human antibody fragment clones specific tetanus toxoid in a bacteriophage-lambda immunoexpression library. *Proc. Natl. Acad. Sci. USA* **87,** 8095–8099.

12. Barbas, C. F., Bjorling, E., Chiodi, F., Dunlop, N., Cababa, D., Jones, T. M., Zebedee, S. L., Persson, M. A. A., Nara, P. L., Norrby, E., and Burton, D. R. (1992) Recombinant human Fab fragments neutralise human type-1 immunodeficiency virus *in vitro. Proc. Natl. Acad. Sci. USA* **89,** 9339–9343.

13. Chester, K. A., Begent, R. H. J., Robson, L., Keep, P., Pedley, R. B., Boden, J. A., Boxer, G., Green, A., Winter, G., Cochet, O., and Hawkins, R. E. (1994) Phage libraries for generation of clinically useful antibodies. *Lancet* **343,** 455,456.

14. Burioni, R., Williamson, R. A., Sanna, P. P., Bloom, F. E., and Burton, D. R. (1994) Recombinant human fab to glycoprotein-d neutralizes infectivity and prevents cell-to-cell transmission of herpes-simplex virus-1 and virus-2 in-vitro. *Proc. Natl. Acad. Sci. USA* **91,** 355–359.

15. Marks, J. D., Hoogenboom, H. R., Bonnert, T. P., McCafferty, J., Griffiths, A. D., and Winter, G. (1991) By-passing immunization—human antibodies from V-gene libraries displayed on phage. *J. Mol. Biol.* **222,** 581–597.

16. Griffiths, A. D., Malmqvist, M., Marks, J. D., Bye, J. M., Embleton, M. J., McCafferty, J., Baier, M., Holliger, K. P., Gorick, B. D., Hughes-Jones, N. C., Hoogenboom, H. R., and Winter, G. (1993) Human anti-self antibodies with high specificity from phage display libraries. *EMBO J.* **12,** 725–734.

17. Hoogenboom, H. R. and Winter, G. (1992) By-passing immunization: human antibodies from synthetic repertoires of germline VH gene segments rearranged *in vitro. J. Mol. Biol.* **227,** 381–388.

18. Nissim, A., Hoogenboom, H. R., Tomlinson, I. M., Flynn, G., Midgley, C., Lane, D., and Winter, G. (1994) Antibody fragments from a single pot phage display library as immunochemical reagents. *EMBO J.* **13,** 692–698.

19. Griffiths, A. D., Williams, S. C., Hartley, O., Tomlinson, I. M., Waterhouse, P., Crosby, W. L., Kontermann, R. E., Jones, P. T., Low, N. M., Allison, T. J., Prospero, T. D., Hoogenboom, H. R., Nissim, A., Cox, J. P. L., Harrison, J. L., Zaccolo, M., Gherardi, E., and Winter, G. (1994) Isolation of high-affinity human antibodies directly from large synthetic repertoires. *EMBO J.* **13**, 3245–3260.

20. De Kruif, J., Terstappen, L., Boel, E., and Logtenberg, T. (1995) Rapid selection of cell subpopulation-specific human monoclonal antibodies from a synthetic phage antibody library. *Proc. Natl. Acad. Sci. USA* **92**, 3938–3942.

21. Hawkins, R. E., Russell, S. J., and Winter, G. (1992) Selection of phage antibodies by binding-affinity—mimicking affinity maturation. *J. Mol. Biol.* **226**, 889–896.

22. Marks, J. D., Griffiths, A. D., Malmqvist, M., Clackson, T. P., Bye, J. M., and Winter, G. (1992) Bypassing immunization—building high-affinity human antibodies by chain shuffling. *Biotechnology* **10**, 779–783.

23. Yanisch-Perron, C., Vieira, J., and Messing, J. (1985) Improved m13 phage cloning vectors and host strains—nucleotide sequences of the m13mp18 and puc19 vectors. *Gene* **33**, 103–119.

24. Vieira, J. and Messing, J. (1987) Production of single-stranded plasmid DNA. *Methods Enzymol.* **153**, 3–11.

25. Garrard, L. J., Yang, M., O'Connell, M. P., Kelley, R. F., and Henner, D. J. (1991) Fab assembly and enrichment in a monovalent phage display system. *Biotechnology* **9**, 1373–1377.

26. Lowman, H. B., Bass, S. H., Simpson, N., and Wells, J. A. (1991) Selecting high-affinity binding-proteins by monovalent phage display. *Biochemistry* **30**, 10,832–10,838.

27. De Bellis, D. and Schwartz, I. (1990) Regulated expression of foreign genes fused to lac-control by glucose levels in growth medium. *Nucleic Acids Res.* **18**, 1311.

28. Carter, P., Bedouelle, H., and Winter, G. (1985) Improved oligonucleotide site-directed mutagenesis using m13 vectors. *Nucleic Acids Res.* **13**, 4431–4443.

29. Gibson, T. J. (1984) PhD thesis, University of Cambridge, UK.

30. Vaughan, T. J., Williams, A. J., Pritchard, K., Osbourn, J., Pope, A. R., Earnshaw, J. C., McCafferty, J., Hodits, R., Wilton, J., and Johnson, K. S. (1996) Human antibodies with subnanomolar affinities isolated from a large non-immunised phage display library. *Nature Biotechnol.* **14**, 309–314.

31. Waterhouse, P., Griffiths, A. D., Johnson, K. S., and Winter, G. (1993) Combinatorial infection and in vivo recombination—a strategy for making large phage antibody repertoires. *Nucleic Acids Res.* **21**, 2265,2266.

32. Gussow, D. and Clackson, T. (1989) Direct clone characterization from plaques and colonies by the polymerase chain reaction. *Nucleic Acids Res.* **17**, 4000.

33. Marks, J. D., Ouwehand, W. H., Bye, J. M., Finnern, R., Gorick, B. D., Voak, D., Thorpe, S. J., Hughes-Jones, N. C., and Winter, G. (1993) Human antibody fragments specific for human blood-group antigens from a phage display library. *Biotechnology* **11**, 1145–1149.

34. Kretzschmar, T., Zimmermann, C., and Geiser, M. (1995) Selection procedures for nonmatured phage antibodies—a quantitative comparison and optimization strategies. *Anal. Biochem.* **224,** 413–419.

35. Holliger, P., Prospero, T., and Winter, G. (1993) Diabodies—small bivalent and bispecific antibody fragments. *Proc. Natl. Acad. Sci. USA* **90,** 6444–6448.

36. Pack, P., Kujau, M., Schroeckh, V., Knupfer, U., Wenderoth, R., Riesenberg, D., and Pluckthun, A. (1993) Improved bivalent miniantibodies, with identical avidity as whole antibodies, produced by high cell-density fermentation of *Escherichia coli. Biotechnology* **11,** 1271–1277.

37. Pack, P., Muller, K., Zahn, R., and Pluckthun, A. (1995) Tetravalent mini-antibodies with high avidity assembling in *Escherichia coli. J. Mol. Biol.* **246,** 28–34.

37a. Hu, S., Shively, L., Raubitschek, A., Sherman, M., Williams, L. E., Wong, J. Y., Shively, J. E., and Wu, A. M. (1996) Minibody: a novel engineered anti-carcinoembryonic antigen antibody fragment (single-chain Fv-CH$_3$) which exhibits rapid, high-level targeting of xenografts. *Cancer Res.* **56,** 3055–3061.

38. Kipryanov, S. M., Little, M., Kropshofer, H., Breitling, F., Gotter, S., and Dübel, S. (1996) Affinity enhancement of a recombinant antibody: formation of complexes with multiple valency by a single-chain Fv fragment-core Streptavidin fusion. *Protein Eng.* **9,** 203–211.

39. Schmidt, T. G. M. and Skerra, A. (1993) The random peptide library-assisted engineering of a C-terminal affinity peptide, useful for the detection and purification of a functional Ig Fv fragment. *Protein Eng.* **6,** 109–122.

40. Neri, D., Delalla, C., Petrul, H., Neri, P., and Winter, G. (1995) Calmodulin as a versatile tag for antibody fragments. *Biotechnology,* **13,** 373–377.

41. Jönsson, U., Fägerstam, L., Ivarsson, B., Johnsson, B., Karlsson, R., Lundh, K., Löfås, S., Persson, B., Roos, H., Rönnberg, I., Sjölander, S., Stenberg, E., Stahlberg, R., Urbaniczky, C., Östlin, H., and Malmqvist, M. (1991) Real-time biospecific interaction analysis using surface-plasmon resonance and a sensor chip technology. *Biotechniques* **11,** 620.

42. Munro, S. and Pelham, H. R. B. (1986) An hsp70-like protein in the ER—identity with the 78 kd glucose-regulated protein and immunoglobulin heavy-chain binding-protein. *Cell* **46,** 291–300.

43. Hochuli, E., Bannwarth, W., Dobeli, H., Gentz, R., and Stuber, D. (1988) Genetic approach to facilitate purification of proteins with a novel metal chelate adsorbent. *Biotechnology* **6,** 1321–1325.

44. Skerra, A., Pfitzinger, I., and Pluckthun, A. (1991) The functional expression of antibody Fv fragments in *Escherichia coli*–improved vectors and a generally applicable purification technique. *Biotechnology* **9,** 273–278.

45. Friguet, B., Chaffotte, A. F., Djavadi-Ohaniance, L., and Goldberg, M. E. (1985) Measurements of the true affinity constant in solution of antigen-antibody complexes by enzyme-linked immunosorbent-assay. *J. Immunol. Methods* **77,** 305–319.

46. Goldberg, M. E. and Djavadi-Ohaniance, L. (1993) Methods for measurement of antibody antigen affinity based on ELISA and RIA. *Curr. Opinion Immunol.* **5,** 278–281.

47. Fried, M. and Crothers, D. M. (1981) Equilibria and kinetics of lac repressor–operator interactions by polyacrylamide-gel electrophoresis. *Nucleic Acids Res.* **9,** 6505–6525.

48. Garner, M. M. and Revzin, A. (1981) A gel-electrophoresis method for quantifying the binding of proteins to specific DNA regions—application to components of the *Escherichia coli* lactose operon regulatory system. *Nucleic Acids Res.* **9,** 3047–3060.

49. Carr, D. W. and Scott, J. D. (1992) Blotting and band-shifting–techniques for studying protein-protein interactions. *Trends Biochem. Sci.* **17,** 246–249.

50. Neri, D., Momo, M., Prospero, T., and Winter, G. (1995) High-affinity antigen-binding by chelating-recombinant-antibodies (CRABS). *J. Mol. Biol.* **246,** 367–373.

51. Neri, D., Petrul, H., Winter, G., Light, Y., Marais, R, Britton, K. E., and Creighton, A. M. (1996) Radioactive labeling of recombinant antibody fragments by phosphorylation using casein kinase II and [γ-^{32}P]-ATP. *Nature Biotechnol.* **114,** 485–490.

52. Tomlinson, I. M., Walter, G., Marks, J. D., Llewelyn, M. B., and Winter, G. (1992) The repertoire of human germline V(H) sequences reveals about 50 groups of V(H) segments with different hypervariable loops. *J. Mol. Biol.* **227,** 776–798.

Index